AF575271

MOVEMENTS OF THE EYES

R H S CARPENTER

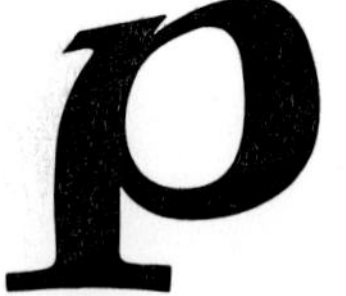

PION · LONDON

MOVEMENTS OF THE EYES

ANDREW E. KERTESZ

RHS CARPENTER

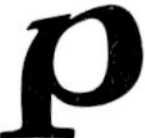

Pion Limited, 207 Brondesbury Park, London NW2 5JN

ISBN 0 85086 063 6

Printed in Great Britain

Preface

It is not hard to see why there has recently been such an upsurge of interest in the systems controlling eye movements. The more we find out about the way in which our eyes seek out and capture objects of interest in the visual world, the more remarkable does its seemingly effortless precision and sophistication appear. At the same time—and this is perhaps why it is increasingly attracting the attention of neurophysiologists—it functions at a level of complexity somewhere between the banality of the spinal reflex and the inscrutability of the voluntary act. One may therefore hope that an understanding of how the eyes are controlled may help us when we seek to understand more complicated motor systems: and indeed it is now becoming apparent that many of what were formerly thought to be unique properties of the eye movement control system have direct parallels even in a system as complex as the control of the hand.

This book has been planned with three classes of reader in mind. First, the medical student who wishes to know rather more about the subject—one that has considerable importance as an aid to neurological diagnosis—than is available to him in more general textbooks. Second, the scientifically oriented physiology or psychology student who is interested in a field in which the application of techniques of systems analysis to neurophysiology has proved particularly fruitful; and lastly but perhaps chiefly, to the research worker in this field who, like the author himself, may well have felt a need for an up-to-date and not wholly clinical reference book that can also be used as a teaching text.

It is divided into three parts, in an attempt to reflect the clear distinction that ought to be made with physiological systems between *performance, structure,* and the notional *models* that are supposed to link structure to performance, and performance to function. Here, part 1 is intended as a description of the phenomena of eye movements, part 2 as an account of the anatomy of the system (including the mechanical properties of the eye ball itself), while part 3 attempts to relate this anatomy to the control mechanisms, and to assess the contribution of eye movements to visual function. Appendices to the text provide a review of techniques for measuring eye movements, and an introduction to linear systems analysis which it is hoped will enable the nonmathematician to follow the mathematical arguments presented in the text.

R H S Carpenter
Gonville and Caius, Cambridge
May 1977

Acknowledgements

I am grateful to Fiona Hake and Peter Starling for help in the preparation of some of the figure material, and to Mrs A J Pine for assistance in finding some of the more obscure references.

I also wish to express my gratitude to the authors quoted in the text for the permissions received to reproduce material from their papers and books, and to the following publishers and organisations for allowing me to use their copyright material:

Academic Press Inc, New York (Bach-y-Rita, Collins, and Hyde, Editors: *The Control of Eye Movements: Experimental Neurology*)

Almqvist and Wiksell, Stockholm (*Acta Oto-Laryngologica*)

The American Institute of Physics, New York (*Journal of the Optical Society of America*)

The American Physiological Society, Bethesda, Maryland (*American Journal of Physiology; Journal of Neurophysiology*)

The American Psychological Association, Washington, DC (*Journal of Comparative Psychology*)

Edward Arnold (Publishers) Ltd, London (Matthews: *Mammalian Muscle Receptors and their Central Actions*)

J F Bergmann-Verlag, Munich (*Experimental Brain Research*)

Butterworth and Co (Publishers) Ltd, Sevenoaks, Kent (Roberts: *Neurophysiology of Postural Mechanisms*)

Elsevier/North-Holland Biomedical Press, Amsterdam (*Archives Néerlandaises de Physiologie, Brain Research*)

The Institute of Electrical and Electronics Engineers, Inc, New York (*IEEE Transactions on Human Factors in Electronics, IEEE Transactions on Systems and Sciences of Cybernetics*)

S Karger AG, Basel (*Bibliotheca Ophthalmologica; Oto-Rhino-Laryngology*)

Henry Kimpton Ltd, London (Duke-Elder: *System of Ophthalmology*)

E and S Livingstone Ltd, Edinburgh (*Quarterly Journal of Experimental Physiology*)

The C V Mosby Co, St Louis, Missouri (Moses, Editor: *Adler's Physiology of the Eye*)

The New York Academy of Sciences, New York, New York (*Annals of the New York Academy of Sciences*)

The Optical Society of America, Lancaster, Pennsylvania (*Journal of the Optical Society of America*)

Pergamon Press Ltd, Oxford (Lennerstrand and Bach-y-Rita, Editors: *Basic Aspects of Ocular Motility; Vision Research*)

The Physiological Society, Cambridge and London (*Journal of Physiology*)

Plenum Publishing Corporation, New York (Yarbus: *Eye Movements and Vision*)

The Psychonomic Society, Austin, Texas (*Perception and Psychophysics*)

The Royal Society, London (*Proceedings of the Royal Society*)

The Royal Society of Medicine, London (*Proceedings of the Royal Society of Medicine*)

Springer-Verlag, Heidelberg (*Experimental Brain Research; Kybernetik*)

Taylor and Francis Ltd, London (*Optica Acta*)

The Wistar Institute Press, Philadelphia, Pennsylvania (*Anatomical Record; Journal of Comparative Neurology*)

In memoriam
D E C

Contents

Part 1

Function

1

The use of eye movements

"The muscles were of necessitie provided and given to the eye, that so it might move on every side: for if the eye stoode fast, and immoveable, we should be constrained to turne our head and necke (being all of one peece) for to see: but by these muscles it now moveth it selfe with such swiftnes and nimblenes, without stirring of the head, as is almost incredible..." [1]

Not all creatures with eyes are able to move them. But—if we ignore winks, *oeillades* and other frivolous tasks—those that do, do so in order to see better. In this first chapter, the intention is to examine very briefly the general relation between vision and eye movements—a topic discussed in more detail in chapter 11—and the ways in which the requirements of sight determine the major classes of eye movement. In subsequent chapters, these various classes are discussed in turn: but for the moment only the most general considerations will be presented. For a more complete account of the teleology of eye movements than space permits here, see Walls (1942).

1.1 Consequences of velocity blur

For a stationary object, the fineness of the detail that can just be resolved is almost entirely a function of such 'physical' factors as the size of the eye, the quality of its optics, the spacing of the receptors, and the degree to which the central pathways from them overlap in their connections. But as soon as the image of the object starts to move across the retina quite different factors come into play. The light falling on any particular receptor is now no longer constant, but fluctuates as different parts of the image pass over its receptive area. The fidelity of the pattern of activity in the receptors to the pattern of light and shade in the original image at any moment will be a function not just of the physical factors mentioned earlier, but also of how good the receptors are at *following* these fluctuations. It turns out that they are in fact rather poor at doing so. Electrical responses in the retina to brief visual stimulation under the most favourable conditions typically show a time course of the order of tens of milliseconds, and flickering lights cannot be seen as such when the frequency of their flicker is more than some 60–80 Hz. The consequent degradation of visual acuity is quite striking: from appropriate published data (for example Robson, 1966; Green and Campbell, 1965) one may calculate that a target movement as slow as $1^\circ\ s^{-1}$—that is, in which any point on the target will take nearly three minutes to cross the visual field —has roughly the same effect on resolution as three diopters of myopia!

Whether for this reason, or simply because of the difficulty of designing a visual system that will analyse and recognise shapes that move as well as

[1] The quotations at the head of each chapter are from Andreas Laurentius (1599).

those that are still, it seems that the first kind of eye movements that evolved were those designed, paradoxically, not to move the eye at all but to hold it still—still, that is, relative to the frame of reference provided by the outside world (see, for example, Walls, 1962). This means that the animal must sense the movement of the head relative to the outside world, and move the eyes in an equal and opposite direction to compensate. Now, since the eyes are only capable of rotation, and cannot displace themselves significantly with respect to the head, it follows that such a mechanism will only provide complete stabilisation against rotations of the head; if the head undergoes translation, no rotation of the eyes can possibly compensate for movements of the retinal images of objects lying at *all* distances from the eyes (figure 1.1).

This may not matter much for animals like man with eyes that face in their normal direction of progress, but for animals with side-pointing eyes —most birds, for example—who are interested in near objects as well as far, it may lead to inconvenience. The only satisfactory solution is to stabilise not the eye but the *head*, which is capable of translation as well as rotation. The result is the slightly comical gait of such birds as chickens, pigeons, ducks, etc, in which the body walks on while the head is temporarily left behind, to be jerked forward again at the next step (figure 1.2) (Dunlap and Mowrer, 1931). But for creatures with heavy heads and short necks this is not a feasible solution, and an animal like the rabbit responds to linear accelerations of the head with rotations of the eyes that are approximately such as to stabilise the horizon (section 2.2). We shall see that in man responses of the eyes solely due to translation of the head have all but disappeared.

There are two essentially different ways in which image-stabilising or *holding* movements of this type can be produced. The most obvious way is simply to use the visual signal itself: we know that one of the kinds of

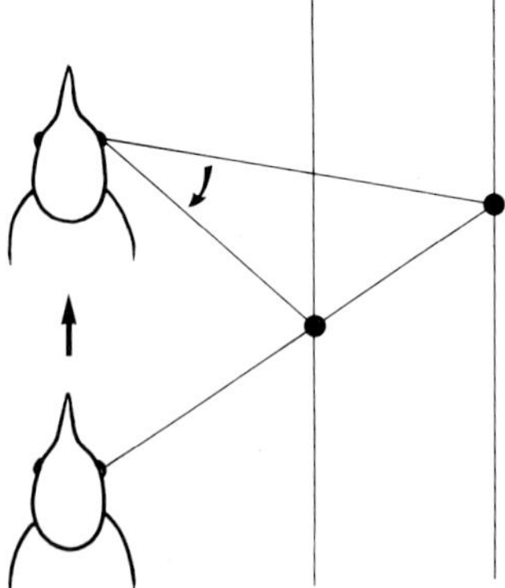

Figure 1.1. Forward movement of an animal with side-pointing eyes leads to different retinal shifts for objects at different distances.

information extracted at an early stage of visual processing is the velocity and direction of 'retinal slip'—movement of the retinal image relative to the retina—and it is easy to imagine how such a signal might be used in a negative feedback system to move the eyes in such a way as always to keep the slip velocity as near zero as possible. Such a mechanism would compensate not only for movement of the head, but also for displacements of the visual objects themselves in the outside world. Movements of this sort are well-known throughout the animal kingdom, having surprisingly similar response characteristics in creatures as different as the crab (Horridge, 1966) and man: similar mechanisms control the head movements of insects (Land, 1969; 1973). Generic names for these responses include *optokinesis* and *smooth pursuit*: they form the subject of chapter 3.

Important as this mechanism is, it has one severe drawback, inherent in all purely visual systems: it is very slow. It takes a fifth of a second or

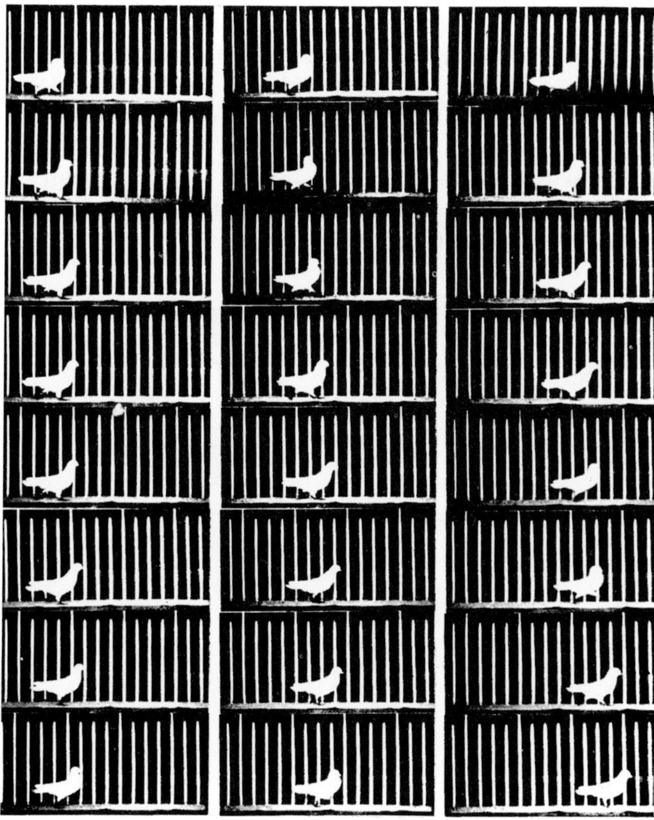

Figure 1.2. Sequential frames ($32\ s^{-1}$) of a film of a pigeon walking, showing 'nystagmus' of the head (reprinted from Dunlap and Mowrer, 1931).

more for the smooth pursuit system to begin to respond to a sudden movement of the head. Fortunately, there are other sources of information about head movement that are a good deal quicker. The most important of these is the *vestibular apparatus*, the system of fluid-filled tunnels and caverns within the thickness of the skull that signals rotational and translational accelerations of the head. In the next chapter, we shall see that powerful and fast reflexes connect this sensory apparatus to the neurons that supply the eye muscles—the *vestibulo-ocular reflexes.* Other sensory pathways that can be used, though probably not to any great extent in man, come from proprioceptors in the muscles and articulations of the neck (section 2.2). These respond to the position of the head relative to the body, rather than to its movement in space.

1.2 Consequences of limited field of view

There is a surprising degree of variation between different species as to how much they can see at any given moment (Walls, 1942; Rochon-Duvigneaud, 1943). The horse, for example, can see almost all round his head (figure 1.3), and, given an adequate system for stabilisation of the retinal image, it is not obvious that it would ever need to make any other kinds of eye movements at all. The reason that it does is that it cannot see *equally well* in all parts of its field. In birds and mammals we find that vision comes in two grades: a luxury grade, with high acuity and often colour discrimination, and an economy grade of low acuity—but often greater sensitivity—and without the added refinement of colour.

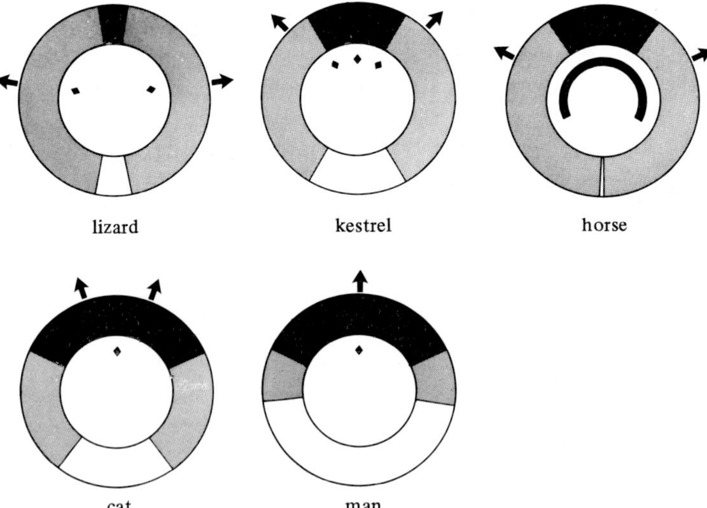

Figure 1.3. Maximum horizontal monocular (shaded areas) and binocular (black areas) fields, directions of optical axes (arrows), and location of the area centralis (inside ring) in different species (data from Walls, 1942).

In the first case, the fine acuity is mostly due to a dense packing of the receptors, and a ratio of the connections between each receptor and the fibres in the optic nerve that approaches one-to-one: in the second, the receptors spread themselves out, and pool their messages before sending them to the brain, resulting in lowered thresholds but poor acuity. In many cases the first type is associated with an abundance of cones, the second with rods.

The reason why the whole visual field is not provided with the luxury grade of vision is presumably partly that under *nocturnal* conditions it cannot function properly because of its relative insensitivity, and partly that the dense packing of the receptors and the one-to-one connections to the optic nerve would lead to the latter becoming unmanageably large. For example, if our entire retina were of the high-quality type, the cross-sectional area of our optic nerve would have to increase by a factor of over two hundred (and no doubt the size of the blind spot would also have to increase proportionately). Thus in practice we generally find that high-quality vision is confined to a special zone in the retina, the *area centralis*, whose position and configuration depends on how the animal normally uses its eyes, and what it particularly wants to see well: there may be more than one such mechanism. Walls (1942) has discussed the configuration of visual fields and specialised areas of the retina in different species with a wealth of interesting detail. Broadly, one finds that predators tend to have a front-facing, compact area centralis, often associated with a local depression in the retina, the *fovea*, while those of their prey often form long horizontal streaks that correspond roughly with the situation of the horizon when the eye is at its normal rest position (horse, figure 1.3).

Whatever its shape, the size of the area centralis in an animal that is not wholly diurnal is only a small fraction of the total field. In man, one can estimate its extent by measurements of visual acuity at different distances from the fixation point (taken to be the centre of the fovea): some observations of this type are shown in figure 1.4 [see also Millodot's

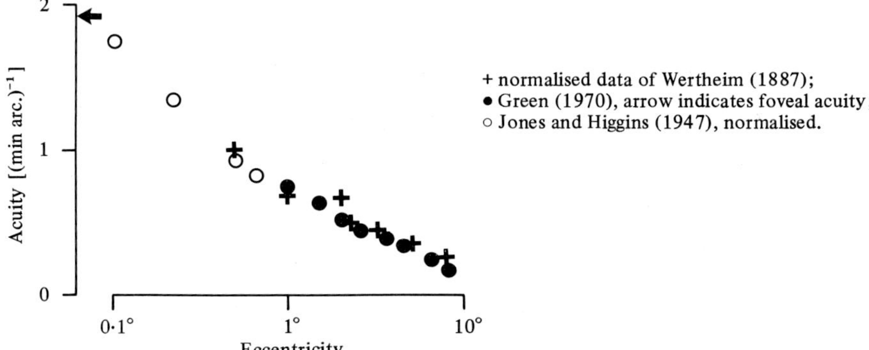

Figure 1.4. Visual acuity as a function of distance from the fovea.

(1972) recent review]. By the time 1 deg from the centre has been reached, visual acuity has fallen by a factor of three or so: the intercone spacing shows a proportionate increase (Jones and Higgins, 1947). In other words, only some ten-thousandth part of the visual field is seen with full clarity: the reason that we are not greatly aware of our loss is that our eyes are continually on the move, pointing this little tunnel of clear vision now here, now there, at whatever we want to see.

The result is that so long as we are prepared to wait the fifth of a second or so that it takes to plan and execute these sighting movements, our vision is as good with our tiny fovea as it would be if most of our retina were packed with the luxury receptors. [Although it must be remembered that in man not all the visual field can be fixated by the eye; the field of fixation is only some 90 deg in its horizontal and vertical extent (Hofmann, 1925; Burian and van Noorden, 1974).] F W Campbell, in an unpublished communication, has put it well:

> "The potential spatial information being continuously supplied to the eye is enormous. A hemisphere has an area 74×10^6 sq. min. Using the argument that a matrix of recognisable letters can be set up each in an area of 50 sq. min., it follows that $1 \cdot 5 \times 10^6$ letters can be displayed in one hemisphere. Say an observer proceeded to read these letters sequentially, taking one second per letter, it would require just over 26 days to identify them, assuming 16 hours of observation were made each day. If the matrix is exposed for 1/10 second, to prevent eye movements, only the 14 letters falling on the central fovea could be identified: this is only 1/100,000 of the total available when eye movements are permitted."

Such ideas perhaps suggest the notion of deliberate scanning of the visual field by the eye, like a radar antenna, or the scanning spot in a television camera. Although this is indeed found in some species with a very small number of retinal receptors [for example the jumping spider (Land, 1969), or the extreme case of *Copilia* with its single retinal unit (Gregory et al, 1964)], it is an unnceccessarily prosaic procedure when there are sufficient low-grade receptors surrounding the fovea to signal to the eye movement system the location of a point of interest in the field that ought to be fixated: and of course localised sounds can be used in the same way. The result is the *catching* movement, either visually evoked or auditory or even purely voluntary, in which a new object of interest is seized by the fovea, and subsequently held there by the *holding* mechanisms introduced in the previous section.

It is apparent that the catching and holding mechanisms are to some extent antagonistic. Catching implies a movement of the eye relative to the visual field: and we saw earlier that a moving eye is an eye that cannot really see. How can these opposite requirements—of displacement without motion—be reconciled? The answer is, by making the catching movements as fast as we can: although the consequent disruption of vision during the movement is that much greater, the period of time for which it occurs is correspondingly reduced. The resulting eye movements—called *saccades*—are actually very fast indeed, with velocities approaching 1000° s^{-1}: they form the subject of chapter 4.

Apart from their role as pure catching movements, saccades also form an inseparable component of the complete holding response. Consider for example the smooth pursuit holding mechanism in circumstances in which the animal is continuously moving in one direction relative to the outside world. It is plain that, although the eye can move at an appropriate rate in the opposite direction to stabilise the retinal image, this compensation cannot go on indefinitely since the eye has only a limited range of travel. What happens in practice is that the slow following movement of the eye is interrupted at intervals by a rapid saccadic movement in the opposite direction, resulting in a sawtooth-like time course called *nystagmus*. Although these saccades are in every respect similar to the catching saccades described above, not all animals that are able to produce them (that is, those animals that show holding of any sort) are also able to produce 'voluntary' target-catching saccades: only those with a developed area centralis do so (Walls, 1962). Vestibular nystagmus—essentially indistinguishable in its time course from optokinetic nystagmus—can equally be evoked by sufficiently prolonged rotation of the head.

1.3 Consequences of binocular vision

With two eyes, it is almost inevitable that there will be at least some degree of overlap of their fields, even when they are essentially sideways-pointing (figure 1.3). But this does not necessarily indicate a need for much cooperation between the movements of the two eyes. In most lizards, for example, best vision occurs in the lateral direction; as a consequence, they are able to enjoy the ability of directing both eyes independently at will to objects of interest in their respective visual fields, although, as in all species, the involuntary holding movements are always fully coordinated in the two eyes. But as soon as there is overlap between the visual fields corresponding to the area centralis of each eye, there is an obvious advantage in binocular yoking of the two eyes in voluntary movements as well. If the foveas overlap, the fineness of their acuity permits the perception of *depth* by comparison of the visual images in the two eyes, each of which sees from a slightly different viewpoint: but this function demands precise control of the relative positions of the eyes. The two eyes thus swivel together as a single unit, the two visual axes pointing in parallel directions.

This arrangement is fine so long as what we are looking at is sufficiently far away: but it is clearly inappropriate as soon as we try to look at objects at different distances from the eye. We then require the eyes to *converge* from parallelity to bring the two images of the object onto corresponding portions of the two retinae. Oddly enough, this ability has only been acquired with difficulty: although man and the primates, and possibly the cat, can converge their eyes in this way, other species with overlapping foveas apparently cannot. Even in man, these *disjunctive* or *vergence* movements are relatively undeveloped, and lack both the precise rapidity of saccades, and their complete voluntary control: it is significant that the diplopias and other disorders caused by malfunctioning of the disjunctive eye movement control system form the largest single group of oculomotor disturbances in clinical practice. Some aspects of the possible evolutionary history of binocular control have been presented in a thoughtful discussion by Walls (1962).

Table 1.1. A classification of types of eye movements.

Catching movements (fast)	
saccades (and microsaccades)	
nystagmus quick phase	
Holding movements (slow)	
vestibular	including nystagmus slow phase
smooth pursuit	including nystagmus slow phase
vergence	

Table 1 summarises the classification of eye movement types presented above. The miniature eye movements have not been mentioned in this chapter because they serve no *obvious* purpose: they are the subject of chapter 6, where their possible teleology is also discussed.

2

Vestibular eye movements

"... for is it not a wittie exploite of nature to close up in so small a hole, a drumme hard laced, having on the hinder part two small strings, and three little bones, resembling a forge, a hammer and a stirrop, three small muscles, and a labyrinth contayning the inward ayre?"

2.1 The vestibular sense organs

2.1.1 Gross anatomy

As its name suggests, the labyrinth of the inner ear is a somewhat complex structure, apparently an elaboration of the apparatus used by aquatic vertebrates to signal movements of the water that surrounds them. In primitive fish the sensory hairs of this mechanism project directly into the external medium and are bent when it flows past them; in higher fishes, these cells lie in protected channels under the scales. In the course of evolution the channels eventually became closed fluid systems containing *endolymph*, and no longer in direct communication with the surrounding fluid. Consequently their function changed from signalling water flow round the fish (which might be due either to absolute motion of the fish, or merely to external water currents) to responding to the eddy movements set up in these canals by the fish's own movements, independently of any external disturbances.

Regions of this system came to be specialised for different functions: parts of the canals came to lie sufficiently close to the surface to respond to vibrations in the surrounding water, while other parts developed into sacs containing calcareous granules. It is probable that these two specilisations correspond to the cochlea and otolith organs of land vertebrates, responding respectively to sound vibrations and to the direction of gravity and other linear accelerations. At the same time, the other parts of the labyrinth have become more specialised for responding to rotational movements, resulting in the standard arrangement of three *semicircular canals* in mutually perpendicular planes which is found universally in land vertebrates.

Thus the labyrinth can be divided into three functionally distinct parts: the cochlea (with which we will not be concerned), the three semicircular canals, and a pair of endolymphatic sacs (the *utricle* and *saccule*), all of which are in communication (figure 2.1). In man, one of the canals is near the horizontal when the head is in a normal erect position, whereas the planes of the others form an angle close to 45° with the sagittal plane (figure 2.2), so that the plane of the right posterior canal is parallel to that of the left anterior one, and vice versa.

The receptor cells in the labyrinth are concentrated together in special regions of the epithelium, the *maculae* of the utricle and saccule, and the *cristae* of the canals. In each case, their hair-like processes project into a mass of gelatinous substance. In the canals, this aggregation of jelly and hairs forms a flap (the *cupula*) that projects across the canal, which is widened at this point to form the *ampulla.* The flap appears to be watertight, so that any displacement of fluid in the canals caused by a turning movement of the head makes the cupula bend to one side, stimulating the receptor cells

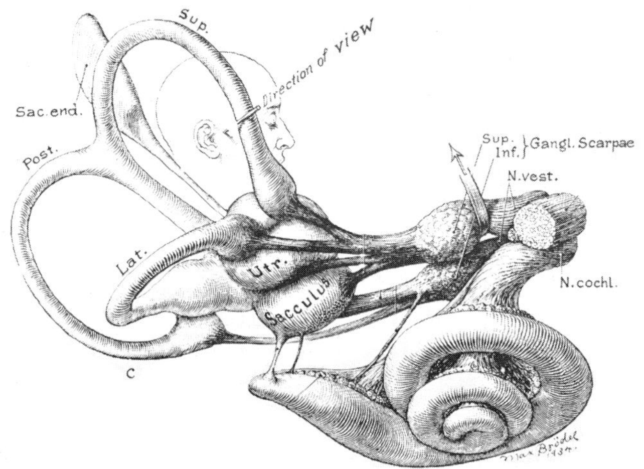

Figure 2.1. The human labyrinth and its innervation (Hardy, 1934).

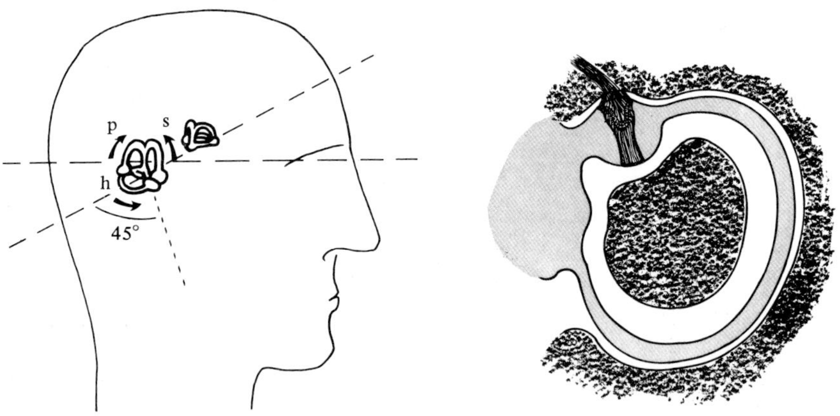

Figure 2.2.　　Figure 2.3.

Figure 2.2. The disposition of the semicircular canals in the head: the arrows show the directions of fluid movement that are excitatory for each canal (s, superior; p, posterior; h, horizontal).

Figure 2.3. Diagrammatic section through a single semicircular canal, showing the membraneous canal containing endolymph (shaded), surrounded by perilymph within the bony canal. At top left, the cupula can be seen effectively blocking the flow of endolymph through the ampulla: associated with it are the hair cells and their sensory innervation.

whose hairs are embedded in it (figure 2.3). In the utricle and saccule—the *otolith organs*—the jelly contains heavy calcareous granules: during movements of the head the whole thing tends to get left behind because of its inertia, stimulating the receptor cells by the bending of their hairs. These same cells also respond to static tilt of the head, because the weight bends them in different directions at different orientations of the head. In fact they respond to gravity no differently than to other linear accelerations, and if the two act together they add vectorially to give a response equivalent to some particular angle of tilt—as would only be expected from a simple inertial system not incorporating the gyroscope principle (figure 2.4).

The structures described so far are contained within the membraneous labyrinth: this in turn lies within a corresponding arrangement of bony tunnels and caves, the bony labyrinth. Between the two is a substantial gap, filled with a fine network of connective tissue and bathed in *perilymph.* Presumably the perilymph also moves about in response to movements of the head: but there is no equivalent to the cupula to impede its flow, and it is thought not to contribute substantially to the responses of the hair cells in the cristae (Dohlman and Kuehn, 1973; McCabe and Ryu, 1973).

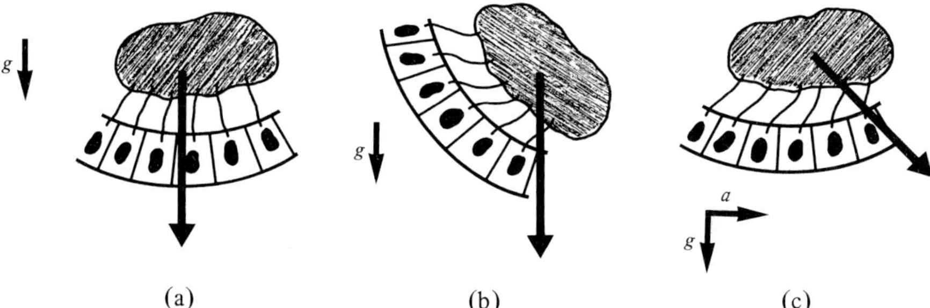

Figure 2.4. The action of the otolith receptors: (a) at rest, (b) with head tilted, and (c) under horizontal linear acceleration. The last two conditions are indistinguishable in their effects.

2.1.2 The receptor cells and their innervation

The sensory cells of the maculae and cristae are closely similar in appearance: their sensitivity to different types of motion is thought to be entirely a function of their relation to the larger structures of which they form a part. In mammals and birds two types of hair cell are generally recognised: a flask- or bottle-shaped *type I* cell, and a roughly cylindrical *type II* cell (figure 2.5), although intermediate types have been described (Wersäll, 1956; Engström, 1965). Both have the same pattern of hairs projecting from their outer surfaces. Two kinds of hair are found: each cell has a single flexible *kinocilium*, originating at the edge of the superficial surface, and some sixty to one hundred stiff *stereocilia*, arranged in a regular pattern and graded in such a way that the longest originate near the kinocilium, and the shortest furthest away (figure 2.5) (Engström et al, 1962).

This gradation of size defines a direction of polarisation for each cell in the epithelial plane, and a striking feature of the cristae is that the vast majority of the cells show exactly parallel orientation. In the horizontal canal the kinocilia face the utricle, whereas in the vertical canals they face away from it. The disposition in the maculae is more complex (Flock, 1964): the directions of individual cells lie roughly parallel with their immediate neighbours, but on a larger scale there are systematic variations of this 'morphological polarisation' in different regions of the macula (figure 2.6) (Spoendlin, 1965). These differences reflect the fact that the semicircular canals are individually one-dimensional receptors, whereas the utricle and possibly the saccule are essentially two- or three-dimensional, signalling the direction of an acceleration as well as its magnitude.

The kinocilium shows a higher degree of internal organisation than do the relatively simple stereocilia, with an arrangement of nine internal longitudinal filaments on the outside and two in the middle that is typical of motile cilia. It seems likely that it is the kinocilium that is the primary sensory element, and that the stereocilia provide a passive mechanism by which the response of the cell is made direction specific: we shall see later that stimulation of vestibular receptors is associated with bending of the kinocilium away from the stereocilia, and that bending in the opposite direction is ineffective. Conceivably the stereocilia simply discourage the kinocilium from bending in their direction.

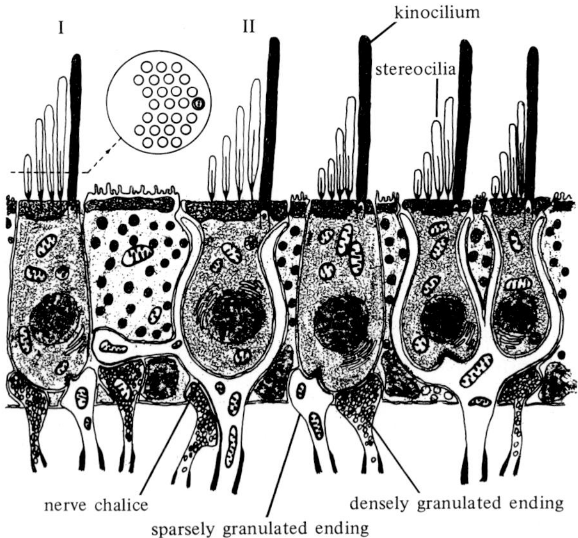

Figure 2.5. Diagrammatic cross-section of vestibular sensory epithelium showing type I and type II cells and their innervation. The inset shows a typical arrangement of the sensory hairs.

The main difference, apart from shape, between the two types of hair cell lies in their innervation. Type I cells are closely enveloped in a single nerve calyx (figure 2.5), from which it is separated by a gap of some 25–30 nm. However, at some points the gap is very much reduced (often in association with synaptic bars): this fact, together with the very large potential synaptic area, has led to the suggestion that the functional connection between receptor cell and nerve fibre may be at least partly electrical in nature. Sometimes two or three receptors may be found within the same enveloping chalice. The type II cells are innervated by at least two different kinds of ending. The first variety is sparsely granulated, and is possibly equivalent to the chalice endings of the type I cells, since collaterals of this type can sometimes be seen innervating both types of receptor. The second type is less common, and forms button-like endings having a dense granulation: these endings are found not only on the bodies of type II cells, but also on the surface of nerve chalices and their collaterals (figure 2.5) (Ades and Engström, 1965), and it is very likely efferent (centrifugal) in nature. Each type II cell receives many endings from independent, branching fibres. Counts of afferent and efferent fibres in the vestibular nerve (Gacek, 1961) show that the number of efferent fibres is very small, perhaps as few as two hundred in the cat; they originate in the lateral vestibular nucleus. Thus, either these fibres must branch very considerably, or alternatively some of the afferent fibres may send back collaterals that terminate as apparent efferents. True centrifugal fibres, despite their small number, have nevertheless been shown

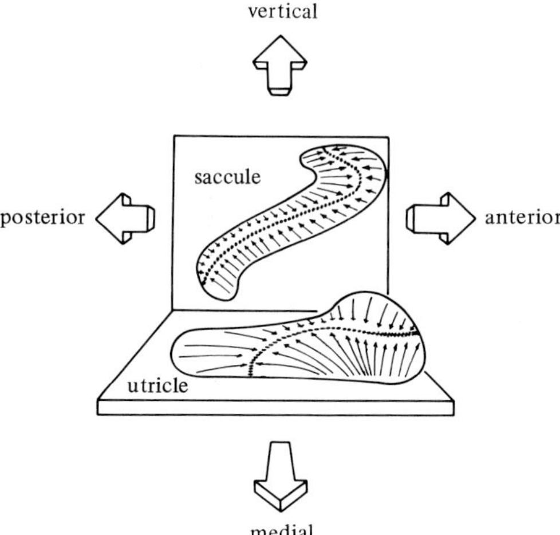

Figure 2.6. Diagrammatic representation of the maculae of the utricle and saccule, in the relative orientation that they occupy in the head. The arrows indicate the direction of functional polarisation of the receptor cells at different points on the surface. Data from Spoendlin (1965).

to have marked effects on the discharge of afferent fibres in the vestibular nerve, particularly during eye movements (Klinke and Schmidt, 1968; Klinke, 1970; Dichgans et al, 1970; Schmidt et al, 1972). The exact nature and function of their influence on vestibular receptors is uncertain.

The cell bodies of afferent fibres innervating vestibular receptors lie in the superior and inferior vestibular ganglion (Scarpa's ganglion) situated close to the labyrinth. The central course of these fibres constitutes the vestibular nerve, which together with the auditory nerve forms the eighth cranial nerve (nVIII). They project to the vestibular nuclei and also directly to the cerebellum: these projections are discussed in chapter 9.

2.1.3 Electrical responses to angular accelerations

Löwenstein and Sand (1940) appear to have been the first to record the relation between movements of the head and activity in the vestibular fibres. Adrian (1943) showed that the otolith organs of the cat gave a slowly adapting and somewhat nonlinear response to tilt of the head, and characterised the directions of rotational acceleration that were excitatory for the different canals (figure 2.7). It can be seen that these excitatory directions correspond with the direction of polarisation of the hair cells of the cristae. Vestibular fibres show a certain amount of variation in their resting rate of discharge, some being spontaneously active and responding to rotational acceleration in different directions by an increase or decrease in their firing rate, whereas others are normally silent and fire only at some threshold degree of stimulation in the excitatory direction. These results have been amply confirmed and extended by many workers since (most recently by Goldberg and Fernandez, 1971). Two questions have received particular attention: they are the nature of the relationship between the time course of rotation of the head and the time course of discharge, and the precise form of the functional nonlinearity relating deviation of the cupula to frequency of firing in individual fibres.

As in so many mechanoreceptors, it turns out that the dynamic response of the semicircular canals is largely determined by the special properties of the mechanical system of which they form a part rather than any

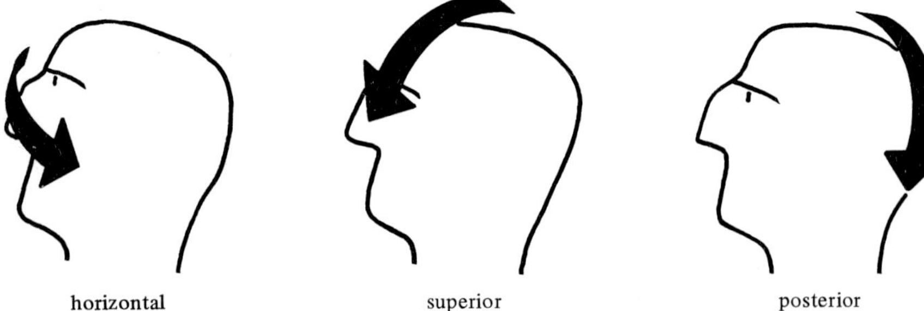

Figure 2.7. Directions of head movement that are stimulatory for the semicircular canals of the left.

intrinsic property of the receptor cells themselves. Thus an analysis of the mechanical behaviour of the endolymph and cupula can provide a surprisingly accurate description of the dynamic characteristics of the neural response to rotations. Steinhausen (1931) was the first to make such an analysis. If an individual canal is taken to be a circular tube of uniform cross-section, filled with an ideal fluid of known density and viscosity, and the cupula is assumed to be perfectly elastic (producing a restoring force proportional to its displacement from the rest position) and watertight, then the system can be perfectly represented by a simple second-order mechanical model such as the one shown in figure 2.8.

The input to this system is the angular position of the head at any moment, θ_{in} (resolved in the plane of the canal), whereas the output is taken to be the corresponding deviation of the cupula, θ_{out}; the whole system behaves like a second-order displacement divider (see appendix 2), and has properties analogous to a damped pendulum. If we use the symbols r, k, and M to represent respectively—in appropriate units—the viscous, elastic, and inertial constants of the system, we can derive the transfer function of the whole arrangement:

$$\frac{\theta_{out}}{\theta_{in}} = \frac{(r\mathrm{D}+k)^{-1}}{(r\mathrm{D}+k)^{-1}+(M\mathrm{D}^2)^{-1}} = \frac{\mathrm{D}^2}{\mathrm{D}^2+\dfrac{r}{M}\mathrm{D}+\dfrac{k}{M}} \;.$$

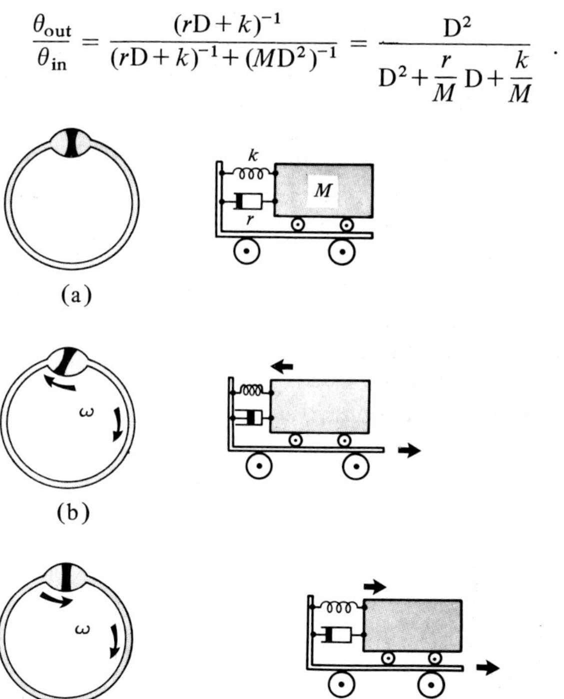

Figure 2.8. The mechanical action of the semicircular canal. Behaviour of the cupula, and of a simple mechanical analogue, (a) at rest, (b) immediately after and (c) some time after a rotation at constant velocity.

Thus only two parameters are needed to describe its behaviour: the ratio r/M, and the ratio k/M. [There is some variation of notation amongst different authors: thus von Egmond et al (1949) and many others use Π, Δ, Θ for r, k, M; Melvill Jones and Spells (1963) use Φ, Δ, I; and Melvill Jones and Milsum (1971) prefer b, k, J. The reader can take his pick! Although an admirable rationalised scheme of notation for this and other aspects of vestibular stimulation has been proposed by Hixson et al (1966), it is not in general use.]

It turns out that the semicircular canals are very highly damped, and so behave like two first-order high-pass units in series:

$$\frac{\theta_{\text{out}}}{\theta_{\text{in}}} = \left(\frac{\mathrm{D}}{\lambda + \mathrm{D}}\right)\left(\frac{\mathrm{D}}{\mu + \mathrm{D}}\right),$$

where $\lambda\mu = k/M$, and $\lambda + \mu \approx \mu = r/M$; thus $\lambda = (k/M)(M/r) = k/r$. The two associated time constants are thus given by M/r (the inertial time constant) and r/k (the elastic time constant). Recent values of these constants for the posterior canal of the squirrel monkey have been obtained by electrical recording from the vestibular nerve at 3 ms and nearly 6 s, respectively (Fernandez and Goldberg, 1971); in the cat, M/r is somewhat smaller, around 1·7 milliseconds (Fernandez and Valentinuzzi, 1968). The time constants can also be estimated by examining the time course of eye movement responses to head rotation, although one must then make the rather unreasonable assumption that the measurements are not obscured by subsequent neural mechanisms. In man, values for the long (elastic) time constant around the 10 s originally reported by von Egmond et al (1949) are found, although it is clear that there is a difference between the horizontal and vertical canals in this respect (Melvill Jones, 1960; Melvill Jones et al, 1964). Gilson et al (1973) recently report time constants of 16 s and 7 s, respectively, and Fernandez and Valentinuzzi (1968) also find differences between the inertial time constants of the different canals of the cat.

The functional significance of these findings can perhaps best be appreciated by considering the response of the semicircular canals to sinusoidal rotations of the head. It is a simple matter to calculate from the transfer function already derived how the gain and phase of the vestibular response will be related to the frequency of such an input (appendix 2). Figure 2.9 shows the frequency response of the mechanical model, with the use of Fernandez and Goldberg's (1971) experimental parameters. At very high frequencies the gain is constant, and there is only a small phase difference between head and cupular displacement, so that in this region the receptors are responding essentially to angular *position* of the head. At intermediate frequencies (that is between about 0·07 and 20 Hz) the response is advanced in phase by some 90° and the gain increases linearly in proportion to the frequency, implying that here the receptors are essentially signalling angular *velocity*.

This can perhaps be seen more clearly if we plot the ratio of cupula displacement to head *velocity* rather than head position (figure 2.9), giving a response which is seen to be flat over the same range of frequencies, with only small phase lags. Finally, at frequencies lower than some 0·01 Hz, the cupula displacement leads head velocity by some 90°, and the corresponding portion of the velocity transfer function increases linearly with frequency: in this region the cupula is responding essentially to the angular *acceleration* of the head. Thus the statement often found in general textbooks, that the semicircular canals are for signalling rotational acceleration, is only true for very slow movements. Over a range of some two and a half decades of frequency, covering what one might call the 'physiological range', the canals are not acceleration transducers but *velocity* transducers.

This can be appreciated by considering the movement of the cupula during a natural spontaneous turn of the head (Roberts, 1967), when the deflection of the cupula follows quite faithfully the time course of the head's instantaneous velocity (figure 2.10). The lower-frequency effects

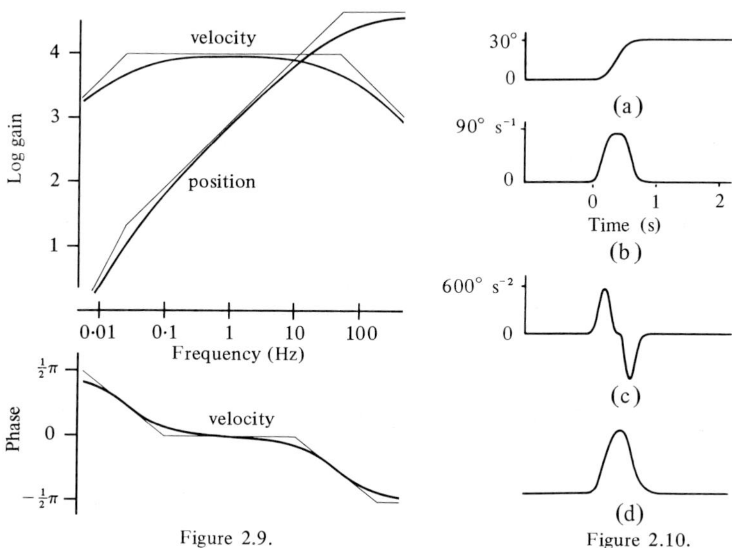

Figure 2.9. Figure 2.10.

Figure 2.9. Gain and phase of the second-order model of the semicircular canal, calculated with the use of Fernandez and Goldberg's (1971) experimental parameters. The 'position' curve is for conditions in which the head is rotated sinusoidally at different frequencies and with constant amplitude of movement: in the 'velocity' case the sinusoidal rotation is of constant peak angular velocity.

Figure 2.10. The canals essentially signal angular velocity under natural conditions. On the left, (a) represents the time course of a typical natural head movement; (b) and (c) show respectively the time course of its velocity and its acceleration; (d) shows the calculated cupular displacement resulting from the same head movement: its similarity to the velocity curve is evident (courtesy of Dr T D M Roberts).

only make themselves felt under the unnatural conditions of laboratory examination with prolonged periods of rotation in one direction at constant velocity, when the cupular response dies away in an exponential manner (figure 2.11), and when an afterresponse of opposite sign occurs at the end of the rotation.

Some evidence that the range of frequencies for which the canals act as velocity transducers is indeed 'tuned' to the speed of natural movements of the head comes from Melvill Jones and Spells' (1963) investigation of the dimensions of the canals in different species. The long time constant of the semicircular canal is in part a function both of its radius of curvature and of its diameter: the authors find that these two quantities show slight but significant changes (corresponding to a lengthening of the time constant) that are related to the mass of the animal to roughly the extent that might be predicted by a consideration of the natural movements of its head. No doubt similar factors underlie the differences between the time constants of the horizontal canals and of the vertical canals, that have already been remarked on.

However, evidence is accumulating that the simple mechanical model discussed so far cannot account for all dynamic properties of vestibular discharges in response to angular rotations, at least at extremes of frequency. Reflex eye movements in response to rotation of the head show an additional component of adaptation over and above the adaptation component associated with the elastic time constant, and intrinsic to the mechanism of the canal (Malcolm and Melvill Jones, 1970; Stockwell et al, 1973; Landers and Taylor, 1975). The time constant of this

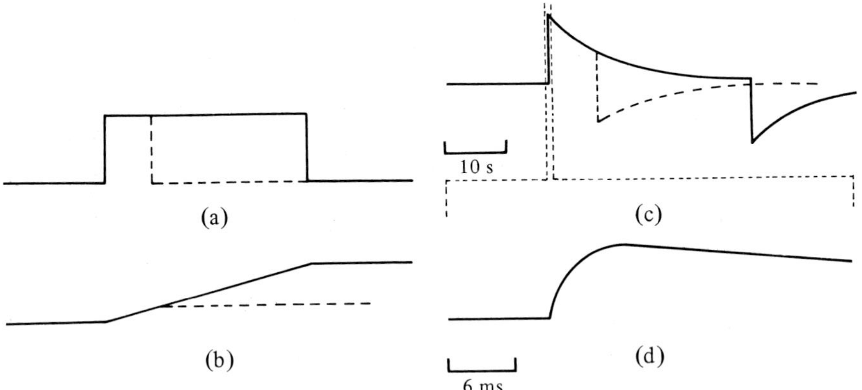

Figure 2.11. Cupular deflection during rotations at constant angular velocity: (a) shows the velocity and (b) the position of the head during a prolonged rotation: the dashed lines indicate a different case, when the movement is stopped relatively soon after it has started; (c) shows the time course of the cupula deviation on the same time scale, while (d) is an expanded representation of the beginning of the response, to show the course of the initial deviation (which depends on the short time constant). In (c) the dependence of the size of the afterresponse on the duration of the rotation can be seen.

component is around 60–120 s (compared with the 6 s to 16 s of the elastic time constant), and so can hardly be said to contribute much to the reflex response under natural conditions of stimulation. Although these observations by themselves cannot distinguish between an adaptation process occurring in the oculomotor pathways from one in the vestibular apparatus itself, Fernandez and Goldberg (1971) find a similar extra component of adaptation in their recordings from squirrel monkey vestibular fibres, with a time constant of some 80 s.

The same authors describe yet another component of the vestibular response seen in some vestibular fibres, that is not anticipated from the mechanical model, and which results in a phase lead at high frequencies. But, like the slow adaptation, it manifests itself at frequencies somewhat removed from those that are significant in the control of eye movements in real life, at least as far as gain is concerned. The observed discrepancy in phase for horizontal movements amounts to some 37° at 8 Hz, equivalent to about 13 ms of prediction, against which must be offset delays associated with passage of information through the vestibulo-ocular system, and in initiating muscular contraction. Uncertainties in these latter factors make the interpretation of phase measurements above 3 Hz or so somewhat metaphysical.

The other problem that has interested workers in this field is the nature of the nonlinear relationship between deviation of the cupula and frequency of firing of the sensory fibres. Although there is great variation amongst fibres as to their resting discharge rate—or whether indeed they fire spontaneously at all—nevertheless these features do not seem to reflect variations in the fundamental form of their response to cupular bending. Groen et al (1952) measured the frequency of firing of individual fibres immediately after impulsive decelerations of different magnitudes, and related these frequencies to the corresponding calculated cupular deflections. They found that individual fibres gave S-shaped response curves as a function of deflection, and that the curves for different units, although similar in shape, were typically displaced by different amounts along the deflection axis, thus accounting for their differing rates of firing at rest (figure 2.12). A possible functional advantage of this arrangement is that the range over which the frequency of impulses in the nerve *as a whole* is linearly related to cupular deflection, is thus considerably greater than the linear range of any one fibre in it. In fact it is difficult to see otherwise why so many sensory fibres are needed to carry information about a single one-dimensional variable.

There is as yet no compelling evidence for a division of fibres into two groups on the basis of their electrical responses, that might correspond with the two morphological classes of receptor cell described in section 2.1.2. It will be recalled that the same sensory fibres are often seen to innervate both types of receptor, so that any differences in their responses are likely to be blurred. Possibly the spread of characteristics that is observed between fibres as to their thresholds for firing and degree of adaptation is simply due to variations in the proportion of each type of receptor that particular fibres innervate. What effect the efferent supply to the vestibular receptors may have on their response curves or dynamic properties has not been established: it is probably predominantly inhibitory (Precht, 1974).

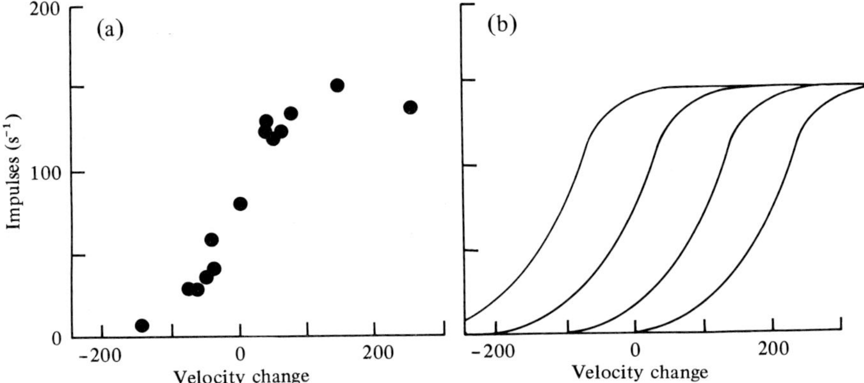

Figure 2.12. Peak firing frequency of vestibular fibres in the ray to sudden angular velocity changes of different magnitudes: one can assume that maximum cupular deviation under these conditions is proportional to the change in velocity, so that there appears to be an S-shaped relationship between cupular deflection and firing frequency. (b) How different units of this type, lying at different points along a scale of cupular deflection, might show the range of tonic activity that is observed (data from Groen et al, 1952).

2.1.4 Electrical responses to linear accelerations

The utricle and saccule have on the whole received rather less attention from investigators than have the semicircular canals. The saccule in particular is still something of a mystery: Ashcroft and Hallpike (1934) could find no responses from saccular fibres in the frog during rotation or tilting, although it appeared to be sensitive to low-frequency vibration. More recent work with mammalian preparations suggests that the saccule may not differ much from the utricle in its adaptation for signalling linear accelerations: electrical stimulation of the saccular macula in the cat can produce vestibuloocular reflexes in the vertical plane (Fluur and Mellström, 1970; 1971).

Löwenstein and Roberts (1949), recording from utricular fibres in the ray, found two classes of fibre. One was essentially static or tonic, and showed no appreciable adaptation in firing frequency for fixed angles of tilt, whereas the other class showed a dynamic or phasic pattern of response that was greater for changes in the angle of tilt, and declined to a lower resting level when the position of the head was fixed. Units of the first kind were found to be preferentially sensitive to different angles of tilt, corresponding no doubt to the variations in the direction of morphological polarisation that is seen in receptors in different parts of the macula. These findings have recently been extended by Loe et al (1973) (figure 2.13), who find that most units are maximally sensitive when the head is in the normal upright position. The rate of discharge for different directions of linear acceleration is a simple function of the component of the acceleration resolved in the direction of maximum response: the relationship may indeed be a linear one (Fernandez et al, 1973).

In these experiments the rate of tilt was sufficiently slow that one can exclude possible effects from the semicircular canals. With faster movements of the head one cannot exclude the possibility that, because of the continuity of the endolymph between the otolith organs and the canals, some kind of mechanical interaction may take place between them. A further possibility is that linear accelerations may distort the semicircular canals and thus lead to modification of the cupular response. Although interactions between linear and rotational accelerations have often been described in vestibulo-ocular reflexes (for example Guedry, 1965; Niven et al, 1966; Benson and Bodin, 1966a; 1966b; Benson, 1970; Bles and Kapteyn, 1973), it is much more probable that these are the result of more central interactions, since it has been clearly demonstrated that convergence occurs in the vestibular nuclei between fibres from the different parts of the peripheral vestibular apparatus (see section 9.1.4).

All the same, Benson et al (1970) were able to show that horizontal canal units in the vestibular nuclei, that were not responsive to linear accelerations in the horizontal plane (and were therefore assumed not to be influenced by otolith organs), could nevertheless be made to fire periodically in response to a rotating linear acceleration vector without rotational acceleration. If the canals do indeed distort significantly under linear acceleration, a rotating vector of this type is the best way to

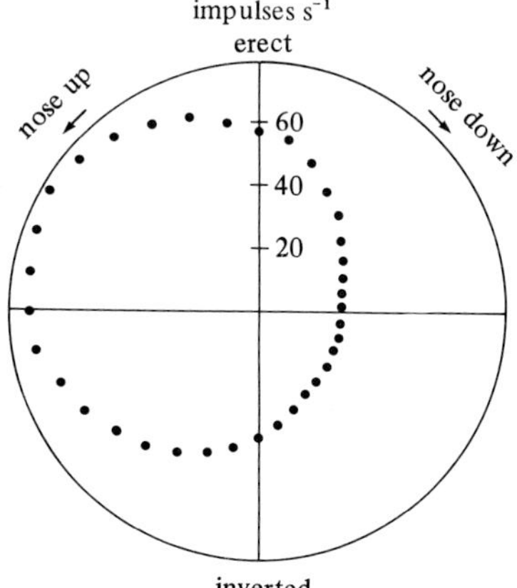

Figure 2.13. The rate of firing of a single fibre from the vestibular nerve of a cat, at different angles of tilt in the sagittal plane (data from Loe et al, 1973).

demonstrate the fact, since the distortion is likely to push the endolymph round the canals in a peristalsis-like manner as it moves in response to the changing direction of acceleration. However, the results of experiments by Correia and Money (1970) in which the response to a rotating linear acceleration vector could still be obtained after blockage of the canal ducts suggest that this cannot, in fact, be the true explanation. Whatever the mechanism of such interactions, they probably in any case play only a minor role in the vestibular control of eye movements under natural conditions.

A simpler kind of interaction is the *positional nystagmus* that can often be observed on tilting the head while 'suffering' from alcohol poisoning. It has recently been suggested (Money and Myles, 1974) that this may result from a change in the relative density of cupula and endolymph brought about by the direct physical effect of the alcohol: the cupula would then act, in effect, like an otolith organ. They observe, in support of this theory, that ingestion of heavy water in suitable quantities can cancel out the density change and prevent the positional nystagmus. It is quite possible that the well-known nauseating aftereffects of alcohol are due to a motion sickness arising from illusory stimulation of this kind.

2.2 Static vestibulo-ocular responses

It is convenient to divide reflex vestibular movements into two classes—static and dynamic—according as they are produced by linear or rotational accelerations. In man and other species with front-facing eyes, the static reflexes are mostly rather weak and easily dominated both by dynamic vestibular reflexes and by vision, but in animals like the rabbit they are easily demonstrated (figure 2.14). If the skull is tilted, the eyes tend to move in such a way as to keep their former orientation in space: This implies that animals with front-facing eyes and those with side-facing eyes will require the contraction of different sets of muscles to compensate for the same head movement. A complicating factor in such demonstrations is the presence of reflex eye movements which occur in response to stimulation of proprioceptors in the neck if the head is moved relative to the body. Thus it is necessary to move head and body together if one

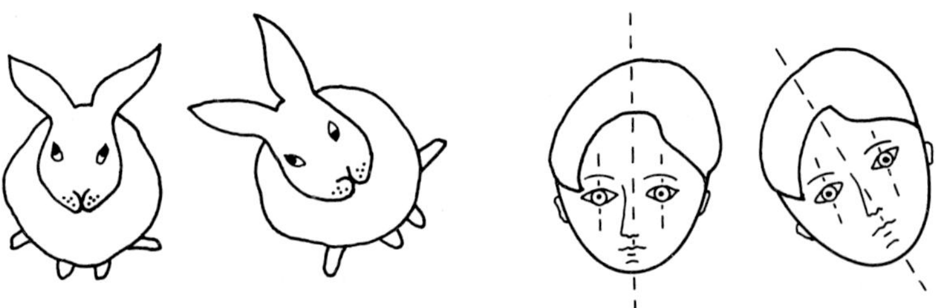

Figure 2.14. Oculomotor responses to tilt of the head compared in the rabbit and in man (after Duke-Elder and Wybar, 1973).

wishes to isolate the vestibular component. In the rabbit, the vestibular contribution to movements of the eyes with the body held still is about 70% (de Kleijn, 1921b), and almost full compensation can be achieved for tilt angles of up to 70° (figure 2.15).

In man, the only static vestibulo-ocular reflex that is not normally completely dominated by vision is the torsion of the eye (that is, rotation about the anterior–posterior axis) that can be observed on lateral tilt of the head (Merton, 1956; Miller, 1962; Belcher, 1964; in the monkey: Krejcova et al, 1973; and in the owl: Steinbach et al, 1974). These counterrolling movements are very small [for example, commonly a maximum of some 7°—as in figure 2.16—although Petrov and Zenkin (1973) report vestibular torsion of up to 18°] and can hardly be said to be compensatory to any significant extent: possibly they represent a vestigial reflex intended for animals with lateral eyes. As in the rabbit, otolith and neck proprioceptor components can be isolated, and there is a further phasic component dying away with a time constant of some two seconds that may well be due to the canals.

This last component can be isolated by having the subject lie on his back, and measuring eye torsion during movements around a vertical axis (Merton, 1956); one cannot assume that this procedure eliminates all otolith contribution, since there is no reason in principle why the maculae of the utricle and saccule could not respond transiently to rotational accelerations as well as to linear. Conversely, as we have seen, experiments involving linear accelerations of changing direction may possibly be due to

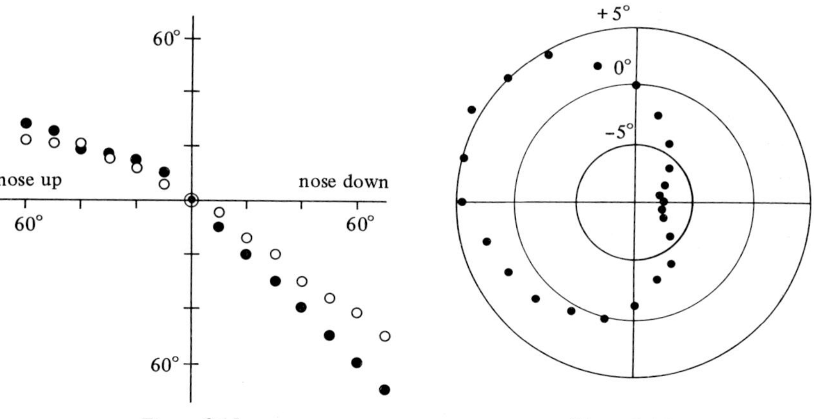

Figure 2.15. Figure 2.16.

Figure 2.15. Compensatory rotation of a rabbit's eye for different degrees of tilt in the sagittal plane (filled circles): the open circles represent observations made when the dorsal roots of the first and second cranial nerves have been cut, that is, when the influence of neck reflexes has been removed to leave a response that is almost wholly vestibular in origin (data from de Kleijn, 1921b).

Figure 2.16. Ocular counterrolling in man: rotation of the eye about a torsional axis measured for different angles of lateral tilt of the head (data from Miller, 1962).

canal as well as otolith function. Using sinusoidal acceleration along a linear track, Baarsma and Collewijn (1975) have measured the frequency transfer function of the 'static' vestibulo-ocular reflex in the rabbit, and find it to fall off rather rapidly with increasing frequency (figure 2.17). The shape of this function is sufficiently different from that of the canal vestibulo-ocular transfer function that it is unlikely that their measurements were contaminated by a canal artefact. The otolith contribution is clearly slow and tonic in nature.

One might expect that a subject with bilateral destruction of the labyrinths and with the head fixed with respect to the body would show no torsion at all on lateral tilt. This is not in fact the case, and such people often show a residual response that may be due to some remnant of labyrinthine activity, to visual cues (see section 3.1), or conceivably to differences in pressure on the two sides of the body (Miller and Graybiel, 1962; Krejcova et al, 1971).

Eye movements in response to movements of the body while the head is kept still seem first to have been described by Barany (1906b). This contribution of the proprioceptors of the neck—mainly joint receptors rather than muscle receptors (McCouch et al, 1951)—is rather small both in the rabbit (figure 2.15) and in man, where the response falls from -10 to -20 dB in the natural frequency range (Young et al, 1966); there

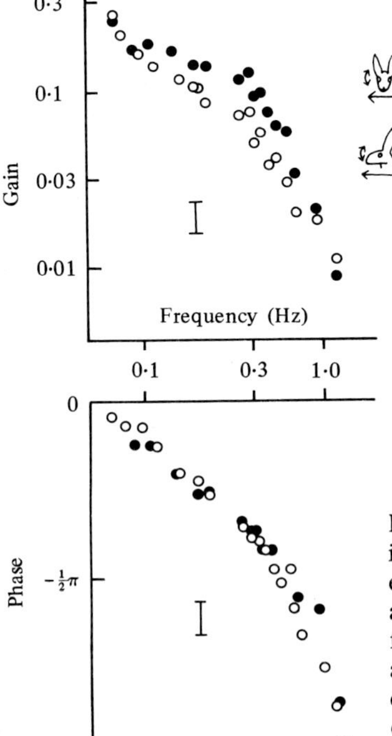

Figure 2.17. Gain and phase of ocular counterrolling in the rabbit in response to sinusoidal variation of the effective direction of gravity by appropriate linear accelerations in the horizontal plane, as a function of frequency. Filled circles are for lateral movement, and open circles for longitudinal: the vertical bar in each graph represents a typical value of the standard deviation of a single observation. After Baarsma and Collewijn (1975).

appears to be very great variability between subjects (Takemori and Suzuki, 1971). in the decerebrate cat it is very difficult to record any response at all to twist of the neck if the labyrinths on each side are destroyed (Carpenter, 1972a). However, the observations of Biemond and de Jong (1961) in the rabbit suggest that cervical effects are in some way dependent on the integrity of the vestibular system: after bilateral labyrinthectomy, the nystagmus formerly provoked by unilateral block of cervical afferents by local injection of procaine is abolished. Recently, however, Dichgans et al (1973; 1974) have shown that, although the neck contribution to responses to head movement in the monkey is normally virtually nonexistent, after bilateral section of the vestibular nerves a certain degree of relearning occurs, so that after some seven weeks nearly all the response is recovered, by an increase in gain of neck reflexes, and by differences in the 'programming' of eye and head movements. Dichgans (1975) has recently reviewed the contribution of afferents from the neck to the oculomotor system.

2.3 Dynamic vestibulo-ocular responses

2.3.1 Vestibular nystagmus

In man, movements of the eyes occur much more readily in response to rotation of the head than to linear acceleration, and indeed form the basis of the commonest clinical tests for vestibular function. We have seen that over a wide range of frequencies the canals signal the angular velocity of the head in different planes; over a large part of this range, vestibulo-ocular reflexes strive to match the velocity of the eye to that of the head, in an attempt to keep the image of the outside world stationary on the retina. However, although with rotating chairs and other laboratory equipment we can rotate the head through as large an angle as we please, the eye obviously cannot go on turning indefinitely in the orbit. In fact, during prolonged rotations the compensatory movements of the eye in the opposite direction are periodically interrupted by fast flicks in the direction of rotation, which thus enable the eye to continue its task of matching *velocity* even though it has reset its *position* in relation to the outside world. Thus a graph of the instantaneous deviation of the eye as a function of time during such a rotation has a characteristic sawtooth or time-base appearance consisting of a *slow phase* in the compensatory direction and a *quick phase* in the anticompensatory direction: the whole pattern of response is what is meant by *nystagmus* (figure 2.18). Vestibular nystagmus has been known for a considerable time: it seems first to have

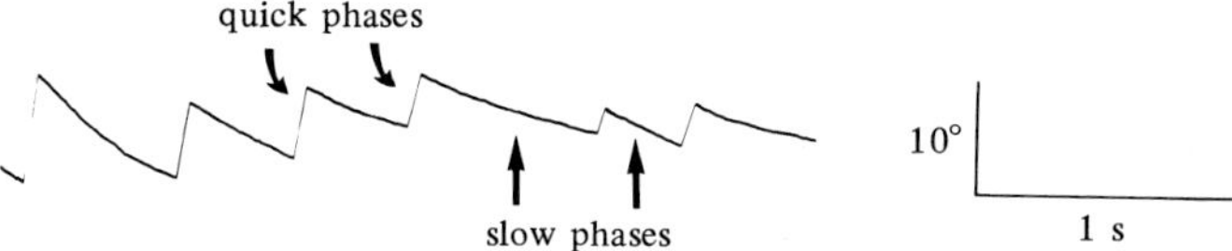

Figure 2.18. A record of human vestibular nystagmus, showing the slow and quick phases.

been described in 1794 by Erasmus Darwin (the remarkable physician, inventor and poet, and grandfather of Charles). Conventionally—and perhaps illogically—nystagmus is characterised not by the direction of the slow phase but by that of the anticompensatory quick phase. Thus a rotation of the head to the right also leads to a nystagmus to the right.

The matching of eye velocity to the signal from the receptors in the cristae is sufficiently faithful that the slow phase of nystagmus during particular patterns of rotation quite accurately parallels the discharge of the vestibular fibres (Henriksson, 1955), although the relationship can be profoundly modified by such factors as arousal (for example Mowrer, 1934) or habituation (see below, section 2.3.2). During a prolonged rotation at constant velocity, for example, the slow phase velocity gradually declines over the course of some 20 s, with a corresponding decline in the frequency of the quick phases (figure 2.19). If the motion is suddenly stopped, a nystagmus in the opposite direction (after- or postrotational nystagmus) is seen, which in its turn dies away with a similar time course. Tests using periods not of constant velocity but of constant acceleration are useful for demonstrating the extra (nonmechanical) adaptational component mentioned in section 2.1.3 (for example Stockwell et al, 1973).

Finally, sinusoidal rotations in the dark at different frequencies can provide useful quantitative descriptions of the dynamic properties of the vestibulo-ocular reflex in terms of its frequency response (Niven and Hixson, 1961; Young et al, 1966; Carpenter, 1972a; Baarsma and Collewijn, 1974; Shinoda and Yoshida, 1974). For small rotations, and in decerebrate animals, the resultant eye movements are sinusoidal; larger movements

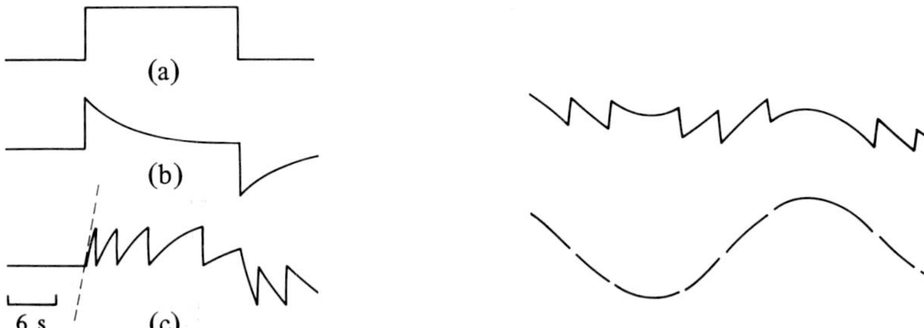

Figure 2.19. Figure 2.20.

Figure 2.19. Vestibular nystagmus during a constant-velocity turn: (a) represents the time-course of the velocity of the head, (b) the resultant deviation of the cupula, and (c)—very diagrammatically—the ensuing vestibular nystagmus: the frequency of the quick phases has been drastically reduced, for clarity. The velocity of the slow phase is approximately proportional to cupular deviation at every point.

Figure 2.20. An illustration of how the quick phases can be removed from a record of vestibular nystagmus to provide a curve showing the cumulative effect of the slow phase on its own.

produce quick phase interruptions which can be removed from the raw records to isolate the slow-phase response (figure 2.20). The result is a quasi-sinusoidal movement, showing asymmetric nonlinearities as the amplitude of the stimulus is increased (Carpenter, 1972a; Mathog, 1972; Shinoda and Yoshida, 1974; Landers and Taylor, 1975). In the linear range, one can proceed to calculate the gain and phase of the system's response at different frequencies: in all preparations studied, the resultant frequency response shows good compensation over a middle range of frequencies, with a falloff of amplitude at frequencies above some 2–6 Hz, and below about 0·05 Hz (figure 2.21).

Measurements of *phase* unfortunately show very much less consistency between different species (figure 2.21): for example, at just under 0·1 Hz, an etherised cat shows nearly 90° phase lead compared with an alert monkey (Sugie and Melvill Jones, 1971; Skavenski and Robinson, 1973). Some of this conflict, particularly at higher frequencies, is undoubtedly due to differences in procedure of phase measurements in the presence of nonlinearities. Another factor that may be relevant is that some of the preparations make quick phases during sinusoidal stimulation (which then have to be removed by the process shown in figure 2.20), whereas in others the quick phases are naturally absent. In the first case, we have to make the assumption that the quick phase is in effect only a brief displacement of the whole record: but it *might* have some disturbing effect on the stretch of record immediately following it, resulting in a distortion of the apparent phase. This is the explanation given by Sugie and Melvill Jones for the large phase advance of the slow phase seen when the depth of anaesthesia of their cats is increased to the point where the quick phases disappear: they suggest that each quick phase consists of a step of displacement followed by an exponential decline with a time constant of about 0·7 s, which is added to the slow phase component.

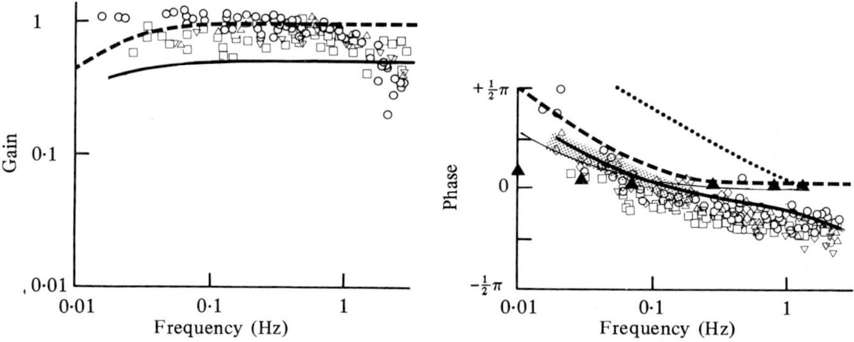

Figure 2.21. Transfer function of vestibulo-ocular reflex in different preparations. Thick line, human (Young et al, 1966); thin line, human (Benson, 1970); shading, human (Niven and Hixson, 1961); dashed line, normal cat (Landers and Taylor, 1975); dotted line, anaesthetised cat (Sugie and Melvill Jones, 1971); open symbols, decerebrate cat (Carpenter, 1972a); solid triangles, normal monkey (Skavenski and Robinson, 1973).

Yet another factor likely to contribute to this variability is the remarkable degree of plasticity shown by the vestibulo-ocular reflex under different adapting conditions (see section 2.3.2), which under extreme conditions can produce phase changes as large as 120° over the course of a week or two.

It has often been suggested that the falloff in gain at lower frequencies is a 'deliberate' feature of the vestibulo-ocular reflex (ter Braak, 1936; Melvill Jones, 1965; Baarsma and Collewijn, 1974). Normally visual reflexes assist the vestibular system in maintaining fixation during head movements, but the visual contribution, though accurate, is very slow both on account of the sluggishness of the visual receptors themselves, and also the many stages of neural processing that must intervene before visual signals can reach oculomotor pathways. As we shall see in chapter 3, the region where the visual component starts to fall off is close to where the vestibular component begins to turn over onto its plateau, so that the two mechanisms working together can by simple addition of effects provide full compensation of head movements right down to zero frequency. The importance of this synergy can readily be seen by means of a simple demonstration (Robinson, 1968b). Hold your hand out at arm's length, and shake it from side to side through a few degrees. Compare the clarity with which you see it with the case when you keep the hand still, but move your head at the same frequency through the same angle: the improvement is striking. One might describe the dynamic vestibulo-ocular reflex as a velocity-matching mechanism for moderate to high frequencies.

The same conclusion—the desirability of a low-frequency falloff in vestibular gain—comes from a consideration of natural head movements. Of course, spontaneous head movements are quite unlike what is experienced in a typical rotating chair experiment; nor, for that matter, are they much like sinusoidal rotations. Furthermore, most head movements are made with the express *purpose* of shifting the gaze. What then is the point of elaborate mechanisms for keeping the eyes still? Here again it is perhaps helpful to distinguish carefully between the control of *velocity* and the control of *position.* Obviously a change in the position of fixation implies that at least for a limited period there must be relative motion between the retina and the visual world: the shorter this period is, the less visual information will be lost during the shift of gaze . But head movements must necessarily be much slower than eye movements, because of the enormously greater moment of inertia of the head in comparison with that of the eye.

The solution then is to use vestibular reflexes to keep the *velocity* of the eye at all times equal and opposite to that of the head, but at some point during the movement to superimpose on this basic response a *position* change in the same direction as the head movement, that is as fast as the oculomotor system can manage. In this way the shift of gaze is achieved with the minimum possible period during which the visual system is out of action. Recordings of eye movements during natural movements of the head confirm that this is indeed what happens (Atkin, 1964;

Morasso et al, 1973) and that, as a consequence, during the head movement the eyes move—relative to the external scene—smartly from one position of steady gaze to the other. One might suppose that the fast anticompensatory movement was simply the same thing as the old quick phase of nystagmus, in a new guise. But a simple experiment makes it clear that the quick part of the response is as it were 'preprogrammed', and is not the result of vestibular stimulation at all (Morasso et al, 1973). If the subject's head is suddenly and unexpectedly restrained at the moment of beginning the head movement, the eye nevertheless moves smartly to the new position of gaze exactly as before; the slow vestibular component is of course abolished (figure 2.22).

In other words, the fast and slow components have quite different origins: both the quick movement and the head movement are *primary* movements, in the sense that they are the direct result of the desire to shift the gaze: but the slow component is *secondary* to the head movement and does not occur if the head is fixed. The quick component may indeed start before the head has moved (Bizzi et al, 1972), although the electrical response from the neck muscles generally precedes that from the eye muscles. All the same, one cannot rule out a vestibular contribution to the quick component, since the same anticompensatory movement is observed when the head is moved suddenly by the subject *without* the intention of shifting the gaze to a peripheral object (Henriksson et al, 1974); while Melvill Jones (1964) found that sudden externally applied turns of the head also produce an anticompensatory flick preceding the slow compensatory component (admittedly with rather large angular accelerations); comparable findings have been published by Barnes (1974). Similar responses have been described as a result of electrical stimulation of the ampullary nerve in the alert monkey, although in this case the quick component follows the slow, and may merely represent an isolated nystagmus quick phase, or the monkey's voluntary effort to refixate what he was looking at before the stimulus (Cohen, Goto, and Tokomasu, 1967; Goto et al, 1968).

One should not forget that the movements of the head relative to the body are also under vestibular control, and at least in some species one can demonstrate nystagmus of the head as a result of this 'vestibulocollic' reflex.

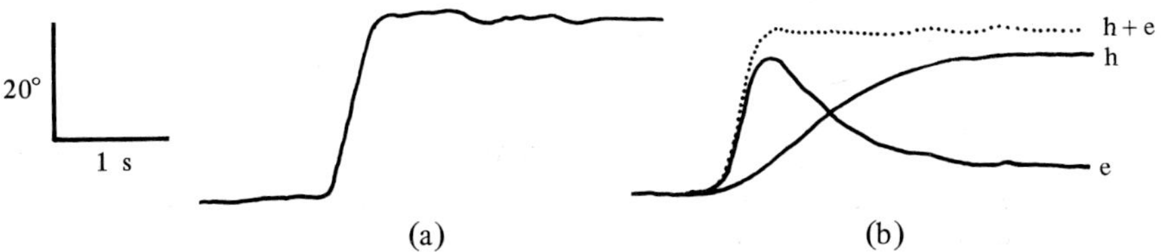

Figure 2.22. Head and eye movements made in looking at novel objects: (a) eye movement (saccade) made in fixating an eccentric target, with the head fixed; (b) head (h) and eye (e) movements made under exactly the same conditions, but with the head free; (h + e) is the sum of the head and eye movements (after Morasso et al, 1973).

There are two reasons why these movements are generally not as prominent as those of the eyes. First, that most animals' heads are mechanically dominated by their inertia, and cannot easily execute high-frequency motion; and second, that the vestibulocollic reflexes have intrinsic negative feedback, in that any compensatory movement of the head necessarily reduces its own stimulus. The prominent head nystagmus of birds when walking was discussed in section 1.1: but this is primarily visual rather than vestibular in origin (Dunlap and Mowrer, 1931). The *quick* phase of head nystagmus is however anticompensatory, and the extra vestibular stimulation it provides may cause a certain degree of synchrony between nystagmus of the head and of the eyes (Hinoki and Terayama, 1966a; 1966b; Outerbridge and Melvill Jones, 1971).

Finally, it is perhaps worth emphasising that, although the great majority of work on the vestibulo-ocular reflexes has been done on horizontal movements of the eyes, nystagmus can equally be observed both in the vertical plane and (with some experimental sophistication: Davies and Merton, 1958; Melvill Jones, 1960; Petrov and Zenkin, 1973) for torsional movements. The decay characteristics of vestibular nystagmus during constant accelerations are markedly different for rotations around different axes, no doubt because of the differences between the mechanical properties of the three canals mentioned above in section 2.1.3; the direction of gravity may also exert an independent effect (Benson and Bodin, 1966b; Benson, 1970).

2.3.2 The nature of the quick phase

There are essentially two ways in which one might imagine the rhythmic movements of nystagmus to be produced. The older notion, expressed for example in some of the writings of Lorente de No (1933 for example) and held by implication if not explicitly by some more recent authors (for example McCabe, 1965) is that nystagmus is the product of a specifically organised neural oscillator—perhaps arranged in a similar manner to an astable multivibrator—that is set running by impulses from the semicircular canals. In Lorente de No's own words (1933, page 289): "Nystagmus is nothing else than an alternating reflex similar to other known rhythmic reflexes. The peripheral labyrinthine stimulation sets into activity a machinery which gives rise to nystagmus in the same way as the spinal cord sets up the scratch reflex as a response to a stimulus produced in the skin." The other view, now more commonly held, is that the slow and quick phases are two quite separate phenomena, the slow phase being a continuous background response to vestibular stimulation, on which the quick phases are superimposed by a different and distinct mechanism.

Perhaps one should not exaggerate the difference between these two concepts, which is largely one of emphasis: Lorente de No himself was fully aware, for example, that there are a large number of different circumstances under which the quick phase can be abolished, leaving the slow phase unaffected. These include brain lesions (for example Holmes, 1938; Wadia and Swami, 1971; Carpenter, 1972a) and sleep (di Giorgio, 1935; Nathanson and Bergmann, 1958); while many drugs have differential effects on fast and slow phases: (Bender, 1955; Rashbass and Russell, 1961; Philipszoon, 1962; Janeke et al, 1969; Melvill Jones and Sugie, 1972; Haliska, 1973). Furthermore, although it is true that the frequency of nystagmus is roughly correlated with the speed of the slow phase, the relation is very far from being the close one that would be expected if both were the product of the same neuronal oscillator (Torok and Derbyshire, 1968; Tibbling, 1969; Sugie and Melvill Jones, 1971). It seems difficult to escape the conclusion that the slow phase is an independent entity from the quick, and that the two are not merely, as it were, the systole and diastole of an *essentially* rhythmic process.

All the same, it is by no means clear exactly what the mechanism is by which the quick phases are repetitively generated during nystagmus. One might expect for example that the quick phase would be triggered when the eye reached a certain limiting deviation in the orbit, perhaps signalled by stretch receptors in the eye muscles. But complete removal of the eye and its muscles from the orbit has virtually no effect on the rhythmic pattern of discharge that can be recorded from the oculomotor neurons during vestibular nystagmus (McIntyre, 1939), and in any case, inspection of records of vestibular nystagmus in response to varying rotational accelerations shows quite clearly that the quick phases are not in fact initiated at fixed deviations of the eye (figure 2.23). Further, Ohm showed in 1936 that if a small-amplitude high-frequency nystagmus were evoked at the same time as a large-amplitude low-frequency one—by two distinct modes of stimulation—the two sets of quick phases showed no interaction (as would be expected if they were generated by the total resultant slow phase component) but behaved exactly as if they were independently generated and added together in a linear manner. The result was thus a large sawtooth waveform with a smaller sawtooth on its edge.

During sinusoidal stimulation one finds that the point at which the quick phase is initiated varies systematically in each cycle, in such a way that the *mean* position of the eye in each phase itself moves sinusoidally, advanced in phase by some 90° relative to the sine wave traced out by the

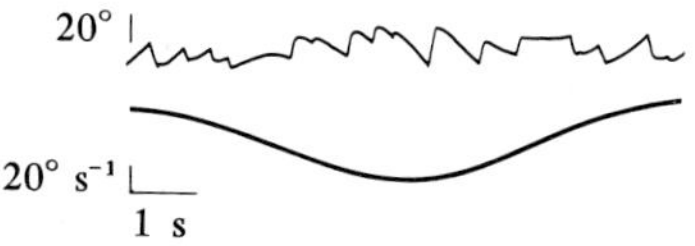

Figure 2.23. Eye movement (upper trace) in response to sinusoidal variation of head velocity (lower trace), showing the lack of regular correspondance between the stimulus and the moments at which the quick phases are initiated (Gonshor and Melvill Jones, 1971).

slow component (Mishkin and Melvill Jones, 1966). This suggests that the quick phase may be triggered when the velocity of the head (and thus the signal from the canals) reaches some fixed threshold value: and it seems also that the size of the quick phase is similarly related to the velocity of the head rather than to the position of the eye. Models of neuronal mechanisms that might underlie this phenomenon are discussed in chapter 12: possibly the mechanism of this phase advance is the same as the one producing the anticompensatory quick phase at the beginning of rapid head movements, discussed in the previous section.

Yet another complicating factor is the observation that the mechanism generating the quick phases also appears to have an inherent *periodicity* (Cheng and Outerbridge, 1974b). When the stimulus is large (and steady) the distribution of intersaccadic intervals (that is, of the intervals of time between successive quick phases) is essentially unimodal. But as the degree of stimulation is increased, the distribution begins to break up into a series of peaks of uniform spacing, about half a second apart. This suggests that the quick phases are generated by a mechanism having an inherent rhythmic tendency with a frequency of about 2 Hz. It is difficult to see what functional advantages such an arrangement might confer; it may possibly be related to the intermittency associated with normal fixation saccades (see below, section 4.2.1).

2.3.3 Habituation, and other aspects of vestibulo-ocular flexibility

Vestibular nystagmus shows an astonishing degree of adaptability in conforming itself to changed circumstances. After damage to the vestibular organs, under repeated excessive vestibular stimulation, and under circumstances when the natural relationship between movements of the eyes and movements of the retinal image has been interfered with, the vestibular response is capable of modifying itself to maintain its usefulness.

Unilateral damage to the vestibular apparatus normally results in a spontaneous nystagmus directed away from the damaged side, together with a tonic deviation of the head and eyes towards it: these effects are presumably due to the loss of the tonic activity of the damaged labyrinth, and the unopposed tonic activity of the sound one (Löwenstein, 1937). After some weeks these effects die away. This apparent central compensation for the sensory asymmetry produced by the original lesion seems widely distributed in the animal kingdom: crabs, for example, show an analogous compensation after unilateral damage to their statocysts (Schöne, 1954). If the contralateral labyrinth is now destroyed, a nystagmus of opposite sign is immediately seen (Bechterew or compensatory nystagmus) which in turn eventually dies away. Simultaneous bilateral destruction of the vestibular apparatus does not of course produce nystagmus: Bechterew nystagmus is presumably essentially a 'rebound' phenomenon whereby the central mechanism that compensates for loss of the first labyrinth suddenly finds after loss of the second that it no longer has anything to oppose.

Some evidence for this view comes from recordings from the vestibular nuclei after unilateral labyrinthectomy (Precht et al, 1966), when it is found that the spontaneous activity on the side of the lesion increases to offset the tonic signal from the other side. Fisch (1973) has recently contrasted this aspect of compensation, which he calls tonic, with the dynamic compensation that must also occur if information from the remaining labyrinth is to be properly used: that is, essentially a decrease in gain. He finds that whereas spontaneous nystagmus has usually disappeared after the lapse of a month or so, imbalance in response to vestibular stimulation takes many months to return to normal, and a permanent depression of the frequency of nystagmus in response to angular accelerations in either direction may be observed (Fluur and Mendel, 1973). One other effect of unilateral damage to the vestibular organs that may be mentioned here is the appearance of a nystagmus when the head is held in a tilted position (postitional nystagmus, see also section 2.1.4): and can be shown to be the result of unopposed operation of the intact otolith organs (Fluur and Siegborn, 1973; Oosterveld, 1973; Uemara and Cohen, 1973).

It is quite possible that a similar mechanism may underlie the habituation of nystagmus that can be observed under certain circumstances of prolonged or repeated vestibular stimulation. Unfortunately there is little agreement amongst experimenters as to exactly what these circumstances are. One difficulty in planning experimental tests of vestibular habituation is that of ensuring that the level of arousal does not change significantly from test to test as the subject becomes accustomed to—and thoroughly bored by—the experimental situation. Arousal strongly modifies vestibular nystagmus (Mowrer, 1934), and the degree of apparent vestibular habituation of nystagmus is greatly reduced in the cat if the animal is maintained in an alert state (Crampton and Schwann, 1961). Yet some decrement in response still remains, even with full arousal (Crampton, 1964).

Further evidence for a specifically vestibular effect comes from experiments in which the habituating accelerations have deliberatly been made asymmetric in intensity in the two directions. Collins and Updegraff (1966) rotated cats and dogs with a programme of accelerations of $3° \text{ s}^{-2}$ in one direction, and $0 \cdot 15° \text{ s}^{-2}$ in the other. Subsequent testing showed a decline in nystagmus provoked by rotation in the same sense as the stronger conditioning acceleration. It would be difficult to maintain that this was only due to a reduction in the level of arousal. Nor could one reasonably hold that such a mild stimulus had caused damage to the cupula, a criticism that is probably valid for some of the early experiments on habituation that used the Barany test: that is, sudden stopping of a chair previously rotating at around $200° \text{ s}^{-1}$ (discussed in Hood and Pfaltz, 1954).

On the other hand, if a stimulus *is* 'physiological' in strength and duration, then *ipso facto* one would hardly expect to be able to demonstrate habituation to it. Gonshor and Melvill Jones (1969) moved human subjects' heads sinusoidally at $0 \cdot 16$ Hz with a peak velocity of $60° \text{ s}^{-1}$ for a total period of an hour (as might be experienced by a spectator at a tennis match!) and found no significant decline in response. Such patterns of rotation are probably nearer to natural head movements than continuous rotations in one direction: Brown and Crampton (1966), using a stimulus (24° s^{-2} for 10 s) that was considerably less intense but also rather less natural, showed quite consistent habituation of nystagmus. All these findings tend to suggest a rather higher level of action of habituation than at the receptor itself, a suggestion reinforced by Hood and Pfaltz's (1954) observation that the very marked habituation exhibited by normal rabbits (figure 2.24) does not develop if they are anaesthetised during conditioning.

All the experiments on habituation described so far were performed in the dark, and can therefore be ascribed wholly to vestibular effects: all the same, it apparently makes rather little difference if the rotations are carried out in objectively stationary visual surroundings (Brown and Crampton, 1966). Rotation under *unnatural* (that is, not objectively stationary) visual conditions reveals an astonishing degree of plasticity in the vestibulo-ocular reflex [in cats and primates, at least: rabbits show virtually no plasticity (Collewijn and Kleinschmidt, 1975)]. The simplest case is that of rotation within a subjectively stationary visual field (that is, rotating with the subject). Under these circumstances vestibular nystagmus is very greatly reduced by vision, and with repeated testing the degree of suppression increases (Takemori and Cohen, 1974a): this is clearly a beneficial adaptation. A similar increase in visual suppression is apparently found in ballet dancers (Dix and Hood, 1969), presumably because their vestibular organs are unable to give them reliable information about the position of the head after gyrations prolonged beyond a period comparable with the elastic time constant of the cupula, so that they have come to rely more heavily on vision. Conversely, one finds that exposure to a

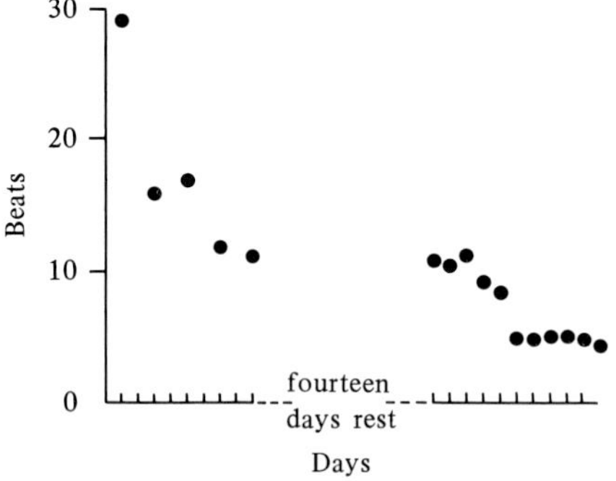

Figure 2.24. Habituation of vestibular nystagmus in rabbits. Decline in the number of nystagmic beats evoked in a standard vestibular test over a period of fourteen days, followed by a further fourteen days in which no vestibular stimulation was given. Nevertheless, no recovery occurred, and the response declined yet further during a final fourteen days of testing (averaged results from four rabbits) (data from Hood and Pfaltz, 1954).

rotating field with the head kept still likewise leads to a reduction in vestibulo-ocular responses (Young and Henn, 1974: but see also Miyoshi et al, 1973). More dramatically, if a subject is made to view the world through reversing prisms, so that his vestibulo-ocular reflexes are anticompensatory instead of compensatory (Gonshor and Melvill Jones, 1971; 1973; 1976a; 1976b), within a matter of days his vestibular nystagmus (tested in the dark) is found to be reversed in direction! In the same way, if the subject wears telescopic lenses that either enlarge or contract the visual scene (so that the vestibulo-ocular reflexes are of inappropriate gain), after a period of habituation it is found that the amplitude of the vestibular eye movements either increases or decreases to correspond with the needs of the visual system (Miles and Fuller, 1974). These results are of extreme interest, in view of the speed and apparent simplicity of the vestibulo-ocular reflex in its classical 'three neuron arc' form (see chaper 9). Unless one believes that a synapse can change in a matter of days from being excitatory to being inhibitory, they imply that such vision-induced reversals of response must be due to changes in pathways other than the fastest ones that link the vestibular organs to the eye muscles. The point is further pursued in chapter 12.

3

Visual tracking

"It is not good to beholde things that move swiftlie, nor yet such as turne round."

This chapter is concerned with the movements of the eyes that are made under visual guidance that hold an object of regard, and follow it when it moves. Such movements have been variously called tracking, or slow pursuit (smooth pursuit), or optokinetic: smooth pursuit is perhaps the most helpful expression, for it emphasises the distinction between this and other kinds of visual mechanisms controlling the eyes. They are rather less reflex in character than the vestibular movements, for they are capable of being modified by an effort of will: but on the other hand, most subjects are quite unable to *generate* them voluntarily in the absence of an appropriate stimulus, and in that respect they are somewhat less 'voluntary' than saccades or vergence movements.

3.1 Optokinetic nystagmus

The easiest way to demonstrate optokinetic nystagmus in the laboratory is to observe the eye movements that are made whilst a subject is viewing a rotating striped drum that fills a substantial part of the visual field. As long as the drum is not moving too fast, the subject tends to fixate a particular stripe and follow it as it moves: as the gaze is carried farther from the primary position, a fast anticompensatory flick is made that brings the point of fixation to some new feature on the drum that is in turn followed. Thus the time course of the movement is of the saw tooth form that we have already seen to result from head rotation (figure 3.1) and is called optokinetic (or sometimes railway-train) nystagmus: Purkinje (1825) seems to have been the first to describe it, in the eyes of a crowd watching a procession of cavalry. Any detailed moving scene will do equally well—the view from a railway carriage window is excellent—and in fact moving patterns of randomly arranged dots have some advantages over stripes for experimental work, because the particular spacing of the stripes strongly influences the pattern of quick phases that is obtained (for example, Cheng and Outerbridge, 1974a). Optokinetic nystagmus occurs with equal facility in horizontal and vertical directions, but not around an anterior-posterior axis: on viewing a visual field rotating in a plane parallel to the frontal plane, one observes not a nystagmus but a steady deviation of the eye, reaching a maximum of some 2° at about 30° s^{-1} (figure 3.2; Kertesz and Jones, 1969).

The form and degree of optokinetic nystagmus is strongly influenced by the subject's attitude to the task, and by the nature of the instructions he is given. Dogs, for example, will not follow moving stripes with their eyes, but may do so if the stripes are replaced by pictures of rabbits: even this may not work if the particular subject does not find rabbits sufficiently interesting (Rademaker and ter Braak, 1948). Human subjects may be instructed either to look at the stimulus, to stare at it (that is without making any effort to follow it with the eyes), or—a more difficult task—to match the velocity of their eyes to that of the target. This last command, paradoxically, produces the poorest correspondence between target velocity and eye velocity, leading to large cumulative positional errors (Puckett and Steinman, 1969). If the subject 'looks' at the drum, his movements are large in extent and his quick phases relatively infrequent: if instead he 'stares' at the drum, the nystagmus is small in amplitude and more frequent (figures 3.1 and 3.3) (Rademaker and ter Braak, 1948).

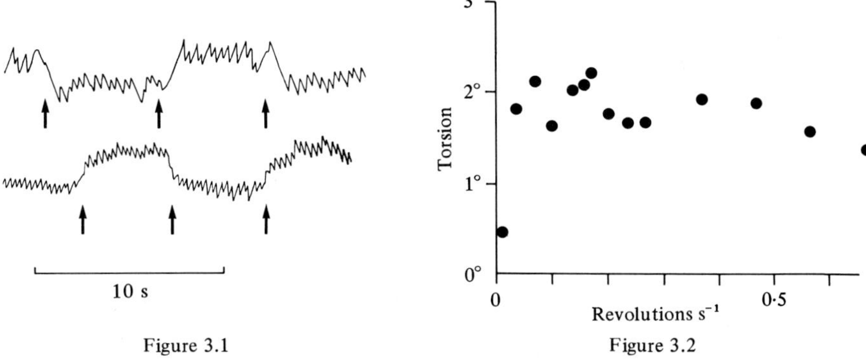

Figure 3.1 Figure 3.2

Figure 3.1. Human optokinetic nystagmus under two different conditions: in the upper trace, the subject was actively trying to follow the stripes of the drum, while in the lower trace the subject was gazing passively at it. The arrows indicate moments at which the movement of the drum was reversed: note the *average* deviation in the direction of drum movement in the first case, and in the opposite direction in the second (Hood and Leech, 1974).

Figure 3.2. Steady torsional response of the human eye to fixation of a field rotating in the plane of fixation at different angular velocities (data from Kertesz and Jones, 1969).

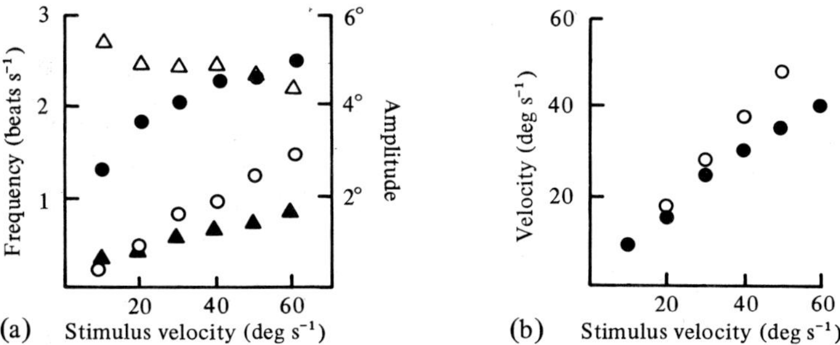

Figure 3.3. Optokinetic responses as a function of stimulus velocity. Filled symbols indicate conditions when the subject was told to *stare* at the drum; open symbols, when he was to *look* at it. In (a) the frequency (circles) and amplitude (triangles) are shown under the two conditions: in (b), the velocity of the slow phase (data from Honrubia et al, 1967).

The velocity of the slow phase is similar in each case, and at moderate speeds (less than some 30° s^{-1}) is close to the speed of the drum (Honrubia et al, 1968). With faster drum speeds, the slow phase lags more and more behind the movements of the drum, until at some 100° s^{-1} the system breaks down completely and only inappropriate movements—if any at all— are made (for example Dodge et al, 1930; Honrubia et al, 1967; and many others).

The smaller the part of the visual field that moves, or the more eccentric it is, the worse the slow phase velocity matches the drum speed (figure 3.4) (Koerner and Schiller, 1972; Easter, 1972): but the relationship between the contributions of the central and peripheral parts of the visual field is a more complicated one than simple summation (Hood and Leech, 1974; Hood, 1975). To see why this is likely to be so, it is helpful to consider the natural circumstances in which visual pursuit is used. Consider for example a cat intent on a mouse that is crossing a patch of undergrowth. The mouse is small, the background immense and detailed. If there were mere summation of effects between the background and the mouse, it is clear that pursuit mechanisms would hold the cat's eyes firmly to the undergrowth, and the mouse would pass with impunity: any attempt by the cat to track it with its eyes would result in apparent movement of the background in the opposite direction, powerfully refixating the eye. Under natural conditions of pursuit, then, there must be some degree of antagonism between the central and peripheral effects of movements of the retinal image: such an antagonism has recently been demonstrated in man by Hood and Leech (1974) and by Hood (1967a; 1975). Patients whose vision is confined to the periphery because of central scotomata actually show *enhanced* optokinetic nystagmus, and can match their slow

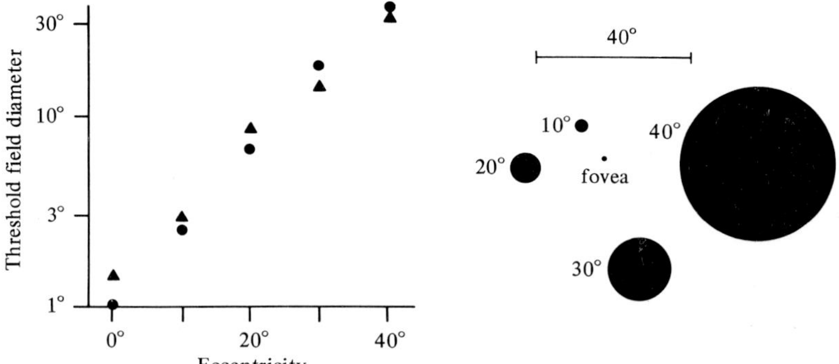

Figure 3.4. Eccentricity and optokinetic sensitivity: the graph shows the minimum area of optokinetic stimulus required to elicit nystagmus at different eccentricities in two monkeys. To the right are shown the same results in diagrammatic form, drawn to scale as regards both the areas of the circles and their eccentricities (data from Koerner and Schiller, 1972).

phase velocity to drum speed at much higher speeds than normal subjects (figure 3.5). Conversely, if the subject's vision is restricted to small central areas, the optokinetic response is considerably reduced (Hood, 1975) (figure 3.5).

Suggestive as these findings are in demonstrating some degree of antagonism between centre and periphery, they do not really provide an answer to the problem of how the eye copes with pursuit against a fixed background, and are in fact directly contrary to what one would have anticipated, that is, a dominance of the centre over the rest. In fact if the relative contributions of centre and periphery are measured not separately, but when both are undergoing optokinetic stimulation, the results are quite different (Hood, 1975). One can arrange for the centre of the field to consist of a stripe pattern moving in one direction while the periphery consists of stripes moving in the opposite direction: one then finds an *enhancement* of the nystagmus response to the centre, as compared to the case when both sets of stripes move in the same direction. It is clear then that no simple notion of addition of effects from different retinal areas can possibly explain the interactions that occur in practice. No doubt the true mechanism is one of selective attention to one or other part of the visual field, rather than a simple 'wired-in' antagonism.

At all events, the fact that optokinetic nystagmus can be elicited despite the extensive loss of retinal or optic tract function makes it a useful neurological tool: some of these clinical aspects of optokinetic (and vestibular) nystagmus are helpfully discussed in Reinecke's (1961) and Jung and Kornhuber's (1964) extensive reviews.

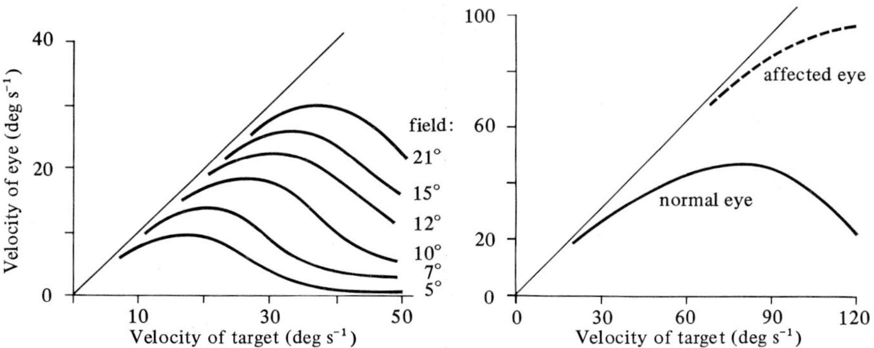

Figure 3.5. Velocity of slow phase of optokinetic nystagmus as a function of stimulus velocity: left, in a normal subject with the visual field restricted to the various visual angles indicated; right, in a subject with unilateral central scotoma (Hood, 1975).

3.2 The quick phase of optokinetic nystagmus

The quick phase of optokinetic nystagmus shares many properties with the ordinary voluntary saccade, and these aspects are left to the next chapter. But a question specifically related to optokinetic nystagmus that may be appropriately considered here is the one that we have already tried to answer in the case of vestibular nystagmus: what *causes* the quick phase to occur at one time rather than another? In this case, the situation is a little more complicated because of the obviously increased importance of volition, a factor which also makes it even harder to believe than in the case of vestibular nystagmus that the slow and quick phases are the product of a common neuronal oscillator (Rashbass, 1961).

There have been two schools of thought about the role of the quick phase in relation to the slow. The older view is that the primary movement is the slow phase, which serves to keep the gaze fixed on the object of regard: the quick phase is then secondary, and shifts the eye to a new object only when the old must be relinquished because it is about to vanish off the edge of the field. But recent evidence supports a different view, proposed originally by Borries (1926), namely that it is the quick phase that is primary, shifting the gaze to new objects appearing in the periphery as a result of the movement of the visual field ('haptation'), while the slow phase merely holds on to the object until a newer and more potent peripheral stimulus again appears. The difference between these two formulations is rather slight once the nystagmus has got going, but each makes different predictions about what will happen when the drum first starts to move. The first notion would lead us to expect that, on setting the drum in motion, the eyes would deviate slowly to follow it, and only subsequently flick back to a new point of fixation; while the second notion would predict that the eyes would first make an anticompensatory quick movement, and only then follow the drum (figure 3.6; cf figure 3.1). The latter is in fact what is observed in normal subjects (Hood, 1967a; Easter, 1972), and results in a mean deviation of the eye during optokinetic nystagmus in the direction *from* which the movement is coming. In dim illumination, however, and in patients with central scotomata, or if the subject is instructed to 'look' rather than 'stare' at the drum, the situation is reversed: it is the slow phase that is primary, and the mean deviation is in the compensatory direction. Perhaps it is more helpful not to think of

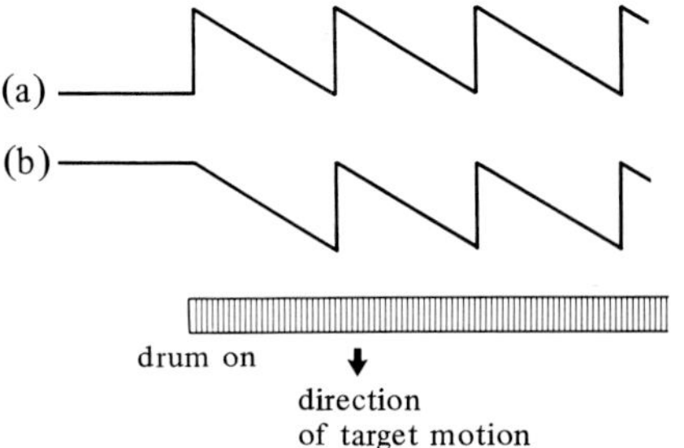

Figure 3.6. The two possible optokinetic responses at the beginning of drum movement (shown by the shaded area at the bottom): (a) haptation, the quick phase comes first; (b) following, the slow phase precedes the quick phase.

the slow and quick phases as primary or secondary to each other at all, but rather as two separate phenomena induced by different aspects of the stimulus and enjoying a measure of mutual independence: the background slow phase striving to maintain the *velocity* of the image over the retina within as small a range as possible, while the quick phases behave in precisely the same way as ordinary saccades, in serving to acquire new objects of interest in the field. The parallel here with what has been said earlier about vestibular nystagmus is obvious: the topic is pursued in section 3.3.1.

Another parallel between the two kinds of nystagmus is the existence of an inherent rhythmicity (Miyoshi et al, 1970; Cheng and Outerbridge, 1974a). Analysis of the intervals between successive quick phases of optokinetic nystagmus shows a similar change from unimodal to multimodal form as the amplitude of the stimulus (in this case drum velocity) is decreased. Cheng and Outerbridge (1974a) find a distinct difference in the distributions if the subjects are instructed to 'look' rather than 'stare' at the stimulus. In the second case the similarity to the vestibular case is striking (with a periodicity of around 3 Hz), whereas in the first there is a natural tendency for the subject to follow a particular aspect of the stimulus until it disappears off the edge, leading to a bimodal distribution in which the longer peak simply corresponds to the time taken for any part of the stimulus to traverse the field.

3.3 The slow phase

3.3.1 Dynamic properties

Pursuit movements under visual control provide a very nice example of a control system with built-in negative feedback. The visual receptors that provide the input to this system must of course move with the eye; so they signal not the absolute position or velocity of a stimulus target, but rather its position or velocity *relative* to the eye itself. Thus the signal from the visual receptors constitutes an *error signal* telling the control system how adequately it is compensating for the movements of the target.

If we assume for the moment that the system that converts this error signal into a corrective movement of the eye is linear, and has a forward gain (relating the velocity of image slip to the resultant eye velocity) of G, then we can represent the whole system in the closed-loop form of figure 3.7. It is a simple matter (see appendix 2) to calculate what the gain of the whole system (that is, from absolute target velocity to eye velocity) will be; it is

$$\frac{G}{1+G}.$$

If the magnitude of G is much greater than unity under some conditions, then it is clear from this expression that the overall gain will then approach unity, so that the eye velocity will be close to that of the target. As we have seen, when looking at targets moving with a constant velocity of less than some $30°\ s^{-1}$ this is substantially true. Under these conditions, a small change in the value of G will make relatively little difference to the overall performance. To take a specific example, if G is simply a pure gain of 20 the gain of the whole thing can be seen to be 20/21, or about 95·24%. If G is increased by a quarter of its value to 25, the overall gain then becomes 25/26, or roughly 96·15%. Thus a 25% increase in the forward gain results here in less than 1% change in the overall performance.

What this implies is that simply looking at the overall performance, that is, the relation between absolute target motion and eye motion under natural (closed-loop) conditions, is likely to tell us rather little about the nature of the control system itself. For the behaviour of the whole thing is more determined by the fact that it *is* closed-loop than by the precise nature of G. The most useful studies of the control system have got round this difficulty by artificially 'opening the loop', converting the system into the form shown in figure 3.8. There are essentially two ways in which this may be done. One can either immobilise the eye that is viewing the target, and record the movements of the other eye (Ohm, 1926) (but one cannot be sure that the lack of normal proprioceptive signals from the fixed eye is not affecting one's results), or one can try to compensate for the eye-movements by moving the target through the same angle that the eye moves, in addition to any extra motion stimulus that one may wish to superimpose on this stabilised background (for

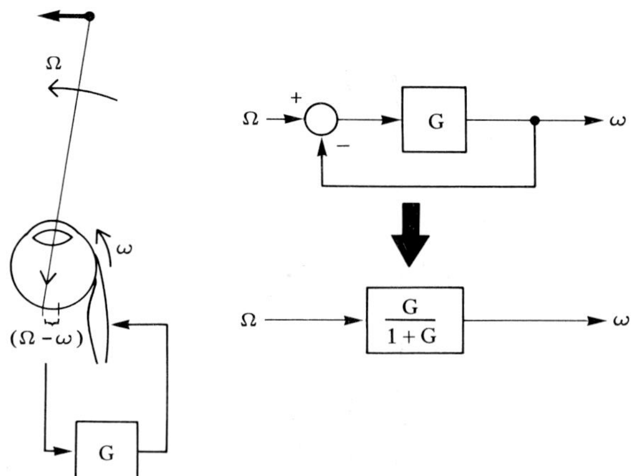

Figure 3.7. The closed-loop nature of smooth pursuit under natural conditions: on the left, an object moving with angular velocity Ω is tracked with an eye velocity of ω. The resultant retinal image movement of $(\Omega-\omega)$ is transformed by the operator G (which represents the central smooth-pursuit mechanism) into the resultant eye velocity (ω). The formal representation of the system is thus as shown at the top right: it is equivalent to a single operator $G/(1+G)$.

example Collewijn and van der Mark, 1972). The two methods in fact lead to similar—and striking—conclusions. If the immobilised eye views a striped drum rotating at constant velocity, the velocity of the slow phase of the resultant nystagmus is found not to be constant in magnitude, but to increase steadily until saturation is reached at some value typically very much greater than the stimulus velocity (for example ter Braak, 1936; Koerner and Schiller, 1972) (figures 3.9 and 3.17), when the angular velocity of the eye may well be as great as $100°\ s^{-1}$. This steady and uniform increase in velocity implies that the forward pathway is performing something like the time integral of the error signal to determine the eye velocity, or in other words that the open-loop gain is actually of the form $k\mathrm{D}^{-1}$: experimentally, it happens that the value of k in the rabbit lies very close to unity (see figure 3.9).

Such a description, attractively simple though it is, can be extremely misleading unless one is very clear about the circumstances in which it may be applied. There are three aspects of the smooth pursuit system that strongly qualify its indiscriminate application: its nonlinearity, its nonstationarity, and the lack of correspondence between its response to target *velocity* and target *position.*

In a simple linear system we would expect to find the closest possible relation between its responses to changes in velocity and its responses to changes in position. For example, if we find that the system's response to

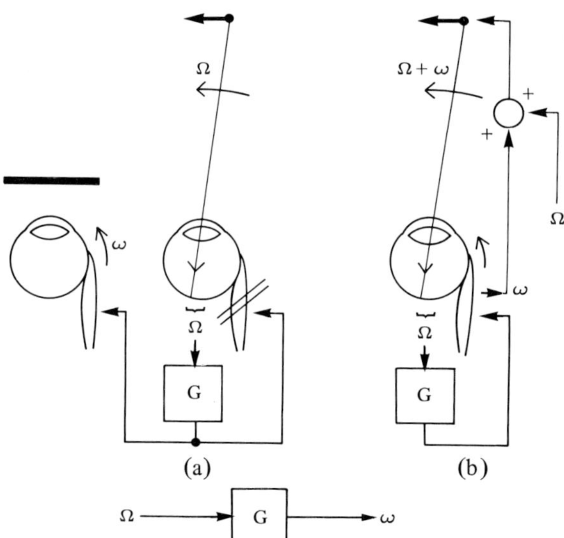

Figure 3.8. Two ways of opening the intrinsic smooth pursuit feedback loop: (a) the viewing eye is immobilised, and the movements of the other are recorded; (b) the target is made to move with an added velocity ω that is arranged to be always equal to the eye's own velocity. In both cases the transfer function of the whole system is simply that of the open-loop operator G.

a step of velocity is—as here—a ramp (a steadily increasing velocity), then we would certainly expect its response to a *position* step to be a position ramp (an output of constant velocity). But this assumes that both position and velocity are processed by the same mechanism, whereas the truth is that from the earliest stages the visual system processes these two quantities in entirely different ways. Position in the visual system is signalled essentially qualitatively, by *which* of the whole array of visual receptors is active at any moment. Velocity is treated quite differently: at a very early stage of the visual process, velocity information is extracted by local 'microprocessing' of firing patterns in small subgroups of receptors, and is thereafter coded *quantitatively*: knowledge of velocity magnitude comes not so much from which fibres are firing as from *how much* they fire. These two kinds of information make very different computational demands on the oculomotor system. The final output is of course of the 'how much' kind—at least, as far as any one eye muscle is concerned. Visual velocity information is already in this form, and it is not hard to devise neuronal circuits that would convert one into the other. On the other hand, positional 'which' information must undergo radical recoding before it can be used to control muscles, and the relative complexity of this task no doubt underlies the slowness of positional oculomotor responses compared with those driven by velocity.

To some extent, in fact, the control of velocity and position are somewhat incompatible, as Rashbass's striking analogy makes clear:

> "Imagine two drivers of the same car, one trying to keep the speedometer at 30 m.p.h. and one trying to keep the car alongside another also travelling at 30 m.p.h. Unless there is communication between the two drivers it is easy to see that the velocity man is going to frustrate the efforts of the position man. Changes in velocity due to the saccades must not be corrected by smooth tracking. Saccadic suppression of vision—the position man putting his hand over the speedometer every time he does something—could account for this..." (Rashbass, 1971).

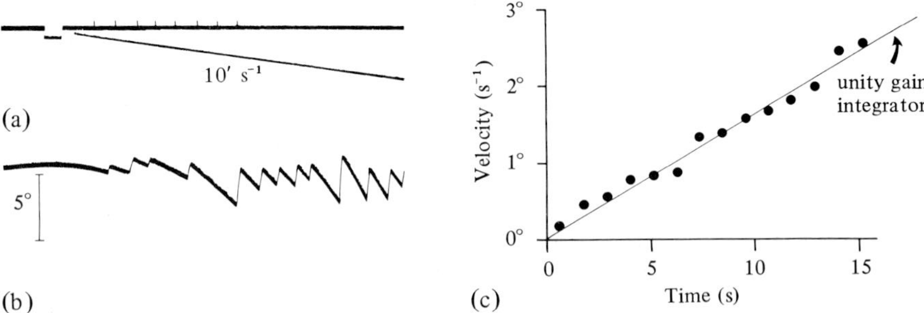

Figure 3.9. Open-loop responses to constant-velocity optokinetic stimulation in the rabbit: (a) timing marks and drum position; (b) resultant nystagmus; (c) the velocity of the slow phase of (b) is plotted as a function of time. It is clear that the velocity rises linearly during the first 15 s; the line is the expectation if the open-loop operator were simply an integrator of unity gain (data from ter Braak, 1936).

Equally, the fact that optokinetic responses break down completely at the kind of velocity levels that are found during saccades would serve the same purpose, without having to suppose a special mechanism of interaction (saccadic suppression is discussed in chapter 11). In practice, the systems are indeed nearly independent, in the sense that positional errors are essentially generators of saccades, while velocity errors produce smooth movements: but even leaving aside Rashbass's point about the kinds of cooperation that must occur for the two systems to coexist in harmony, experiments show that each system is not solely responsive to its own proper input. We shall see in chapter 4 that saccades can be initiated perfectly easily by pure velocity errors, and conversely it is equally clear that pure errors of position can generate smooth movements. This can be demonstrated most easily by arranging to displace a stabilised image through a small angle (for example, Robinson, 1965; Steinbach and Pearce, 1972), or even by viewing a stationary stabilised image—an afterimage will do very well—and concentrating the attention on one or other side of it (Kommerell and Täumer, 1972). The importance of attention suggests a rather high level of development of the response, as does Jordan's (1970) observation that he could 'track' an afterimage of his hand in the dark more smoothly if he actually moved his hand as he did so.

Now we saw earlier that, if the system were linear and essentially unitary, we would expect the response to a step of position to be a movement of constant velocity. In fact this is not at all what is observed: step displacements give rise to movements whose velocities increase steadily (figure 3.10) (Robinson, 1965), and whose magnitudes are not particularly dependent on the size of the original step (Steinbach and Pearce, 1972). It is quite clear, then, that linear operators like $k\mathrm{D}^{-1}$ cannot possibly be used to describe this kind of behaviour, which fortunately is only revealed under the extremely unnatural conditions of stabilised images. In real life it is the saccade that corrects for any positional errors that may arise, and, if slow responses do occur in response to static errors, they are small enough to be considered as part of the drift component of the micromovements (discussed in chapter 6).

Nonlinearities are also prominent in the smooth pursuit system. Two kinds of stimuli are capable of generating large signals at one or another part of the system, and hence of revealing nonlinear behaviour: they are on the one hand stimuli having a large instantaneous velocity at some point in their time course, and on the other hand, stimuli of moderate magnitude that are unidirectional and prolonged. The first kind of signal overloads the input to the system: with input velocities greater than some $100°\ \mathrm{s}^{-1}$ the optokinetic response breaks down completely (see section 3.1), suggesting that the nonlinearity at the input is not merely a saturation but actually shows a decline in output with increasing stimulus velocity. This decline can be observed directly in the velocity-sensing neurons themselves (for example Oyster, 1968). We saw earlier that such behaviour might be useful in making the smooth pursuit system insensitive to saccadic movements of the eyes. Saturation must also inevitably occur if an integrator is presented with a constant input for a prolonged period: its output cannot increase indefinitely, and somewhere a limit will be reached.

Under normal closed-loop conditions the efficiency of the slow pursuit mechanism means that prolonged visual slip does not occur; or if it does occur, as when following an object against a steady background, the optokinetic response is suppressed. Saturation can readily be demonstrated under open-loop conditions (figure 3.11): at low input velocities the output saturates at a value proportional to the input velocity (and some hundred times greater); above about 0·1° s^{-1} the level of saturation itself levels off in the region 10–100° s^{-1} (it is striking that quantitatively similar results have been found in the fly optomotor response: Mittelstaedt, 1964). It is impossible from experiments of this kind to disentangle effects due to saturation at the input from effects due to saturation at the output; in any case the relationship at low input velocities shows that a simple description in terms of saturation at input and output is inadequate: one must also suppose that the integrator is somewhat leaky. It is perhaps worth emphasising that nonlinearities of this kind are in no sense 'faults' in the system, irksome though they can be to the experimenter trying to investigate it: the optimum controller in a closed-loop system like the smooth pursuit mechanism is almost always nonlinear in behaviour, since faster responses can be achieved by always using maximal control signals.

In order to avoid both the Scylla of transient input saturation, and the Charybdis of prolonged output saturation, may experimenters have used

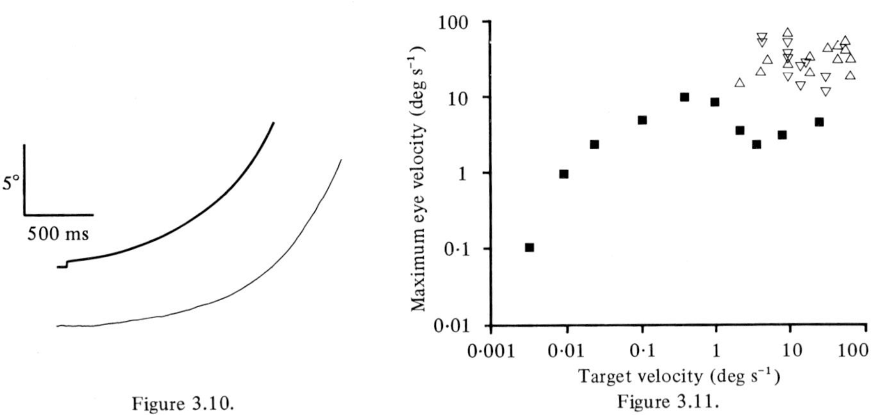

Figure 3.10. Figure 3.11.

Figure 3.10. Human open-loop responses to a small step displacement of the target. The thick line represents target position, the thin line eye position: the approximately parabolic nature of the response is evident (after Robinson, 1965).

Figure 3.11. Open-loop response to constant target velocity: the graph shows maximum eye velocity as a function of target velocity in the rabbit (squares: Collewijn, 1969) and in two monkeys (triangles: Koerner and Schiller, 1972). The gain is very high at low velocities, but saturates when the target moves at more than some 0·5° s^{-1}.

sinusoidally moving targets to investigate the pursuit system. As in the case of the vestibular system, sinusoidal inputs are likely both to be more 'physiological' from this point of view, and also to provide more detailed information about the system's dynamic properties. Unfortunately, the use of repetitive and therefore predictable stimuli brings problems of its own. It turns out that the pursuit system in man [but not in monkeys (Fuchs, 1967b)] is capable of learning to improve its response to such stimuli with practice, so that, although a subject's performance at the task is at first poor, with many corrective saccades, in quite a short time his eye movements smoothly match the movements of the target. One might say that he is learning to *predict* where the target is going to be by the time the movements he initiates take their effect. St Cyr and Fender (1969c) suggest that this is an unjustifiable description: it is not so much that the system predicts the position of the target, but rather than it can learn to reduce the delay with which it responds. Whichever form of words one prefers, the fact is that the phase lag between target and eye is greatly reduced—particularly at higher frequencies—as a result of practice. It is the unpracticed response that is the more interesting as far as our understanding of the mechanism of pursuit is concerned, since natural movements of the visual world are more often unpredictable than not.

One might suppose that this requirement would effectively rule out the possibility of making measurements of the frequency response of the system, but this is not so. If we take a number of sine waves that differ only slightly in frequency and add them together, the resultant waveform will in general only repeat itself at a frequency very much lower than that of the sine components of which it is made, and, if the components are properly chosen, such a waveform is to all intents unpredictable. But since the component frequencies are close together on the frequency axis, measurement of the response of the eye to a number of such clusters, centred on different frequency bands, will enable the experimenter to plot a frequency response for the system, though with rather less resolution than is possible with single sinusoids. This does not result in much loss of information in practice, since the frequency responses show little by way of fine structure. Another way of achieving the same result is to start with a source of random Gaussian 'noise', and pass it through broadly tuned filters centred on various frequencies: again, a signal is achieved that, though unpredictable, is concentrated in a narrow frequency range. The predictability of these signals can be varied by altering the width of the filter, or in the case of multiple sine waves, by using a larger or smaller number of individual components (Michael and Melvill Jones, 1966; St Cyr and Fender, 1969b; 1969c).

With either method it is found that the phase lag of the eye behind the target is directly related to the predictability of the stimulus in the region around 0·3–1 Hz: above this range the response appears to be limited by other factors (which must include, for example, the mechanical properties of the eye), while at lower frequencies the performance is equally good whether or not the stimulus is predictable (figure 3.12). St Cyr and Fender (1969c) find that the relationship between phase lag and predictibility is roughly compatible with the idea that there is a delay in the system that increases in proportion to the quantity of information carried by the signal: similar relations between reaction time and information transfer have long been known to experimental psychologists (see for example Edwards, 1969).

Investigation of the dynamics of two-dimensional tracking has led to interesting findings (Goodwin and Fender, 1973a; 1973b). If a target is moved sinusoidally in the horizontal direction, and randomly in the vertical direction, tracking is found to be essentially independent in the two channels (in the sense that very little extra power at the sinusoidal frequency is observed to leak into the vertical eye-movement component): similarly, little interaction is observed between saccades and slow pursuit in perpendicular meridians (Feinstein and Williams, 1972b). Furthermore, it is found that the usual reduction in phase lag for the sinusoidal stimulus occurs (relative to that for the random stimulus) even if the two axes are tilted away from the horizontal and vertical. Thus it is clear that this independence of processing of the two components is not the result of a fixed division into horizontal and vertical vectors, but rather the result of

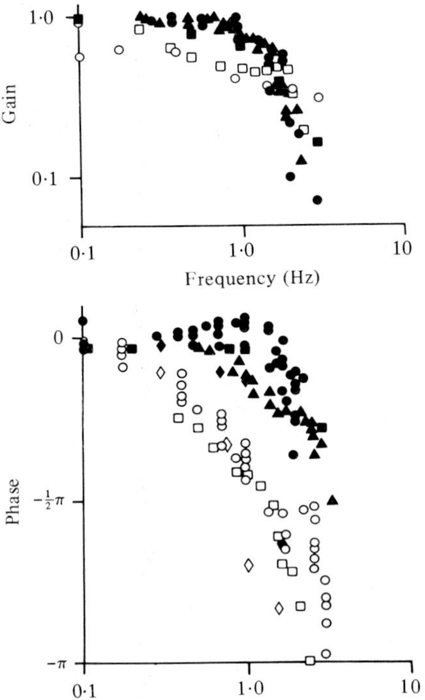

Figure 3.12. Closed-loop transfer functions for smooth pursuit of targets moving sinusoidally (solid symbols) and unpredictably (open symbols) by human subjects. The sources of the data are: triangles, Fender and Nye (1961); circles, Stark et al (1962); squares, Dallos and Jones (1963); lozenges, Michael and Melvill Jones (1966). The results have been normalised for a sinusoidal gain of unity at frequencies near 0·2 Hz.

the ability of the pursuit system to seek out for itself, and adapt itself to, a predictable component of the two-dimensional motion, whatever its orientation in space. This conclusion may not be valid for species like the rabbit in which the velocity-sensing units are densely clustered round retinal orientations corresponding with the lines of action of the muscles (Oyster, 1968).

Although these experiments with stimuli of varying predictability are of great interest for understanding the adaptive properties of the system, being performed under closed-loop conditions they are less useful as far as our main purpose here is concerned, which is to describe the short-term dynamics of the forward pathway. Unfortunately, those experimenters who have studied open-loop preparations have so far limited their stimuli either to single sinusoids or to the classical stimulus of a target moving indefinitely at constant velocity. While it is true that such studies have on the whole produced consistent results, it is not so clear that they have much relevance to the way in which the system behaves under conditions that are natural in the sense of being unpredictable.

Perhaps the most dramatic demonstration of the ability of the system to tailor its performance to the type of stimulus it is given is the fact that, if one looks at the response to each of the separate components within a small cluster of sinusoids, the gain of the system is found actually to *increase* with frequency within the group; if one group is compared with another, the relation is the expected one of falling gain with rising frequency (figure 3.13: St Cyr and Fender, 1969b). Such two-faced behaviour is no doubt advantageous to the system, but makes life difficult for the experimenter, who would prefer to have to deal with a system

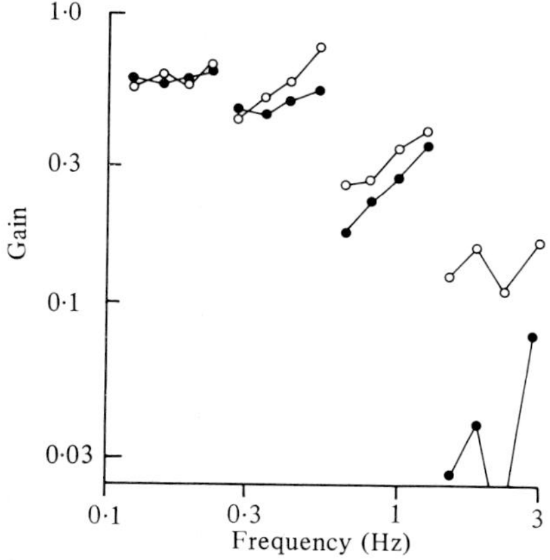

Figure 3.13. Closed-loop frequency response of smooth pursuit of complex target motion by two subjects, in limited frequency bands. The motion consisted of four closely spaced sinusoids: it can be seen that for each of the two subjects, gain tends to *rise* with frequency when comparing the responses to each individual component within the band, but that the overall response comparing one band with another is similar to that of figure 3.12 (data from St Cyr and Fender, 1969b).

the pursuit mechanism and the vestibular reflexes (figure 3.15); Ohm had previously shown in 1922 that vestibular and optokinetic nystagmus were roughly additive. At the beginning of a turn of constant velocity, with the eyes shut, the velocity of the compensatory movement gradually declines because of vestibular adaptation. On the other hand, if the eyes are open and the head still, and the visual surroundings are suddenly set into rotation at a constant speed, the velocity of the compensatory movement is small at first but gradually rises to give virtually complete compensation if the stimulus velocity is not too great. So under natural conditions, with the visual surroundings objectively stationary and the animal's eyes open, the decline of the vestibular response more or less corresponds to the growth of the visual response, so that a nearly constant slow-phase velocity of the correct magnitude results (see figure 3.15).

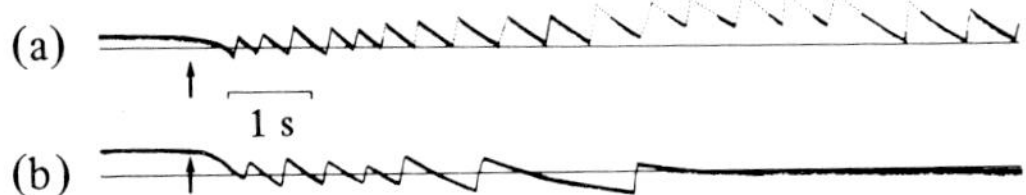

Figure 3.15. Nystagmus responses in the rabbit during rotation at constant velocity in stationary visual surroundings with the eyes open (a) and covered (b). In the first case, vestibular and optokinetic influences add to give a nearly constant slow phase throughout the movement, despite the decline in vestibular response demonstrated in (b) (after ter Braak, 1936).

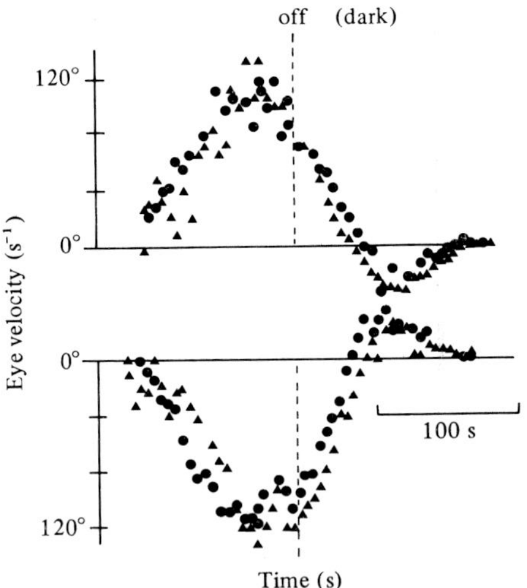

Figure 3.16. Open-loop slow-phase velocity responses to pattern movement of constant velocity (▲, $16^\circ\ s^{-1}$; ●, $3{\cdot}6^\circ\ s^{-1}$) in two opposite directions in the monkey. At the instant marked by the broken line, the pattern movement was stopped and all illumination extinguished. It is clear that the eye velocity builds up more or less linearly during stimulation until saturation, and that it gradually declines in the dark (optokinetic afternystagmus) with a distinct overshoot in which the direction of nystagmus is reversed (after Koerner and Schiller, 1972).

Similarly, at the end of such a turn, the vestibular afternystagmus is in the opposite direction to the optokinetic afternystagmus, resulting in near cancellation of the unwanted responses.

However, although it is true that in the monkey open-loop preparation an afternystagmus can be observed on cessation of the stimulus motion (figure 3.16), only if the room lights are simultaneously switched off is it prolonged for more than a second or two (Krieger and Bender, 1956; Koerner and Schiller, 1972); under these conditions durations as long as two minutes have been reported (Mackensen and Wiegmann, 1959). (Afternystagmus with optokinetic stimuli seems first to have been noticed in man by Fox et al in 1931.) In any case, the complete response when the eyes are open is not simply the sum of the responses when the eyes are shut and when the head is still and the visual surroundings are moved, because whereas the first response comes from an intrinsically open-loop system (the vestibulo-ocular system), the second response is of an intrinsically closed-loop system (figure 3.17).

If we represent the transfer function of the vestibular component by its low-frequency approximation, $\mathrm{D}/(\mathrm{D}+\lambda)$ (where λ is the reciprocal of the long time constant), and the open-loop pursuit transfer function by $k\mathrm{D}^{-1}$, then the overall closed loop response is *not* given by

$$\frac{k}{k+\mathrm{D}}+\frac{\mathrm{D}}{\mathrm{D}+\lambda}=\frac{k(\mathrm{D}+\lambda)+\mathrm{D}(k+\mathrm{D})}{(k+\mathrm{D})(\mathrm{D}+\lambda)}$$

as one might expect (in which case one would anticipate that $k=\lambda$ would give a perfect overall response), but by:

$$\frac{[\mathrm{D}/(\mathrm{D}+\lambda)]+k\mathrm{D}^{-1}}{1+k\mathrm{D}^{-1}}=\frac{\mathrm{D}^2+k\mathrm{D}+k\lambda}{\mathrm{D}^2+(k+\lambda)\mathrm{D}+k\lambda},$$

for which (if we were free to manipulate it) k should be as large as possible for optimum performance. Since this is clearly not the case (if it were, we should expect that moderate steady inputs would under open-loop conditions cause the output to rise immediately to its saturating

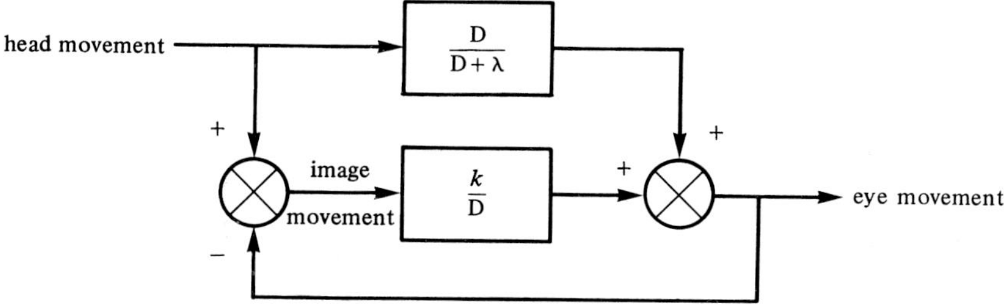

Figure 3.17. The way in which the vestibulo-ocular system (upper pathway) and the smooth pursuit mechanism (lower pathways) interact during head movements with stationary surroundings, assuming linear summation of the two mechanisms.

velocity instead of taking its time to do so: for example at least 15 s in the case of figure 3.9), we cannot really say that the vestibular and optokinetic systems are matched in this way at all: the fact that k and λ are of the same order of magnitude is a misleading coincidence. In any case, careful measurements of vestibular and optokinetic eye movements in the rabbit (Collewijn and Kleinschmidt, 1975) show that the effects of these two modes of stimulation in fact add in a nonlinear manner. Furthermore, it was emphasised in the previous chapter that most head movements are *voluntary,* implying that in principle information is available to the oculomotor system in advance of the intention to move the head. Although direct evidence that such information can actually be used to improve eye movements is lacking, the importance of this kind of 're-efference' in general can easily be demonstrated. Steinbach (1969) showed that subjects were better at tracking targets that they moved themselves than ones that were moved in a similar manner by other people. As usual, the firmest conclusion we can draw is that the system is more complex than we would like to think.

3.4 Visual pursuit with altered feedback

A little more can be learnt about the control system for visual pursuit by extending the experimental method in which movements of the eye are cancelled out by moving the target through the same angle. The same apparatus can be modified to create any feedback relation that we wish, in addition to the two cases already considered of unit negative feedback (that is, natural intrinsic feedback) and zero feedback (or open-loop conditions). All real feedback systems are at best conditionally stable (see appendix 2); if the loop gain is steadily increased, there must eventually come a point when the gain associated with the frequency for which the phase lag round the loop is 180° exceeds unity, resulting in spontaneous oscillation at that frequency. This is in fact precisely what is observed, although one must be careful to separate saccadic corrections from those

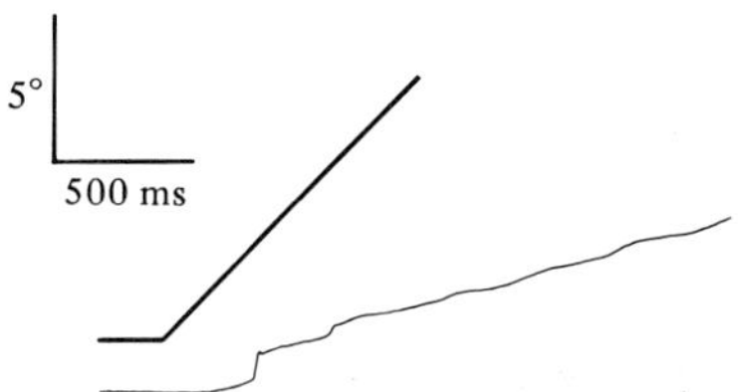

Figure 3.18. Human pursuit of a target that suddenly moves off with a velocity of $10^\circ\ s^{-1}$, under artificial feedback conditions: the feedback gain for smooth pursuit is arranged to be -4, but to be -1 for saccades. The thick trace is the open-loop stimulus, the thin trace is the response of the eye. After a pair of initial saccades, irregular oscillations of the eye record are evident, with a frequency of some 2·9 Hz and peak velocity deviation of $1{\cdot}25^\circ\ s^{-1}$ (after Robinson, 1965).

due to smooth pursuit, for the nature of their potential instability is different. Robinson (1965) arranged to filter any saccadic movements out of the electrical signal representing the eye movements: this signal was then fed back to move the target, after a stage of amplification of variable gain. With an initially stationary target, the system is found to be stable until the feedback gain is increased from -1 (that is, natural conditions) to -8, when spontaneous oscillations begin at a frequency near 3·3 Hz. However, it is still possible to trigger transient oscillations in response to the onset of target motion (figure 3.18), even when the feedback gain is only -2, a reminder again that we are not dealing with a simple linear system.

A striking feature of the oscillations with these intermediate values of feedback is that their amplitudes wax and wane during the stimulus, finally dying out not in the exponential manner that might be expected, but considerably more abruptly. A possible reason for this phenomenon comes from a consideration of the differences in phase lags already noted as between unpredictable (Gaussian) and predictable (sinusoidal) stimuli. Presumably, after a few cycles of the oscillation the system parameters adjust themselves to correspond with the predictability of the stimulus: the phase lag is then reduced, and consequently the stability of the system increased (Robinson, 1965). These results suggest that the gain of the system is just about as large as it can be without the danger of instability: the difference between a feedback gain of -1 and one of -2 is not very great. One might expect to find transient oscillations in response to sudden accelerations of the visual field even under natural conditions, although the saturation of the input in response to high angular velocities would tend to reduce such an effect. It may be that the intermittent discontinuities of velocity that have sometimes been described in the oculomotor response to changing-velocity stimuli (for example Westheimer, 1954b; Puckett and Steinman, 1969) really represent an oscillational instability superimposed on the basic smooth response. Certainly the interval between these periods of apparent change of velocity (some 200 ms) is of the right order of magnitude to be consistent with such oscillations. Another kind of instability can be induced if the feedback is arranged to be positive instead of negative, so that any corrective movement made by the eye makes the error larger instead of smaller. As might be expected, only a small amount of feedback of this kind (for example a feedback gain of around $+0·3$) is needed to induce this type of instability (Fender and Nye, 1961): it does not tell one much about the system.

4

Saccades

"To be short, they be wholly given to follow the motions of the minde, they doe change themselves in a moment, they doe alter and conforme themselves unto it in such maner, as that *Blemor* the Arabian, and *Syreneus* the Phisition of Cypres, thought it no absurditie to affirme that the soule dwelt in the eyes..."

In the strictest sense, saccades are the fast movements of the eyes that serve to bring a new part of the visual field to the foveal region. They are essentially voluntary, and indeed are the only voluntary eye movements that an unpracticed subject can make. However, some other fast eye movements, less voluntary in character, share many properties with voluntary saccades, and are probably generated by the same mechanism. These include the 'quick phase' of vestibular or optokinetic nystagmus (Dichgans, Nauck, and Brooks, 1969), and the microsaccades which can be observed during fixation, to be described in chapter 6. The word 'saccade' appears to have been introduced by Landolt (1891): Westheimer (1973) has briefly reviewed the historical development of ideas about voluntary eye movements.

4.1 The time course of voluntary saccades

Saccades are remarkably stereotyped movements: for a particular subject, the time course of a saccade of a given amplitude is largely independent of the means by which it is evoked, whether voluntarily to a visual target, or involuntarily in response to its sudden appearance; the *latency* of the movement may however be subject to apparently random variation. Neither practice nor extra voluntary effort appear to influence the time course. Unlike smooth movements, saccades are so fast that there is no time for visual feedback to guide the eye to its final position. The saccade control system must therefore calculate in advance a pattern of muscle activation that will throw the eye exactly to the desired position. The resultant movement is thus preprogrammed or *ballistic* (the same property that distinguishes ballistic missiles from guided missiles). The way in which the time course of this movement 'package' varies for different saccade amplitudes can tell us something about how the control system performs what is, on the face of it, a complex calculation in which distances across the retina have to be converted into temporal patterns of muscle activity.

4.1.1. Amplitude-velocity-duration relationships

Figure 4.1 shows the time courses of a number of horizontal saccades of different amplitudes, in man: saccades in other meridians do not differ in their essential characteristics (Gurevich, 1961), nor is much interspecies variation observed (for example, for very similar results in the goldfish, see Hermann and Constantine, 1971; Easter, 1975). A notable feature of such records is the magnitude of the velocities that are observed, often more than 700° s^{-1} for large amplitudes. Not all recording technqiues are suitable for measuring such high velocities: slippage of contact lenses may lead to underestimates of saccade velocites (Byford, 1962), as does electro-oculography (Byford, 1963; Stryker and Blakemore, 1972; Boghen et al, 1974). It can also be seen that the duration of the complete movement is not constant, but increases with increasing amplitude (figure 4.2); the duration of saccades larger than some 5° in amplitude is roughly given by 20–30 ms plus about 2 ms for every degree of amplitude (Dodge and Cline, 1901; Hyde, 1959; Robinson, 1964).

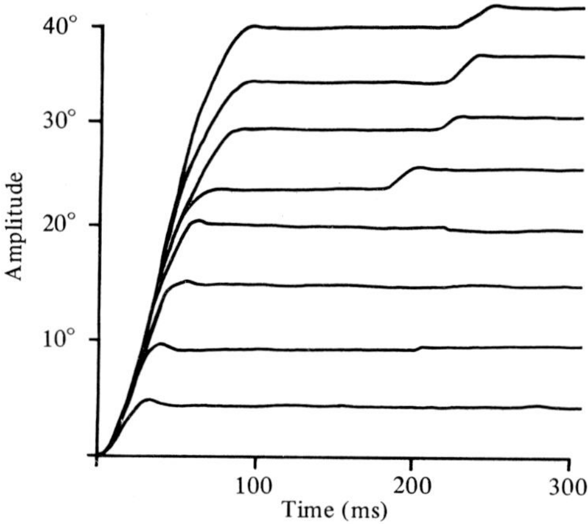

Figure 4.1. Human saccades of different sizes. The traces have been superimposed so that the beginning of each movement is at time zero. The dependence of the duration of the saccade on its amplitude can be seen, as well as 'corrective' second saccades at around $t = 200$ ms (Robinson, 1964).

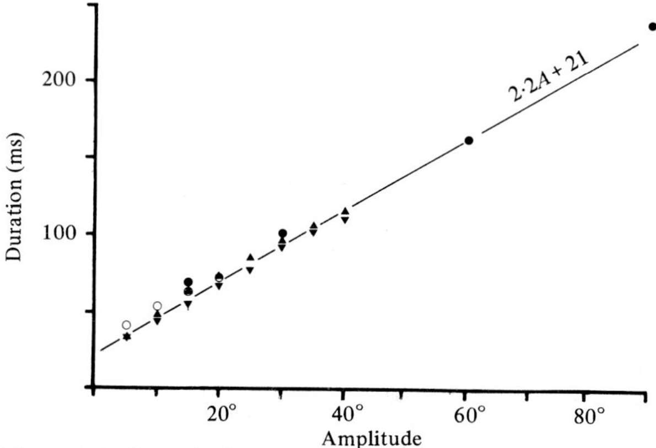

Figure 4.2. Saccade duration as a function of amplitude: ▲ nasal saccades and ▼ temporal saccades, Robinson (1964): ○ Yarbus (1956); ● calculated from Hyde's records (1959). The line represents the function $(2{\cdot}2A + 21)$ ms, where A is the saccade amplitude in degrees.

This dependence of duration on amplitude is commonly—and misleadingly—taken to imply that the system is in some sense nonlinear. But it is impossible to say whether a system is linear or nonlinear simply by looking at a sample of its output: we must also know what the corresponding input was that produced it. The implicit assumption here is that the input that produces saccades of different sizes is a step function of varying height: if this were true, then differences in response duration would indeed imply a nonlinearity. But we know now that the fast rising part of the saccade is generated not by a step of activity of variable height, but essentially by a pulse of constant height whose *duration* determines the amplitude of the saccade (see section 7.5.5). Such a pulse, acting on a linear model of the mechanical properties of the eye, produces amplitude-duration relationships very similar to those observed in actual voluntary saccades (Robinson, 1964). For saccades less than some 5° in amplitude, the pulse is very short and the response is dominated by the mechanical properties of the eye, resulting in the more nearly constant duration associated with small saccades; under these circumstances the peak velocity varies in proportion to the amplitude. The situation is rather like that of a man falling through the air: if his drop is a long one, the duration of his fall will be in proportion to its height, since for most of the way he will be falling at his terminal velocity. In shorter falls, acceleration will dominate his performance, and his peak velocity will depend on the distance he falls. In either case, his initial trajectory will be the same: in the case of the eye, one can observe almost identical patterns of acceleration at the *beginning* of the movement, whatever its amplitude (figure 4.3). [Yarbus' (1956) description of saccades in terms of sinusoidal pulses of angular velocity may be convenient for approximate calculations, but tends to obscure the basic physical mechanisms underlying the saccadic trajectory.]

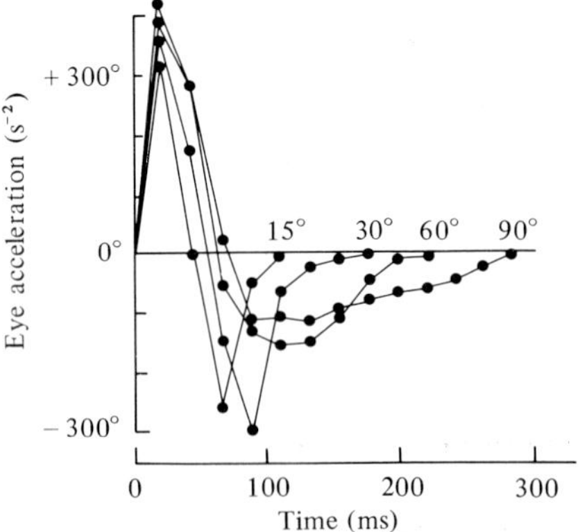

Figure 4.3. Time course of acceleration of the eye during saccades of different extent. It can be seen that the initial pattern of response differs very little in the four cases, and certainly is not scaled to the saccade amplitude (after Hyde, 1959).

Very similar relationships between amplitude, duration, and velocity have been reported in the quick phase of nystagmus (Mackensen and Schumaker, 1960; Ron et al, 1972), lending weight to the notion that the quick phase is not essentially different in nature from the ordinary saccade. Under 'natural' conditions—the subject moving freely in his normal surroundings—the frequency of fast eye movements (taking saccades and quick phases together) as a function of their amplitudes is not bimodal, but appears to follow a simple exponential function with a characteristic amplitude of some 7·6° (Bahill et al, 1975a). Thus more than 85% of natural saccades have amplitudes of less than 15° [as is also the case for the rabbit (Collewijn, 1970b)], and again, saccades and quick phases seem to fall into a single statistical population.

Some subjects appear to show a slight degree of overshoot at the end of a saccade (for example Westheimer, 1954a; Thomas, 1961): in monkeys, Fuchs (1967a) found a roughly constant 0·5° overshoot on saccades greater than some 25°. It is not always easy to be sure that some of the overshoot is not introduced by the recording method (or, for that matter, that a genuine overshoot has not been attenuated by a method such as electrooculography which has a limited frequency response), and it appears that there is considerable variation from one subject to another, and in one subject on different occasions, as to the degree to which overshoot—or indeed the converse, 'undershoot'—actually occurs (Yarbus, 1967; Fleming et al, 1969) (figure 4.4). At one time the existence or otherwise of overshoot was thought to have some theoretical importance in relation to the mechanical properties of the globe, but now we know that the eye is heavily overdamped, the idea that overshoot is due to mechanical 'ringing' of the globe cannot be held. It seems that overshoot

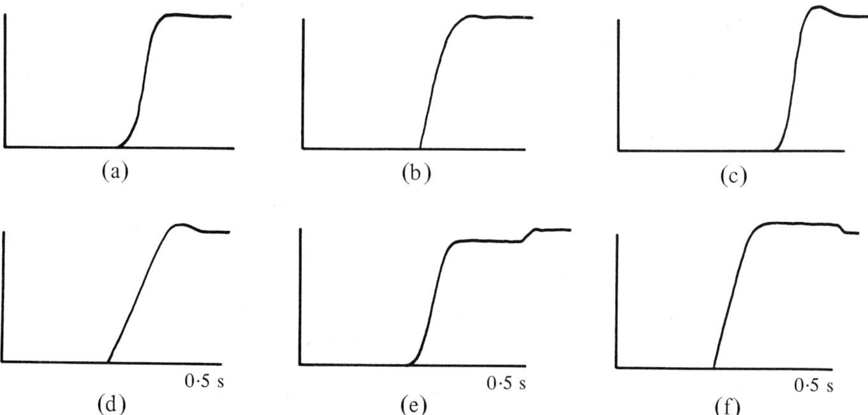

Figure 4.4. Idiosyncratic variations in the saccadic time course in different subjects under similar conditions: (c), (d), and perhaps (b) show an overshoot; (e) and (f) illustrate secondary corrective saccades (from Fleming et al, 1969).

or undershoot is due to slight mismatching between the sizes of the phasic and tonic components of the pattern of activation of the muscles during a saccade (see chapter 7).

Finally it is perhaps worth noting that, although these amplitude–duration relationships vary rather little under different stimulus conditions for movements in any one direction, differences in the velocity of saccades made in *different* directions have sometimes been noted, though not always consistently (for a summary see Fuchs, 1971). Reduced velocities have been observed when the subject is under the influence of alcohol or sedatives, or fatigued (Aschoff, 1968; Becker and Fuchs, 1969; Franck and Kuhlo, 1970; Gentles and Llewellyn Thomas, 1971; Wilkinson et al, 1974). Voluntary saccades made in the dark are considerably slower than those made in the light (Riggs et al, 1974; Körner, 1975).

4.1.2. Latencies of saccadic eye movements

The complexity of the calculation necessary to transform retinal distances into eye movements is reflected in the rather long reaction times associated with saccadic movements. In a simple stimulus arrangement commonly used, the subject fixates a stimulus light that is suddenly switched off while a nearby light is simultaneously switched on: the saccade he then makes to the new target typically does not begin until about a fifth of a second later. This reaction time increases to some extent with increased saccade amplitude, for example by some 40 ms for a 40° movement (figure 4.5) (White et al,

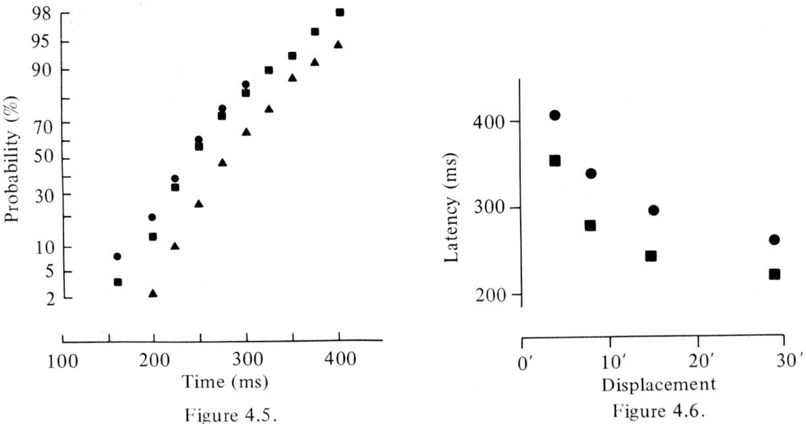

Figure 4.5.

Figure 4.6.

Figure 4.5. Statistical properties of the timing of saccades of different amplitudes. Each point shows the probability of a saccade having occurred in response to target movement, within the time shown on the abscissa: the cumulative probability scale is such that a Gaussian distribution of saccade latencies would give a straight line. Results for three amplitudes are shown: ● 10°; ■ 20°; and ▲ 40° (data from White et al, 1962).

Figure 4.6. Average latencies (for two subjects) of saccades in response to rather small target displacements, as a function of their size (data from Wyman and Steinman, 1973b).

1962; Bartz, 1962). Paradoxically, it also increases if the required amplitude is very *small* (figure 4.6) (Wyman and Steinman, 1973b): it seems that the probability (per unit time) of making the saccade falls sharply if the size of the positional error is very small. It is probably true to say that no target displacement is so small that a saccade will not eventually be made towards it: certainly saccades can be repeatedly elicited by target movements rather less than 10 min of arc in amplitude (Timberlake et al, 1972; Wyman and Steinman, 1973a; Haddad and Steinman, 1973). Reaction times for saccades are also increased under conditions of low retinal illumination (figure 4.7) (Wheeless et al, 1967), although the effects here are not very marked until the luminance of the target is actually below foveal threshold, introducing an obvious difficulty of interpretation!

If the subject knows in advance where the target is going to appear, he may anticipate and show spuriously low reaction times: but if the number of possible target positions is increased beyond two, the reaction time is apparently not correspondingly increased (Saslow, 1967b). Saccadic reaction times thus differ in this respect from what is found in other reaction-time experiments as the number of possible responses is increased (see for example Edwards, 1969). If the subject knows both where and *when* the stimulus is to appear—as for example in tracking a spot that is jumping back and forth at regular intervals—his performance rapidly improves, and after a few cycles he can produce saccades that are virtually in synchrony with the stimulus movement (Westheimer, 1954b; Dallos and Jones, 1963; Stark et al, 1962; Fuchs, 1967b) (figure 4.8). As already noted for sinusoidal tracking, monkeys are apparently unable to make use of this kind of redundancy in the input, and the saccades they make to repetitive stimuli of this kind show no improvement with time (Fuchs, 1967b).

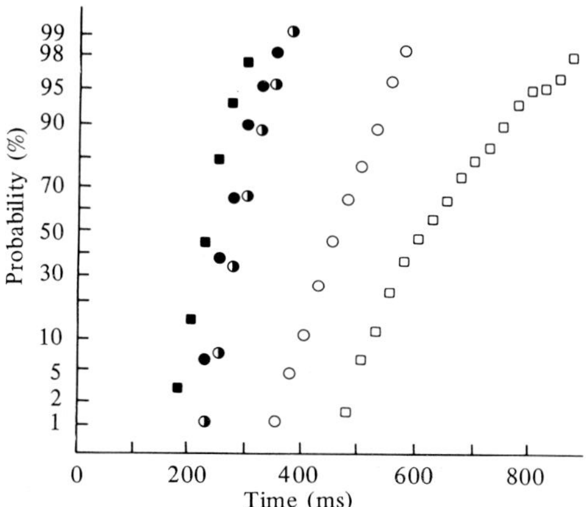

Figure 4.7. Saccade latency and luminance: cumulative latency proabilities are plotted as in figure 4.5 for five different luminance conditions: ◑ target luminance equal to the foveal threshold; ● 1 log unit, ■ 2 log units above foveal threshold; ○ 1 log unit, □ 1·5 log units *below* foveal threshold (data from Wheeless et al, 1967).

Another factor influencing the latency of saccadic movements is the apparent *refractoriness* that is observed after a saccade: in normal circumstances one saccade cannot follow another with an interval of less than some 150 ms. This can most easily be demonstrated by arranging for the visual target to switch back to the centre again after the initial displacement, providing a brief pulse of displacement rather than the step used in conventional saccade measurements (figure 4.9). If the length of this displacement pulse is less than some 150 ms, one of two responses may occur: either the eye simply ignores the brief excursion, and does not move, or it makes a full saccade to the eccentric target, followed by a return movement. The return movement is not separated from the excursion by a time equal to the width of the pulse, as would be expected from a simple delay, but by a relatively fixed interval of some 150–200 ms (Westheimer, 1954b). It makes little difference if the second saccade is in a different meridian from the first (Feinstein and Williams, 1972a).

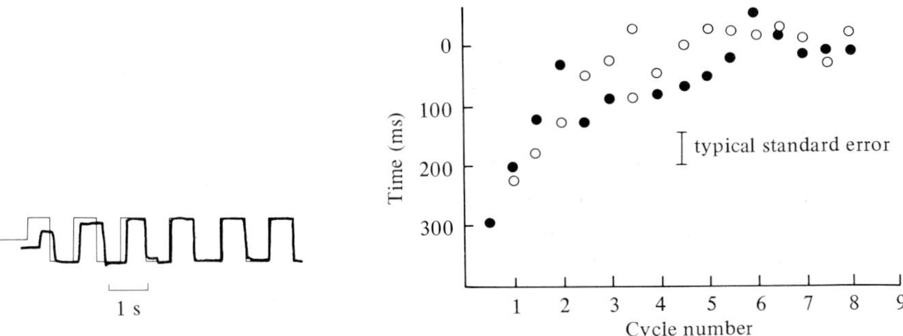

Figure 4.8. Progressive reduction in saccade latency with square-wave targets: left, human eye-movement response (thick line) to target jumping from side to side at a frequency of 0·8 Hz; right, progressive reduction of latency as a function of the number of cycles of such a stimulus of 0·5 Hz (●) and 0·8 Hz (○) (after Fuchs, 1967b).

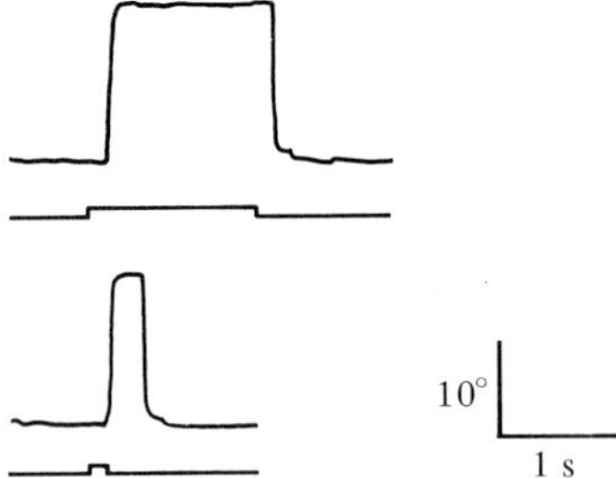

Figure 4.9. Saccadic responses to long and short pulses of displacement. In the second case it is clear that the initial saccadic response is unaffected by the fact that it is completely inappropriate—the target has already returned to its starting position—and the latency of the return saccadic is very greatly increased.

A similar refractoriness is observed in the microsaccades of fixation (Nachmias, 1959), a fact which raises a doubt as to whether conventional measurements of saccade latencies really measure reaction times at all. For if, in the course of fixating the central target, the subject happens to have executed a microsaccade very shortly before the target movement occurs, the saccade will be delayed by an interval representing the refractory period, rather than the true reaction time. Indeed, one could imagine a microsaccade occurring up to one reaction time *after* the moment of target motion (correcting for where the target *was*), resulting in a maximum latency of one refractory period plus one true reaction time. The minimum possible latency is of course the reaction time. Some evidence that previous microsaccades can influence saccade latencies has been given by Saslow (1967a) (see also Becker, 1972), who arranged that the time of extinction of the central fixation light, and of illumination of the eccentric one, could be independently varied. If the central light is turned off more than 200 ms before the eccentric light is turned on, the latency (measured relative to the latter event) is reduced from an average of some 200 ms to an average of about 150 ms, presumably because the frequency of microsaccades is reduced in the absence of a visible fixation point (figure 4.10). Microsaccades cannot be completely abolished by these means, however, and the true reaction time is thus probably rather less than 150 ms.

Some light could be shed on this question by examining the detailed statistical distribution of reaction times: if the variability in latency that is a feature of saccades were due to an effect of the type just described, then one would expect to find a flat distribution of latencies between the expected minimum and maximum, that is, 100–150 ms and 300–350 ms. Unfortunately, few experimenters have been primarily concerned in measuring the exact shapes of frequency distributions of latencies. All the same, it is clear from what data there are (for example White et al, 1962; Wheeless et al, 1966; Fuchs, 1967a) that the actual distribution is peaked and not flat; but equally, it is significantly different from a Gaussian distribution (as can be seen in the cumulative distributions of figures 4.5 and 4.7). Measurements are dominated by variability between subjects, and in particular subjects from day to day [as may be seen in comparing

Figure 4.10. The possible consequence of extinguishing a saccade target before it moves. If latency under normal conditions (left) is dominated by refractoriness (R) to a previous fixational microsaccade, extinguishing the target just before it is moved (right), by reducing the frequency of microsaccades, may reveal the true saccadic reaction time t.

the distributions for identical stimulus conditions in Wheeless et al (1966; 1967)] and it does not in fact seem possible to make quantitative deductions from them. In particular, it is not clear whether the distributions are compatible with the hypothesis of a fundamentally 'flat' process of the type suggested, modified by an additional, more rounded, source of variability.

Finally, one can demonstrate refractoriness of the quick phase of nystagmus after voluntary saccades (Judge, 1973), underlining once again the probable identity of these two movements. However, a quick phase does *not* apparently delay a subsequent saccade in the expected manner, perhaps because a novel visual stimulus in some way suppresses the more primitive nystagmus mechanism.

4.1.3. Corrective saccades

In man large visually evoked saccades almost invariably fall short of their targets, and are followed—after the expected refractory period—by second, corrective, saccades (figure 4.1): making a saccade to a target is thus not unlike taking a hole at golf. The greater the distance of the target from the original point of fixation, the greater is both the probability of a corrective saccade occurring, and its magnitude if it does occur (B Clark, 1936); and if the saccadic error is different in the two eyes, a slow, disjunct, corrective movement may also be observed (see for example Weber and Daroff, 1972). However, it has been suggested (for example Easter, 1973) that these slow movements are not so much corrective as the result of the settling of the slower elements of the eye's mechanics (see chapter 7), and may not be related to disjunctive errors at all. All the same, it is clear from the behaviour of the vergence control system that, if disjunctive errors *did* occur as the result of asymmetric saccades, the movements would be of comparable time course to those actually observed.

Similar corrective saccades may be observed sometimes after smaller movements as well, and may be in either the same or the opposite direction to the original saccade. One might suppose that, after the first saccade has finished, the position of the eye is compared with that of the target, and a second saccade initiated if there is a sufficient discrepancy between the two. In the case of the largest saccades, which can last 100 ms or more, this would imply a very short reaction time (rather less than 100 ms) for the generation of the corrective saccades, though one that is not completely incompatible with Saslow's (1967a) shortest latencies. Indeed one might see here the explanation for having a refractory period at all: the system must obviously ensure that the eye has stopped moving at the time the estimate of the error is made, and this could perhaps be arranged most easily by holding up the calculation until some fixed time has elapsed after the beginning of the last one, long enough to allow for even the largest eye movements. One might suppose that it would be more efficient to allow more settling time for larger saccades than for smaller: but this does not seem to occur. The latency of the correction as measured from the *end* of the main saccade is greater, the smaller the size of the original movement (Becker, 1972); but the latency as measured from the *beginning* of the main saccade is roughly constant whatever its size.

However, a number of experiments indicate that the notion that corrective saccades of this type are the result of monitoring a visual error is erroneous. Corrective saccades are still observed after large voluntary saccades made in total darkness, when of course no visual monitoring is possible (Becker and Fuchs, 1969); in the same way, extinguishing the target just before the main saccade does not abolish them (Pernier et al, 1969; Barnes and Gresty, 1973). In any case, the characteristics of the error in the first saccade do not suggest that the system is doing its best to get it right first time: if this were so, we might expect that the endpoint of the first saccade would be randomly distributed about the target, whereas in fact the first saccade nearly always *under*shoots, by an amount that has an almost linear relationship to the size of the first saccade, and which is itself subject to comparatively little random variation (Becker, 1972). Nor is it simply that the eye is incapable of executing a single saccade of more than a certain amplitude: a saccade of 30° is executed in two stages, even though the first component of a 40° saccade is itself a saccade of more than 30° (figure 4.1). Just why large saccades have to be made in this clumsy way remains a mystery.

There is no reason to doubt that corrective saccades following *smaller* movements are the result of sensing an error of fixation. One way of demonstrating this is by opening the intrinsic visual feedback loop (in the manner described in the previous chapter) so that every time the eye makes a saccade toward the target, the target simultaneously jumps away from the eye by the same amount. One then finds that the response of the eye to an initial step displacement consists of a regular series of saccades of equal amplitude, forming a staircase in which the treads are

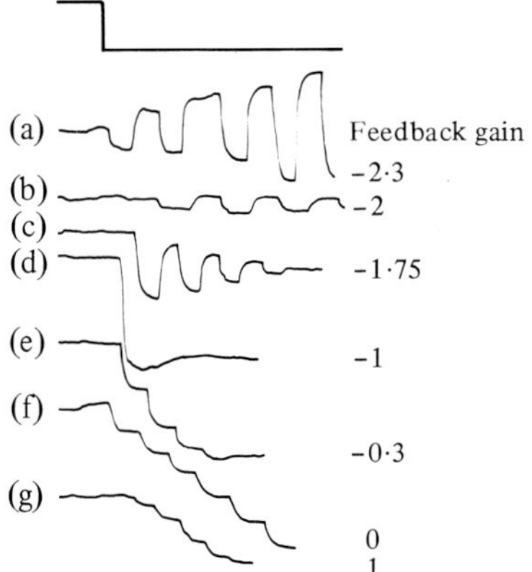

Figure 4.11. Saccadic responses to a step of target position (top trace) under different artificial feedback conditions: −1 is the natural condition (after Young and Stark, 1963).

some 200 ms long [figure 4.11 (f)] (Young and Stark, 1963; Robinson, 1965; Fuchs, 1967a; Fleming et al, 1969). If the negative feedback is increased beyond its natural value of -1, a step displacement of the target produces oscillations (again, as in the case of the smooth pursuit mechanism) which either die away or increase in amplitude, depending on the value of the feedback gain [figure 4.11, (a)-(c)]: for a gain of -2 they neither grow nor shrink, and the result is a stable oscillation. This is of course only what would be expected if the saccade size is matched accurately to the perceived target error, and tells us nothing new about the system beyond confirming that small corrective saccades are indeed normally the result of visual feedback.

4.2 The control of saccades in relation to the visual stimulus

4.2.1 Visual sampling

The fact that saccades are discrete, prepackaged, events does not of itself imply that the visual information used to generate them needs to be obtained in a similarly discontinuous manner. But the existence of intrinsic feedback, by which the visual scene is shifted by the eye movements themselves, puts certain bounds on the periods of time preceding a saccade during which visual information about the position of a target is actually useful. On the one hand, information obtained before a previous saccade is clearly out of date; on the other, information acquired within one reaction time of the saccade itself is too late to influence it. These limits to the period in which visual information is of any use do not necessarily apply to *velocity* information, which is not rendered out-of-date by an intervening saccade (this question is considered in the next section). But for positional control, it follows from this that an ideal system would make use of, or sample, the visual input only during the period between the end of one saccade and one reaction time before the beginning of the next. [It is true that for *flashed* targets, information acquired during or even before a prior saccade might be better than none at all (see for example Hallett and Lightstone, 1976a;1976b; and section 11.1). But the argument presented here concerns 'natural' continuously visible visual objects.]

The information gathered during this interval is not all equally useful, however: clearly more weight ought to be attached to the most recent information. In fact, in a noise-free situation (in other words, where the target is not subject to relatively fast random motion, and where the monitoring device has perfect certainty of the target's position at any instant) the best strategy is to make a very short sample of the visual information, at the last possible moment. The greater the noise in the system, the longer this sampling interval will have to be for accurate performance. A simple way of meeting all these requirements would be to sample the visual scene at regular intervals of time, the intervals being chosen to be greater than the sum of the reaction time and the duration of the longest saccades, that is, of the order of 200 ms. Is this in fact what happens?

The experiments that best demonstrate the existence of intermittent sampling are those that involve pulses of target displacement, of the kind described above in connection with the demonstration of the refractory period (for example Westheimer, 1954b). If the sampling pulse happens to coincide with the brief displacement of the target, the system would be expected to respond with a saccade; if not, no movement would be expected. This is exactly what is observed: on some trials, a full saccade is made, corresponding in amplitude with the displacement of the target, while on others, nothing happens at all. It is significant here that the response is 'all-or-none', in the sense that one very seldom observes saccades of intermediate size. This implies either that the sampling period is extremely short, of alternatively that the information acquired during it is *not* subject to some kind of averaging process, but rather that, if faced with a target that occupies two different positions during the sample, it chooses one or other position as its goal rather than a compromise somewhere between the two.

Similar results have been obtained by using a slight modification of this arrangement, namely the 'pulse-step' stimulus (Wheeless et al, 1966; extended by Komoda et al, 1973). Here the target first jumps to one side of a central fixation spot, and then after a brief interval jumps to the other side of it and stays there (figure 4.12): to prevent learning changes, this stimulus is randomly alternated with suitable controls. The resultant response is again found to be probabilistic, the eye making a saccade either to one or to the other side of the centre. As the duration of the pulse is increased, the probability of the initial saccade being in the same direction as the pulse also increases (figure 4.12). This is exactly what would be expected if brief samples of the visual input were being made at regular intervals: the longer the pulse, the greater the probability that the

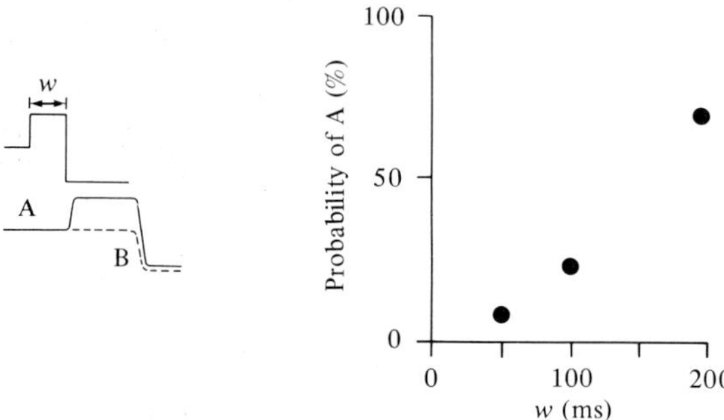

Figure 4.12. The pulse-step experiment. On the left, the upper trace shows the target movement: it steps to one side for a duration *w* ms, then steps back to the same distance on the other side of the midline. The eye (lower trace) either follows it back and forth (A), or only moves in the final direction (B). The graph shows the probability of A as a function of *w* (data of Wheeless et al, 1966).

sample will happen to fall within it. Even with a pulse lasting 200 ms, only some 70% of responses follow it, suggesting a sampling interval somewhat longer than 200 ms: this may also explain the unusually long latencies observed in these particular experiments (some 280 ms).

But, if we examine the *distribution* of the latencies for the different types of response, we find some features that cannot be explained by a simple sampling model. Consider first what are our expectations: if the only source of variation of latencies is the random occurrence of the stimulus sample with respect to the stimulus itself, the expected distribution of latencies for a simple *step* stimulus will be a rectangular function, flat in the region t_r to $t_r + s$, where t_r is the reaction time of the system, and s is the intersample interval (figure 4.13). If now a pulse-step stimulus is presented, with a pulse of width w, then all responses whose latencies lie in the region t_r to $t_r + w$ will follow the pulse, while those in the region $t_r + w$ to $t_r + s$ will follow the step, resulting in two nonoverlapping distributions for the two responses. If other sources of variation exist (as they certainly must) the difference between the two distributions will blur, but the argument is otherwise unchanged.

Looking now at the actual distributions that are found in this experiment (figure 4.14), we see a significant departure from our expectation. Although the number and distribution of pulse-following responses agree well with the model (as can be seen by comparing their cumulative distributions with those for the simple step stimulus) the distribution of latencies for the responses that follow the step is markedly shifted to the right, by some 130 ms. Now if the only information available to the system about the position of the target was obtained by a series of samples more than 200 ms apart, there is no way in which the system could possibly know that the step had been preceded by a pulse in the opposite direction. Yet it must in fact know that these are not just normal steps, for it responds to them with latencies that are enormously increased.

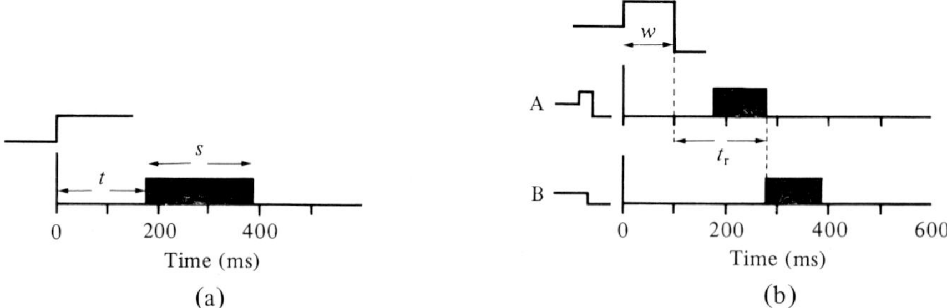

Figure 4.13. Expected distributions of reaction times in the Wheeless experiment, on the very simple hypothesis of regular sampling at an interval s (uncorrelated with the stimulus) and a simple reaction time t_r: expected distribution (a) in response to a step of position, and (b), for each of the two kinds of response to the Wheeless stimulus; w is the duration of the stimulus pulse.

One is therefore forced to conclude that the system does *not* rely solely on intermittent brief samples in calculating its saccades, and that in the pulse-step experiments the presence of the step can in some way cancel the pulse response that would otherwise have occurred, and conversely that the presence of the pulse can profoundly modify the response to the ensuing step. Rather similar effects were shown by Becker and Fuchs (1969), using stimuli consisting of a large step followed by a smaller step. If the interval between the two is large enough for the second step to take place after the saccadic responses to the first, extremely large latencies—again of the order of 400 ms—are observed in the second saccade.

Observations of this kind do not rule out the notion of intermittent sampling altogether: but they imply that visual input can be used in a continuous manner to cancel saccades that are in the course of elaboration and which are realised to be inappropriate. A hypothetical system of this type is represented in figure 4.15. After suffering a delay v, visual information is used in two ways: it is intermittently allowed access as data to the process that calculates the next saccade, and it is also able to cancel any calculation that is in progress. One might suppose that the second pathway was activated if the rate of change of position of the target

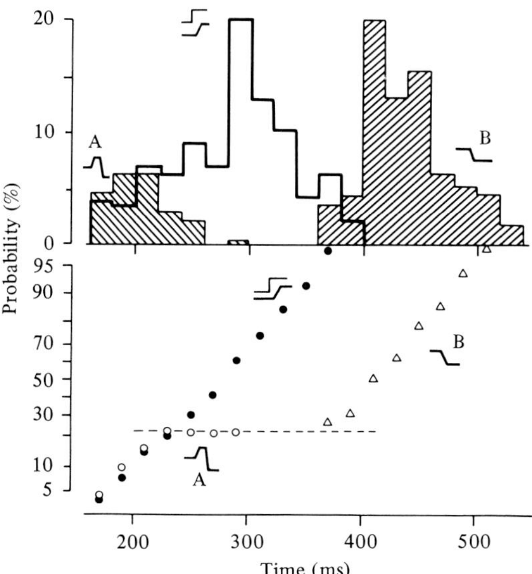

Figure 4.14. Statistical properties of the latencies in the experiment shown in figure 4.13. Above, the shaded areas show the observed latency histograms for two kinds of response, A and B: the unshaded histogram is for a simple single step of the same amplitude under identical conditions. Below, the same data are plotted in the form of cumulative probabilities, showing that the type A responses lie on the curve for ordinary single-step saccades, whereas the latencies for type B responses are as if the single-step distribution were cut in two at around $t = 230$ ms, and the later responses delayed as a whole by some 130 ms (data from Wheeless et al, 1966).

200 ms) the longer is the interval between the two saccades—as would be expected if the second response latency were effectively uncorrelated with the first—while longer values of the determinant time interval tend to lead to single saccades that jump immediately to the final position of the target. Intermediate values can produce saccades of an amplitude intermediate between those appropriate for the first and second stimulus steps. They interpret these results as suggesting that the system uses efference copy of the first saccade to calculate in advance the requisite size of the second, a notion that fits nicely with a model of the saccadic pulse generator presented in chapter 12.

A model of the saccadic mechanism that is conceptually rather different from those presented so far has been suggested by Robinson (1973), and is specifically intended to explain some of the statistical properties of the response to double-step stimuli. In essence, Robinson proposes an array of independent processors acting in parallel and corresponding to different points on the retina. Each takes a certain time to reach its 'decision' about the command to be issued, and when the decision is reached, it both initiates a saccade, and cancels any decisionmaking activity that may be going on in the other units. The time needed for any particular unit to make its decision is subject to random variation: thus if—as in the Wheeless experiments—one unit is activated only a short period of time after another, it may nevertheless complete its operations sooner and thus produce a saccade that jumps immediately to the final target position. By choosing plausible probability functions for the decision times of the individual units, it is possible to make quantitative predictions of many kinds of double-step responses, without having to postulate the existence of a regular sampling process.

4.2.2 Saccadic responses to targets in continuous motion

We saw in the previous chapter that visually guided tracking movements exhibit large phase lags with even moderately high frequencies of target motion: more simply, the smooth pursuit mechanism is distinctly sluggish. In the case of a step change in target velocity, as for example occurs when a target initially stationary moves off with constant velocity, this sluggishness implies that in the absence of any other mechanism, although the eye quite soon reaches the same *velocity* as the target, it does so with a permanent error in *position* (figure 4.18). In practice, however, what happens is that the saccadic system intervenes, generating a saccade that is of exactly the right size to correct the positional error. The astonishing thing is that this corrective saccade is typically initiated long before the positional error is fully manifest (Westheimer, 1954b; Rashbass, 1961). One is forced to conclude that the saccadic control system must estimate from the velocity of the target how large a correction is going to be required: in doing so it must also of course allow for the dynamic properties of the slow pursuit mechanism. It appears that this estimate is added to any other step displacement that may be required: if at the moment of moving off, the target is also simultaneously displaced, the resultant saccade is still of exactly the right magnitude to correct the total positional error (figure 4.19). In particular, if the target is displaced backwards by a suitable amount at the start, no saccade at all is necessary—and none occurs. If the target is extinguished shortly before the first response, a saccade still takes place to the point where it would otherwise have arrived, and the eye continues for some 200 ms with the previously appropriate velocity (Westheimer, 1954b).

This seemingly intelligent behaviour could in fact be produced by quite a simple mechanism. All the system needs to do is to monitor the velocity of the target, and generate a saccade that is proportional in amplitude to this velocity, since (if linear) the permanent positional lag of the pursuit system will vary directly with the velocity of the stimulus. One could conceive of a more sophisticated system that took into account not only the velocity of the target but also any acceleration it might have, to form a better estimate of its future position. But experiments with targets moving off with constant acceleration show that this does not in fact occur, and that in these circumstances the extra error due to the acceleration remains uncorrected (figure 4.20) (Fleming et al, 1969). If the target velocity is very high, so that there is still a residual *velocity* error by the time the saccade has taken effect, one or more additional saccades may be made to correct for the positional lag that will result from it (Fleming et al, 1969). One might perhaps expect that in these circumstances the system would simply have arranged for the whole ultimate error to be cancelled at a stroke; but this would result in a larger mean deviation of the eye

Figure 4.18. Response to a target moving off at constant velocity: left, response of smooth pursuit system alone leads to a permanent positional lag because of time required for the eye to approach the target velocity; right, diagrammatic representation of how a saccade of appropriate size can eliminate any positional errors of this kind.

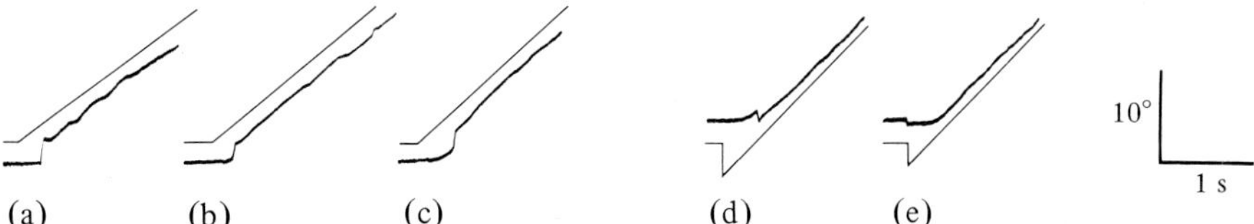

Figure 4.19. Monkey eye movements in response to ramp and ramp-step target motion: (a)-(c), ramps of 10° s^{-1}, showing clear saccadic components; (d), (e), ramps of 13° s^{-1} combined with backwards steps: the saccades are reduced or eliminated (Fuchs, 1967a).

over the whole movement than piecemeal correction by a number of smaller saccades. It may in any case be the result of the saturation nonlinearity of the smooth pursuit mechanism.

This particular mechanism also shows a certain degree of adaptive plasticity; if monkeys are repeatedly trained at one ramp velocity, on switching to a different ramp velocity they tend to persevere with the (inappropriate) previous saccade size (Barmack, 1970a). A similar observation in man is that, if the target velocity is altered at the moment of the saccade, so that the eye movement has an inappropriate velocity, with training the eye learns to move with a velocity matched to the second target velocity rather than to the first (figure 4.21) (McLaughlin and Kelly, 1968). This experiment is further discussed in chapter 11. Attention can also be used to select one moving target rather than another. If while tracking one moving spot across an oscilloscope screen, one is required to shift the gaze to another spot moving with a different velocity in a different part of the field, a saccade of appropriate magnitude is generated to reach it despite the powerful and misleading visual slip signal being generated by the objectively stationary surroundings (Atkin, 1969).

It was argued in the last section that intermittent sampling of the velocity of visual targets was unnecessary, since velocity information is not rendered out of date by intervening saccades. A simple experiment (Barmack, 1970b) shows that velocity information is indeed continuously monitored, even though it is used to control saccades. If we arrange for a target to move off at constant velocity from an initial stationary position (as in the previous experiments), but then suddenly reduce its velocity shortly after it has set

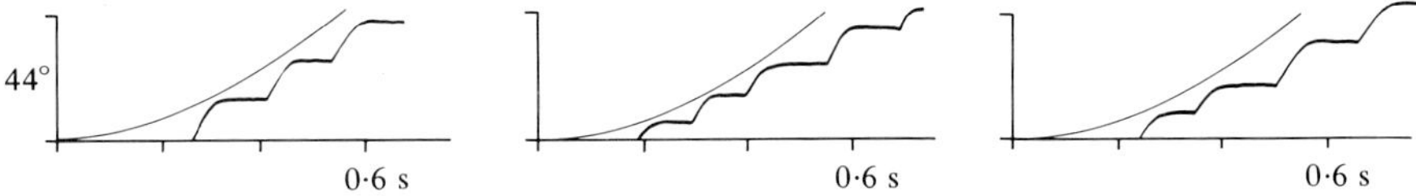

Figure 4.20. Human responses to targets moving off with constant acceleration, showing gradually increasing error despite a sequence of corrective saccades (after Fleming et al, 1969).

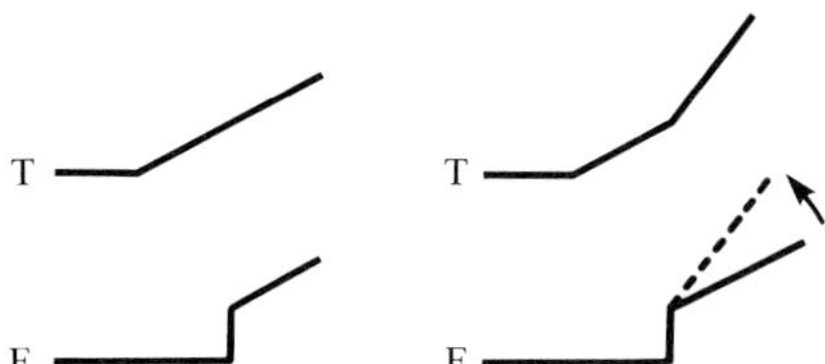

Figure 4.21. Schematic representation of McLaughlin and Kelly's (1968) experiment. On the left, the normal response to a target ramp; on the right, the experimenter arranges for an increase in target velocity at the moment of the saccade: the response is initially the same as before, that is, appropriate for the former velocity, but with practice the eye velocity approaches the final velocity of the target.

off, the resultant saccade is found to be correspondingly reduced, by exactly the right amount to bring the eye finally on to the trajectory of the target, so long as the change in velocity occurs more than some 50 ms before the saccade (figure 4.22). One cannot avoid the conclusion that all the velocity information gathered for a considerable period of time before the saccade is capable of influencing its size, and that the latency for using such information is very much shorter than that for positional information. The latter conclusion is perhaps not very surprising, bearing in mind the difference in complexity between velocity and position control that has repeatedly been urged in previous chapters.

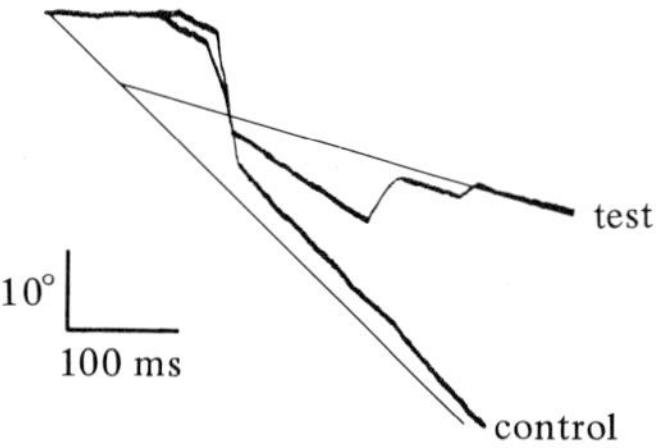

Figure 4.22. Latency of responses to altered target velocity. Thin lines show target movement, thick lines show the eye response. In the control experiment the target moves off at constant velocity and the eye responds in the usual way with a saccade of appropriate size. In test runs, the target velocity is altered soon after it has started to move: nevertheless the saccade size is correctly modified, with considerably reduced latency (after Barmack, 1970b).

4.2.3 Scanning stationary visual scenes

Visual scanning is obviously a rather high-level phenomenon in man, and its adequate treatment involves a consideration of topics like perception and attention that are well beyond the scope of this book. The subject has considerable applied interest, and much work has been done by psychologists on patterns of eye movements made when viewing for example the control panel of an aeroplane, or a promotional display in a supermarket. A more physiological question that is of considerable interest is how, out of all the possible points on a particular visual object, the oculomotor system selects *one* point as the target for a saccade. Suppose for example that a subject is looking at a fixation spot on a screen, and that we instruct him to look at any visual target we may flash on the screen, a few degrees to one side. If the target we present consists simply of a small spot, then we know that his gaze will jump accurately onto it. But if we give him a larger object such as a triangle, it is not clear *a priori* whether he will fixate its centre, or an edge, or even one of the points. If we believe that the system behaves mechanistically, it must presumably have built into it some algorithm for converting two-dimensional retinal images into a single point which is the desired endpoint of saccades used for looking at it. Elucidation of this process would undoubtedly be an important step towards an understanding of a point of some conceptual difficulty.

Unfortunately, although many experimenters have been interested in determining what features of a scene attract the gaze (for example Mackworth and Mackworth, 1958; Yarbus, 1967; Stark, 1971), their interests have tended to lie at an altogether higher level of control. Although it is interesting, for example, that the amplitudes of the eye movements made in scanning the pair of intersections of the Müller–Lyer illusion figures show the same metrical changes as the perceived illusion itself (figure 4.23) (Yarbus, 1967), it would be useful from the physiologists's point of view to know more about the saccadic responses to simpler figures. Some preliminary experiments of this type have been reported by Kaufman and Richards (1969; see also Richards and Kaufman, 1969), who examined not so much the initial eye movements made in response to a figure suddenly presented, as the relative popularity of various parts of figures as resting places for the eye, measured by the relative amount of time spent there.

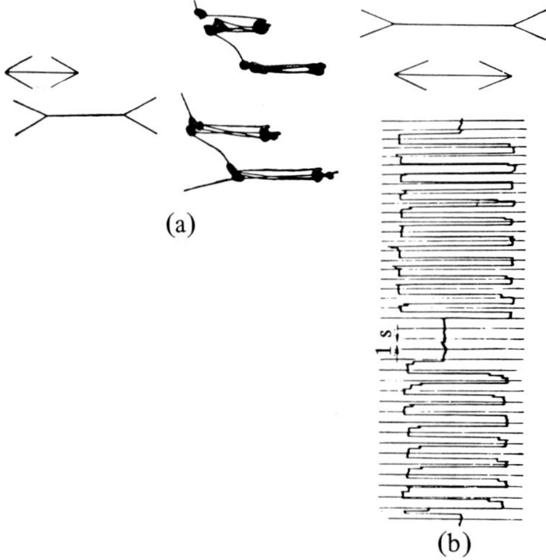

Figure 4.23. (a) Two-dimensional records of eye movements made in viewing Müller–Lyer illusion figures, showing that the amplitude of the eye movements corresponds on the whole to the illusory size. The comparison can be made more easily in (b), which shows the time course of the horizontal eye movements made by a subject instructed to scan his eyes between the intersections of each figure (Yarbus, 1967).

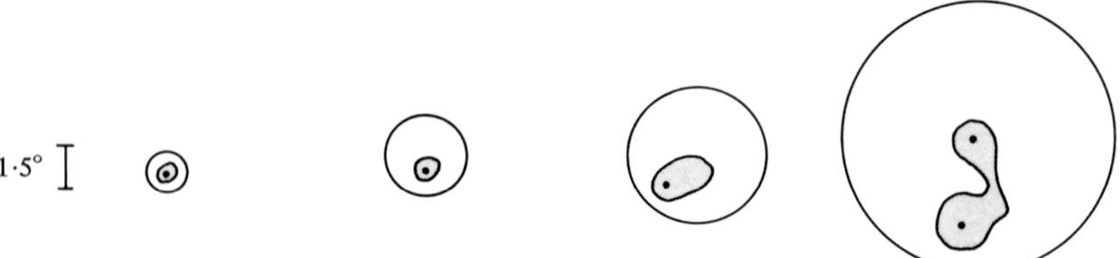

Figure 4.24. Fixational tendencies in prolonged viewing of extended objects: the shaded areas include 86% of recorded fixations by two observers, and the dots show mean fixation positions (after Kaufman and Richards, 1969).

They find that the centre of gravity is attractive, as are also the edges and corners (figure 4.24): similar findings have been presented by Levy-Schoen (1973). Gould and Peeples (1970) claim that a subject's *interpretation* of a simple figure has no effect on the eye movements he makes when viewing it, and that it is only its 'physical attributes' that determine the movements. It is plain, however, that this cannot be true of targets more complex such as photographs of faces, where the eye movements are obviously strongly influenced by the high-level perception of such 'attractive' features as the eyes and mouth.

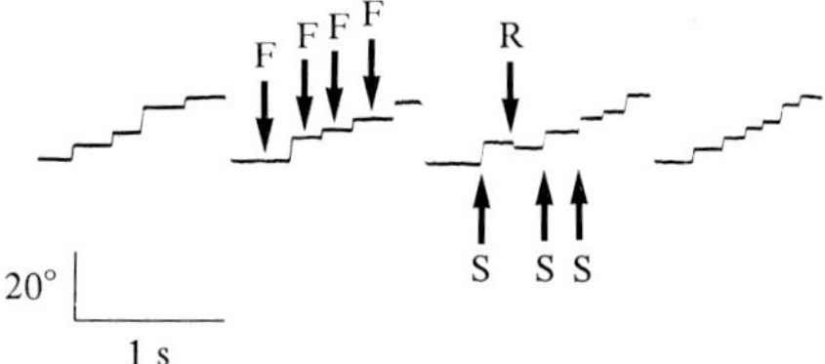

Figure 4.25. Typical eye movements made while reading, showing fixational pauses (F), interfixational saccades (S), and a regressional movement (R).

One special and important case of visual scanning occurs of course in reading. Normal eye movements made while reading consist of a sequence of saccades along the text, at intervals of some 250 ms, with an amplitude and a frequency that depend on the skill of the reader and the difficulty of the reading matter (for example Hering, 1879a; Erdmann and Dodge, 1898; Vernon, 1931; Gruber, 1962) (figure 4.25). Bouma and de Voogd have recently (1974) shown that reading can be performed quite adequately if the subject fixates a stationary point, while the whole text is stepped sideways in a saccade-like fashion at an appropriate regular rate, suggesting that the saccades made in reading do not have to be particularly closely tailored to the visual stimulus for comprehension to be possible.

5

Vergence

"These two eyes, although they bee farre enough separated the one from the other, have such a fellow-feeling, and doe so well agree the one with the other in their actions, as that the one of them cannot move without, or otherwise than the other: for it is not in our abilitie, to looke up with the one and downe with the other, or els to stir the one and hold the other still."

So far, we have considered only *conjugate* movements of the eyes, movements which are closely similar in amplitude and direction in the two eyes and thus obey Hering's principle of 'equal innervation' (Hering, 1868). The requirements for binocular visual fusion as the gaze is transferred from one distant object to another clearly demand that this should be so. But if the image of an object that is near the eyes is to be brought to the fovea of each retina, it is equally clear that the lines of sight of the two eyes must be brought to converge from the parallelity they assume for very distant objects. Horizontal vergence movements are thus a consequence of overlap between the visual fields of the two eyes, and are prominent only in those species that have forward-facing eyes: otherwise movements of the two eyes may be essentially uncoordinated (Walls, 1942; 1962). Although commonly said to be restricted to the primates, cats at least can also be shown to converge on occasion, though rather infrequently under natural conditions (Hughes, 1972; Stryker and Blakemore, 1972). Perhaps because of their relatively recent evolution, disturbances of vergence movements—resulting in double or unilaterally suppressed vision—are amongst the commonest clinical ophthalmological symptoms; and it is a common experience that it is these movements that are first affected by fatigue, and alcohol and other drugs, sometimes long before any other behavioural manifestations.

The simplest way to specify a particular degree of horizontal vergence is by the angle between the two lines of sight, that is, the angle subtended by the interocular distance at the point of binocular fixation (neglecting the fact that the line of sight may not pass through the centre of rotation).

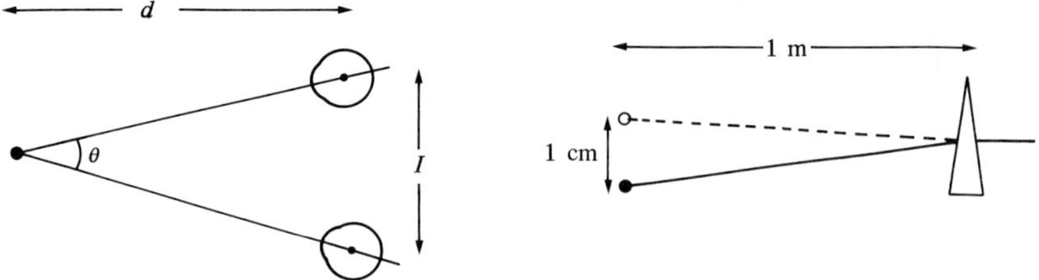

Figure 5.1. Defining angles of convergence: on the left, I is the interocular distance, d the distance of the point of fixation from the base-line, and θ is the angle of convergence. On the right, a prism whose power is one prism diopter (1 Δ) deviating a light ray by 1 cm at a distance of 1 m.

In clinical practice, it is usual to express this angle in *prism diopters* (Δ): a prism of 1 Δ deviates a light ray by 1 cm (measured tangentially) at 1 m (figure 5.1). Thus for a point of fixation at a distance d m from the base line, in the sagittal plane, the angle of convergence in prism diopters is given by I/d, where I is the interocular distance in centimetres: but this definition is not applicable to very close objects. A similar objection applies to the use of the *metre angle* (given by the reciprocal of d: see the discussion in Alpern, 1969c, page 110), and physiological studies of vergence are made simpler if the angle of vergence is specified directly in degrees or radians.

5.1 Sensory stimuli for vergence movements

People vary enormously in the degree to which their vergence movements are susceptible to voluntary control. Many find great difficulty in converging on command onto the rather artificial targets—for example, points of light in a darkened room—that are commonly used in the laboratory, while others can converge and diverge at will. Sir James Barrett (1921) describes a patient who could voluntarily diverge either eye whilst keeping the other still: he "had been able to do this all his life and... it was just the same thing to him as moving the hand". Yet this is by no means a difficult feat, if—like him—one is allowed the use of a fixation point. I myself can hold my left eye fixed, while moving my right eye at will through a range of about 25° inward to 8° outward for parallelity. Again, it is commonly said that one cannot voluntarily diverge the eyes in the absence of a suitable visual target: yet I can do it with ease, and so can quite a number of my students. The voluntary control of vergence is probably not a profitable field of enquiry.

Vergence movements are of course normally performed unconsciously in response to visual objects that are closer or farther away. Fixation of a near object induces not only convergence, but also accommodation of the lens and constriction of the pupil: these three together constitute the *near response* (triple response or near reaction). Now there are many ways in which the nearness of an object can be recognised: these include binocular retinal disparity, the degree of accommodation required for optimum focusing, and a number of factors such as perspective, size of known objects, overlap, etc, than can be classed together as 'psychic' or high-level cues (Maddox, 1907). There is ample evidence that the first two sources of information are capable of generating large vergence movements on their own. The higher-level cues have not received as much attention, although it is clear that they can contribute both to vergence and to accommodation (for example Hofstetter, 1942; Ittelson and Ames, 1950; Alpern, 1958). Indeed, Landolt suggested in 1886 that the eye strain frequently resulting from the use of optical instruments like microscopes, especially by inexperienced users, might be due to inappropriate vergence and accommodation responses caused by the subject's awareness of the proximity of the eyepiece. The next two sections consider the relative contributions of disparity and accommodative information to the evocation of horizontal vergence.

5.1.1 Disparity vergence

It is a simple matter to show that disparity information alone can generate compensatory vergence movements. If, while a subject is binocularly fixating a visual target, a weak horizontal prism is suddenly introduced before one eye, the disparity which results from the shift of the image of the target in that eye leads to a vergence movement of which the subject is generally unaware (figure 5.2). Clearly there is no stimulus to accommodation in this situation. Similarly, in the stereoscope—where different parts of the binocular scene have different disparities, to give an illusion of depth—the observer performs vergence movements as he shifts his attention from one part of the field to another. Again, the actual distance of the visual plane remains unchanged, and so accommodation can play no part in evoking the movements. On the other hand, the degree of accommodation is itself influenced by pure disparity information of this sort (Fry, 1937; 1939), as may also be pupil size (Knoll, 1949; Marg and Morgan, 1949; 1950).

In natural visual surroundings, just as in the stereoscope, different parts of the visual field will show different degrees of binocular disparity: and we would certainly expect to find—as in the case of smooth pursuit—that there is some mechanism for selecting one area rather than another as an input to the vergence system. A simple way to do this would be if only the fovea were capable of eliciting disparity vergence, so that one would automatically converge on what one was looking at. Ludvigh and McKinnon (1966; see also Ludvigh et al, 1965) showed that disparity in the fovea was indeed more effective than disparity in the rest of the visual field, although extensive objects in the periphery could override the fovea if of sufficient contrast and detail. There is certainly also a purely voluntary attention component, as the reader can demonstrate for himself. Fixate a point on a distant wall, and hold a pencil up near the face a few degrees to the left of the line of sight of the left eye: with a little practice the binocular images of the pencil can be fused *without* having to fixate it, and with the gaze still in the original direction.

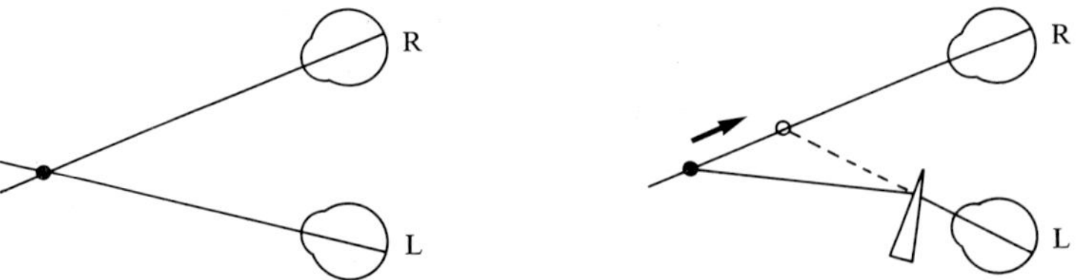

Figure 5.2. Prism vergence: introducing a weak prism in front of one eye when both are binocularly fixating necessitates unilateral vergence to bring the two retinal images back into correspondence.

One question that is of some interest from the point of view of elucidating the sensory mechanisms of disparity vergence is how similar the retinal images in the two eyes must be to provoke compensatory fusional movements. It is clear for example that slight optical blur of one of the images does not matter much, since subjects with an uncorrected refractive error on one side can nevertheless perform such movements quite adequately. Westheimer and Mitchell (1969) made a systematic investigation of the tolerance of the fusional mechanism to such differences between the two retinal images, presenting the images in brief flashes so that actual fusion could not occur: what was measured was the initial vergence response of the system. They showed that the mechanism was startingly indifferent to a lack of similarity between the two images (figure 5.3). Short disparate lines separated in the *vertical* direction by as much as 4° could still initiate vergence, as could such grossly dissimilar targets as a vertical and a horizontal line, or a circle and a cross. Neither dimming of one of the figures by a factor of thirty, not even reversal of its light and dark areas, prevented the correct vergence responses from being elicited. The conclusion must be that disparity information is tapped off the visual pathway at quite an early stage, before any coding of information into channels representing recognised objects (the existence of 'disparity units' in the visual cortex is discussed in chapter 9).

However, there are limits to the system's tolerance, and in clinical practice a Maddox rod (Maddox, 1907) can be introduced in front of one eye to disable the disparity vergence system. This consists of one or more small red horizontal transparent cylinders arranged side-by-side in a frame: a point source of light viewed through it is drawn out into a vertical red streak which is sufficiently dissimilar from the source itself not to evoke fusional movements. Under these circumstances, or indeed if one eye is covered or if the binocular scene is completely blank, the eyes assume the 'physiological position of rest', in which their visual axes may or may not be parallel. If they are not, the condition is described as *heterophoria,* a state of tonic convergence or divergence. This important clinical topic

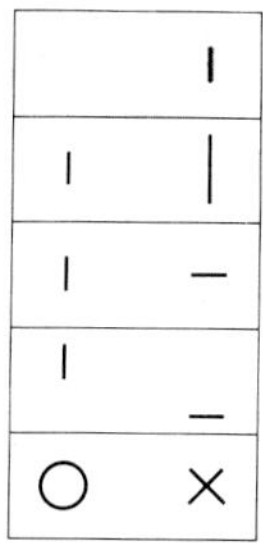

Figure 5.3. Examples of pairs of dissimilar binocular targets which when presented one to each eye can nevertheless initiate vergence movements (after Westheimer and Mitchell, 1969).

lies beyond the scope of the present account, and the interested reader should consult a standard textbook of ophthalmology (for example Duke-Elder and Wybar, 1973; Burian and von Noorden, 1974) for further information.

Although horizontal disparity vergence movements are by far the most important, since the disparities that generate them result naturally from the relative positions of the two eyes in the head, under artificial conditions other kinds of vergence may also be demonstrated. If a weak prism is put before the eye in a suitable position to provoke ordinary horizontal vergence, and then slowly turned through a right angle so that its base is horizontal, fusion can still be maintained: the vertical disparity has produced a state of *vertical* disjunction (Helmholtz, 1909). One might hope in the same sort of way to be able to generate *torsional* vergence movements, by allowing one eye to view a scene that is twisted relative to the other about an anterior–posterior axis. Such a situation is not as unnatural as it sounds, for a consequence of the torsional movements made when the eye is in tertiary positions (the movements described by Listing's Law; although it is doubtful whether the law is actually strictly obeyed in these circumstances: see chapter 7) is that when near objects are viewed in extreme tertiary positions, a state of torsional disparity must exist between the two retinal images. Although it is certainly true that an observer can learn to fuse pairs of images having rotational disparity (by 'cyclofusion': see Ogle and Ellerbrook, 1946), it is only recently that it has been possible to make sufficiently accurate objective measurements of the corresponding eye movements. It turns out (Kertesz and Jones, 1970) that one cannot in fact record any torsional vergence at all during cyclofusion: the fusion must be the result of a high-level mingling of the neural signals from the eyes, rather than a physical rotation to bring the two retinae into correspondence. Neural fusion of disparate images is of course well-established for horizontal disjunction: the limit of disparity for which neural fusion is possible ('Panum's fusional area') is about 6′ under normal conditions, but may be as large as 20° if measured with binocularly stabilised images (Fender and Julesz, 1967). It follows that one cannot confidently make accurate *subjective* measurements of vergence by comparison of binocular images.

5.1.2 Accommodation vergence

In a classical experiment, Johannes Müller showed that accommodation by itself can produce vergence movements (Müller, 1826). If one eye is covered while the other fixates a target, and then a negative lens is suddenly introduced before the seeing eye, the other responds by converging (figure 5.4). The only possible origin of this vergence in this experiment is the accommodative effort made in refocusing the target. Many experimenters have investigated the relationship between the magnitude of the accommodative stimulus and that of the resultant accommodation and accommodation convergence: the ratio between these last two quantities is often called the AC/A ratio, and may be measured in prism diopters per diopter (Δ/D); it actually has the dimensions of length, and ought more properly to be expressed in centimetres. One cannot of course assume that the actual degree of accommodation is necessarily exactly what is required to cancel the negative lens, and strictly speaking one should also distinguish between stimulus AC/A and response AC/A; but in practice, the differences are usually small, of the order of 8% (Alpern, 1969c). For fairly small accommodation stimuli (less than some 5 D), vergence in most subjects is effectively a linear function of accommodation (figure 5.5) (Flom, 1960, part 1) and the AC/A ratio is constant at around 3–4 Δ/D, with considerable variation between subjects (figure 5.6) (Morgan and Peters, 1951; Emmes, 1949; Morgan, 1944; Flom, 1960, part 2). Now it is easy to verify by simple geometry that a perfect accommodation vergence response (that is, one that generated exactly the amount of vergence corresponding to the apparent movement of the fixation point) would show an AC/A ratio equal to the interocular distance in centimetres, for relatively distant targets. Since this distance in adults is around 6 cm (Hofstetter, 1972), it is clear that the accommodation convergence component in fixating near objects is substantial, accounting for rather more than half the total response.

Many writers have speculated on the origin of accommodation vergence: in particular, on whether the relationship is a fixed one, present at birth, or whether on the other hand (as Helmholtz suggested in 1909) the two responses to nearness become linked with each other by association through being always simultaneously evoked under natural conditions.

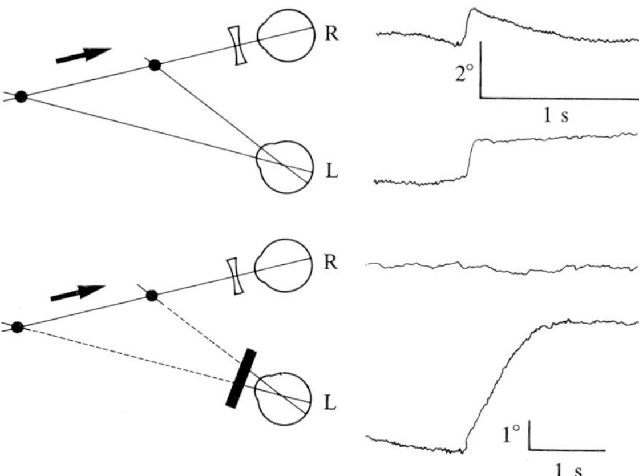

Figure 5.4. Asymmetrical convergence: above, under normal binocular viewing conditions, movement of the fixation point along the line of sight of one eye results in a mixed conjunct and disjunct movement of both. Below, if the eye which has to move is covered, then it alone moves in a simple monotonic manner: this is pure *accommodation convergence* (data from Alpern, 1957; Alpern and Ellen, 1956).

The relationship is perfectly reciprocal in that changes in vergence can also elicit accommodation. In the words of Porterfield (1759):

> "... it is evident, that there is a necessary Connection and Dependence established between those Motions, whereby the Conformation of our Eyes is changed, and certain corresponding Motions in our Axes of Vision, which make it impossible for us to direct our Eyes to any Object within the limits of distinct Vision, without at the same time giving them that Disposition that is necessary for seeing distinctly at that Distance...".

If these close associations are really the result of a learning process, we might expect to be able to modify them by suitable training programmes. For example, we might hope to change a subject's AC/A ratio by the use of stimuli in which the natural relation between accommodation and disparity was severed, as for example by the use of cyclopegics such as homatropine, that enormously increase the AC/A ratio (Flieringa and van der Hoeve, 1924; Morgan, 1954). Yet steady use of such preparations over long periods of time has apparently no observable lasting effect on the ratio (Alpern, 1969c). On the other hand, direct intensive visual training over a period of two months was found by Flom (1960, part 3) to induce a significant but rather short-lived increase in AC/A. The question appears to be an open one, and perhaps is only of rather academic interest. The whole question of the relation between accommodation and vergence has been comprehensively reviewed by Alpern (1969c).

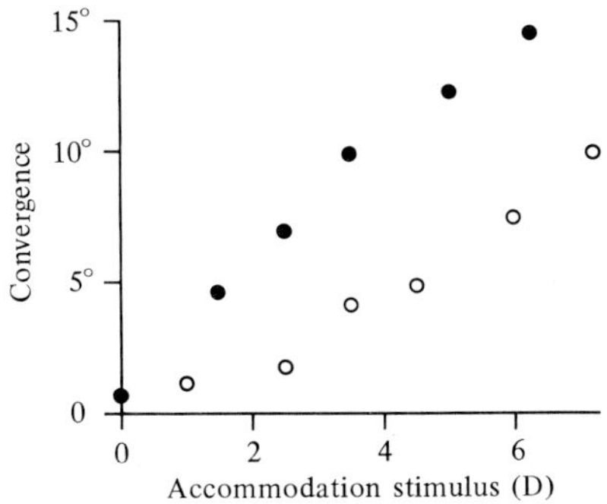

Figure 5.5. The relationship between accommodation and convergence in two subjects, showing the effectively linear relationship in each case, with individual differences in slope (data from Flom, 1960, part 1).

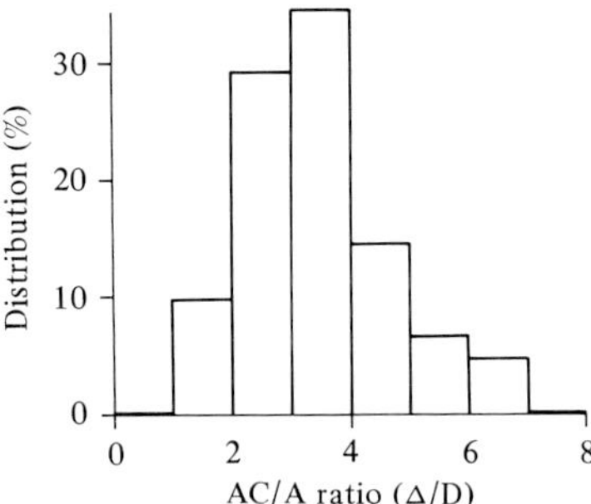

Figure 5.6. A measured distribution of AC/A ratios amongst 104 subjects (after Ogle and Martens, 1957).

5.2 Dynamics of vergence movements

5.2.1 The time course of vergence movements

Vergence movements are necessarily rather small (in fixating an object that moves from one metre away to two, each eye moves through less than a degree), so that quantitative studies of the control of vergence movements have had to wait for the development of sensitive and accurate methods of measuring small eye movements (see for example Riggs and Niehl, 1960; Rashbass and Westheimer, 1961a).

Disparity vergence control can best be investigated by arranging for each eye to view separate and independently moveable visual targets: in this way, visual stimuli can be presented whose disparity can be varied at will. In response to a step change in disparity, after a reaction time of some 160 ms the eyes move smoothly and comparatively slowly to their final positions, in a roughly exponential manner (figure 5.7: Westheimer and Mitchell, 1956; Riggs and Niehl, 1960; Rashbass and Westheimer, 1961a): the whole movement may take nearly a second to complete. The latency of accommodation vergence is similar (some 150–200 ms): the time course is also comparable but possibly somewhat slower, being typically only 90% complete after 1·2 s (Alpern and Ellen, 1956; Robinson, 1966). By analysis of covariance between random fluctuations of accommodation and of vergence, it is possible to show that most of this delay arises in pathways that are common to both phenomena, that is, essentially in the visual system itself (Wilson, 1973a). In the case of disparity vergence, the movements are extremely accurate, in the sense that the final positions of the eyes are within at most a minute or two of the vergence required to reduce the disparity to zero. This is only to be expected of a system with intrinsic negative feedback, and it is an easy matter to show that these movements are guided rather than ballistic, by using pulses of disparity instead of steps.

In chapter 4 we saw that the saccade control system responded to pulses of displacement by generating either a full-sized saccade or none at all: the response of the vergence system is quite different (figure 5.8). One reaction time after the beginning of the pulse, the eyes begin their vergence movement; and one reaction time after the end of the pulse, the eyes start to move back to their original positions. Thus it is clear that these movements are not ballistic, and also do not exhibit the refractory behaviour that is characteristic of saccades. If the disparity is caused to

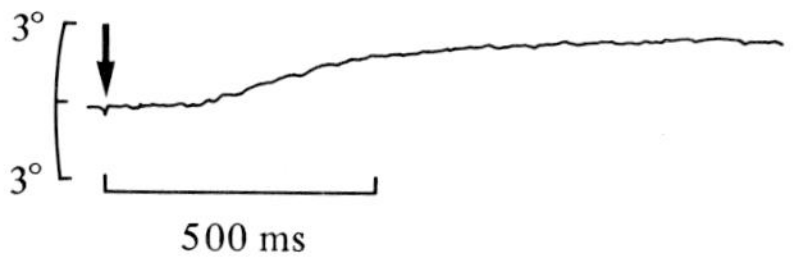

Figure 5.7. Vergence response (recorded from one eye) to a sudden step of disparity applied at the moment indicated by the arrow: closed-loop conditions (Rashbass and Westheimer, 1961a).

vary sinusoidally, the resulting vergence is found to track it quite accurately so long as the peak velocity of the stimulus is not too great. Adequate tracking can be observed until the stimulus frequency increases to around 1 Hz, when the response begins to break down: the gain is reduced to less than 1% before 4 Hz is reached (Richards, 1972); in this respect they clearly resemble smooth pursuit movements. Another point of similarity is in their reaction to barbiturates: with even quite moderate doses of sodium amytal, disparity vergence responses are considerably slowed (Westheimer and Rashbass, 1961); accommodation vergence is similarly affected (Westheimer, 1963). Smooth movements behave in a similar way (Rashbass, 1959).

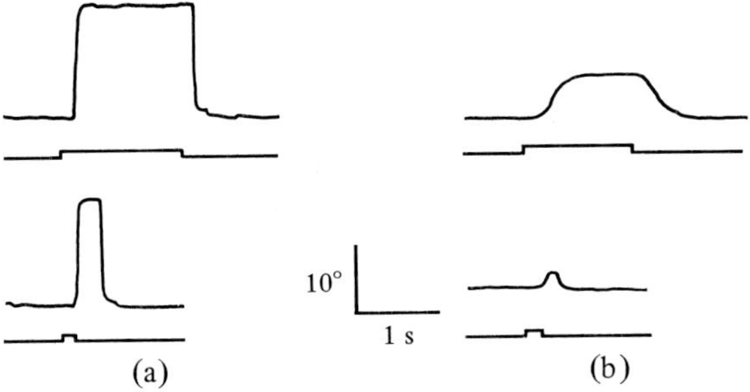

Figure 5.8. (a) Demonstration of the ballistic behaviour of saccades when a subject is presented with a short pulse of target movement; (b) simple additivity of vergence responses to a short pulse of disparity. The total response is in each case approximately the sum of the responses to the rising and falling edges of the disparity pulse, and there is no refractory period.

5.2.2 Open-loop studies of the vergence control system

As in the case of the smooth pursuit system, the disparity vergence mechanism embodies intrinsic feedback, in the sense that any vergence movement made immediately alters the disparity stimulus, under natural conditions. Accommodation vergence on the other hand is intrinsically open-loop in nature; but the interaction between accommodation and disparity vergence discussed in section 5.1 implies that each of the two systems must partake of some of the properties of the other. For example, a purely accommodative binocular stimulus—for example suddenly introducing a negative lens in front of each eye—will induce a vergence movement: but this is immediately opposed by the disparity vergence system, which in turn, as we have seen, may generate an associated accommodation response. Even in the classical demonstration of accommodation vergence, in which one eye is covered, one cannot be sure to what extent the vergence response itself modifies the accommodation effort and thus induces second-order effects. Indeed it is not clear whether the accommodation vergence is more closely related to the actual accommodation of the eye, or only to that part of the accommodation that is due to defocusing of the retinal image rather than other potential sources such as disparity. At all events, it is clearly desirable to remove at least some of this obscurity by 'opening the loop' and arranging for the disparity stimulus, at least, to be independent of any vergence movements that may be made.

If the disparity stimuli are generated by means of moveable spots on the faces of a pair of cathode-ray tubes, with suitable arrangements to ensure that each eye sees only its own spot, one can arrange for an electrical signal proportional to the difference in angular position between the two eyes—that is, proportional to the vergence—to be continuously added to whatever input disparity signal is used (figure 5.9) (Rashbass and Westheimer, 1961a; Zuber and Stark, 1968). If the gain of this artificial external feedback loop is correctly adjusted, it cancels out the effect of the intrinsic loop, and the response of the system then corresponds only to the forward part of the control pathway. If a step of disparity is now applied, it is found that after the usual reaction time of about 160 ms the vergence of the eyes starts to increase at a steady rate. Thus the

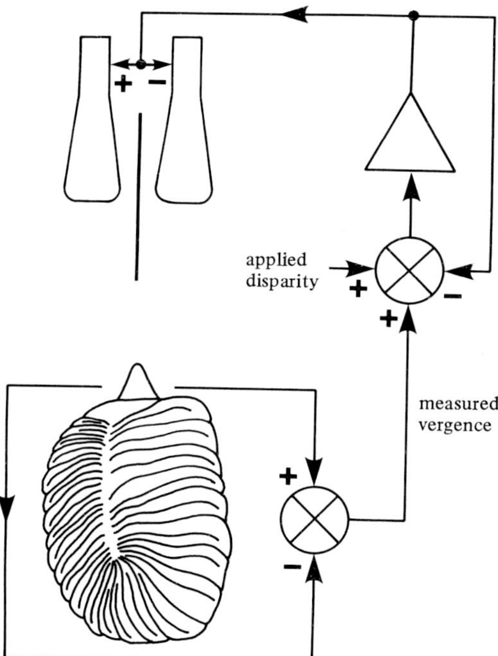

Figure 5.9. A method of opening the feedback loop in the control of disparity vergence. The movement of each eye is measured separately: the difference between these signals (proportional to the vergence) is added to the applied disparity stimulus and used to generate reciprocal movements of the spots on two cathode-ray tube screens such that the subject's vergence responses are cancelled out. Disparities may thus be applied and 'clamped' at any desired value.

response to a square-wave disparity input is a triangular-wave vergence output (figure 5.10) in which the slope is directly proportional to the amplitude of the input, up to some 4° of disparity (figure 5.11). This suggests, as in the case of the smooth pursuit system, that the input signal is being integrated with respect to time to generate the vergence response. If this were true, we would expect that the amplitude frequency-response for sinusoidal disparity inputs under open-loop conditions would also be characteristic of an integrator, namely a straight line with a slope of −1 in logarithmic coordinates. This is found to be the case, at least for a moderate range of frequencies (figure 5.12), but the phase response is more puzzling. A pure integrator would be expected to show a phase lag

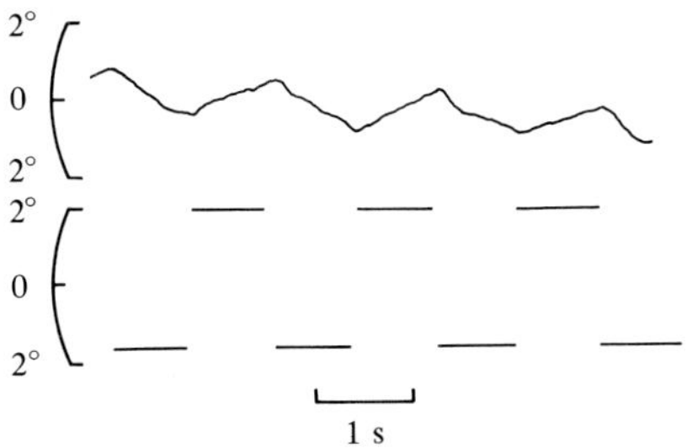

Figure 5.10. Open-loop vergence response (upper trace) to applied square-wave modulation of disparity (lower trace). The integrator-like response of the eye is clearly seen (Rashbass and Westheimer, 1961a).

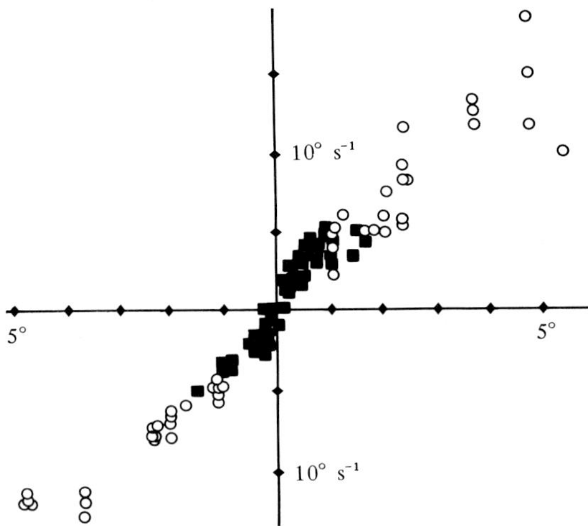

Figure 5.11. Open-loop disparity vergence: the relation between disparity and rate of change of vergence for different applied disparities: the relation is evidently a linear one until disparities of around 5° are reached (data from Rashbass and Westheimer, 1961a).

of 90° at all frequencies, while the observed reaction time of 160 ms would add to this a component increasing with frequency, amounting to an extra 90° of lag at about 1·5 Hz.

The actual phase lags that are observed do not correspond with this expectation at all (figure 5.12), and are consistently smaller than would be anticipated from the amplitude response, assuming the system to be minimum-phase apart from the constant 160 ms delay. Now we saw in the case of the smooth pursuit system that such unusually small phase lags were associated with adaptive behaviour to repetitive stimuli, whereby the system effectively learned to predict where the stimulus was likely to be. However, there is no evidence that the vergence control system can change the parameters of its behaviour in this way, and the response to repetitive stimuli does not show any improvement with practice, under open-loop conditions. But it was argued when considering the predictive properties of the smooth pursuit system that if the modification of the response to suit a particular type of stimulus were achieved by parametric

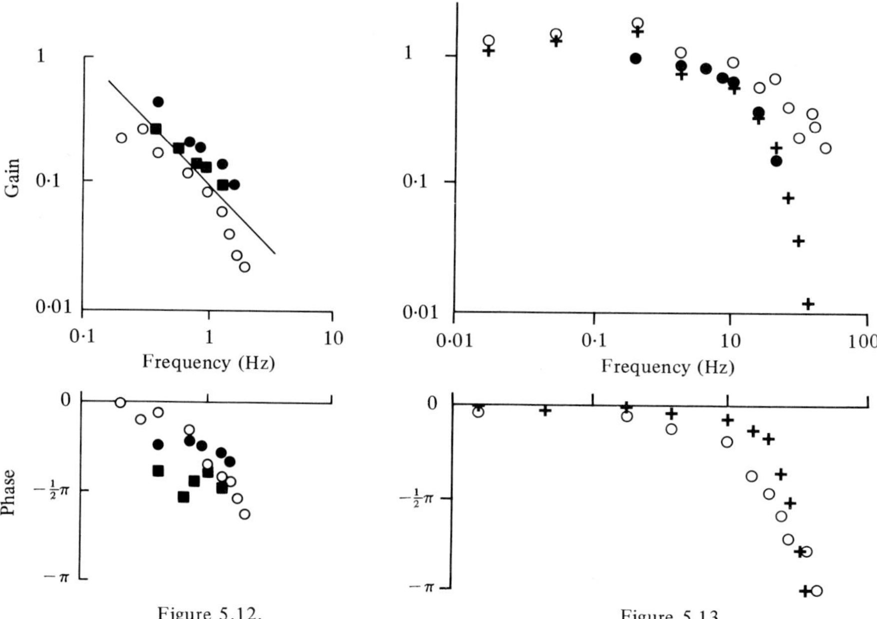

Figure 5.12. Frequency response of open-loop vergence responses to sinusoidal variation in applied disparity: ○, Zuber and Stark (1968); ● and ■, two subjects from Rashbass and Westheimer (1961a). The line in the gain plot shows what would be the expected response from a simple integrator.

Figure 5.13. Frequency response of closed-loop vergence responses to sinusoidal variation in applied disparity: ●, Yoshida and Watanabe (1969); +, Zuber and Stark (1968). The open circles show the latter authors' measurements, using summed sinusoidal components, for unpredictable target motion.

feedback, with the use of a long-term comparison of input and output, then we would not expect to be able to observe it under open-loop conditions. Zuber and Stark (1968) have in fact shown that prediction of repetitive stimuli *does* occur under natural closed-loop conditions, and that the system gain is greatly reduced if less predictable stimuli are used (figure 5.13).

Even under open-loop conditions, prediction of a rather different kind can occur: the system often exhibits an unexpectedly short response time to some brief stimuli that are presented only once, as for example the ramp-step combination of figure 5.14 (Rashbass and Westheimer, 1961a). The vergence movement is of the parabolic form expected as a result of integrating the ramp: but the turning point of the parabola, which would not be expected until some 160 ms after the moment when the stimulus passes through zero disparity, actually *anticipates* this moment by at least 100 ms. One possibility is that information about *rate of change* of disparity, as well as disparity itself, is used to predict the future degree of vergence required. Certainly Ludvigh and McKinnon (1968) found that the rate of change of disparity under natural (closed-loop) conditions influenced the size of vergence movements that could be made: but it is difficult to see why if such a component exists it does not show up in the observed amplitude frequency-responses.

Another problem with trying to represent the disparity vergence system in linear form is that the closed-loop responses to steps of disparity are markedly nonlinear: convergence is considerably more rapid than divergence (figure 5.15) (Zuber and Stark, 1968). Again, there appears to be a discrepancy here between closed-loop and open-loop behaviour, for the latter shows no non-linearities of this magnitude (see figure 5.11).

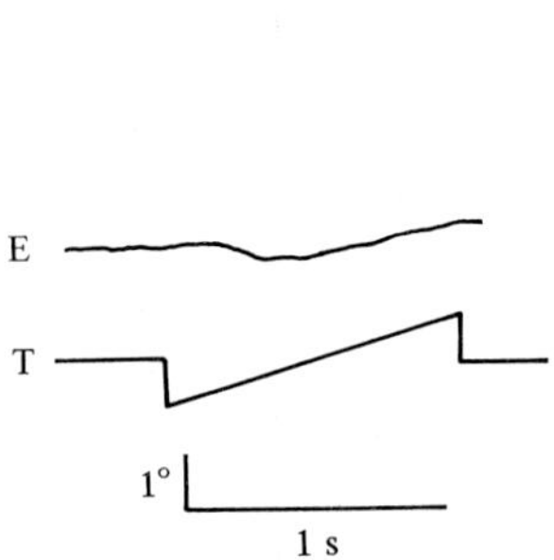

Figure 5.14. Anticipatory vergence response to ramp-step of disparity: see text.

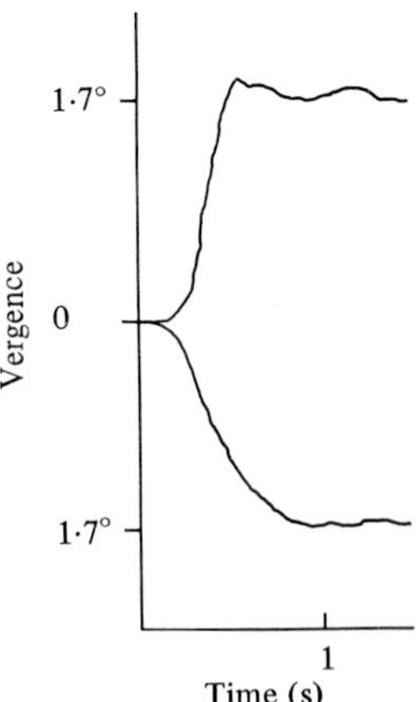

Figure 5.15. Differences in the time course of convergence and divergence responses of the same amplitude (after Zuber and Stark, 1968).

Conceivably the more complicated behaviour of the system under closed-loop conditions reflects the intrusion of linked accommodation responses in the manner suggested earlier. Another complicating factor is the influence of higher visual 'recognition' functions on the fusional response: it is a common experience when viewing difficult stereograms that fusion may be hard to achieve at first, but gets progressively easier over the course of a minute or so, as the various depth relationships in the figure are recognised and understood (see for example Helmholtz, 1909).

One curious aspect of natural disparity vergence that invites speculation is its slowness: not the latency of 160 ms or so, which is after all slightly better than what is achieved by the saccadic system, but the leisurely fashion in which the movement gradually slows to a halt over a period of a second or more. A possible explanation comes to mind from consideration of the stability of the closed-loop system. The slowness of the response is simply a function of the gain of the open-loop integrator, whose transfer function we may write as $k\mathrm{D}^{-1}$. If k is large, the system will respond to small errors of disparity with a large corrective vergence velocity that will smartly restore the error to zero: if speed were the only consideration, k should be made as large as possible. But if there is also some intrinsic delay round the loop, then if k is too large there will be no time for the information that the error has been reduced to zero to be transmitted to the input of the integrator and turn off its output: the result will be an overshoot, and a subsequent 'hunting' oscillation as the eyes swing back and forth about the correct degree of vergence.

It is a relatively straightforward matter to calculate, for a particular loop delay, how large k may safely be (see section 2.8 of appendix 2): on the assumption of pure integration in the forward pathway, k must have a value of less than about 10 s^{-1} to prevent oscillation of this kind, and nearer half this figure if transient instabilities are to be avoided. The value of k in man can be deduced from the results shown in figure 5.11: it is somewhere between 4 and 5 s^{-1}. In other words, the system is about as fast as it can be if it is not to be unstable. However, the fact that the measured phase delays are considerably shorter than would be expected from a simple integrator and a delay in series suggests that the calculated maximum value for k is on the conservative side, and it would be interesting to determine by direct experiment (by appropriate manipulation of the external feedback loop in an arrangement such as Rashbass and Westheimer's) how far the open-loop gain may in fact be increased with safety. Of course, one is still entitled to ask why the vergence system chooses to operate as a feedback, guided, system at all, and not go for ballistic control as the saccadic system has done. The answer may be that the vergence system is still young, and has not yet had time to evolve the rather more sophisticated mechanisms needed to achieve ballistic control: possibly its rather puzzling predictive properties are the fruits of its first tentative steps in that direction.

The dynamics of accommodation vergence do not appear to be markedly different from those of disparity vergence. The vergence response to sinusoidal modulation of an accommodative stimulus is broadly similar to that of sinusoidal disparity vergence (figure 5.16), although there is some disagreement as to the magnitude of the system gain. Like disparity vergence, accommodation vergence also demonstrates a certain degree of predictive behaviour (Krishnan et al, 1973).

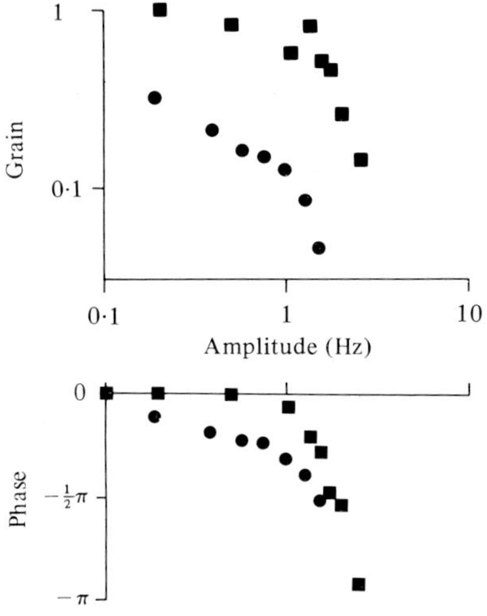

Figure 5.16. Frequency responses of vergence response to sinusoidal variations of accommodation: Data from: ■, Troelstra et al (1963); ●, Yoshida and Watanabe (1969).

5.3 Mixed vergence and version

The natural movements made in looking successively at different objects in space normally of course involve components both of vergence and of version, and it is reasonable to ask whether the eye control system makes any attempt to coordinate their separate requirements, or whether on the other hand the two systems issue independent commands that merely summate in the final common path. A critical experiment that helps to answer this question is that of unilateral prism vergence (Alpern, 1957), when Müller's demonstration is performed without the other eye being covered (figure 5.4). Only the eye that receives the prism needs to move: and one might expect that the other eye would remain motionless throughout the operation, maintaining steady fixation on the target. This is not in fact what happens at all. After the usual 160 ms or so, both eyes participate in a symmetrical vergence movement: but shortly after it has begun, a conjunct *saccade* is superimposed that brings their mean position of gaze in line with the target, the vergence movement meanwhile proceeding to completion. The same pattern of movements—a slow vergence movement with a saccade superimposed in the middle—is seen under more natural conditions when a subject shifts his gaze between objects situated at different distances and different directions (figure 5.17) (Yarbus, 1957a; 1967).

In each case it can be seen that the versional component of the movement obeys Hering's principle, in that the two eyes move equally in the same direction: and at the same time, in the vergence component, it can be seen that the two eyes move by roughly equal amounts in *opposite* directions. The contribution of each eye to vergence movements is, however, probably not *exactly* equal, but depends on the relative dominance of the two eyes; the conjunctive component in asymmetric vergence of this kind tends to bring the eye to a point lying on the line joining the target to not the midpoint of the base line, but to the *binoculus*, or subjective sighting centre, which tends to lie to the side of the more dominant eye (figure 5.18) (Pickwell, 1972). This need not imply a violation of Hering's principle during the saccadic component.

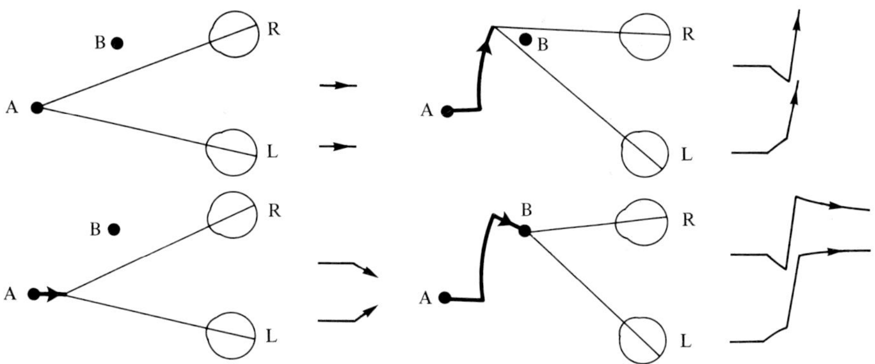

Figure 5.17. The sequence of events in a mixed vergence and version movement. The thick line on the left in each diagram shows the locus traced out by the point of fixation; on the right, the time course of the movement of each eye is plotted separately.

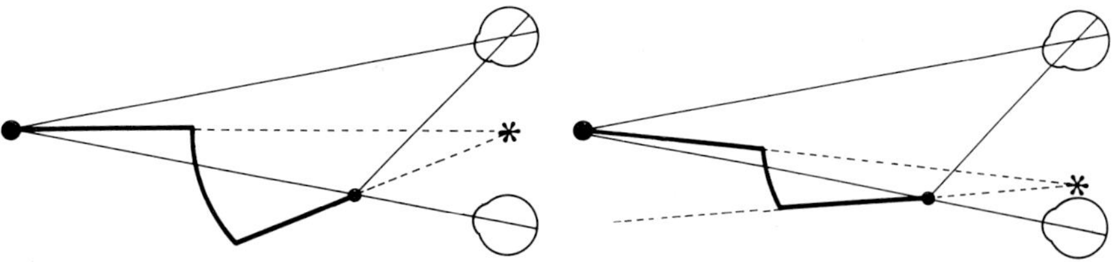

Figure 5.18. Mixed vergence and version with unequal contributions of the two eyes. On the left, the fixation locus (as in figure 5.17) when the eyes contribute equally to vergence: on the right, when the left eye is dominant and contributes less to vergence. The asterisk shows the position of the binoculus in each case.

It appears from these observations that there is little cooperation between the two systems, even, as in the case of prism vergence, when their independence leads to unnecessary motion. The degree of independence of the two systems, for smooth pursuit as well as saccades, has been thoroughly investigated by Rashbass and Westheimer (1961b), who found no circumstances at all in which any kind of interaction other than simple linear addition could be seen. The only exception to this rule seems to be when one eye is covered, as in the case of Müller's classical demonstration of accommodation vergence, already referred to: under these circumstances the seeing eye remains stationary and only the occluded eye moves (Alpern and Ellen, 1956), suggesting that the normal relationship depends in some way on the presence of natural visual feedback.

A division of this kind, into movements that are purely conjugate and purely anticonjugate, leads to the notion of an 'oculomotor map' of visual space, divided by lines of equal version (in the sense that any point on such a line may be reached from any other point on it by means of a pure vergence movement) and lines of equal vergence. The latter—which could be called *isophores*—correspond exactly with the Vieth-Müller circles (see Shipley and Rawlings, 1970a; 1970b) that link lines of equal disparity when the visual axes are parallel and horizontal: in a horizontal plane including the base line, they consist of a series of circles passing through the centres of rotation of each eye (figure 5.19). The lines of equal version—which one might call *isotropes*—form a series of rectangular

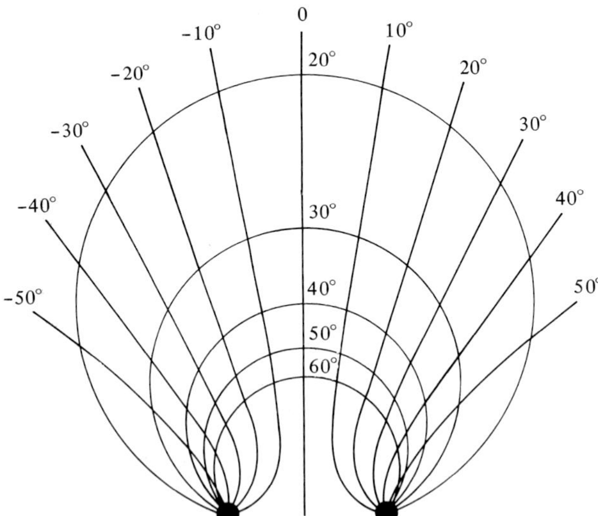

Figure 5.19. A horizontal section through a system of space coordinates based on lines of equal vergence and lines of equal version. The two dots are the notional centres of rotation; the circular arcs are isophores (lines of equal vergence), and the rectangular hyperbolae are isotropes (lines of equal mean version) (after Luneburg, 1948).

hyperbolae whose centre is the midpoint of the base line and which pass through the two centres of rotation. Similar hyperbolae were introduced by Hillebrand (1893) to describe the perceived geometry of visual space. Any movement of the eyes from one point to another on such a map can be resolved into its versional and vergence components along these coordinates. That a similar system of coordinates is also appropriate for perceptual space has been convincingly argued by several authors (for example Luneburg, 1948; 1950; Leibovic et al, 1971), and no doubt stems from its utility in the calculation of three-dimensional eye movements.

6

Miniature movements

"... but I assure you... the eye standeth not still but moveth incessantly."

All the classes of movement considered so far confer some obvious benefit on the visual system: they either serve to move the point of regard from one place to another, or alternatively they hold or help to hold the image of a visual object in place on the retina, despite any movement it may make relative to the head. But normal subjects make a number of other, less prominent, types of eye movement whose usefulness, if any, is not so obvious. These movements are an order of magnitude smaller than anything that has been considered so far, and can be observed best when a subject is attempting to hold his fixation on a stationary object (figure 6.1): they can be described as *micro-* or *miniature* movements, or as movements of fixation. Because of their small amplitude, exact knowledge of their characteristics has had to wait for the development of recording techniques exquisitely sensitive to eye movement, but unresponsive to head movement: Barlow (1952) gives a good idea of the heroic methods that may be necessary to achieve this aim.

Discussion of the controversial question as to whether these movements do or do not assist the visual system in some way is deferred until chapter 11.

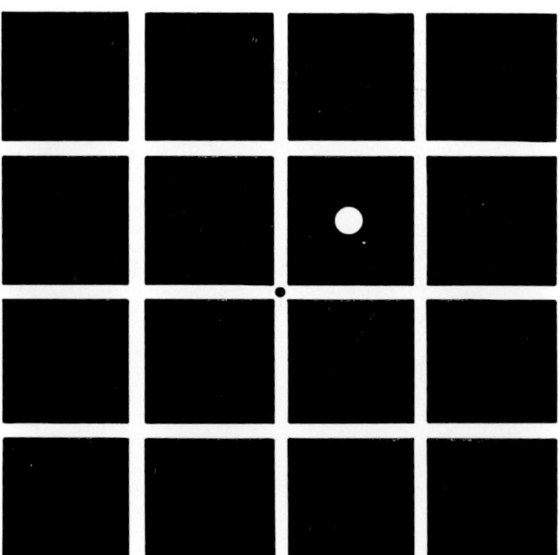

Figure 6.1. Verheijen's demonstration of the micromovements of fixation (Verheijen, 1961). The reader should first fixate the centre of the large white dot, and then after a time sufficient to get a good afterimage—some 20 s—fixate the small black dot. Small displacements of the afterimage relative to the figure itself are then made strikingly obvious, and it should be possible to see the slow drifting movements of the eye as well as the microsaccades that tend to refixate it.

The whole topic of miniature eye movements, including methods of measurement and visual considerations, has recently been comprehensively discussed by Ditchburn (1973).

6.1 Characteristics of miniature eye movements

Descriptions of miniature eye movements have been given by (among others) Adler and Fliegelman (1934), Lord and Wright (1948), Ratliff and Riggs (1950), Barlow (1952), Ditchburn and Ginsborg (1953), Nachmias (1959) and Yarbus (1967). It is generally agreed that in man there are essentially three different components of the miniature eye movements: tremor, drift, and microsaccades (figure 6.2). Ratliff and Riggs (1950) also describe slow random movements in a frequency range of about 2–5 Hz and with amplitudes of the order 1–5′, which they consider to be separable from slow drift. The same classes of movement have been described in the cat (Hebbard and Marg, 1960; Pritchard and Heron, 1960): their characteristics are broadly similar to those observed in man, except that microsaccades are rather less frequent, and the amplitude of the drift component somewhat larger. The miniature eye movements of birds show some striking differences. Tremor is undetectable in the pigeon, but both here and in the owl one can record short bursts of oscillation, with frequencies in the region of 20–30 Hz, and with comparatively large amplitudes, in the region of 2° or more (Nye, 1969; Steinbach and Money, 1973); it is not known what initiates these bursts, or what function they may have.

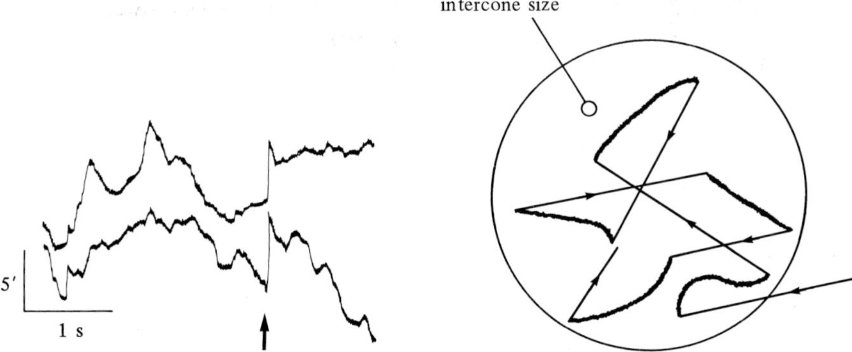

Figure 6.2. Simultaneous records of the miniature movements of the two eyes. The small-amplitude high-frequency component is the *tremor,* the large and relatively slow excursions are *drift,* while at the arrow both eyes execute a *microsaccade.* It can be seen that drift movements are essentially dissociated in the two eyes, whereas the microsaccade is virtually exactly conjugate (after Yarbus, 1967).

Figure 6.3. Schematic representation of the kind of two-dimensional motion of the fixation point consequent on the miniature movements. The large circle has a diameter of 10′ (after Pritchard, 1964).

The effect of tremor, microsaccades, and drift together is to move the retinal image about, irregularly and incessantly, so that it traces out a path on the retina whose dimensions are considerably larger than that of the foveal receptors (figure 6.3).

6.1.1 Tremor

It can be seen in figure 6.2 that the amplitude of tremor is substantially smaller even than that of the other miniature eye movements, and is in fact of the order of the diameter of the smallest cones (some 24″). Estimates include Ratliff and Riggs's (1950) median of 17·5″, Ditchburn's (1955) range of 5–15″, and Yarbus' (1967) of 20–40″. Probably the smaller estimates are nearer the truth, since experimental difficulties are likely to increase rather than decrease the estimated amplitude. Most of the movement occurs in a bandwidth of some 90 Hz: measurements of the power spectrum of ocular tremor show a function that falls essentially monotonically with increasing frequency above 10 Hz, until the level of background noise is reached, typically in the 150–200 Hz region (figure 6.4) (Fender and Nye, 1961; Bengi and Thomas, 1968b; Findlay, 1971; St Cyr, 1973). It may be that there are significant resonance bumps on the curve, particularly in the regions around 40 and 80 Hz (Bengi and Thomas, 1968b), but these are not consistently reported: the possibility that they may be due to resonance in the contact lens attachments used for the measurements, or even in the globe itself, cannot be completely ruled out (Boyce and West, 1968).

St Cyr (1973), discussing the rate of decline of the power spectrum with increasing frequency, distinguishes two possibilities: the fall-off may either be due to the intrinsic frequency characteristics of the noise source itself, or it may be the result of filtering a flat (white) noise with a

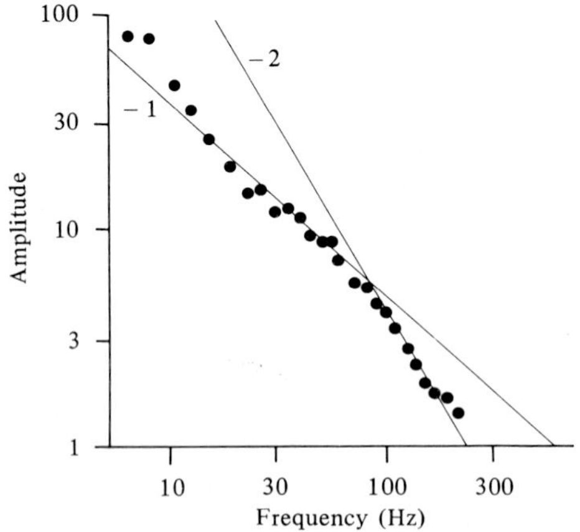

Figure 6.4. Amplitude frequency spectrum of the tremor component of the miniature movements. The two lines show amplitudes that fall off with the reciprocal of the frequency, and with the square of the reciprocal (data from Findlay, 1971).

peripheral low-pass filter. He suggests that the observed rate of decline is what would be expected if the noise spectrum were essentially determined by the mechanical properties of the eye (assumed to be dominated by *inertia* at small amplitudes). But it is equally compatible with a white-noise generator passed through a central integrator and then further filtered by the more commonly accepted *viscosity*-dominated eye mechanics, a notion that is in some ways more attractive (see chapter 12). D Wilson (1973b) has similarly suggested that the decreased high-frequency noise in accommodation vergence (as compared with that of accommodation itself) may also be the result of differential peripheral filtering.

Binocular measurements of tremor indicate that it is uncorrelated between the two eyes (Riggs and Ratliff, 1951), suggesting a rather peripheral origin. There is no evidence that the amplitude of tremor can be influenced by the visual conditions, or by efforts of the will.

6.1.2 Drift

Drift movements are comparatively large and slow, having velocities in the region of $1'\ s^{-1}$, and median amplitudes of around $2-5'$ (Ditchburn, 1973, has an exhaustive list of previous measurements). Boyce (1967) has published statistical analyses of the frequency of occurrence of drifts of various extents, showing a roughly exponential decline in frequency with increasing amplitude. Since each drift movement is necessarily terminated by a microsaccade, such distributions really reflect the statistical behaviour of the timing of the microsaccades, rather than any property associated with the mechanism underlying drift. Drifts in the two eyes are apparently uncorrelated (Krauskopf et al, 1960), although it has been suggested that over shorter time spans periods of significant *negative* correlation—corresponding in other words to randomly fluctuating waves of vergence—may be observed (Ditchburn and Ginsborg, 1953). However, such periods are only to be expected from time to time on a purely random basis, balanced by a comparable number of periods of positive correlation, and arguments based on such 'runs of luck' do not seem very convincing.

The question as to whether or not the direction and amplitude of drift movements are related to the position of the target relative to the fovea is complicated to some extent by the fact, as we shall see, that the micro-saccades that terminate the drifts are on the whole such as to bring the visual target nearer the fovea. If the drift movements were entirely independent of the visual input, this fact would *still* lead us to expect a correlation between drift amplitude and direction and the position of the fixation target on the retina: for if on average the endpoint of a micro-saccade is nearer the target than was its point of initiation, the converse must necessarily follow for drifts. And on average, this is—as it must be—precisely what is observed (Nachmias, 1959; 1961). But the possibility still remains that particular subclasses of drift movement (for example, in particular directions) may be corrective in nature, whereas others are anticorrective: and in fact many experiments (Nachmias, 1959; 1961; Boyce, 1967) have shown that, under particular circumstances, drifts in the compensatory direction may be observed. Thus one of Nachmias's subjects showed compensatory drift near the vertical meridian, but none elsewhere.

A further complicating factor is introduced if random errors in vergence are considered. Such errors are the inevitable consequence of independence of drift movements in the two eyes: and we saw in the previous chapter that mechanisms exist that generate slow corrective vergence movements in response to small changes in disparity, and which would therefore act to oppose drifts of opposite sense in the two eyes. However, if the vergence errors to be corrected are themselves the result of drift, the presence of such a mechanism, though effectively reducing the size of anticorrective drifts, *cannot* make the average direction of drift revert to the compensatory direction. Yet St Cyr and Fender (1969a) found that on average, in binocular fixation, the position of the eyes was nearer to the target at the ends of horizontal (but not vertical) drift movements than at the beginning. One must conclude from this, contrary to the suggestion of Krauskopf et al (1960), and to Easter's (1971) finding in the goldfish, that from the point of view of the control of *vergence,* saccades are not on average corrective at all, but anticorrective. Finally, if there were a corrective component to drift, the information for which were derived from the visual input, one would expect that the mean rate of drift would increase in the dark. Such an increase was observed by Ditchburn and Ginsborg (1953) and by Nachmias (1961), but not by Cornsweet (1956); fixation movements in the dark seem to be especially idiosyncratic, in respect of both drift and microsaccades, and a subject may even learn to use quite unrelated sensations to control his eye position (e.g. artificial auditory feedback: McLaughlin et al, 1968). Becker and Klein (1973) report that drift in the dark is on the whole directed to the primary position, even when eccentric fixation is attempted, suggesting a source of error information derived from a sense of eye position obtained from muscle stretch receptors or by monitoring motor commands: these possibilities are further discussed in chapter 10.

But whatever the source of the information used to generate these hypothetical corrective drift components, observation of long stretches of drift (possible in the dark because of the reduced frequency of micro-saccades) should be able to tell us whether in fact such correction is taking place at all. For, if the direction and amplitude of drift is wholly random with respect to the position of the desired direction of gaze in the field, the trajectory of the direction of gaze will be of the 'random walk' form: in particular, the mean square of the deviation from the initial position will grow linearly with time. This is not in general true if the gaze is also subject to a correcting influence tending to pull it back to the origin. Actual experiments indicate that in fact the mean square rule is followed quite accurately, and that, although significant deviations may occur, they are relatively small (figure 6.5) (Riggs et al, 1954; Matin et al, 1970; Findlay, 1974). Skavenski and Steinman (1970) similarly found that any corrections in the dark were made by microsaccades and not by drift. The consensus seems to be therefore that drifts taken as a whole are not corrective: and the fact that the movements in the dark can be well described by a random walk model suggests once again that the source of the noise that produces drift lies central to an integrator of some kind.

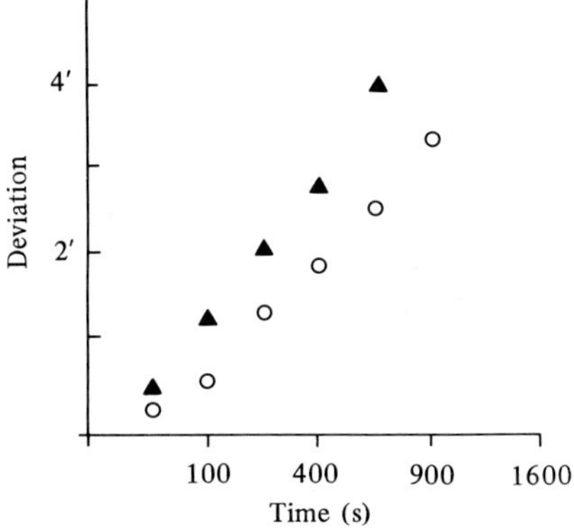

Figure 6.5. Drift in the dark. The open circles show measurements of median eye deviation of the eye from the original fixation point for different periods of time in the dark: the triangles show measurements of the accuracy of perceiving the position of a flashed object under similar circumstances, and indicate a distance that could be discriminated correctly 75% of the time. The time axis is such that, if the data followed a 'random walk' model, it would lie on a straight line (data from Findlay, 1974).

6.1.3 Microsaccades

Since microsaccades have broadly the same function as ordinary gross saccades—that of bringing a visual target to the centre of the fovea—one might perhaps hope that they would be found to share the same control mechanisms. Some evidence that this is the case comes from a comparison of the time course of ordinary and microsaccades of different amplitudes. Figure 6.6 (Zuber et al, 1965) shows the peak-velocity–duration relationship for microsaccades plotted together with the same relationship for voluntary saccades: it is quite clear that the microsaccades fall convincingly on an extrapolation of the main curve. Similarly, Ginsborg (1953) was able to show that the *mean* velocities of microsaccades also lie on an extrapolation of the corresponding curve for ordinary saccades. The implication is that the same temporal pattern of activation is generated in the ocular muscles to produce the two kinds of saccade, from the smallest microsaccades of around 1–2′ (Nachmias, 1961) to the largest voluntary saccades having amplitudes some six thousand times larger.

The main difference between microsaccades and gross saccades apart from size is that the former show a very much greater degree of random variation both in direction and amplitude relative to the desired target, and in the time of onset of the movement. The statistical properties of these parameters have been investigated by many workers, and are summarised by Ditchburn (1973, pages 84–85) in tabular form. Median saccade amplitudes show great intersubject variability, ranging from about 1′ (Nachmias, 1961) to nearly 23′, while mean intersaccadic intervals vary from about 300 ms to 5 s or more. Microsaccades are predominantly corrective in nature, and the probability of their occurrence increases on average with the distance of the visual target from the centre of the fovea (figure 6.7) (Cornsweet, 1956; Boyce, 1967): the same mechanism no doubt underlies the greatly increased saccade latency associated with very small target displacements (cf figure 4.5).

But since these movements take place on a background of continuous slow drift, it is not easy to disentangle a process in which the probability of a saccade depends essentially on the distance of the visual target, and one in which it merely depends on the time lapsed since the last saccade. Some evidence for the latter view is provided by the fact that the frequency of microsaccades does not increase in the expected manner when the drift rate is artificially increased by having the subject accommodate (Nachmias, 1959). Since the effect of drift is on average to cause a steady increase in the fixation error as time passes after a microsaccade, one would expect the frequency distribution of intersaccadic times to show a rather steeper falloff than is the case for a strictly Poissonian process in which the probability is

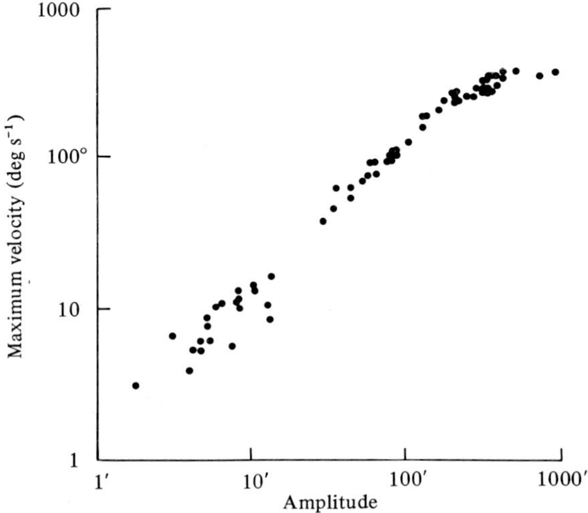

Figure 6.6. Maximum velocities of saccades and microsaccades as a function of their amplitudes, showing the essential continuity in the properties of the two kinds of movement (after Zuber et al, 1965).

stationary with respect to time: such published data as there are (Ginsborg, 1953) contain too few observations for exact comparisons to be made, but indicate that such a model is too simple, and that at least in some subjects there are other factors that strongly influence the probability of microsaccades. It is now well established, for example, that microsaccades can be greatly influenced by volition: an increase in attention (as for example in fixating a fresh object) is associated with an increased frequency of microsaccades (Barlow, 1952). Subjects can also learn to reduce the frequency of their microsaccades at will, or even abolish them altogether for limited periods (Fiorentini and Ercoles, 1966; Steinman et al, 1967): this is not achieved merely by relaxing the accommodation to degrade the quality of the retinal image (Steinman et al, 1969).

Recently, Steinman and his colleagues (1973) have suggested that microsaccades may be the result of the artificical circumstances of the laboratory, in which deliberate and unnatural fixation of objects is demanded for periods of time that far exceed their intrinsic interest. Microsaccades are apparently not observed in natural viewing, as for example in the

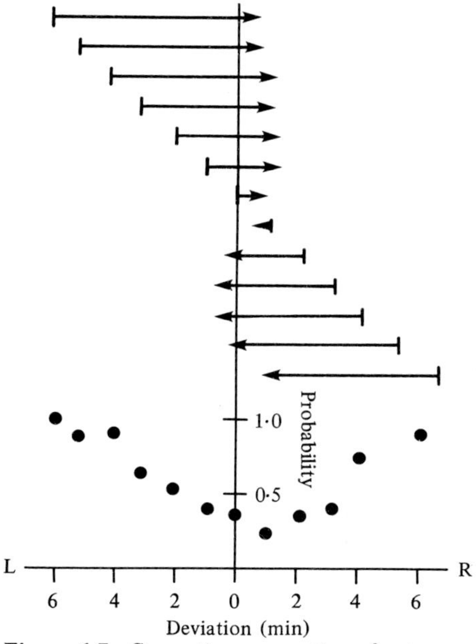

Figure 6.7. Corrective properties of microsaccades. Below, probability of a microsaccade occurring in a period of 1 s, when the eye is at various deviations from the long-term mean fixation position. Above, the arrows show weighted mean amplitudes of microsaccades from various initial deviations. The length and direction of each is given by (mean absolute microsaccade amplitude) × ($p_R - p_L$), where p_R and p_L are respectively the probabilities of a microsaccade being directed to the right and to the left, at any particular initial deviation. It can be seen that in each case the effect of microsaccades is, on average, to bring the point of fixation close to its long-term mean (data from Cornsweet, 1956).

fixational pauses of reading (Cunitz and Steinman, 1969); but it is perhaps debatable whether reading can really be considered a 'natural' pattern of activity. They suggest that microsaccades represent tiny searching or scanning movements, although this view conflicts to a certain extent with the fact that these movements are so strongly corrective in nature, as may be seen from figure 6.7, or from the evident correlation between the directed magnitude of a microsaccade and the visual error immediately preceding it (figure 6.8) (Nachmias, 1959). The notion of deliberate small-scale scanning is considered further in the next section.

The level of illumination and colour of the target have little influence on the mean intersaccadic interval, within the phototopic range (Boyce, 1967; Steinman, 1965): since the fovea is relatively ineffective at scotopic levels, one would expect a considerable alteration in the pattern of microsaccades, and this is indeed observed (Steinman and Cunitz, 1968). Under these circumstances, the saccades are found on average to move the target not *into* the fovea, but *out* of it. In complete darkness, as we have seen, the eye gradually drifts away from its initial position—as much as 1–2° away after two minutes (Skavenski and Steinman, 1970)—and deviations of this magnitude are tolerated without correction by the saccadic system (Ditchburn and Ginsborg, 1953). Under *intermittent* illumination, particularly at frequencies in the range 3–4 Hz, the intersaccadic interval is significantly reduced (West and Boyce, 1968): the explanation for this phenomenon is obscure.

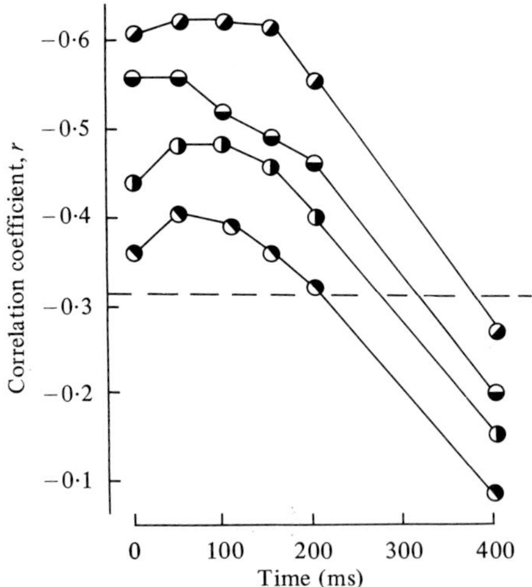

Figure 6.8. Correlation between fixation errors and microsaccades. The graph shows correlation coefficients (r) between directed magnitudes of saccade components and projected retinal image positions at different times before the beginning of the saccade: the directions used are indicated by the orientation of the bisections of the circles. The broken horizontal line shows the smallest value of r which is significant at the 1% probability level (data from Nachmias, 1959).

6.1.4 Statistical properties of the point of fixation

If we ignore the distinction between the three components of fixational noise, we can describe their combined effects simply as if the point of intersection of the visual axis and the plane of fixation were subject to random perturbations around the fixation spot. We can then proceed to make an analysis of the two-dimensional statistics of these disturbances using as data the coordinates of this point at successive instants of time, and paying no particular attention to the velocity of the eye movement, or indeed to any other aspect of their actual detailed time course. If the plane of fixation is divided up into a number of small equal areas, one can reduce this data to a two-dimensional histogram showing the total period spent by the point of regard in each of the sampling areas over some specified time interval: if these areas are small enough the results may be displayed as contour maps (Bennet-Clark, 1964) (Figure 6.9). (The whole process may be automated by reflecting a beam of light off the eye and on to a photographic plate, when the density in any area will be proportional to the fraction of the time that the eye has spent in the equivalent direction.) Histograms of this sort, if derived from data collected over a period of around half a minute, are typically close to a bivariate normal distribution, that is, a distribution of which any cross-section is a normal one-dimensional distribution (Nachmias, 1959; Steinman, 1965). Thus one may make a further reduction of the data by describing such a distribution in terms of its mean, maximum and minimum standard deviations, and orientation to the horizontal. Since the maximum and minimum standard deviations are generally significantly different, the observed contour maps are distinctly elliptical in shape: the same directional preponderance is also observed in the angular distribution of microsaccades and drift (figure 6.10) (Nachmias, 1959). The reader can observe the directionality of his own miniature eye movements by steadily fixating the centre of a figure like that of figure 6.11: moiré fringes generated by the relative movement

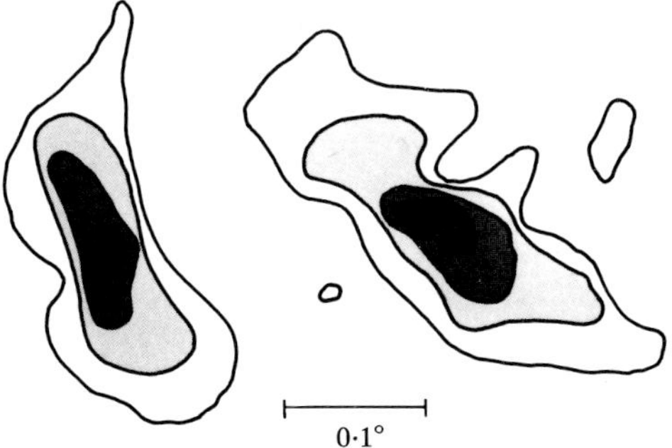

Figure 6.9. Two typical spatial distributions of fixation dwell times. The contours define areas within which the point of fixation was to be found 25%, 50%, 75% and 100% of the time, in order from darkest to lightest (after Bennet-Clark, 1964).

of the afterimage of the figure against the figure itself make directional preponderance particularly obvious.

A further simplification of the statistical description can be made by calculating the standard deviation of the distance of the point of fixation from the mean point of fixation, without regard to direction: if we call this quantity σ, then

$$\sigma^2 = \sigma_1^2 + \sigma_2^2,$$

where σ_1 and σ_2 are the maximum and minimum standard deviations. The first measurement of σ was made by Barlow (1952), although he confined himself to disturbances due to drift and tremor: his value of 15″ is considerably smaller than those of later authors (extensively reviewed in Ditchburn, 1973), who considered all three components. Typical values of σ lie between about 1·5 and 4′, and depend to some extent on the nature of the fixation target (Steinman, 1965; Boyce, 1967; Sansbury et al, 1973; but see also Murphy et al, 1974), and its position in the visual field. This implies that for over 60% of the time, the point of regard lies within an area of about one hundredth of a square degree, surrounding the visual target.

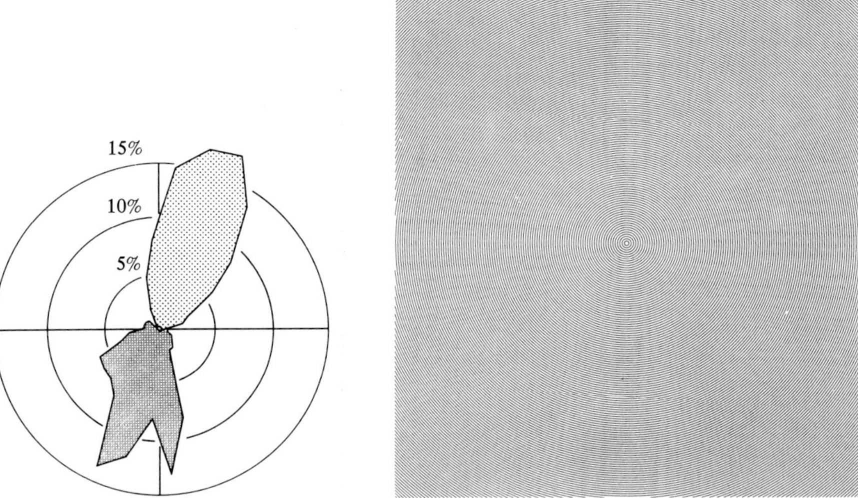

Figure 6.10 Figure 6.11.

Figure 6.10. Relative frequency of drift and microsaccades in different directions. The graph shows the percentage of drift and microsaccades made in particular 10° sectors by a single subject (subject J A, Nachmias, 1959). The upper, dotted area is for microsaccades, and the lower for drift.

Figure 6.11. A subjective demonstration of directional preponderance in the micro-movements. If the reader fixates the centre of the pattern, micromovements will become apparent as moiré fringe patterns between the afterimage of the pattern and the pattern itself: the number of lobes in the pattern can be used to estimate the amplitude of the miniature movement.

All these methods of data reduction make the implicit assumption that the process giving rise to the disturbance is a stationary one; that is, that its statistical properties do not vary with time. One such possible time-dependent factor that has sometimes been suggested (for example Barlow, 1952) is that the retinal point of fixation (that is, the point on the retina to which visual objects are brought) might be moved about within a small area from time to time, and that this might in some way be beneficial to the visual system, perhaps by allowing different sets of receptors to examine the image, and possibly akin to the mechanism by which the attention can be directed to different parts of stabilised images (see Pritchard, 1958). The unimodal character of distributions obtained over periods of half a minute or so suggests that such adjustments are either rather small in comparison with the other disturbances, or that they occur over much longer time scales. Boyce (1967) used a 'cumulative sum' technique (calculating, in effect, the time integral in two dimensions of the eye position) and claimed to be able to show that slow changes of this type do in fact occur. However, the method of cumulative sums is somewhat tendentious, in that it amplifies low-frequency spectral components in proportion to their period and thus gives them a misleading and unnatural prominence. Strict statistical analysis has so far failed to provide evidence for slow adjustments in the retinal point of fixation, nor for slow small-scale scanning of extended visual targets (to which it is equivalent).

Part 2

Structure

7

Statics and dynamics of the eye

"If the sence of sight be wonderfull, the member or instrument serving for the same can not but goe beyond all wonder: for it is framed so cunningly, and of such beautifull parts, as that there cannot be the man, which is not ravished with the consideration of the same..."

If one were to ask an engineer to make a movable artificial eye, one might be surprised if the lens were not lined up with the line of sight, if it wobbled as it rotated, and if the mechanism for elevating its gaze also made it twist to one side: yet all of these are features of the eyes that nature has given us. None is exactly a defect, nor are the discrepancies very large, but they are properties of the eye that necessarily make the task both of the eye movement control system and of the visual system considerably more difficult than they might otherwise be: from that point of view they are probably worth discussing. They may also serve to remind one that it is one thing to know the exact position of a subject's eye, but quite another to deduce from that exactly where he is looking: it is only too easy to slip into the assumption that the two things are equivalent.

7.1 Terminology

Discussion of the geometrical relationships between the various parts of the eye unfortunately requires the use of a certain amount of technical jargon: it is particularly important to be as precise as possible in terminology when one is making distinctions between entities (such as visual axis and line of sight) that are very commonly treated as though they meant exactly the same thing.

7.1.1 Optical terminology

Any refracting image-forming system consists of one or more refracting surfaces, which can be treated as if they were spherical in form if the angles of incidence are sufficiently small. One can thus define a *centre of curvature* for each surface, such that every point on the surface is at a distance from this centre given by the *radius of curvature*. If there is more than one refracting surface in the system, the extended line joining the two centres of curvature constitutes the *optical axis*: if more than two, the various centres of curvature may or may not lie on the same straight line. If they do—as in most man-made equipment—then this is the optical axis of the whole assembly; if not, no single optical axis can be defined.

Rays of light impinging on an imaging optical system, parallel to the optical axis, will be brought to a point, the *focal point*; a second focal point will correspond to similarly parallel rays coming from the opposite direction. A pair of *nodal points* on the optical axis can also be defined, such that any ray directed to one nodal point will emerge from the other in a direction parallel to its original direction, and vice versa. If the system consists of a single surface, the nodal points are identical, and lie at the centre of curvature. But in more complicated arrangements like that of the eye as a whole, the two points are distinct, though often close together. The centre of the pupil is another useful reference point: one cannot of course observe the pupil itself, but only its image after refraction in the cornea. This image is called the *entrance pupil.* One may define a *pupillary axis* as a line joining the centre of curvature of the cornea to the centre of the entrance pupil. The positions of some of these lines and points are shown for a relaxed and an accommodated eye in figure 7.1: good accounts of geometrical optics in relation to the eye can be found in Helmholtz (1909) and Bennet and Francis (1969).

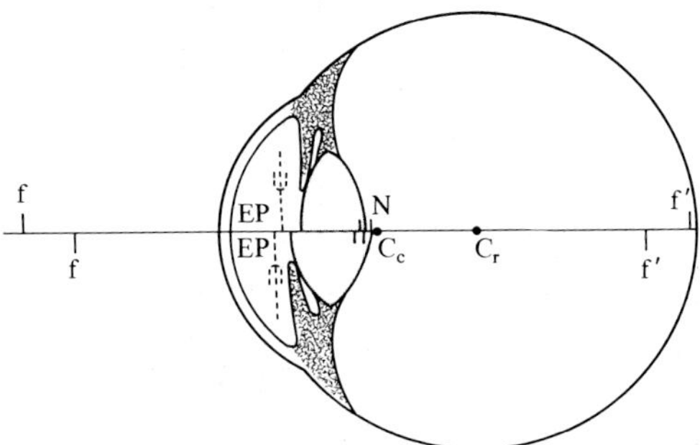

Figure 7.1. Geometrical optics of the eye: a schematic cross section under relaxed accommodation (upper half) and full accommodation (lower half), showing the positions of: the anterior and posterior focal points (f and f′), the two nodal points (N), entrance pupil (EP), approximate centre of rotation (C_r), and centre of curvature of the cornea (C_c).

7.1.2 Geometrical terminology

Any movement of a rigid body can be described as a series of infinitesimal rotations about a constantly moving axis (that may lie outside the body itself), although if the object is undergoing predominantly linear translation —like a tram—this is not a very helpful procedure. But in the case of the eye, whose movements are almost entirely rotations, this notion of an *instantaneous centre of rotation* can be useful. From the hemispherical shape of the posterior surface of the eye, and its tight fit in the orbit, we might hope that its centre of rotation would be a point fixed with respect to the head. As we shall see, this is not in fact true. However, the discrepancies are not large, and one can proceed to define a *base line* joining the centres of rotations of the two eyes, giving a reference axis in the skull to which eye movements may be referred. Another useful construct is the *face plane,* tangent to the chin and to the eyebrows and providing a more easily determined axis of reference fixed relative to the head.

7.1.3 Terminology of visual geometry

When a person with normal vision wishes to examine an object, he directs his eye so that the object's image falls centrally on the *fovea* of his retina, a small central area subtending only some 0·5° of arc at the nodal points and specialised for the discrimination of visual detail. A line joining the point he is looking at to the first nodal point of his eye will then be parallel with a line joining the second nodal point to the centre of the fovea: this direction can be called the *visual axis*, or visual line. It happens that the nodal points are both very close to the centre of curvature of the cornea (see figure 7.1), so that visual lines are always nearly perpendicular to the cornea's surface. In practice, the visual axis is difficult to determine precisely because the position of the nodal points has to be derived by calculation, and it is simpler to use another indicator of the direction of regard called the *line of sight*. This is a line joining the centre of the entrance pupil to the object of regard, and can easily be found by direct observation. Although the entrance pupil is situated a millimetre or two anterior to the nodal points, any errors introduced are very small because of the proximity of the visual axis, optical axis, and pupillary axis. We can also define a *plane of regard* containing both the base line and the object of regard. This plane will not in general also contain the line of sight, because this line does not always pass through the centre of curvature: but again, deviations are usually insignificant. One way of removing these imprecisions—but an inelegant one—is simply to define the centre of rotation as a point some fixed distance (for example, 13·5 mm) behind the cornea along the line of sight (Alpern, 1969a). But even this can lead to theoretical difficulties, since it is not in general true (as will be seen later) that a point can be found on the line of sight that is fixed in space as the eye moves (that is, is a *sighting centre*), or even fixed relative to the eye! Further points that can be

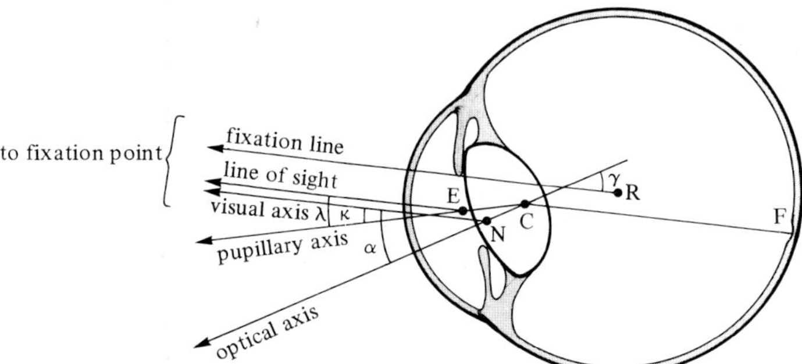

Figure 7.2. Cross section of eye with grossly displaced lens, to clarify the definition of certain axes and lines, and the angles between them. E is the centre of the entrance pupil, N the notional single nodal point, C the centre of curvature of the cornea, R the notional centre of rotation, and F the *fovea centralis*.

defined by reference to the line of sight are the *anterior* and *occipital poles,* where this line crosses the anterior and posterior surfaces of the eye.

Finally, there are two ways of defining a 'straight-ahead' position of the eye: the *straight-forward* position is when the line of sight is perpendicular to the face plane, while the *primary position* indicates the position of the eyes in the skull when the head is held in a natural erect position and the line of sight is horizontal, and perpendicular to the base line. This latter definition is obviously imprecise: a better definition from this point of view is to define it as the position from which purely horizontal or vertical deviations of the eye are not accompanied by a change in the vertical meridian of the eye relative to absolute vertical. This definition relies, as we shall see, on the validity of Listing's Law, and on the fixity of Listing's plane within the head, which is by no means certain. In any case, the magnitude of the expected tilt for small deviations from the true primary position is very small, and it is doubtful whether in fact this definition is any more precise than the classical one.

7.2 Measurements of the eye's functional geometry

7.2.1 Determination of the optical and pupillary axes

There are four refracting surfaces in the optical system of the eye: they are the anterior and posterior surfaces of the cornea, and the anterior and posterior surfaces of the lens. Apart from refracting the light that is incident on them, they also reflect some of it back: since the surfaces are curved, they thus form secondary images of the source. These images are called, in order, the first, second, third, and fourth *Purkinje images* (P1, P2, P3, P4). The first three are formed by surfaces convex to the incident light, and are thus real and erect, while the last is virtual and inverted. Their appearance and position in the eye are shown in figure 7.3. The positions of these images will depend not only on the position of the eye relative to the source (for which reason P1 in particular provides a useful way of measuring movements of the eyes—see appendix 2), but also on the radii of curvature and centres of curvature of the optical surfaces. If the Purkinje images appear colinear (figure 7.3) this implies that the centres of curvature are also colinear, that is, that an optical axis can be defined for the whole system. The position of this axis can best be found by using a pair of small sources equidistant from a sighting tube (figure 7.3): when the Purkinje images appear symmetrically disposed around the sighting marks, the tube must lie along the optical axis of the eye. In this way one can measure the angle between the optical axis and the visual axis or pupillary axis. The former quantity is often called the *visual angle,* α, and typically has a value of around 4–7°. The visual axis is usually directed inward of the optical axis, and most frequently a degree or two upwards, although there is considerable personal variation. However, for some subjects it is impossible to align the Purkinje images under any conditions, and in this case no visual angle can be defined. Generally in these cases it is found that the axis of the lens is slightly higher than that of the cornea. Other angles (γ, δ, κ, λ) can be defined in analogous ways (figure 7.2) (see Howe, 1907; Lancaster, 1943).

The use of the pupillary axis rather than the optical axis avoids this difficulty by ignoring the existence of the lens and its associated Purkinje images altogether: the relation between the pupillary axis and the line of sight (the angle λ) can be measured with no apparatus more complicated than an ordinary torch. The experimenter holds the torch just below his own viewing eye—the other being shut—and observes its reflection in the cornea of the subject's eye while the subject monocularly fixates a stationary target. The experimenter then moves his head until this image seems to be centred in the subject's entrance pupil (figure 7.4); it can easily be verified that he is then looking directly along the pupillary axis,

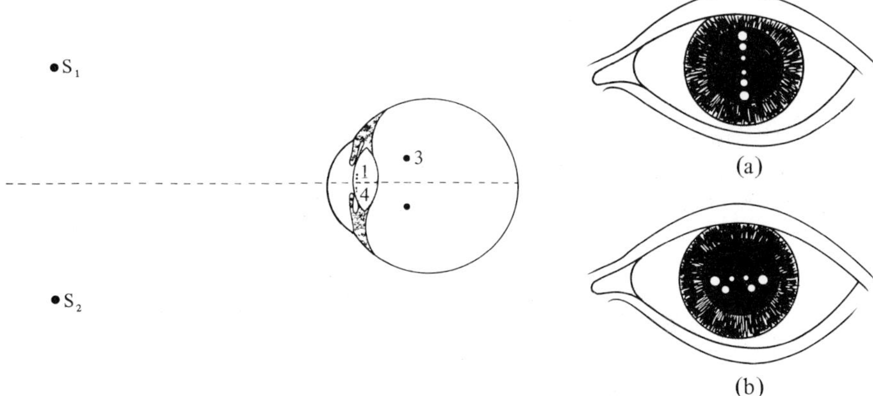

Figure 7.3. Purkinje images. Left, position of the Purkinje images when viewing a symmetrical pair of point sources S_1 and S_2: 1, 3, and 4 represent respectively the positions of the first, third, and fourth Purkinje images, while the second is very dim, and close to 1. Right, the appearance of the eye when illuminated as above: (a) is a normal eye, in which the three brightest images are aligned, (b) is for an eye in which no optical axis can be defined and the images cannot be brought into colinearity.

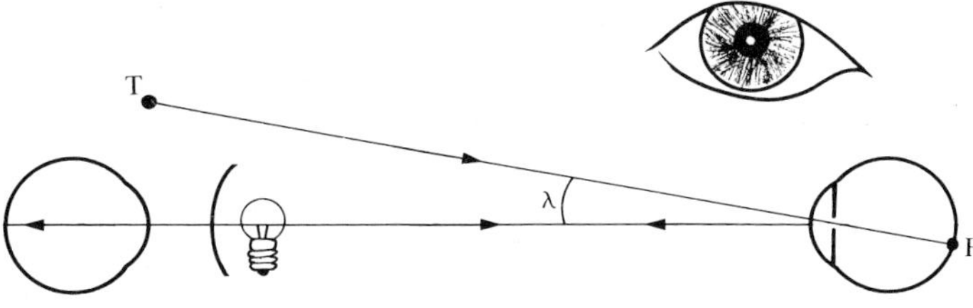

Figure 7.4. A simple method of finding the angle λ, explained in the text. T is the target at which the subject directs his gaze; when correctly aligned, the image of the light bulb is centred in the subject's entrance pupil, as in the inset.

and the angle λ between this axis and a line joining the target to the centre of the entrance pupil can readily be obtained. Park and Park (1940), using a photographic variation of this method, showed that the angle λ (called by them the 'physiological angle') not only varied considerably from subject to subject, but in any one subject showed continual variation, in the form both of drift and of random movements. Such movements could be due to two possible mechanisms: either to motion of the lens within the eye, or possibly to a continual change in the virtual point of fixation on the retina, in the manner discussed in section 6.1.4.

Related effects are seen in prism vergence (Peckham, 1934): after the introduction of 10° prism before one eye, a subject can re-fuse his disparate images by a version movement. Yet the necessary angle of version for fusion (measured by reflection from the cornea) is often less than half the expected angle—a difference of 5°. It is of course quite true that some of this discrepancy may be accounted for by neural fusion at a higher level in the visual system, as we saw must be the case for cyclofusion (Kertesz and Jones, 1970) (see section 5.1.1). Nevertheless, Park and Park (1940) found that aphakic subjects did *not* show these large fusional discrepancies, and further that, in reading text of fixed-length lines, the total amplitude of the horizontal excursions of the aphakics' eyes were much larger than those of normal subjects' eyes. This suggests that the lens may be capable of changing its axis relative to the pupillary axis, and that this movement may be used as an adjunct to movements of the whole globe: possibly the ciliary muscles give a fine adjustment of the direction of regard.

Such an idea is so contrary to present assumptions about the relation between movements of the globe and movements of the visual image that it seems strange that the question has not been taken up more recently. The ingenious measuring device of Cornsweet and Crane (1973), which is capable of tracking both the first and the fourth Purkinje images (see appendix 2), ought to be suited to this purpose. One implication of such movements—if they really exist—is that estimates of the standard deviation of the point of regard in fixating a point, derived from a study of the eye movements alone, may be rather smaller than the standard deviation of the deviation of the retinal image from its mean position (see section 6.1.4). Yet estimating the latter by a subjective method that would therefore include both sources of variance (Barlow, 1952) produced, as we have seen, the lowest estimate of all. A possible explanation might be that the observed random movements of the eye as a whole are in fact partially *compensating* for random movements of the lens, although there is absolutely no direct evidence for such a mechanism.

7.2.2 Determination of centres of rotation

The ophthalmometric observations described in the previous section can be applied not only with the eye in the straight-forward position, but equally when it is deviated in the orbit. From such measurements the instantaneous centre of rotation at any deviation can be found. From observations of this kind, Park and Park (1933) showed that the centre of rotation was not fixed, but moved in a systematic way along a curved line fixed in space, the space centrode: (figures 7.5 and 7.6). If this same line is plotted as a curve on axes that move *with* the eye, we obtain a second curve which may be called the body centrode: the whole movement of the eye can thus be described as a rolling of the body centrode on the space centrode. Over the entire range of horizontal movements the centre of rotation is found to move relative to the eye through a distance of some two millimetres in the posterior–anterior direction, and approximately a third of this distance horizontally. Despite this complex motion of the globe, they found that

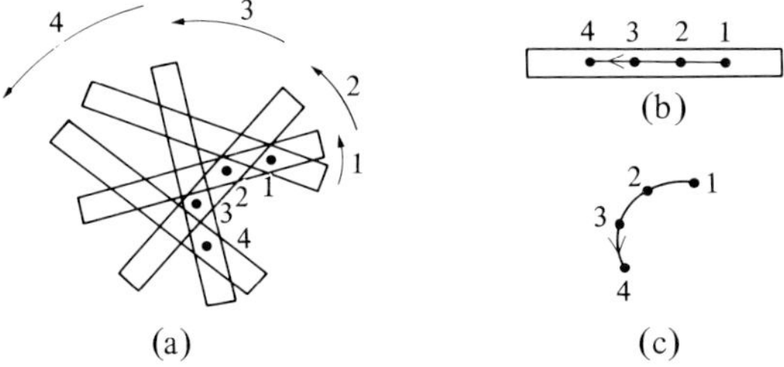

Figure 7.5. Body and space centrode. (a) shows the five successive positions taken up by a body after rotation about each of the points 1, 2, 3, 4 in turn, as shown; (b) shows the *body centrode,* that is, the locus of these points of rotation relative to the body itself; (c) shows the *space centrode*, the locus of the succession of the same points in space.

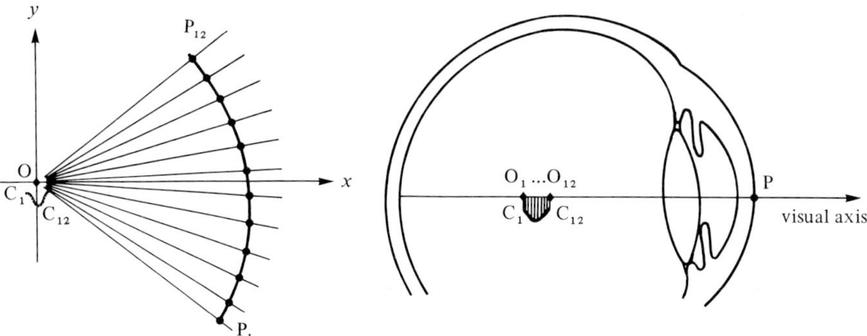

Figure 7.6. Body and space centrodes of the human eye. Left, the radiating lines are the subject's visual axes as he looks in different directions: in each case, P_1–P_{12} are the projected positions of the anterior pole P on this line. The visual axes are found to meet at a point fixed in space, O. C_1–C_{12} are the calculated positions of the centre of rotations corresponding to P_1–P_{12}: together they form the space centrode of the movement. Right, O_1–O_{12} show the positions of the point O relative to the eye for the same set of conditions, and C_1–C_{12} show the successive positions of the centres of rotations, again plotted relative to the eye itself: they thus form the body centrode of the movement.

the visual axis for any horizontal deviation always passed through a point fixed in space (the sighting or viewing centre).

This confirmed much earlier observations by A W Volkmann (1869), Woinow (1870), and others, that the visual axes of the eye as it looked in different directions always intersected at a point; the easiest way to do this is to line up pairs of pins by eye for different directions of regard. More recent work, however (Fry and Hill, 1962; Davis and Fernald, 1963; Grolman, 1963), with more accurate measurements of the visual axis have shown that this is not exactly true, and that for many subjects the visual axes do not meet at a point, but sometimes form a series of tangents to a small circle of fixed radius whose centre is fixed in the eye. One might therefore assume that the centre of this circle must also be a centre of rotation of the eye: but, because of movements of the lens in the way suggested earlier, this is by no means a necessary conclusion if we allow the possibility that the visual axis may not be fixed in the eye. Indeed in most of these more recent experiments it was in fact not the visual axis but the pupillary axis that was measured, the assumption being made that the two are a constant angle apart. As we have seen, such an assumption is not in practice justified, and systematic axial displacements would be expected to produce exactly the kind of tangential results that are observed, if in fact the sighting centre *were* fixed in space. The findings of Fry and Hill (1962) are not, however, open to this kind of criticism: again, the problem might be finally resolved by accurate measurements of all four Purkinje images. Shipley and Rawlings (1970a; 1970b) have suggested that these peculiarities of the rotational properties of the eye, particularly the lack of fixity of the centre of rotation, may actually be useful to the visual system in that they can help compensate for distortions introduced, in near vision, by the fact that the nodal points are far from the centre of the eyeball.

Finally, it was shown long ago by Berlin (1871) that rotations of the eye in the horizontal plane are accompanied by a vertical translation. This can be demonstrated by lining up two horizontal threads at different distances from the eye while looking straight ahead, and then observing their relative displacement as the eye is rotated horizontally; this displacement can only be due to vertical movement of the nodal points. These displacements along the axis of rotation have been called *screw movements,* and can be demonstrated for vertical and oblique rotations with equal ease. Fry and Hill (1963) have made accurate measurements of these displacements and find that they may reach as much as 0·4 mm for extreme rotations.

7.3 Kinematics of eye rotations

To specify the situation of a rigid body in space in general requires six parameters: three of these can describe the position of some defined point in the body, and the other three can represent possible rotations about axes through this point. For the eye, as we have seen, particular rotations *determine* its position within the orbit: thus the first three parameters are superfluous. If we also choose to ignore the translations associated with rotation, and regard the centre of rotation of the eye as fixed in space and in the eye itself, then the three rotational parameters are a perfectly complete description of its disposition within the head. It is convenient to refer the three rotational axes to the primary position: an axis for vertical movements (the base line); an axis for horizontal movements perpendicular to the first axis and also to the line of sight; and an axis for torsional movements along the line of sight. As soon as the eye moves away from the primary position, we have to choose whether (as in the case of the body and space centrodes) to indicate the direction of subsequent rotations relative to axes fixed in the head in the positions they had when the eye was in the primary position, or alternatively to make them move with the eye. To make the difference between these two possibilities a little clearer, consider what happens when the eye is deviated, say, 45° horizontally to the right. What is *then* meant by a vertical movment? According to the first system, it would imply a rotation of the globe about the base line: according to the second, a rotation about a horizontal line at 45° to the base line. In practice, as we shall see, both methods are in use, and in fact the commonest coordinate systems use one method for horizontal movements and the other for vertical movements. A similar ambiguity about the method of specifying *torsional* rotations has led, as will become apparent, to nearly a century of controversy and confusion about the existence and nature of Listing's Law.

Observation of actual rotations of the globe during natural movements shows that the eye does not in fact make use of all three of its degrees of rotational freedom. In the absence of head tilt, and with stationary visual surroundings, the degree of torsion measured relative to any system of axes is uniquely determined by the degree of horizontal and vertical rotation, and is the same for any particular degree of rotation about the other axes, regardless of the manner in which the eye arrives at it (Donders' Law; Donders, 1847). [This does not necessarily mean that it is equally rigidly determined *during* a movement: Westheimer and McKee (1973) present some evidence that it is not.] Leaving aside for the moment the question of exactly what form this fixed relationship has, a consequence of this fact is that the situation of the eye needs only two, and not three, parameters to be fully described. This in turn means that the eye's rotations can be represented completely by points on a (two-dimensional) graph: and by choosing a suitable form of graphical representation, consideration of the otherwise somewhat mind-bending problems associated with rotation in three dimensions can be greatly clarified. It turns out that a highly appropriate representation of such movements is in the form of a stereographic projection (Helmholtz, 1909).

7.3.1 Stereographic representation of eye movements

Suppose a sphere of unit radius and centre C touches a plane surface at a point O (figure 7.7), and that the pole P is at the opposite end of the diameter through O. Then for any point A on the surface of the sphere, we can define a corresponding point A′ on the plane such that PAA′ is a straight line. In this way we can form a *stereographic* mapping of the surface of the sphere on to the plane, a method dating back at least to the second-century astronomer Ptolemy, and commonly used as a map projection: useful information on this and other spherical projections may be found in standard books on cartography, for example, that of Steers (1953). Such a projection has the property that *small* areas are mapped with the same shape as the original, a property known as orthomorphicity. Thus if two lines meet at an angle θ at a point on the surface of the sphere, then at the corresponding point on the plane the projection of the lines will also meet at an angle θ. All circles on the sphere that pass through P are mapped as straight lines: other circles map as circles. Great circles—that is, circles with unit radius—through P map as straight lines through O (figure 7.8).

To represent eye movements with this projection, we can let C be the notional centre of rotation of the eye and O be the intersection of the fixation line with the cornea, with the eye in the primary position. Then movements of the eye from the primary position in purely horizontal and vertical directions will be represented on the plane by straight horizontal and vertical lines through O: points on these lines represent *secondary positions* of gaze. It is convenient to imagine a small cross with vertical and horizontal arms fixed on the anterior pole of the eye: because the projection is orthomorphic, it will always project as a cross with perpendicular arms, and its orientation will be related to torsion of the eye (figure 7.9).

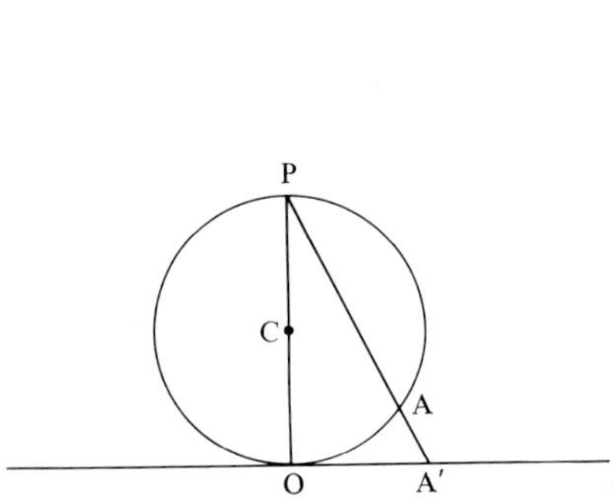

Figure 7.7. The basis of the stereographic projection: see text.

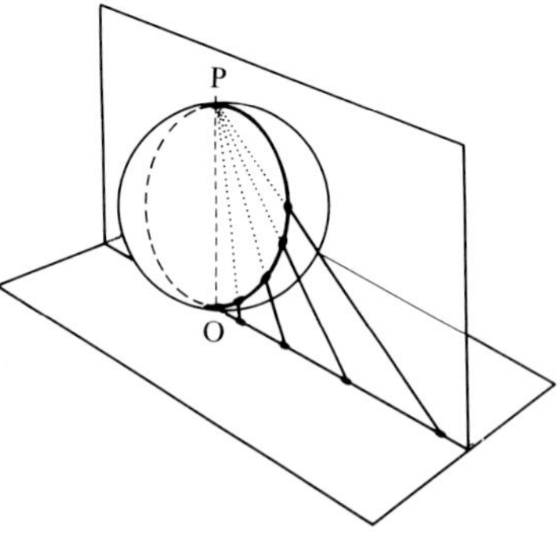

Figure 7.8. Great circles on the sphere project as straight lines on the stereographic plane.

We now have to consider the problem of what system of coordinates to use to describe a particular position of the eye, whether fixed in the head or moving with the eye. This problem does not arise when secondary positions of the eye are being described, because they involve rotation about only one of the primary axes. A movement with rotation about both horizontal and vertical axes brings the eye to a *tertiary position* (figure 7.9). Let us suppose that such a movement can be decomposed into an initial horizontal component, and a subsequent vertical component. At the end of the horizontal movement the position of the eye is specified unambiguously, because the plane of rotation is exactly the same whether considered relative to the eye or to the head. But this is not at all true of the ensuing vertical movement, as was noted in the earlier example: the vertical plane of rotation as fixed in the eye has now moved relative to that fixed in the head, so that it now matters a great deal about which of the two possible axes the next component is considered to occur.

The usual convention in the case of such tertiary positions is to use an axis that moves with the eye: this is equivalent to treating the eye as if it moved in gimbals (figure 7.10). In this system—sometimes called Fick's

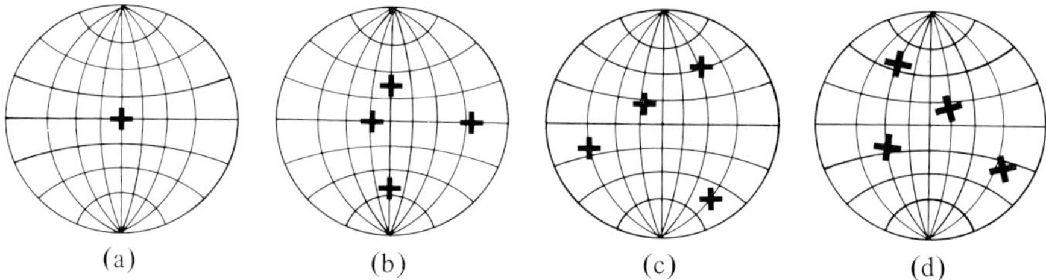

Figure 7.9. Eye movements in stereographic projection: (a) shows a stereographic net for deviations of up to 90° from the primary position at intervals of $22\frac{1}{2}$°: the cross marks the position of the eye in the primary position; (b) shows some secondary positions of gaze, and (c) some tertiary positions. In (d) the eye is shown in tertiary positions with different degrees of added torsion.

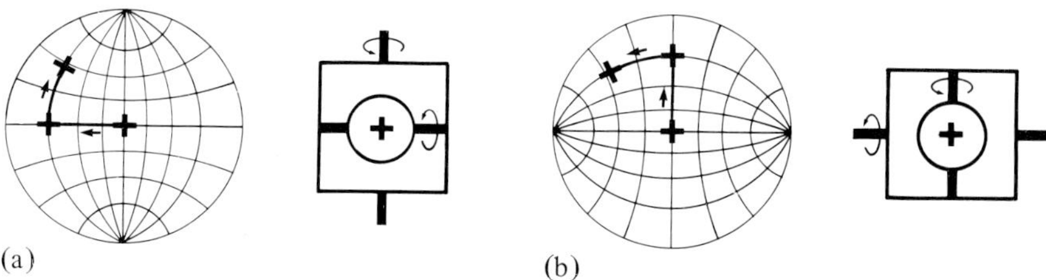

Figure 7.10. Two possible ways of specifying tertiary positions. (a) Fick's system: the horizontal (*longitude*) component is specified first, followed by the vertical (*latitude*) component, as in the equivalent gimbal arrangement on the right. (b) Helmholtz's system: here the *elevation* is specified first, and then the *azimuth*. It can be seen from the final orientation of the cross in the two cases that they lead to different notions of *torsion*.

system (Fick, 1854)—a tertiary position is effectively described in terms of its *latitude* and *longitude*, the longitude corresponding to the horizontal movement, and the latitude to the subsequent movement along a vertical meridian. A set of coordinates for the Fick system is shown in elevation and sterographic projection in figure 7.11. An unsatisfactory feature of this method is its asymmetry with respect to horizontal and vertical. We could have chosen to do it the other way round, taking the vertical component of the rotation before the horizontal. If we do this we obtain a different set of coordinates (Helmholtz's), in which the eye is assumed first to move vertically through an angle of *elevation*, and then to rotate in the plane of regard through an *azimuth* angle (figures 7.10 and 7.11). This gives rise to a set of coordinates at right angles to the first, and is in fact preferable to Fick's system for two reasons. The first (Helmholtz, 1909, § 27) is that the straight-forward position is much less exactly defined in the vertical direction than in the horizontal. If some correction has to be made on this account, in the Helmholtz system only the elevation components of tertiary positions need to be modified (simply by adding to them the actual amount of the error), whereas in the Fick system, such an error will affect both the apparent latitude *and* the apparent longitude, by an amount that is a complicated function of both. The second reason for preferring elevation and azimuth comes from a consideration of binocular movements (Putnam and Quereau, 1951). If both eyes are fixating an object, by definition each fixation line lies in the same plane of regard and so each will have the same elevation component.

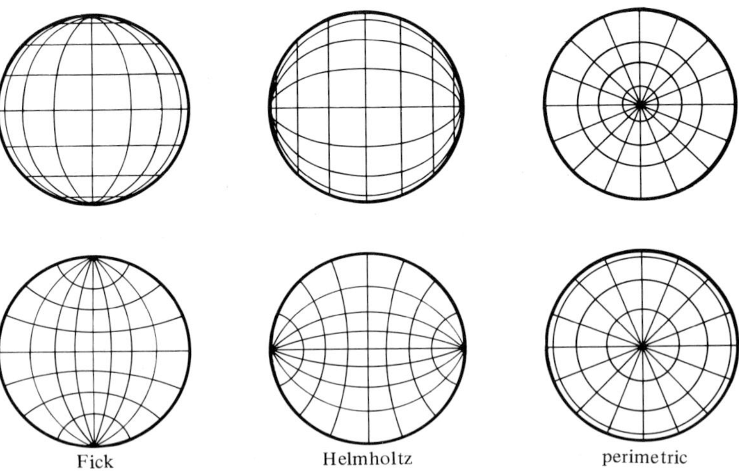

Figure 7.11. Three coordinate systems in elevation (above) and stereographic projection (below). The first two are those of Fick and Helmholtz; the last is the perimetric system which specifies eye positions in terms of meridional angle and eccentricity.

The angle of vergence will then be given by the difference of their azimuths. But in Fick's system, each eye will have different latitude components, and the angle of vergence will be an awkward function of both latitude and longitude.

A third possibility, which removes the asymmetry implicit in both the foregoing systems, is to use, in effect, axes that are fixed in the head, and that specify the angular distance of a tertiary position from the primary position (its *eccentricity*), and the angle that a great circle going through both the tertiary position and the primary position makes with the horizontal (the *meridional* angle). Its elevation and stereographic projection are also shown in figure 7.11. Although, as we shall see in the next section, this system corresponds more closely than the other two with the way in which eye movements are actually elaborated, it is inferior to Helmholtz's in dealing with binocular movements and in practice is hardly used except in perimetry and similar work where the main interest is in the visual rather than the oculomotor system.

7.3.2 Torsion and Listing's Law

Exactly the same problem of deciding whether to use axes fixed in the head, or axes that move with the eye, arises in the case of torsion, and a lack of clarity in this matter has been the cause of endless confusion. Consider what happens to the stereographic projection of a cross on the anterior pole as the eye moves to a tertiary position by successive pure horizontal and vertical movements, as in Fick's system (figure 7.10). After the horizontal component, the arms of the cross remain of course horizontal, and they are still horizontal after the vertical component. But, if we take the horizontal and vertical components in the opposite order, the result is quite different (figure 7.10). Again, after the first (vertical) movement, the arms are horizontal: but the second component, the rotation in the plane of regard, shifts them out of the horizontal. (To see that this is so, consider what would happen if the second component were a rotation of 90°: the eye will then find itself in the same position as if it had simply moved 90° in the horizontal direction from the primary position, but the cross will be inclined at an angle to the horizontal given by the original angle of elevation.) Thus the orientation of the cross clearly depends not only on the final position of the eye at the end of the complete movement, but also on the route by which it got there.

Since the final position of the eye is the same in each case, it is reasonable to suppose that this difference in orientation is due to some kind of torsion. But in which case has the torsion occurred? Or have *both* manoeuvres generated torsional components that are different relative to some other absolute standard? It is at this point that the confusion starts. Everyone is agreed that torsion must be measured around an axis that moves with the eye, namely, the anterior–posterior axis. What is in doubt is whether the reference direction for measuring

rotation about a single axis in a plane fixed in the orbit perpendicular to the fixation line in the primary position (the equatorial plane, or *Listing's plane*). Such movements plot as straight lines through the origin in stereographic projection (figure 7.13), resulting in the corneal cross retaining its orientation in the projection, wherever it is situated: an added benefit of this method of representing eye movements. Comparison of the upright of the cross with the vertical meridians of the Fick coordinates enables one to read off at any position what the magnitude of the tilt will be.

The expected degree of tilt can be calculated from Listing's Law without much difficulty (Helmholtz, 1909; Lamb, 1919; Westheimer, 1957). This is done most easily if the eye position is specified by means of the third, perimetric, system of coordinates, which in any case corresponds closely with Listing's notion of rotation about a single axis in Listing's plane, whose direction is variable: the meridional angle corresponds to the direction of this axis, and the eccentricity to the extent of the rotation itself. The problem is tiresome to solve by conventional methods—even Helmholtz takes three pages over it—but it lends itself to the use of quaternions, rotational operators that embody in themselves the mutual interactions between rotations about different axes that generate relationships like Listing's Law. For an eccentric angle w, and a meridional angle c, the calculated tilt from the vertical is given by

$$\tan^{-1}\frac{\tan c\,(1-\cos w)}{1+\tan^2 c\cos^2 w}\,.$$

This function is plotted in figure 7.14: it can be seen that quite substantial degrees of tilt are produced by comparatively modest eccentricities of gaze in tertiary positions: for example, if c and w are both 35°, the resultant torsion amounts to more than 5°.

Listing's Law is strictly only applicable when the head is erect and stationary, under monocular conditions with the gaze at infinity, and even under these conditions is probably not accurate to more than a degree or so. If a near, central, object is viewed binocularly, it is clear that Listing's Law demands torsions in opposite senses in the two eyes, which ought to

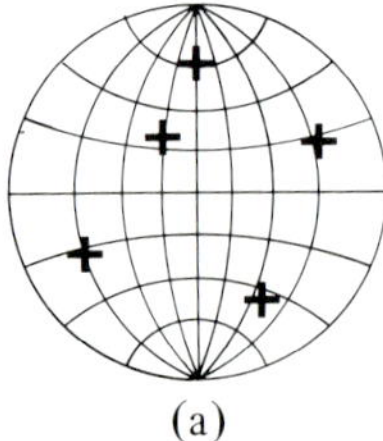
(a)

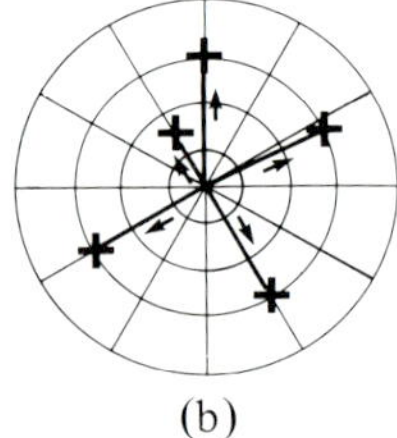
(b)

Figure 7.13. Listing's Law in stereographic projection: (a) torsion of the eye in tertiary positions is such that the eye retains its primary orientation in stereographic projection; this amounts to saying that it is as if the eye moved directly from primary to tertiary positions with no torsion at all, relative to axes moving with the eye (b).

result in a rotational disparity in the two retinal images. In practice, such a disparity is not readily apparent (Hering, 1868; Allen, 1954; and others), but it is not clear whether this is due to compensatory ocular counter-rolling, or to a mechanism of visual fusion. The question of whether cyclofusion is an oculomotor or a perceptual mechanism has already been discussed (section 5.1.1): we saw that recent investigations (Kertesz and Jones, 1970) lend support to the idea that cyclofusion is not accomplished by cyclotorsion, so that Listing's Law may not give rise to apparent binocular disparities. Both Helmholtz (1909) and Hering (1868) suggest reasons why it might be desirable for the eye to obey Listing's Law rather than some other torsional rule (as, for example, keeping verticals in the outside world always vertical on the retina). Of the two, Hering's argument is perhaps more compelling: a consequence of Listing's Law is that of the self-congruence of retinal images of oblique lines in the outside world as the gaze travels along them. In other words, no matter what point on a straight line is fixated, the line's image will always fall along the same set of retinal receptors (and hence presumably trigger the same set of cortical line-orientation detectors). For further discussion of this point see Westheimer and Blair (1972b).

As Nakayama has emphasised, from the point of view of the oculomotor control system the effect of Listing's Law is to reduce the number of degrees of freedom for each eye from three to two—as in the 'golf ball' of certain typewriters, where each letter is constrained to be vertical when it hits the page. But unlike the typewriter, the eye is not *mechanically* constrained to do this and it is clear that Listing's Law is the result of an active neural mechanism—one that is lost, for example in sleep (Nakayama, 1975).

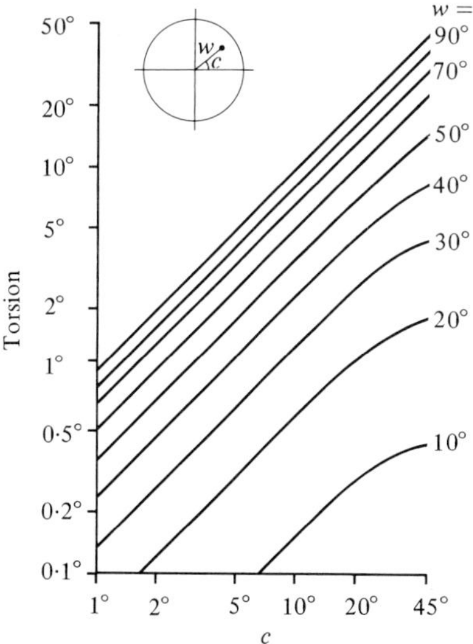

Figure 7.14. Calculated Listing torsion of the eye for different meridional angles (c) and eccentricities (w). Ordinate and abscissa are both logarithmic.

7.4 The action of the eye muscles

So far we have treated rotations of the globe in a rather abstract way, defining axes of reference to suit our analytical treatment. But the fact remains that eye movements only occur because of changes in the tensions exerted by the six extraocular muscles, and from the point of view of the system that controls the position of the eye, the rotational axes defined by the actions of these muscles are perhaps rather more relevant. We need to know not only what directions these muscular axes assume when the eye is in the primary position, but also whether, and to what degree, they move when the eye itself moves. So while the simplest description of rotations of the eye is in terms of rotations about a varying axis in Listing's plane, it is not at all clear that such a description will suit the muscles as well.

7.4.1 Gross anatomy of the eye muscles

There are three pairs of extraocular muscles to each eye: the medial and lateral recti, the superior and inferior recti, and the superior and inferior obliques (figure 7.15). All of them except the obliques originate in a common ring-shaped tendon at the apex of the orbit (round the optic foramen) called the annulus of Zinn, as does a further muscle—the levator palpebrae—that raises the upper eyelid, and will not be further discussed. These muscles terminate in an orderly fashion on the annulus, and diverge as they extend forward in the orbit to insert on the globe. In the case of the four recti, their course is uneventful and they pass through Tenon's capsule to join the sclera as tendons with insertion widths of around 10 mm, terminating some 5–7 mm from the border between the cornea and the sclera. In the case of the lateral and medial recti, the lines of insertion are both approximately centred on a horizontal plane passing through the

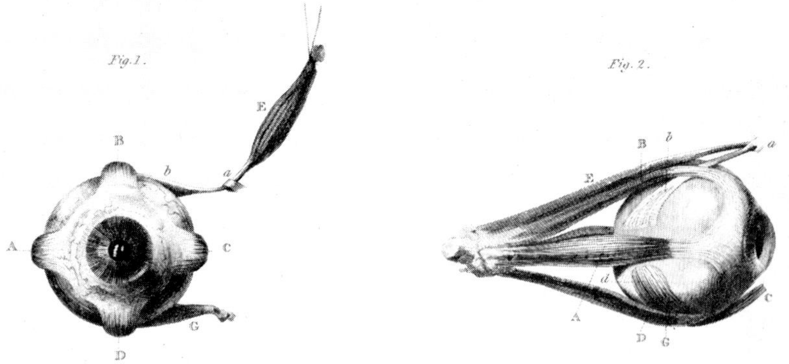

Figure 7.15. The extraocular muscles of the human eye. A, lateral rectus; B superior rectus; C, medial rectus; D, inferior rectus; E, superior oblique, acting via the trochlea, *a*; G, inferior oblique (from Bell, 1823).

notional centre of rotation, so that the effect of their contractions is of almost pure horizontal rotation. But in the case of the superior and inferior recti, the lines of insertion are displaced in a medial direction: figure 7.16 shows a stereographic projection of the lines of insertion of the four rectus muscles. Consequently the lines of actions of the superior and inferior obliques are inclined—by about 23°—to the visual axis in the primary position (figure 7.17).

The course of the superior oblique is quite different: from the annulus of Zinn it runs to a loop of cartilage—the trochlea—through which the tendon of the muscle is inserted; the tendon then changes its direction (the trochlea thus acting as a pulley), passing laterally under the superior rectus to insert along an arc some 10 mm in length, running obliquely to the posterior-anterior direction, with the inner end close to the sagittal vertical meridian. Its line of action (from the insertion to the trochlea, not the annulus of Zinn) thus forms a large angle—around 53°—with the primary direction (figure 7.17). The inferior oblique does not originate in the annulus of Zinn at all, but rather in the orbital surface of the superior maxilla, near the opening of the nasolacrimal duct. Like the superior oblique, it passes laterally and posteriorly, over the inferior rectus but under the lateral rectus, inserting in an oblique line in the inferior lateral surface of the globe. The posterior end of the insertion is only a few millimetres from the optic nerve, rather further back than that of the superior oblique: thus the axes of rotation associated with these two muscles

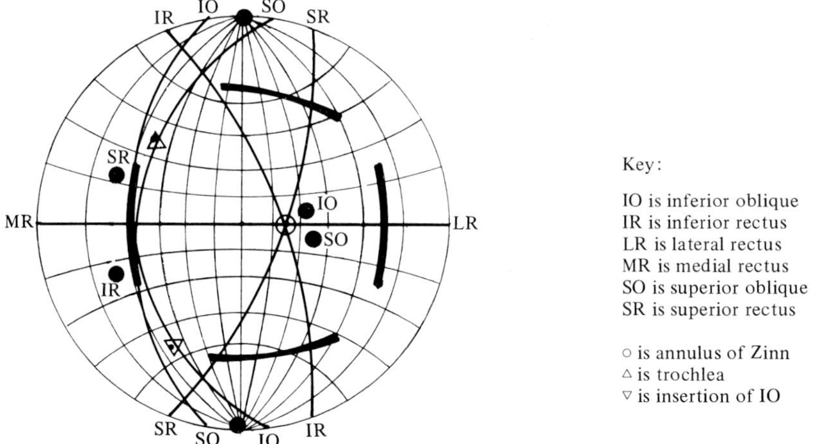

Figure 7.16. Geometry of the eye muscles in stereographic projection. The thick lines show the lines of insertion of the rectus muscles; the open symbols show the central terminations of the muscles, as shown in the key. The filled circles show the axes of rotation from the primary position for each muscle acting independently, and the thin lines show corresponding planes of action. In the case of features such as the Annulus of Zinn that lie behind Listing's plane, it is their antipodes that are represented (data from Helmholtz, 1909; Duke-Elder and Wybar, 1973).

are not exactly coincident. Alpern (1969a) summarises measurements of human extraocular muscles and their insertions, and should be consulted for a more complete account than space allows here.

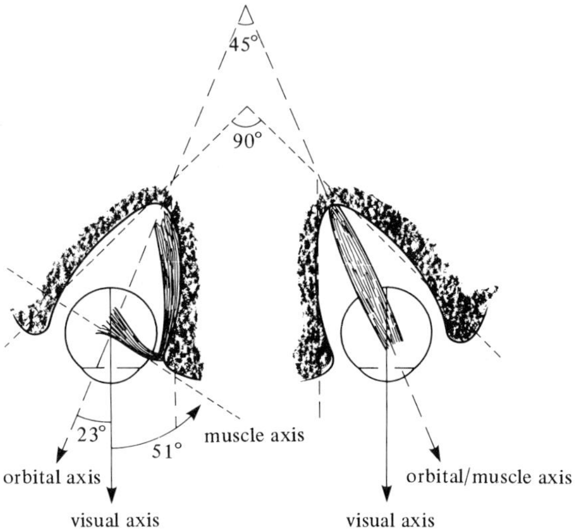

Figure 7.17. Some of the angular relationships between the visual axes, the superior rectus and oblique, and the orbit.

7.4.2 Lines of action of the muscles

If we suppose that the muscles are free to slip over the globe beyond their insertions [an assumption that cannot be true for deviations vary far from the primary position (Robinson, 1975a)], under tension they will take up positions on the globe corresponding to arcs of great circles—since such arcs represent minimum distances between points on the surface—in a plane called the *plane of action* that is defined by the two ends of the muscle and the centre of rotation. Corresponding to this plane of action is an axis, perpendicular to it and passing through the centre of rotation. Figure 7.16 shows the planes of action and axes of rotation of the six muscles with the eye in the primary position. The actions of the various muscles will be further complicated if the globe starts from any position other than the primary, because of the resultant changes in the positions of insertion: but for the moment this problem will be ignored.

The horizontal movement produced by the lateral rectus is directed temporally (*abduction*: hence its alternative name of *abducens*), while that of the medial rectus is nasal (*adduction*): the main actions of the superior and inferior obliques are respectively *elevation* and *depression*; and those of the superior and inferior obliques, *intorsion* and *extorsion*. But the superior and inferior obliques also produce a slight degree of adduction, together with an intorsional component from the superior rectus, and an extorsional component from the inferior rectus. These effects can be deduced from figure 7.16, but are probably more easily appreciated in the drawings of figure 7.18. Activation of the vertical recti is thus associated with rotation about all three axes, although of course the vertical effects predominate. In the same way, the superior oblique has a secondary component of depression, while the inferior oblique's is of elevation, and both cause secondary abduction (because their insertions lie posterior to the centre of rotation).

These various actions can be summarised conveniently on Hering's classical diagram (figure 7.19) (Hering, 1879a), which shows the locus of

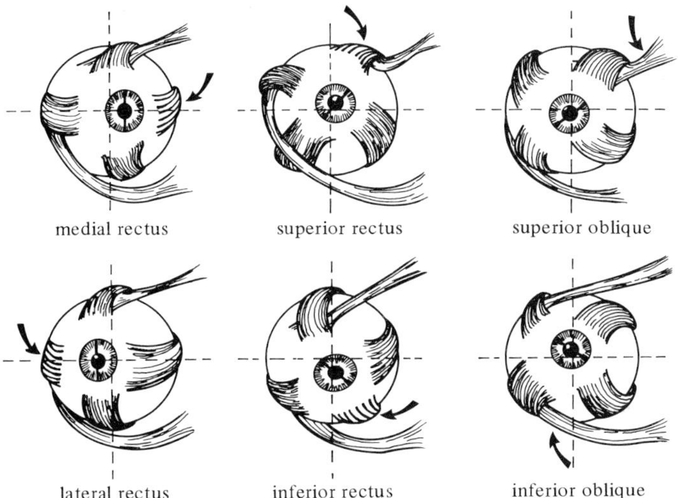

Figure 7.18. Schematic pictorial representation of the action of each extraocular muscle acting on its own (after Moses, 1970).

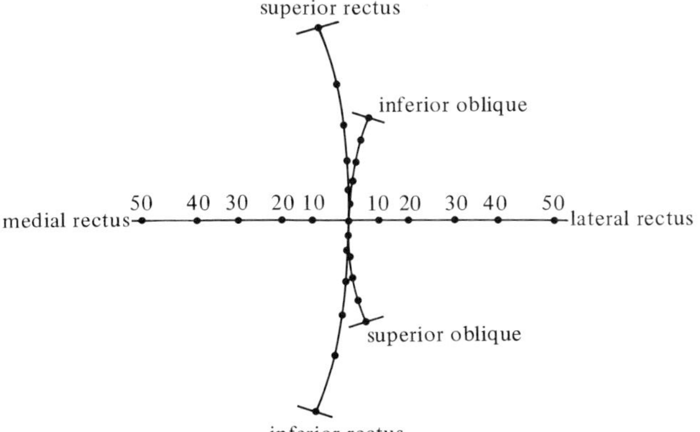

Figure 7.19. Hering's representation of the individual effect of different degrees of activity in each muscle on the projection of the line of sight on a frontal plane: the orthogonal lines indicate associated torsion.

view, this is much more interesting, and enables better diagnoses to be made of paralysis and other disorders of individual muscles, from examination of the resulting squints. It turns out, for example, that contrary to the classical ideas presented earlier in this section, the superior rectus does *not* have more innervation on looking up from abduction rather than from adduction, because much of the innervational effort is used in balancing the effects of other muscles, rather than causing direct changes in length. There is no doubt that this work will form the foundation for a much more precise understanding of the genesis of squints.

7.4.3 Actual muscular cooperation

It is important to emphasise that the curves described in the last section are essentially theoretical, and based only on measurements of the geometrical relations between the centre of rotation and the insertions of the muscles, and that there are many complicating factors that may lead to discrepancies between theory and observation. Perhaps the most serious source of error is the assumption that the muscles act at a point on the globe: in fact, as we have seen, all the muscles have very long lines of insertion, so that one cannot dismiss the possibility that a muscle might be able to alter its effective point of action on the globe by activating some fibres rather than others. Consider for example the fibres of the lateral rectus when the eye is elevated: because of the resultant rotation of the line of insertion, the lower fibres in the muscle are likely to be stretched more than the upper and thus may well exert more tension. This would in effect lower the point of action, and correspondingly reduce the anticipated degree of secondary elevation: no compensation of this type will work in the case of torsional movements, however.

Certainly the measured mechanical properties of the eye muscles are of the right magnitude: their approximately linear length–tension relations (see below, section 7.5.3) mean that the expected shift of the virtual point of insertion is linearly related to rotation, if small. The deviation is in fact given by $r^2\theta/3k$, where r is half the length of the insertion, θ is the angle of rotation, and k is the extension of the muscle that is necessary to double its tension in the primary position: it has the value of approximately 3 mm in man (Collins et al, 1975), and r is also some 5 mm, as we have seen. For this mechanism to correct perfectly for elevation, the quantity $r^2/3k$ should be equal to the anterior displacement of the insertion relative to the centre of rotation: in fact the former comes to nearly 3 mm, while the latter is rather more than 5 mm (von Kries, note to Helmholtz, 1909, § 27). Thus, although the proposed mechanism is not able to compensate entirely for the effect of elevation, it is able to reduce the secondary effects by more than half. Evidence that this sort of effect does actually occur in practice has been presented by Jampel (1966) for the superior oblique in the monkey, by recording the rotation arising from electrical stimulation of the trochlear nerve for different horizontal deviations. He found that the axis of the rotation changed very little despite the horizontal movements [although Tokumasu et al (1965) came to the opposite conclusion—in the cat—but with rather less precise measurements].

It is a pity that more work has not been done along these lines, for it has important theoretical implications with regard to the eye movement control system. If it were true that the effect of any one eye muscle depended markedly on the degree of excitation of every single one of its companions, it is clear that the complexity of the task of the peripheral oculomotor system would be enormously increased (Robinson, 1968b). In the case of the vestibulo-ocular reflex, for example, not only would each canal have to be connected to every muscle, but the degree of activity in each path would have to be modified in response to that of the others. If, on the other hand, the muscular axes were fixed—albeit not in purely horizontal, vertical, and torsional axes—commands for rotation about the three muscular axes could be processed in separate and independent channels (figure 7.23). All the same, one should not minimise the potential of the central nervous system for performing complicated calculations: one need only think of the intricate problem in three-dimensional ballistics that is solved every time one throws something into a wastepaper basket!

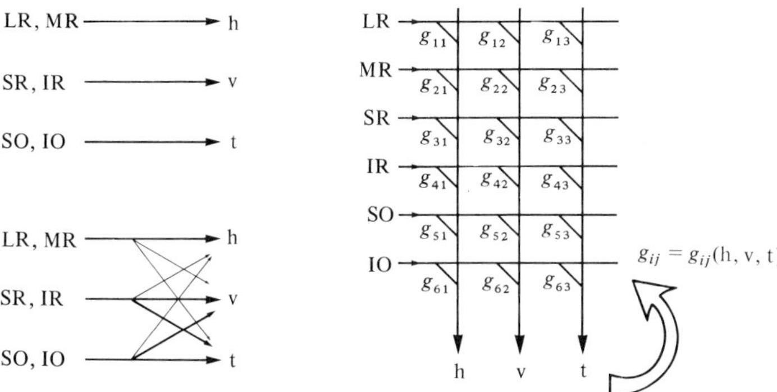

Figure 7.23. Schemes of cooperation between the eye muscles. Top left, an over-simple arrangement in which pairs of muscles have a fixed contribution to one of each of the horizontal (h), vertical (v) or torsional (t) components of movement. Below, an improved scheme in which each muscle contributes something to each component of motion, but the contributions are still fixed. Right, a scheme that is nearer reality: each muscle contributes to each component of movement with a weighting *g* that is not fixed, but a function of the position of the eye at any moment (bottom right).

7.5 Kinetic properties of the eye

So far we have considered only what might be called the *kinematic* properties of the globe—the positions it will assume under different degrees of muscular action when sufficient time is allowed for all transient effects to settle down. But in practice this ideal state of affairs is seldom achieved—if only because of the incessant micromovements—and to describe completely the behaviour of the eye during rapid changes in muscular activity (as for example in the saccade) we must also take account of its kinetic or dynamic properties. Ideally, we would like to be able, given complete information about the time course of activity in each of the extraocular muscles, to predict the resultant position of the eye at every moment: the techniques of systems analysis provide the methods for doing this. In what follows, an elementary acquaintance with these methods is assumed; those readers who are not already familiar with them may perhaps find the elementary introduction in appendix 2 of some use.

7.5.1 The basic mechanical model

Analysis of the mechanical properties of the eye is greatly simplified if only one axis of rotation is considered at a time: it is then a simple matter to calculate complex rotations involving all three axes, with the use of no new mechanical principles beyond the kinematic properties already discussed. Because they produce nearly pure horizontal rotations, and because horizontal rotations are on the whole easier to measure than those in other meridians, the medial and lateral recti have been studied far more often than any of the other muscles.

Before discussing the results of actual experimental determinations of the mechanical properties, it is perhaps worthwhile first to consider the basic skeleton of a model representing the mechanical interactions between the eye, the orbit and the eye muscles. Now, of all the moving elements in the orbit, only the globe itself performs rotations: indeed it cannot execute any other motion at all, if we neglect the small movements of the centre of rotation. So the mass of the eye will only enter into our calculations in the guise of its moment of inertia about the centre of rotation. Now if, as is the case with the eye, we have a spherical body free to rotate only about its centre and acted on by a force F tangential to the surface (figure 7.24), then the couple exerted by the force and the reaction at the centre of rotation must equal the product of the angular

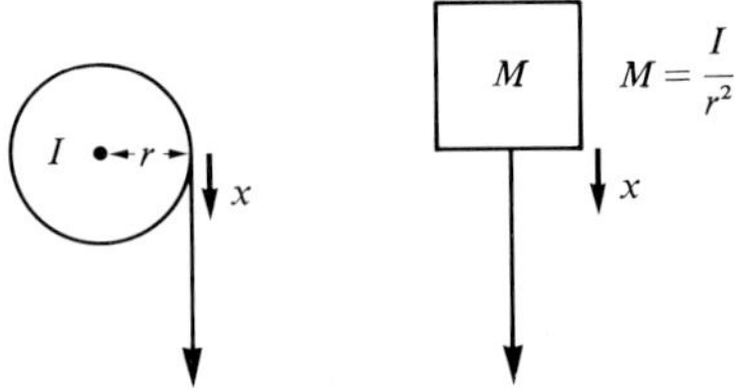

Figure 7.24. The movement of the eye in response to forces acting only at its surface is as if its moment of inertia I were considered to be a mass (I/r^2) concentrated at its surface. In this way the mechanics of eye rotations can be treated as if they consisted of linear displacements of this equivalent mass (right).

acceleration $D^2\theta$ and the moment of inertia I:

$$Fr = ID^2\theta,$$

where r is the radius of the sphere. If we rewrite this equation in terms of the displacement x of the surface, rather than in terms of the angle of rotation ($x = r\theta$), we obtain:

$$F = \frac{I}{r^2} D^2 x,$$

which is identical in form to the equation,

$$F = MD^2 x,$$

describing the force–displacement relation for a simple mass moving in a straight line. Since all the other forces apart from inertia act on the surface of the globe, this means that we can reduce the mechanical system of the globe and muscles to a system of colinear motion by treating the globe as a simple inertial element of mass I/r^2 (figure 7.24).

These other forces concern the way in which the globe is mechanically coupled to the orbit. It is helpful to divide this coupling into two classes: those forces that are transmitted through the muscles, and whose properties may be expected to vary under different conditions of muscular activation, and those that are not (figure 7.25). In the second class come frictional forces between the eye and the orbit, and elastic coupling (for example through the optic nerve and its surrounding vessels), and may be represented by the familiar spring and dash-pot symbols as in figure 7.26. Parallel

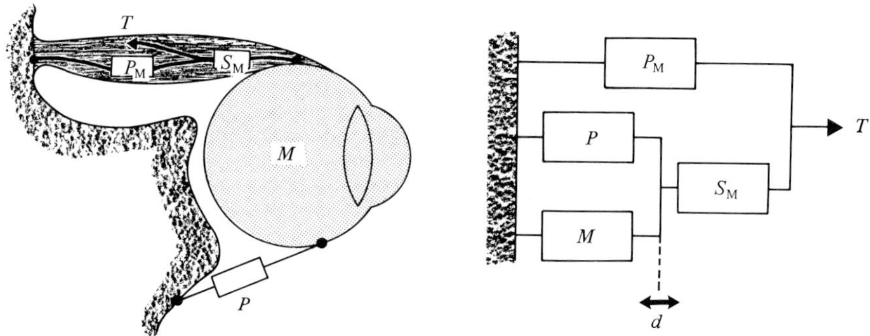

Figure 7.25. The mechanical elements of the globe: general considerations. Left, the mechanical elements consist of those that are embodied in the muscle (S_M and P_M), respectively in series and in parallel with the active tension T which moves the eye), and those whose origin lies outside the muscles, such as the inertia of the globe, M, and the various elastic and frictional forces that couple the globe to the orbit in a passive manner (P). Right, the formal network corresponding to this arrangment is shown: the input is the force T, the output is the resultant displacement d. In practice, of course, the mechanical properties of more than one muscle must be considered.

combinations of viscous and elastic elements—together forming a Voigt element—are often used in series combinations to represent the mechanical properties of tissues (for example Buchthal and Kaiser, 1951; Pringle 1960): we shall see later that there is direct experimental evidence that they are equally appropriate in this case. These mechanical elements not associated with the muscles themselves are sometimes collectively known as the *passive* or *globe-restraining* elements. The inertia of the globe does not strictly fall into this category, because it is the globe's rotation relative to an inertial frame of reference fixed in space rather than in the orbit that is relevant: the distinction might become important when considering movements of the eye in response to head movements, when the globe's inertia would, in principle, actually *help* the eye to respond efficiently. But it turns out that the inertia of the eye is only of consequence at frequencies very much higher than those involved in the vestibulo-ocular reflex, and so the distinction is perhaps somewhat academic.

The mechanical properties of the muscles are likely to be complex, if only because they are in part dependent on the degree of overlap of the sliding filaments at different degrees of contraction. At the very least they will contain a relatively fixed series element representing in part the tendons and other tissues transmitting force from the sliding filaments to the scleral insertions, and viscous and elastic elements in parallel with the active contractile process. The properties of these elements cannot easily be disentangled from the length dependency of the contractile process itself, and the normal procedure is to pretend that the parallel elastic element has properties that depend only on the degree of extension of the muscle, and not on its activation. Together with the series elastic element, they form the *passive elasticity* of the muscle: the total muscle tension at any moment is the sum of the *passive tension* generated by the elastic

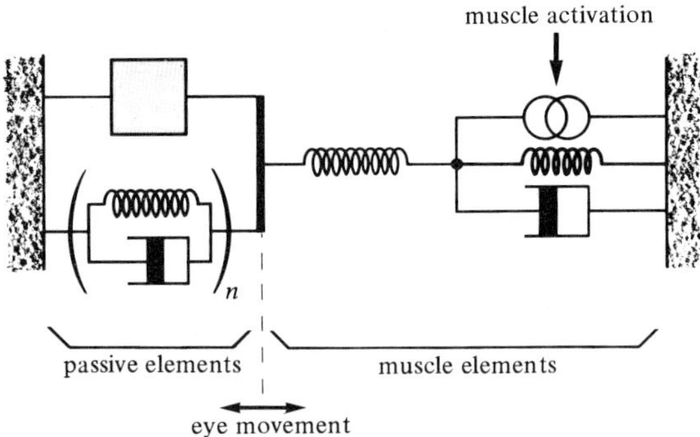

Figure 7.26. Schematic representation of the mechanical elements of the eye after transformation into a system of linear displacements as in figure 7.24, and showing only one of the extraocular muscles. On the left, the passive components: mass (inertia) in parallel with a viscoelastic element (or a series of them) to represent the globe-restraining tissues. On the right, the active element of the muscle (here considered as essentially a force generator), with a parallel viscoelastic element and series elastic element.

and viscous elements—the contribution of the latter being nil when the muscle is at rest—and the added *active tension* produced by the contractile mechanism when it is activated. Some authors (for example Collins et al, 1969) prefer to think of the contractile elements as primarily length changers rather than tension generators. The known internal mechanical properties of muscle fibres (see Hill, 1970, for a review) suggest that both views are considerably oversimplified: but the first approach corresponds more simply with experimental procedures. It is clear from inspection of the resultant mechanical model (figure 7.26) that the system as a whole is likely to be at least second order in form (because of the presence of all three types of mechanical element), and that we may therefore expect it to exhibit some kind of resonant behaviour unless the contribution of the viscous (damping) components is sufficiently great: in other words, only *quantitative* consideration of the various components will enable us to determine even the *classes* of behaviour that the system will show.

7.5.2 Experimental measurements of mechanical properties

The mechanics of the eye have been investigated in two quite distinct ways. In the first, the subject tries to keep his eye fixed in direction while the experimenter measures the force then necessary to deflect it through a given angle, or at a given angular velocity. The second type of procedure is to record the movement of the eye as a function of time during some standard pattern of behaviour (for example a saccade, or during pursuit or vergence movements), and then to measure the force required to keep the eye stationary—that is, the isometric tension—during the same pattern of movement. Alternatively, the eye may be loaded or impeded in other ways, and the influence that this has on its trajectory during the same movement observed. A possible criticism of both procedures is that they both assume that the degree of excitation of the muscles is not affected by the fact that actual position of the eye does not correspond with where the oculomotor system intends it to be: one might expect, for example, that some sort of feedback system might use the error signal derived from this discrepancy to modify the activity in the oculomotor nerves to correct it. Such a response would not be distinguishable, on these experiments alone, from the purely mechanical properties of the muscle. But we shall see later that there is an abundance of evidence that, despite the presence (in most species) of receptors in the muscle capable of providing this kind of feedback information, in practice, proprioceptive error signals are *not* used in this way, and that nothing equivalent to the stretch reflex of skeletal muscles can be elicited from extraocular muscle. However, one cannot rule out longer-term effects that might arise from parametric feedback, or from the subject's knowledge of whether the eye is free or hindered on any particular occasion, and well-designed experiments arrange for random intermingling of test and control trials, unknown to the subject.

In principle, of course, if one knew *a priori* what the pattern of muscle tension was during some standard response like a saccade, one could tell from the time course of the movement what the mechanical properties of the system were. Westheimer's (1954a) pioneering observations were of this type. He observed the time course of the deviation of the eye during a lateral saccade; but rather than measure the associated muscle tension, he simply assumed it to increase in a step-like manner from its initial to its final value. Thus the observed motion was taken to represent the step response of the mechanics; arguing, along the lines already presented, that the mechanics were likely to correspond in simplified form to a second-order system, he deduced from the step response what the values of the two describing parameters would be. Because his recordings happened to show a pronounced overshoot, he calculated that the whole system was underdamped, with a resonant frequency around 20 Hz. As will be seen later, it is now clear that muscle tension does *not* increase in a step during a saccade, and we have already seen that overshoot is a somewhat variable phenomenon by no means universally present in saccades. Nevertheless, Westheimer's preliminary work in this field showed how powerful the methods of systems analysis could be in handling the problem of eye dynamics, and pointed the way to fuller analyses, described in the three sections that follow. It is convenient to start with experiments in the first of our two categories, that is, where the subject attempts to hold the eye still.

7.5.3 Experiments with static applied disturbances

One of the simplest experiments on the mechanical properties of the eye is to measure the steady force required to rotate the globe to various fixed lateral deviations, when the subject tries to keep it still and in a fixed position. If sufficient time is allowed for the system to come to equilibrium, the observed force–angle (or force–muscle-length) relationship reflects only the elastic components, with no contribution either from inertia or from viscosity. Figure 7.27 shows the result of such an experiment in the anaesthetised cat (Collins, 1971), before and after detachment of the

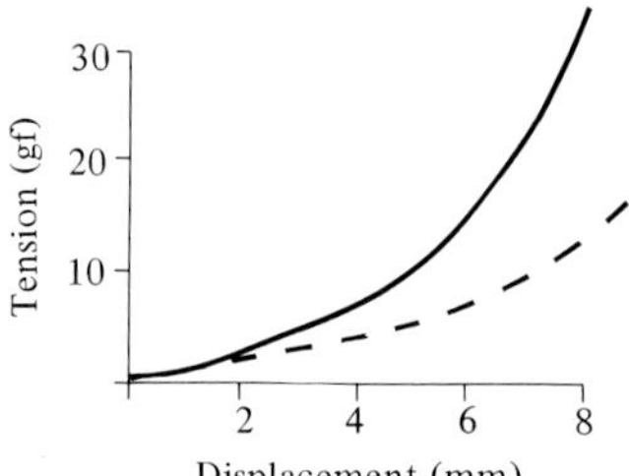

Figure 7.27. Tension–displacement curves for an anaesthetised cat eye in the horizontal plane. Solid line, with the muscles intact; broken line, with horizontal muscles removed, revealing the contribution of the passive globe-restraining tissues (after Collines, 1971).

horizontal recti from the globe. The difference between the two curves thus represents the contribution of the elastic elements of the muscles (presumably the passive elastic elements, if there is no neural activation of the muscles). It can be seen that in both cases the relationship is noticeably nonlinear beyond about 25° of deviation, with progressively increasing stiffness, and that in the approximately linear region the combined stiffness is some 0·3 gf deg^{-1} (1 gf = 9·81 x 10^{-3} N).

Further information can be found by finding the length–tension relation for individual muscles under different degrees of neural activation. This can be done either by stimulating the appropriate motor nerve at different rates (for example Robinson, 1964, in the cat), or in man by fixating a moveable target with the unoperated eye, and relying on the accuracy of Hering's Law of equal innervation (for example Robinson et al, 1969; Collins et al, 1975). In spite of the species difference, and the slightly different procedure, the sets of results are qualitatively in good agreement (figure 7.28), and show that increasing activation shifts the curves horizontally in a roughly parallel manner, as would be expected if the main source of the elastic nonlinearity were in the parallel element of the muscle (P_M, figure 7.25) rather than in the series element (Collins, 1975). From the human length–tension curves we can read off the lateral

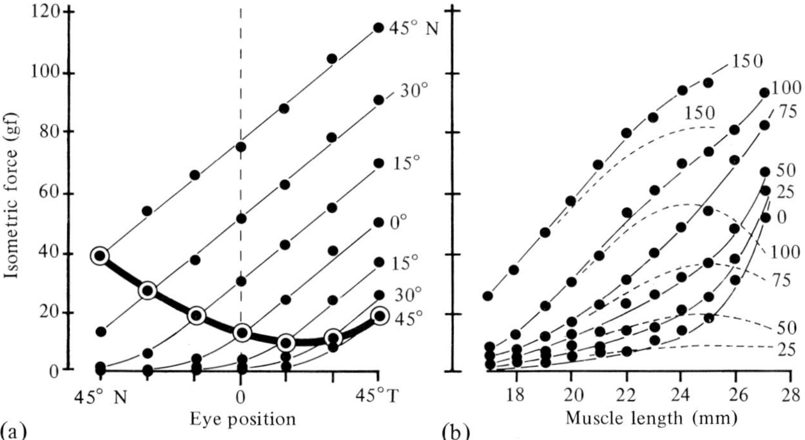

Figure 7.28. Length–tension relationships for extraocular muscle, at different degrees of activation: (a) in conscious human subjects, and (b) in an anaesthetised cat. In (a) the different degrees of innervation were achieved by having the subject fixate at different angles in the nasal (N) and temporal (T) directions: the thick line joins points that correspond with the deviations that would thus result under natural conditions. The data are the means of observations on four subjects, partly from lateral rectus and partly from medial rectus. In (b) the lateral rectus was stimulated electrically at the different rates shown: the curve for zero stimulation represents the passive mechanical properties, and if it is subtracted from each of the others, the resultant curves (dashed) can be said to represent the active tension added by the different degrees of stimulation (data of Collins et al, 1975; Robinson, 1964).

rectus tension used to hold the eye at any particular deviation [the thick line in figure 7.28(a)]: the result is a roughly parabolic curve with a minimum at about 15° in the medial direction. The relationship has recently been confirmed by the implantation of miniature strain gauges in series with the eye muscles of human subjects (Collins et al, 1975). The linearity of these length–tension curves is the result of a happy cooperation between the passive and active elastic properties of the muscle. The former are of course represented by the relationship for zero activation (in the case of the cat), and by subtraction of this passive curve from the others, the active contribution for different stimulation frequencies can be found, resulting in the dashed curves of figure 7.28(b) (Robinson et al, 1969). These curves rise to a maximum and then fall off again at extreme degrees of stretch, in the fashion to be expected of the sliding-filament mechanism: these extreme stretches do not of course represent a situation that could actually occur in real life.

In practice, of course, the lateral rectus does not work on its own but in partnership with the medial rectus. If we assume that this muscle has the same kind of length–tension curves, then we can calculate their joint effect at different deviations of the eye. To do this, we must take the curves in pairs (10° left for the medial rectus with 10° right for the lateral rectus; 15° left and 15° right; and so on), and add their opposed contributions. [Figure 7.29(a) shows the result of this operation for one such pair; figure 7.29(b) for a number of pairs.] It is a property of two

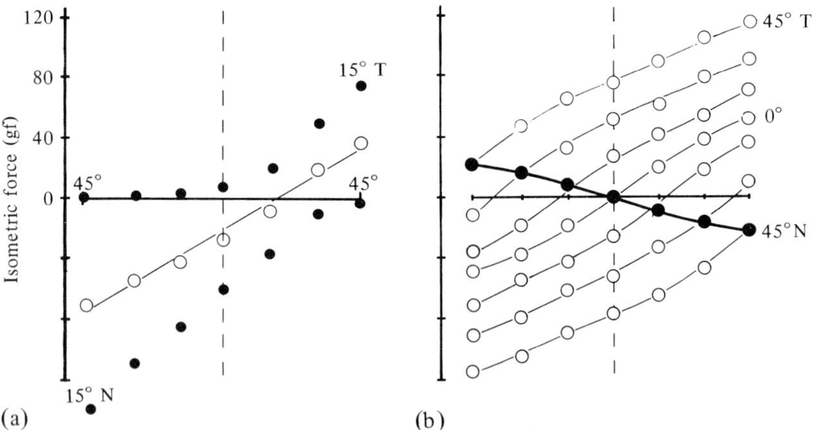

Figure 7.29. Eye deviation and tension under natural conditions: (a) how pairs of data sets from results such as those of figure 7. 28 (a) can be combined to calculate the joint deviation-tension curve for the two rectus muscles acting in cooperation, by simple addition (open circles); (b) a series of such curves is shown for various intended directions of gaze: the thick line joins points for which the intention is realised, and thus must represent the combined elasticity of the elements not forming part of the horizontal recti.

similar curves added together back-to-back in this way that certain kinds of nonlinearities are greatly reduced: more precisely, *even* nonlinearities that are common to both functions cancel each other out to leave a predominantly linear function. (The same principle underlies the linearisation achieved by a 'push–pull' output stage in an amplifier.) Consequently, as can be seen in figure 7.29(b), the functions relating the total muscular force acting on the eye at different deviations form a series of roughly parallel straight lines for different degrees of innervation. In this figure the points representing the natural equilibrium states (that is, for which the actual deviation of the eye matches the desired deviation) are represented by filled circles: these also lie on a straight line, through the origin. This last function must of course represent the passive (globe-restraining) elastic elements, because the sum of the force exerted by the passive elements and the muscle elements must necessarily be zero when the globe is at equilibrium. Near the origin the slope of this line agrees quite well with the results of direct measurement on the cat, but at greater deviations shows a decrease rather than increase in stiffness: the reason for this discrepancy is unclear. Other estimates of the passive stiffness have ranged from 0·5 to 1·5 gf deg^{-1} (Robinson, 1964; 1965; 1966; Childress and Jones, 1967; Collins et al, 1969; Robinson et al, 1969).

7.5.4 Experiments with transient disturbances

Once we have some idea of the static mechanical properties of the eye, observation of the time course of its response to transient disturbances can provide information about the time-dependent mechanical components: inertia and viscosity. If the eyeball were a solid and rigid body, it would be possible simply to calculate its moment of inertia from its distribution of mass: in fact, there is evidence that during rapid eye movements the contents of the eye may lag behind the rest (Hilding, 1954), resulting both in a reduction in the apparent moment of inertia, and also in further complications on account of the nature of the coupling between the globe and its contents. In the dog, Stone et al (1965) found that the measured inertia of the globe was about 10% less than its calculated inertia, possibly for this reason: Robinson (1964) calculates a value of about 4 gf cm^2 for the human eye, and applies a 50% correction for the same reason. Converting this into an equivalent mass (see section 7.5.1) gives a value of about 1·4 gf, since the radius of the human eye is some 12 mm. It turns out, as we shall see, that at moderate frequencies the moment of inertia of the eye plays little part in determining its mechanical properties, and that its precise evaluation is probably not important.

If the eye is deviated to one side by a steady tension, and the tension is suddenly removed, the resulting time course of the eye's movement represents the step response of the passive mechanical elements (Robinson, 1964; Childress and Jones, 1967). Such responses show at least two components: a fast phase lasting some 10–20 ms, and a much slower component which may take nearly a second to reach completion (figure 7.30). However, one cannot immediately assign these two components to particular elements in the basic mechanical model of figure 7.26. One might take the fast component to represent the shortening of the series muscle element, and the slow to represent equilibration of the globe restoring forces against viscous forces in the orbit (Childress and Jones, 1967). But equally, it might be that one cannot adequately describe the globe restraining tissues with only one Voigt element, and that the fast and slow components represent two separate fast and slow viscoelastic elements connected in series. By repeating the experiment with removal of the muscle attachments, one can show that the latter is the true explanation, and that the time constants are (for the cat) about 10 and 800 ms (Collins, 1971); indeed Childress and Jones's own experiments showed that the fast component remained after retrobulbar anaesthesia. Robinson's (1964; 1965) investigations in man are not precisely comparable as to their conclusions because he does not distinguish between the elastic components in the muscles and those outside; he finds it necessary to describe their lumped mechanics as consisting of three Voigt elements in series, having time constants of 8, 285, and 500 ms.

It is perhaps worth emphasising at this point that there are any number of possible ways in which one can represent the various mechanical elements that make up the system (see for example Thomas, 1967); *all* are wrong, to the extent that the real system is continuous and not lumped. Which one is chosen depends on the taste and expectation of the experimenter: since investigators tend to adjust their models' parameters empirically by matching the model's performance with that of the actual system, these variations are likely to give rise to apparent quantitative discrepancies between one model and another. But there is no substantial disagreement about the facts that these models are meant to explain.

A complicating factor in these procedures is that any nonlinearities, either of viscosity or elasticity, will tend to confuse the results. A better experimental procedure from this point of view is that of Collins (Collins, 1971; Collins et al, 1969), in which the force required to displace the eye

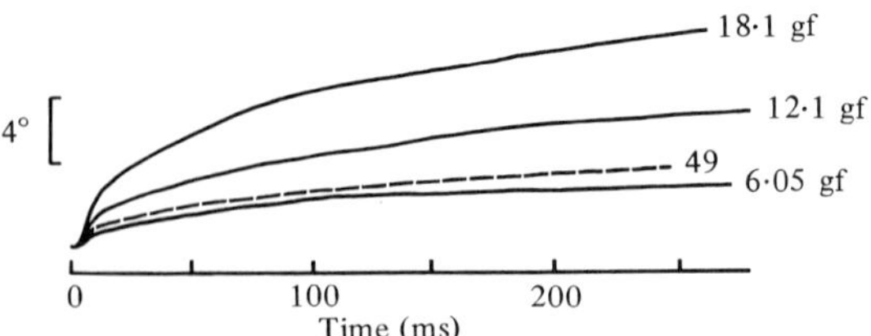

Figure 7.30. Release of the eye from externally applied tension. The tensions used are indicated on the right: the solid lines are from Robinson (1964); the broken line is from Childress and Jones (1967), and was determined under conditions of retrobulbar anaesthesia.

at different velocities is measured. For any particular deviation of the eye, the force required to do this is the sum of that needed to overcome elastic forces (that is, to hold the eye at that position) and that needed to overcome the viscous resistance. Figure 7.31 shows some raw data of this type from isolated cat eye muscle: the lowest curve effectively represents the purely elastic length–tension relationship—with increasing velocities it can be seen that the force required increases. If the lowest curve is subtracted from the others, one can obtain graphs of the type shown in figure 7.32, showing the additional force as a function of rate of stretch, at a number of deviations. The fact that for any deviation the force is proportional to the velocity (within this moderate range) indicates that the viscous properties are Newtonian (that is, constant for different velocities) but depend on the degree of stretch, as would be anticipated from the effect of overlap between the sliding filaments. It turns out that in the cat the nonlinearities in elasticity and viscosity increase in a more or less parallel fashion, so that the associated time constants remain nearly constant. Collins has also recorded the time course of tension in the isolated lateral rectus after a sudden small decrease in length: this technique enables one to distinguish between the series and parallel elements of the muscle, and so complete the viscoelastic description of its behaviour.

It is quite clear from the work of all the authors mentioned so far that these viscous forces are extremely important in determining the behaviour of the eye at natural frequencies, to the extent that the eye is heavily overdamped and incapable of exhibiting much in the way of resonance phenomena; below some 10 Hz it behaves very much like a first-order low-pass filter (see figure 8.16). However, a very different conclusion was reached by Thomas (1967), who preferred to work not with transient

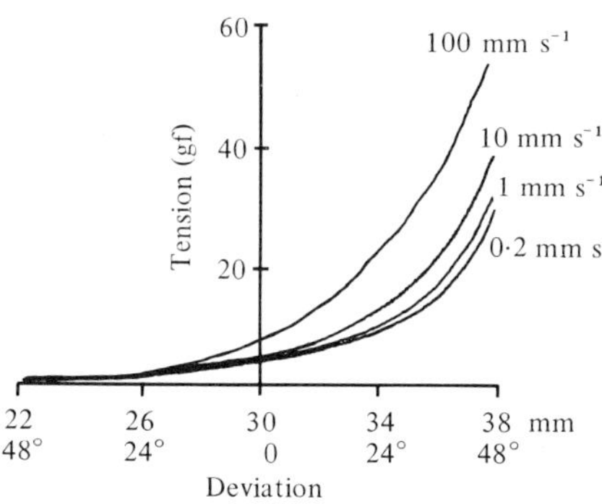

Figure 7.31. Effect of rate of change of stretch: cat passive lateral rectus length–tension curve, traced out at the rates of stretch indicated on the right, showing the additional forces required at higher rates of stretch (after Collins, 1971).

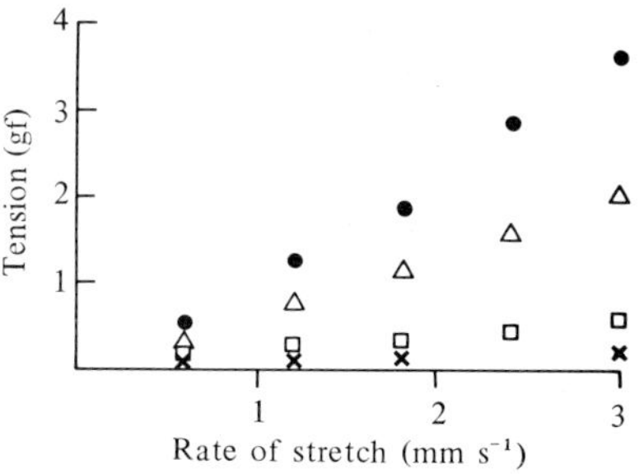

Figure 7.32. Linear relation between velocity and tension at low rates of stretch: added tension required at various muscle lengths (●, 36 mm; △, 34 mm; □, 30 mm; ×, 27 mm) as a function of rate of stretch. This linear relation is not observed at higher velocities (after Collins, 1971).

disturbances, but with external forces that varied sinusoidally. In this technique, a contact lens is fitted with a piezoelectric accelerometer and a small iron armature, and subjected to sinusoidally varying forces by means of a modulated magnetic field. Since the transducer only responds to acceleration, the recording method is only useful in a rather high frequency range, between about 10 and 80 Hz. In the middle of this range, centred on between 30 and 40 Hz, Thomas finds a pronounced peak in the frequency-transfer function relating maximum velocity to applied torque, which leads him to suppose that the system is not overdamped, but resonates with a natural frequency of some 37 Hz for horizontal movements, and rather lower for vertical: similar results have been found in the dog by Stone et al (1965) using a similar technique. However, the method of plotting maximum velocity against frequency tends to exaggerate the importance of such peaks, and if the data is replotted in more conventional form (figure 7.33) it can be seen that the bump on the curve, though undoubtedly present, is far from sharp, and in fact only some 3 dB in height. In agreement with their prediction, but directly contrary to the observations that have already been described (for example figure 7.30) they find that a step of force applied to the eye gives a movement with a distinct transient oscillation.

When one is faced with such a direct conflict of observation, it is hard to be convinced that all possible sources of artefactual resonance have been removed: suspicion falls most heavily on contact lens assemblies with stalks of the type used in these investigations, since Boyce and West (1968) have shown them to be intrinsically prone to resonance in the 50 Hz region upwards. However, it is important not to exaggerate the difference between an 'underdamped' and an 'overdamped' system: the mechanics of the eye are actually of rather higher order than second, and it is quite possible for high-order systems of this type to be 'overdamped' with respect to one particular mode of oscillation, and 'underdamped' with respect to another,

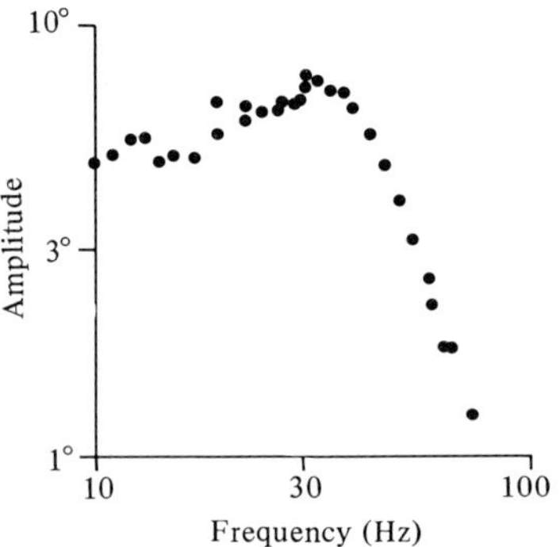

Figure 7.33. Frequency transfer function (gain only) relating eye movement amplitude to peak applied torque, when the latter is sinusoidally modulated, showing the maximum in the region of 40 Hz (data from Thomas, 1967).

particularly when substantial nonlinearities are present. Thus Robinson's (1964) results may be summarised by a transfer function linking external forces to displacement of the form:

$$\frac{0\cdot7(0\cdot22D+1)(0\cdot02D+1)}{(0\cdot3D+1)(0\cdot06D+1)(10^{-5}D^2+0\cdot0042D+1)},$$

which in the high-frequency region investigated by Thomas simplifies to:

$$\frac{0\cdot16}{(10^{-5}D^2+0\cdot0042D+1)},$$

while in the same region, Thomas's transfer function approximates to:

$$\frac{0\cdot16}{(0\cdot7\times10^{-5}D^2+0\cdot0027D+1)},$$

which is not so very different (Robinson, 1968b).

7.5.5 Experiments with stereotyped patterns of activation

Experiments of this type have mainly been carried out by Robinson, initially using saccades as reproducible stereotype movements (1964) and then with following movements (1965) and vergence movements (1966). Since all three studies used very similar methods, and arrived at nearly identical results, only the saccade experiments need be described here in much detail. Several different procedures were used, including not only the measurement of isometric tension by sudden unexpected clamping of the eye, but also the effect of loading the eye with added inertia on the time course of the movement, and two other procedures which have already been described in the previous sections.

During isometric measurements the eye is fixed, or nearly so, and the passive mechanical elements linking it to the orbit contribute nothing to the observations, nor does the inertia of the eye: the measurements thus reflect only the properties of the muscle mechanics. The high-inertia saccades simply serve to demonstrate how highly damped the eye is, and thus that the moment of inertia of the contact lens used for the measurements—and indeed that of the eye itself—is quite unimportant: what is found is that no sign of resonance occurs with increasing inertial load until the total inertia is nearly *one hundred* times greater than that of the eye itself (figure 7.34). The damping is in fact so great that the rapid

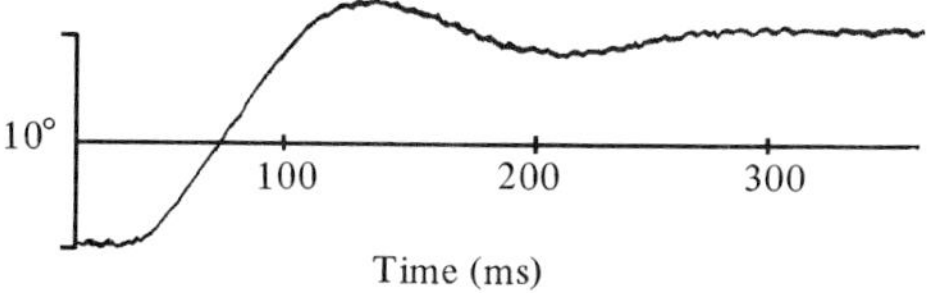

Figure 7.34. Record of the time course of an attempted saccade when the moment of inertia of the eye is artificially increased by a factor of roughly 100, showing a slight transient oscillation (Robinson, 1964).

time course that is typical of the saccade could not possibly be achieved if the muscles merely increased their active tension in a step-like manner: and if one makes a recording of the isometric tension during a saccade (figure 7.35) one observes an extra peak of tension at the beginning of the saccade, to move the globe rapidly against the overwhelming viscous forces, and that it finally drops at the end of the movement to the much lower tension necessary simply to hold the globe in place against the relatively weak elastic forces.

Now the isometric tension is itself a filtered version of the active tension generated by the contractile elements of the muscle: from the experiments previously described that enable one to measure the viscous and elastic properties of the muscle itself, one can work backwards from the isometric tension to calculate what time course the active tension must have during a saccade to generate the isometric tension that is observed. It turns out that a good approximation to this time course takes the form of a step of tension just sufficient to hold the eye at its final position, with an added rectangular pulse of force (about 40 ms in duration for a 10° saccade) superimposed at the beginning (figure 7.35).

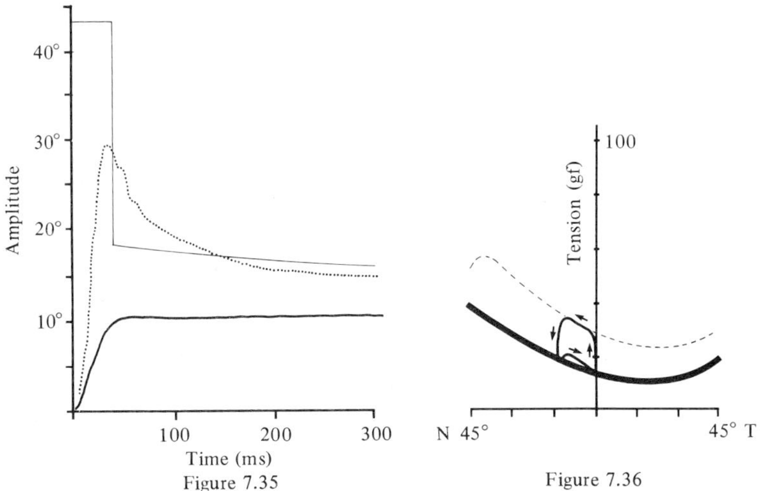

Figure 7.35. Tension and position during a saccade: the thick line shows the time course of a typical human 10° saccade, and the dotted line the corresponding isometric tension. The thin line is the calculated time course of active tension that would be required to generate the other two curves (after Robinson, 1964).

Figure 7.36. Human medial rectus length-tension curve during voluntary saccades. The heavy line is the same as in figure 7.27, and represents the normal locus for slow position changes. During saccades there is an added tension, resulting in the locus shown as a broken line above it. The counterclockwise loop shows the actual locus during a sequence in which the subject made a 15° nasal saccade from the midline, and then another saccade back to the origin. The area between the full and broken lines represents the normal operational region (after Collins, 1975).

(The presence of nonlinearities in the mechanics of the eye makes it difficult to calculate the exact shape of this burst of activation.) An interesting feature is that, as larger and larger saccades are executed, the height of the pulse remains fixed but increases in *duration*, thus accounting very well for the amplitude–velocity–duration relationship for saccades that is actually seen: this point has already been anticipated in section 4.1.1. It was also suggested in that section that the overshoots and undershoots that are often seen in saccades (for example Fleming et al, 1969) might be due to a mismatch between the duration of the pulse and the height of the step. If the duration is too long, the eye will overshoot: if too short, the eye will undershoot, in the sense that it will move only slowly to its final position after the termination of the first fast component.

One consequence of the existence of this added pulse is that the trajectory of saccades when plotted on a length–tension curve is a stereotyped one lying between the 'natural' length–tension relationship of figure 7.28(a), and the same curve displaced upward by the height of the added pulse of muscle tension (about 30–40 gf; Collins et al, 1975) (figure 7.36): it is fortunate for the systems analyst that this working region of the muscle happens to lie entirely within the area in which the length–tension curves enter their straight sections. Finally, the area within the loop formed in such a plot as the eye makes a saccade to an eccentric point and back again is equal to the mechanical work done during the movement: it amounts to some 0·6 erg deg^{-1}. Clearly the energy expended even in what are normally considered very tiring oculomotor tasks is very small: to read the whole of this book, for example, requires—even if a generous allowance is made for the inefficiency of the ocular muscles—an energy consumption about equal to that needed to raise a glass of beer from the table to one's lips!

The most direct evidence for 'preemphasis' of this kind comes both from electromyographic studies (for example Miller, 1958), and from observations of the firing patterns of oculomotor nerve fibres during saccades, which belong more properly in the next chapter. The existence of this pattern of firing has very great theoretical interest in relation to modern ideas of the basic principles of the control of eye movements, and is discussed in this light in chapter 12. Finally, it is perhaps worth pointing out that the models of the mechanisms of the oculomotor apparatus that can be derived as a result of the work described in this chapter are now sufficiently accurate and complete that one may calculate in advance the precise effects of particular operative procedures in cases of ocular palsies, squints, and the like, and thus greatly increase their chance of success. With small computers easily available and relatively cheap, there is no reason why such quantitative procedures should not become routine clinical practice.

8

The extraocular muscles and their innervation

"The other couple of sinewes march on unto the muscles of the eyes, and serve to help their motion: their dividing of themselves is pretie, full of kindnes, for they send to every muscle as it were a little fine thred."

8.1 The structure of the extraocular muscle fibres

Unhappily for the student of eye movements, there is probably no other set of muscles in the body whose structure is the subject of as much confusion and controversy as that of the six extraocular muscles. The reasons for this are perhaps partly that these muscles seem to show an unusual degree of variation as one compares species with species, and also that it is only comparatively recently that electron microscopy has demonstrated how very inadequate were the classical descriptions of extraocular muscle tissue. Two questions currently remain unanswered. The first relates to the number of types of motor fibre that are observed: there is as yet no agreement on the number of different types that can be distinguished, even in the comparatively well-studied eye muscles of man. Still less has it been possible to associate different functional roles to the types that are observed, or to trace different patterns of innervation to them from the central nervous system. The second question, in active debate for at least a century, is concerned with the proprioceptive elements in eye muscle: although it is now clear that some sort of sensory receptor (not necessarily a classical muscle spindle) occurs in virtually every species studied, we are really still in the dark as to what function these receptors may actually serve in the control of eye movements.

Both these questions of course have the most profound significance for an understanding of the oculomotor system: if it is true that different populations of fibres within the muscle are used for different kinds of movements, or possibly at different times in a single movement, then we can say goodbye to any hope of finding unifying mechanisms common to different types of movement at a more central level of the central nervous system. And as far as the proprioceptors are concerned, it obviously makes a great difference to the nature of a control system if it does or does not use some kind of feedback of information about its performance to modify its behaviour, and the presence or absence of such information will profoundly influence the kinds of signal processing that are appropriate for the forward pathway. But at the time of writing it is simply not possible to synthesise simple answers to either of these problems, and what follows must necessarily be either confusing, or if not confusing, misleading. The author is painfully aware of these deficiencies, and with limited space has tried to err towards oversimplification rather than the opposite. Fortunately, detailed reviews of some of these problems have appeared within the last few years (Peachey, 1971; Alvarado and van Horn, 1975), which the reader who is unsatisfied with generalities may find useful.

8.1.1 Gross anatomy of the fibres

The four recti are broadly similar in their properties, having lengths of around 40–50 mm, and between twenty and thirty thousand fibres in each muscle (Kato, 1938): the equivalent figure for the obliques is probably just under twenty thousand. In respect of the types and distribution of their fibres—although recent critical comparisons are lacking—it is probably safe to assume that the six muscles are comparable. As we have seen, because of their complex synergistic action in executing actual movements, one cannot associate any one particular class of movement with particular pairs of muscles: all contribute simultaneously, so we need not expect to find very great differences between them in respect of functional anatomy.

The cross-sectional areas of the muscles being of the order of 20 mm^2, the fibre counts suggest that extraocular muscle fibres are unusually fine: measurements of human superior rectus (quoted in Alpern, 1969b) suggest that cross-sectional areas of individual fibres may average around 150 μm^2, while the very smallest fibres may be only some 5 μm in diameter. However, as will be seen in the next section, it is clear that there are several distinct populations of fibres of different sizes (the largest being some 40–50 μm in diameter) and that these are arranged in roughly semicircular layers running from the outside (orbital) surface to the inner central region (Kato, 1938). There is rather less agreement about the longitudinal arrangement of the fibres. Cross sections made at different distances from the proximal origin reveal differences in the relative numbers of fibres of different sizes: on the whole the most distal portion has smaller fibres than the central region, although there is some disagreement about the most proximal part (Hines, 1931; Cooper and Daniel, 1949; Cooper et al, 1955). There are two ways in which this appearance might arise: either the larger fibres are shorter than the muscle itself and terminate in the body of the muscle before the distal end is reached, or alternatively they run the whole length of the muscle but get smaller as they approach the end.

Hines (1931) favoured the former arrangement, having observed in the rabbit that some of the larger fibres do indeed seem to end abruptly before reaching the distal tendon. Cooper and Daniel (1949) and Lockhart and Brandt (1938) were less certain that such premature endings could be found, and preferred the notion of tapering fibres that run the whole length of the muscle. Modern electron miscroscopy techniques allow more accurate measurements to be made: in the inferior oblique of the cat it appears that most of the small-diameter fibres are shorter than the whole muscle, and that some large fibres may extend from tendon to tendon (Alvarado and van Horn, 1975). The problem is a difficult one to solve simply by looking at cross sections through the fibres, and must still probably be considered unresolved. Peachey (1971) has pointed out that a tapering muscle fibre would presumably exert different forces at different points along its length: a useless arrangement that would lead to mechanical instability under load. But if the other arrangement is the true one, it means that one must be careful not to generalise from a cross section at a particular point in a muscle about the properties of the fibres taken as a whole.

8.1.2 Types of motor fibre

There are many criteria apart from size by which it is possible to classify the extraocular muscle fibres on the basis of their microscopic appearance: most of them provide a two-fold classification, often with rather vague boundaries (for example, 'more mitochondria' versus 'fewer mitochondria'). One might suppose that the fibres would form a continuum of variation, and that separation into classes would be more a function of the observer's preconceived notions than a reflection of a true specialisation of function: but Peachey (1971) has argued, as many previous experimenters have tacitly assumed, that there is a sufficient degree of correlation between some of the various criteria that a small number of different classes—perhaps four or five—can provide a realistic description of the fibre population. These criteria include: diameter; position in the muscle (that is, surface or interior); size and arrangement of the fibrils; biochemical features such as succinate dehydrogenase activity and glycogen content: number of mitochondria; degree of elaboration of the sarcoplasmic reticulum; fine structure of the fibrils, for example, presence or absence of the 'M' line; and type of innervation, whether single or multiple.

Now some of these criteria evidently relate to the same direction of functional specialisation, along a continuum of which one might take the classical 'twitch' and 'slow' fibres to be extremes. A two-fold classification of this sort was probably first proposed for extrafusal fibres by Cilimbaris (1910) on the basis of their appearance, and functionally established by Peachey and Huxley (1962), who succeeded in correlating the two morphological types with the electrophysiological 'fast' and 'slow' properties first described by Kuffler and Vaughan Williams (1953a; 1953b). Very briefly, the electrophysiological observations were that while some frog striated muscle fibres (twitch fibres) showed the usual all-or-nothing propagating response to electrical stimulation, others (the slow fibres) showed graded contractions in response to graded stimulation, without propagation. What Peachey and Huxley showed was that fibres classified in this way exhibited well-marked *morphological* differences. The fast fibres had a well-developed sarcoplasmic reticulum in intimate contact with regularly spaced-out fibrils [Krüger's *Fibrillenstruktur* (1929)], and large single nerve endings ('en plaque') on each fibre. The slow fibres on the other hand had a poorly developed sarcoplasmic reticulum, with irregular masses of bunched-up fibrils (*Felderstruktur*), and multiple endings ('en grappe') having relatively unspecialised subsynaptic regions.

This correlation is rather what would be expected: if the fibre is to be activated quickly, then it clearly makes sense for the information represented by the action potential that passes over its surface to be passed as nearly simultaneously as possible to all the individual fibrils in the fibre, by means of an extended and intimately penetrating sarcoplasmic reticulum. In the slow fibre, multiple innervation must spread activation over the surface in the absence of an action potential, and an elaborate system for conveying information rapidly to the interior is no longer required, and is indeed taking up valuable space that could be devoted to extra fibrils. In the same way, the steady, unremitting energy requirements of the slow muscles must be met by the larger number of mitochondria with their high oxidative enzymatic activity (for example succinate dehydrogenase activity), while the more acute needs of the fast fibres can be taken care of by drawing on glycogen stores that can be built up during periods of rest. In the frog, then, we seem to have a happy correspondence between structure and function. But when we turn to the eye muscles, the situation is not so simple.

It is certainly true that fibres can be found in mammalian eye muscles that are very similar in appearance to frog slow muscles (Hess, 1961), with similar endings 'en grappe' (Dietert, 1965; Namba et al, 1968; Harker, 1972a), and that corresponding electrophysiological properties can also be found that divide extraocular fibres into 'fast' and 'slow' types. But it is now clear that in most mammalian eye muscles, and certainly in man, a simple morphological division of fibres into '*Fibrillenstruktur*' and '*Felderstruktur*' is not enough to cover the variety of types that actually occur. Apart from the slow fibres, which are comparatively easy to distinguish, there are at least two, and probably as many as four different classes of fibre that fall into the 'fast' category (Cheng and Breinin, 1966; Miller, 1967; Mayr, 1971; Peachey, 1971; Maier et al, 1972; Nowgrodska-Zagórska, 1974; Alvarado and van Horn, 1975). The distinctions are made essentially by size and position in the muscle, and also, more significantly from the functional point of view, in terms of their mitochondrial and enzymatic content. At the same time, associated differences may be observed in the elaboration of the sarcoplasmic reticulum, the fibril grouping, the fine structure of the fibrils, and the pattern of innervation (Teräväinen, 1968). Thus Peachey's (1971) four 'fast' fibre types comprise two small types of cell (5–20 μm) from the surface, one 'red' (that is, with large numbers of mitochondria) and one 'white' (with few mitochondria), and two types from the interior, one a moderately large red fibre and the other a large (25–50 μm) white fibre. Table 8.1 summarises a possible classification along these lines [but see Durston (1974) for a somewhat dissident view]. It is important to emphasise that although it is fairly certain that the morphologically 'slow' fibres are also *physiologically* 'slow', we still have rather little idea about the different functions associated with the other fibre types (see below, section 8.2.1): it may be that some of them—perhaps the red fibres with larger fibrils—are not actually 'fast' at all, but functionally 'slow', and Peachey urges that these terms should not be used to describe extraocular muscle until they are firmly justified by electrophysiological investigation. But purely anatomical terms like *Felderstruktur* and *Fibrillenstruktur* are hardly better, because they represent only one of many possible criteria that could be considered (Zenker and Anzenbacher, 1964).

In part 1 of this book we saw that a basic distinction can be made between 'fast' and 'slow' *movements*, and it is naturally tempting to suppose that these two modes of action correspond to 'fast' and 'slow' fibres, saccades, for example, being executed by twitch fibres, and convergence movements by slow fibres (for example Alpern and Wolter, 1956). In particular, the apparently unnecessary slowness of vergence movements clearly invites the suggestion that it is the result of some peripheral limitation of this type. An alternative hypothesis might be that the slow fibres are used for tonic deviations of the eye, and the twitch fibres provide the extra burst of activity that we saw in the previous chapter to be associated with the saccades that move the eye from one position to another. Such ideas were probably more attractive when it was thought that the muscles contained only two types of fibre: we are now faced with something of an *embarras de richesse*, and it is not easy to think of five distinct functions that could be associated with five different types of muscle fibres. However, the most direct evidence on this question comes from a study of the discharge patterns of oculomotor fibres during different kinds of movement, and so the point is taken up again in section 8.3.4.

Table 8.1. Extraocular fibre types (adapted from Peachey, 1971).

	Location	Description	Fibrils	Sarcoplasmic reticulum	Innervation
Fast	surface	small 'red'	larger, indistinct	moderate	single
		small 'white'	smaller, indistinct	moderate	multiple
	interior	moderately large 'red'	small, distinct	much	single
		large 'white'	small, distinct	much	single
Slow	interior	medium	large, indistinct	little	multiple

8.1.3 Sensory endings in extraocular fibres

Two kinds of mechanoreceptors are classically described in striated muscles: the *Golgi tendon organ*, essentially in series with the contractile fibres and thus responding more to the tension they develop than to the stretch of the muscle, and the *muscle spindle*—effectively in parallel—

which responds to stretch rather than tension (figure 8.1). Further specialisation of function is evident in the spindles themselves: each spindle contains several thin striated muscle fibres which seem to be of two distinct types. The shorter and thinner fibres have a single chain of nuclei at their centre (nuclear chain fibres), while the longer and fatter fibres have their numerous nuclei bunched together (nuclear bag fibres): both were described by Barker (1948). Two different kinds of sensory innervation can be seen in the spindles: large afferent fibres—primary afferents—provide branching spiral endings in the nuclear bag region (annulospiral endings), while smaller (secondary) afferents terminate on each side of the central region in complicated spray-like endings (flower-spray endings: figure 8.2). Very fine motor fibres also enter the spindle (γ efferents) and end on motor endplates on the striated fibres, and may also be divided into two types. Electrical recordings from primary afferents show that they give a phasic or rapidly adapting component in their

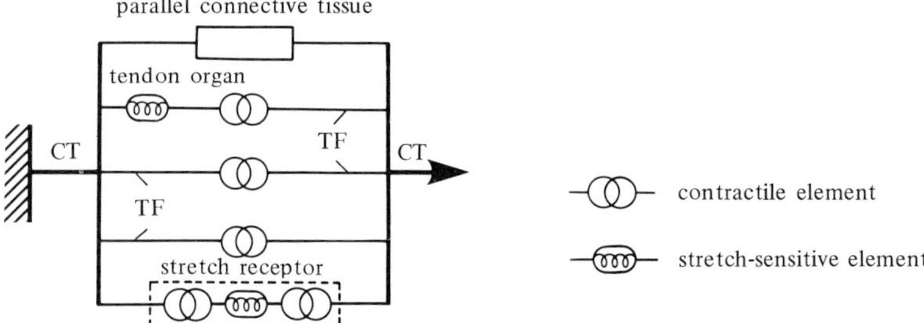

Figure 8.1. Schematic representation of the arrangement of contractile and stretch-sensitive elements in extraocular muscle. CT is the common tendon of the muscle, TF are the tendinous fascicles; the structure within broken lines is a spindle-like stretch receptor, and its two contractile portions would be innervated separately from other contractile elements.

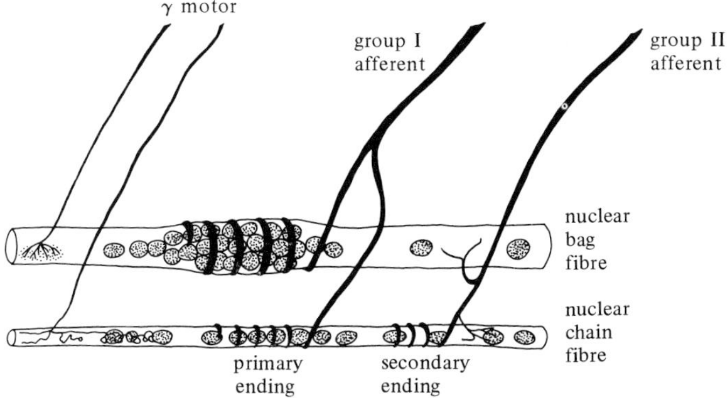

Figure 8.2. Simplified representation of typical spindle fibres. Above is shown a nuclear bag fibre, below a nuclear chain fibre, with their sensory and motor innervation (after Matthews, 1972).

response to stretch, or in other words that they respond partly to the instantaneous degree of stretch, and partly to its rate of change. The secondary fibres are qualitatively similar in their response, but are rather less rate-sensitive than the primary fibres and thus show less adaptation. Stimulation of γ fibres, which presumably deforms the sensory region in much the same way as an externally-applied stretch, increases the rate of firing of the afferent fibres; the γ fibres may differ amongst themselves in the degree to which they elevate the phasic or tonic sensitivity of the sensory fibres. The structure and function of muscle spindles have been admirably reviewed recently by Matthews (1972).

The Golgi tendon organs have been less intensively studied. At first it was thought that their very high threshold to externally applied forces meant that they could play little part in normal physiological processes, but it is now clear (Houk and Henneman, 1967) that they fire quite readily if the fibres to which they are attached are undergoing active contraction. This is sometimes taken to mean that they are more sensitive to 'active' than to 'passive' stretch: but of course under externally applied stretch the total tension is divided amongst all the tendons of the muscle, so that each receptor experiences only a fraction of the total. There is no evidence that an individual receptor responds any differently to the same degree of tension, whether exerted from outside the muscle or by the activity of the fibre to which it is joined.

Both classical types of receptor have been described in extraocular muscle in many species, while in some others they are conspicuously absent. Cilimbaris (1910) found spindles in the eye muscles of ox, deer, sheep, goats, and chimpanzees, but not in horses, dogs, cats, rabbits, hares, foxes, rats, or macaques: he also found tendon organs in ox, man, monkeys, horses, dogs, and cats (see also Huber, 1900). Subsequently, spindles were found in mice, pigs, and man (Daniel, 1946; Cooper and Daniel, 1949), and were confirmed to be absent in many birds (Maier et al, 1971). It is difficult to discern any particular pattern in this miscellaneous menagerie as between those animals that do or do not possess extraocular spindles: the distinction is in any case a little arbitrary, as many species that do not have classical spindles do nevertheless have stretch receptors of very similar properties (for example the cat: Bach-y-Rita and Ito, 1966b), and some of the accepted spindles have features, particular in regard to their patterns of innervation, that are not normally seen in 'classical' spindles (for example in man: Buzzard, 1908; Daniel, 1946; Sas and Appeltauer, 1963). Even so, at least one species (squirrel monkey: Ito and Bach-y-Rita, 1969) appears to have neither spindles, nor—from electrophysiological recording—any other kind of stretch receptor.

The spindles of human extraocular muscle are rather small (some 20–100 μm diameter) with a thin capsule, and are found mostly in the proximal and distal thirds of the muscle (Merillees et al, 1950; Voss 1957).

The intrafusal fibres do not show clear nuclear bags (Cooper and Daniel, 1957), and the sensory endings are not directly comparable with the annulospiral and flower-spray endings of classical muscle spindles (Daniel, 1946), while several other types of ending not commonly seen elsewhere can be observed (Wolter, 1955). Sas and Appeltauer (1963) also describe spiral endings not associated with spindles, but innervating small muscle fibres near the surface, and it may well be that the stretch responses recorded by Bach-y-Rita and Ito (1966b) in the cat—which has no spindles—were from endings of this type. The fine γ fibres with which these muscles are multiply innervated would then play an analogous role to the γ fibres of ordinary muscle spindles (Bach-y-Rita, 1971).

8.2 The physiology of extraocular muscles

8.2.1 Electrical properties of motor fibres

We saw in section 8.1.2 that several different types of fibre could be distinguished in extraocular muscle—on purely morphological grounds—and that these features would be likely to be associated with physiological specialisation of the various fibres. In particular, one might expect that single endplates would be associated with propagated impulses, and multiple endings with slow junctional potentials. However, actual electrical recordings show that such a view is overoptimistic. Although it is certain (Matyushkin, 1961; Hess and Pilar, 1963; Ozawa, 1964) that at least in cats and rabbits the largest, single-endplate fibres do indeed show propagated action potentials on stimulation, there is less agreement about the multi-innervated fibres. Although these authors found that the multi-innervated fibres could show the expected slow potentials on stimulation, Bach-y-Rita and Ito (1966a) found in the cat that the small superficial fibres with multiple innervation in the superior rectus were *also* capable of carrying propagated action potentials under suitable conditions; a result which Pilar (1967) was not able to confirm fully, although he agreed that such behaviour was in principle possible.

Some reasons why their results were in conflict have been discussed by Bach-y-Rita, and include that of electrode damage to these very small fibres: such injuries are likely to produce electrical leakage which will reduce the membrane potential and also lead to overstability. This effect will make itself more felt in small fibres than in large. A further suggestion (Bach-y-Rita and Ito, 1966a) is that some of these fibres may be innervated by more than one nerve fibre, in a manner similar to that demonstrated for cat skeletal muscle spindles by Hunt and Kuffler (1951). If this were so, one might imagine a dual mode of functioning for these fibres: if spatial summation between the endings was possible, then while the response to stimulation by a single nerve fibre might result in slow, graded local contractions, simultaneous activation by all the innervating fibres might generate a propagated action potential and fast twitch.

However, attractive though this notion is, more recent experiments (Bach-y-Rita and Lennerstrand, 1975) suggest that polyneuronal innervation is actually unimportant, if indeed it exists at all.

8.2.2 Active contractile properties of muscle fibres

The eye muscles are the fastest of all the muscles in the body: in the cat, Cooper and Eccles (1930) measured contraction times for medial rectus of the order of 7·5–10 ms, compared with 40 ms for medial gastrocnemius; the corresponding fusion frequencies being of the order of 350 Hz and 100 Hz respectively (figure 8.3). Other authors have reported even higher fusion frequencies (for example 450 Hz; Bach-y-Rita and Ito, 1966a), but this may be due in part to a lack of consensus about the precise definition of 'fusion'. A single maximal shock to the nerve gives a twitch whose decay is disproportionately long in relation to the very rapid rise. By selective denervation of the muscle, it can be shown that this is due to slower contributions from fibres other than the very fastest twitch fibres, presumably in fact from the small multi-innervation fibres [although recent attempts to provide direct mechanical evidence for slow fibres in whole muscle has failed (Barmack et al, 1971; Close and Luff, 1974)]. These fibres show a rise time of some 25 ms (Bach-y-Rita and Ito, 1966a) and thus contribute little to the initial peak of tension, but are probably responsible for the slow approach to maximum tension that is observed under tetanic stimulation near the fusion frequency. In the sheep superior oblique it is possible to stimulate slow fibres in isolation: they have a contraction time of some 20–50 ms, and cannot contribute more than about 5% of the total muscle tetanic tension (Browne, 1976).

A clearer separation of the properties of the two broad categories of fibre can be made by observing their response to depolarising blocking agents: the depolarisation induced by such an agent will tend to block the activation of single-endplate fibres, but also *induce* contractures of the multi-innervated ones (Kern, 1965). This is certainly the explanation for the observation (Duke-Elder and Duke-Elder, 1931) of slow tonic contractions of extraocular muscles in response to acetylcholine and other agents that are not blocked by atropine, as Kern (1965) was able to show

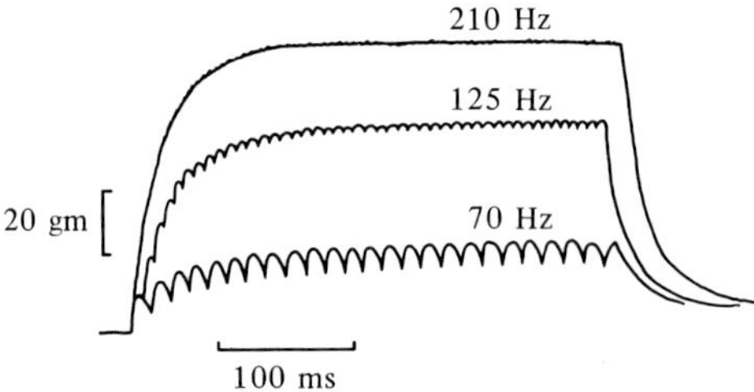

Figure 8.3. High fusion frequency and slow rise time of cat medial rectus isometric tension, when the third nerve is stimulated electrically at different frequencies (after Cooper and Eccles, 1930).

by pharmacological stimulation of isolated slow fibres from rabbit eye muscles. This contribution from slow fibres can apparently reach as much as one-third of the muscle's maximum tetanic tension (Bach-y-Rita and Ito, 1966a). The fact that a depolarising blocker like succinyl choline will also deactivate the fast fibres can be used very effectively to isolate the two components in single twitches (Katz and Eakins, 1966a; 1966b) or during tetanic stimulation (Bach-y-Rita and Ito, 1966a). A discussion of the effects of other blocking agents is really beyond the scope of this section: Eakins and Katz (1971) provide a useful review of this and other related pharmacological aspects of extraocular muscle.

8.2.3 Responses from stretch receptors

Many of the early recordings from proprioceptive afferent fibres were made in the goat, which has prominent spindles (Cooper et al, 1951; 1953a; a useful review of earlier work is that of Whitteridge, 1960). The recordings made by these workers were typical of those that can be obtained from skeletal muscle spindles, and showed the same division of types into phasic, with marked rate sensitivity, and tonic, with less adaptation (figure 8.4). The distinction is not a sharp one, and in the sheep, at least, one sees a continuum of responses between the two extremes (Browne, 1975). The afferent fibres are large, with conduction velocities in the region of 100 m s^{-1}, and may fire at frequencies of up to 400–500 Hz (Cooper et al, 1951). Again like skeletal muscles, γ fibres could be found by subdivision of the motor nerves, which on stimulation increase the sensitivity of the stretch receptors (Whitteridge, 1958; 1959; Bach-y-Rita and Lennerstrand, 1974) (figures 8.5, 8.6), in a way comparable to what is commonly found in skeletal muscle: the effect is apparently more marked on the tonic than on the phasic components of the response to stretch.

Subsequently, it was shown that quite similar responses could be recorded from the afferent fibres of animals like the cat that do not have ordinary spindles (Cooper and Fillenz, 1955; Bach-y-Rita and Ito, 1966b). A difficulty in interpretation of results in such species soon becomes apparent, however. As we have seen, a tendon organ in series with a small multi-innervated motor fibre can behave in many ways like a classical

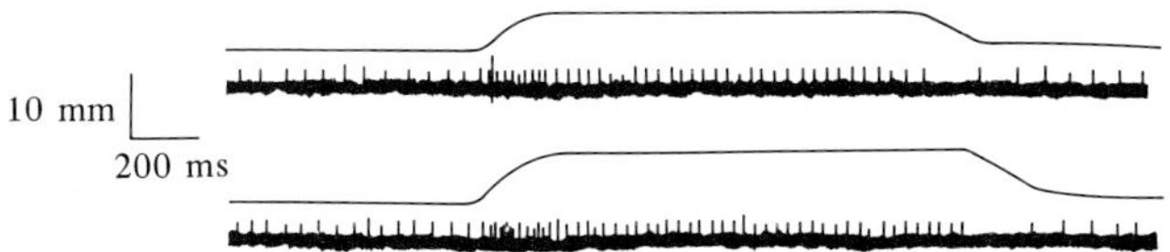

Figure 8.4. Stretch receptor responses from extraocular muscle. The spike trains are recorded from the nerve supplying the inferior oblique of the goat: stretching of the muscle is indicated by the upper trace in each of the two cases, a 0·6 mm stretch (above) and a 0·85 mm stretch (below). The relatively greater increase in firing rate immediately following the onset of stretch, indicating a marked phasic component in the response, is noticeable, as is also the corresponding pause at the end of stretch (Cooper et al, 1951).

spindle component, and the usual distinction between mechanoreceptive elements considered to be in parallel with the motor fibres, and those considered to be in series can no longer usefully be made. Thus Cooper and Fillenz attributed their high-threshold, adapting responses to tendon organs, while Bach-y-Rita and Ito, describing what appeared to be the same types of response—although they used tension rather than actual stretch as the input variable—simply ascribed them to a second type of stretch receptor in a *parallel* arrangement. The observation that the rate of discharge fell during stretch when the nerve was maximally stimulated may merely indicate that the particular motor fibre in series contracted less than its neighbours. These latter authors also found that the dynamic index (a measure of the relative responsiveness to rate of stretch rather than stretch itself) increased as the fibres were stretched, and also that some of the fibres were spontaneously active. Conduction velocities seem to be lower than in the goat, in the region of 10–50 m s^{-1}. In the squirrel monkey (Ito and Bach-y-Rita, 1969) the same authors found no afferents that could be considered primarily sensitive to stretch; and on the basis of cooling experiments, and the effect of the application of adrenaline, concluded that such afferents as there were came from the walls of blood vessels and were not directly concerned in eye movements at all. The question of what function, if any, extraocular stretch receptors may have in the control of eye movements is postponed until chapter 10.

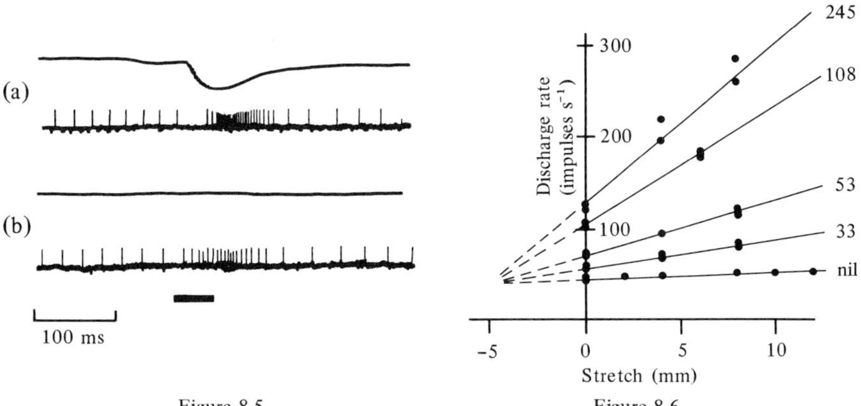

Figure 8.5. Figure 8.6.

Figure 8.5. Demonstration of γ fibres innervating the superior oblique of the goat. The spikes in the two cases are recorded from the same afferent branch. In (a), a small number of fibres from the motor nerve were stimulated (black bar), resulting in an increase in tension (upper line) and in the rate of afferent discharge. After further division of the efferent branch, it was possible (b) to obtain the increase in firing frequency on motor stimulation, unaccompanied by an increase in tension (after Whitteridge, 1959).

Figure 8.6. Effect of γ fibre stimulation on afferent response to stretch, in a preparation like that of figure 8.5. The rates of efferent stimulation are shown on the right: the effect of γ stimulation is clearly to increase the sensitivity of the receptor (after Whitteridge, 1959).

8.3 The nerve supply to extraocular muscles

8.3.1 Efferent pathways

The classical motor innervation of the extraocular muscles is from three cranial nerves, the third, fourth, and sixth: it is convenient to refer to them as nIII, nIV, and nVI, and the corresponding nuclei in the brainstem from which they originate as N.III, N.IV, and N.VI. The superior, inferior and medial recti, as well as the inferior oblique are supplied by nIII; nVI supplies the lateral rectus (and the retractor bulbi, where present); while nIV, unique amongst the oculomotor nerves in that it is crossed, runs dorsally at first to decussate in the medullary velum and supplies the superior oblique. Other names for these nerves are *oculomotor* for nIII, *trochlear* for nIV, and *abducens* for nVI: but, as the use of 'oculomotor' in this sense deprives one of a useful word for denoting the whole set of nerves and their nuclei, as well as for the eye movement control system as a whole, I shall be referring to nIII by number rather than by name and use 'oculomotor' in the more general sense.

While no one doubts that these nerves represent the paths taken by the larger fibres [innervating the larger muscle fibres (Woolard, 1931)], it is not quite so certain that the smaller muscle fibres receive their innervation via the same routes. One possibility that has been suggested from time to time is that some of these fibres might, like the *intra*ocular muscles, be innervated by branches of the autonomic nervous system (for example Boeke, 1926). Destruction of the cervical ganglion does not cause degeneration of the smaller fibres (Woolard, 1931), nor does stimulation of the cervical sympathetic system either induce contractions of extraocular muscles, or influence the amplitude of contractions evoked in other ways (Brecher and Mitchell, 1957). On the other hand, stimulation of the ciliary ganglion *can* apparently cause extraocular muscle contractions (Armaly, 1959), and its destruction can result in degenerating fibres in at least some of the extraocular muscles (Kure et al, 1927). However, we shall see in the next section that in some species there is convincing evidence that proprioceptive fibres may pass partly through the ciliary ganglion on their way to the fifth nerve nuclear complex, and if this is the case the preceding observations are open to other interpretations. In any case, such fibres must be very few in comparison with the large numbers of small fibres found in the 'classical' motor pathways: thus Donaldson (1960) found that nearly 30% of fibres in the goat were of gamma type, around 5 μm in diameter (observed also in rabbit and sheep: Fernand and Young, 1951; Browne, 1976), and Steinaker and Bach-y-Rita (1968) demonstrated further that in the cat nVI there was little significant difference in the spectrum of fibre sizes measured near the brain stem and at the lateral rectus, although they failed to confirm the second prominent peak in the 13–16 μm region that Donaldson found in the goat. In the sheep, selective stimulation of the small nerve fibres does indeed produce slow contractions (Browne, 1976).

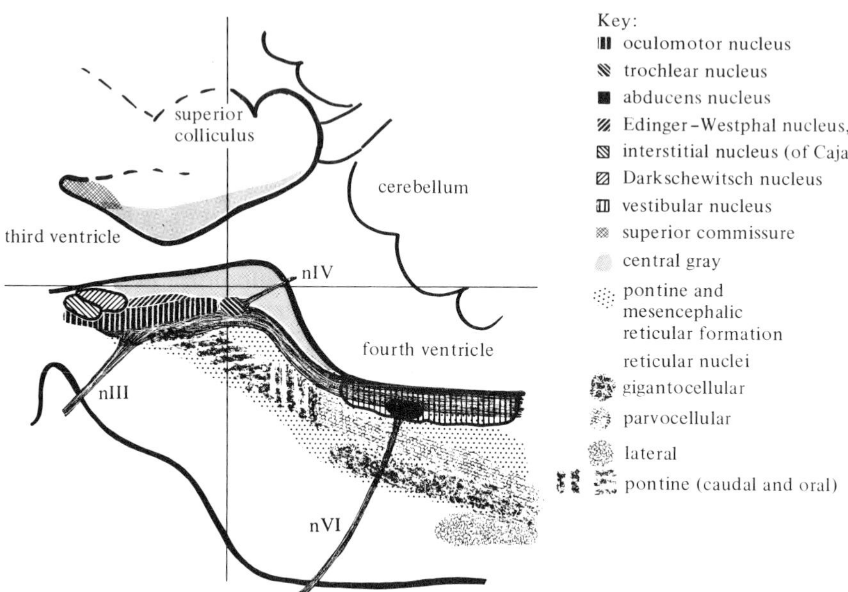

Figure 8.7. Topography of some areas associated with eye movements in the cat; the structures are shown laterally projected on to the sagittal plane: the axes show the position of the Horsley-Clarke A-P and H planes. (Data mainly from Snider and Niemer, 1961.)

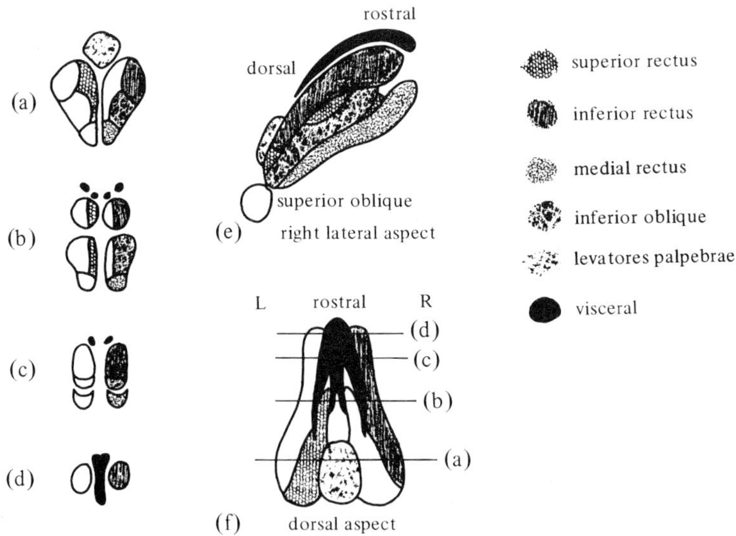

Figure 8.8. Schematic topography of the oculomotor nuclei: (a)-(d) show sections at the points indicated in the dorsal view, (f); (e) shows the right lateral aspect (after Warwick, 1964).

by Tarlov (1972) and Tarlov and Tarlov (1971), with some disagreement that may represent a species difference between cat and primate. [See van Biervliet (1899) for an early degeneration study in the rabbit that also showed a division into strips]. Antidromically evoked responses can also be helpful, but seem to give less precise results (Highstein, 1971). Stimulation experiments, however carefully performed (Bender and Weinstein, 1943; Danis, 1948) are always open to objections on account of current spread, and stimulation of fibres rather than cell bodies, and have often led to wildly contradictory conclusions about the order of representation of muscles in the nucleus, and even whether they are crossed or uncrossed. It appears that in fact only the superior rectus has a fully crossed innervation (like the superior oblique), while the levatores palpebrae, whose fibres originate in the caudal central nuclei, are partially crossed: some confirmation for this has been given by Szentágothai (1942) in the cat.

A particular source of disagreement has been the nature of the other central nuclei in the complex, especially the nucleus of Perlia. Although long considered to be a 'nucleus for convergence' (Brouwer, 1918) on rather uncompelling comparative and clinical grounds, and firmly established as such in some textbooks, it is clear now that not only does possession of this nucleus not correlate particularly well from species to species with the enjoyment of binocular vision (Le Gros Clark, 1926), but that even in species where it does appear it is often extremely ill-defined (Crosby and Woodburne, 1943), and is frequently completely absent in particular specimens (for example in some 80% of macaques: Warwick, 1955). Finally, the anteromedian nucleus appears to be wholly parasympathetic, like the Edinger–Westphal nucleus with which it is probably continuous: the fibres from both are entirely ipsilateral.

8.4.2 Adjacent structures

The eye muscle nuclei are embedded in the reticular formation of the brain stem: as will be described in the next section, the firing of some neurons in the reticular formation is strongly correlated with movements of the eyes. Although connections between the reticular formation and the abducens nucleus were demonstrated by Lorente de No in 1933, Carpenter et al (1963) could not find the expected retrograde degeneration of cell processes in the pontine or medullary reticular formation after lesions in N.VI, and so there must still be some doubt about the nature of the connections. Fuchs and Luschei (1972) suggest that their 'long-lead' units (see below) probably synapse with the 'medium-lead' ones, which in turn may project directly to the motor nucleus itself. Only twenty-seven out of 187 units described were of the latter type, so it is possible that the number of projections of this type might be very small. At least some of the units in the rostral pons are responsive to large-field directional visual stimulation, often with very short latencies, and might conceivably be concerned in some aspect of visual control of eye movements (Baker et al, 1976).

There are three other nuclei situated near the oculomotor complex that seem at least partly to be concerned with eye-movements: they are the *nucleus of Darkschewitsch*, the *interstitial nucleus of Cajal,* and the *nucleus of the posterior commissure*. The first (Darkschewitsch, 1889) lies just dorsal and lateral to the third nerve nucleus, and is often rather indistinct. It appears to receive fibres from the medial longitudinal fasciculus (Carpenter and Hanna, 1962) but not to send to it (Pompeiano and Walberg, 1957). It is possible that both this nucleus and the interstitial nucleus relay impulses from the superior colliculi to the eye muscle nuclei (Szentágothai, 1950; Altman and Carpenter, 1961). The interstitial nucleus (Cajal, 1908), outside the central gray, also lies close to the rostral end of the oculomotor nucleus (figure 8.7), but is separated from it by the the medial longitudinal fasciculus, from which it receives both afferent and efferent connections (Pompeiano and Walberg, 1957; Markham et al, 1966; Markham, 1968). The nucleus of the posterior commissure is found dorsal to (and outside) the central gray between the level of the middle of N.III and the posterior commissure itself, with which it is associated. Lesions of the posterior commissure produce degenerative changes throughout the oculomotor complex and its associated nuclei (except in the ventral nuclei of the somatic columns, in the trochlear nucleus, and in parts of the superior colliculus, yet not in the medial longitudinal fasciculus below the level of N.IV (Carpenter, 1971).

The functional roles of these areas are not understood: relevant physiological findings are presented in chapter 9 in the course of discussion of afferent pathways to the oculomotor nuclei from other parts of the brain.

8.4.3 Patterns of discharge in the nuclei

The earliest (indirect) observations of discharging ocular motor neurons were made by means of electromyographic recordings from whole muscles: once reliable methods of amplifying and recording small electrical signals had been developed, electromyography could be used to investigate many basic questions about the gross coordination of activity in the extraocular muscles. Thus Miller (1958; 1959) was able to demonstrate the extra burst of activity associated with the fast rising phase of the saccade, as well as confirming the existence of reciprocal innervation for these fast movements, as Sherrington had demonstrated more directly for slow movements some sixty years before (Sherrington, 1894; see also Theopold and Kommerell, 1974). A question much discussed in this period was whether under certain conditions coactivation of antagonist muscles might supercede the usual reciprocal relationship. The two circumstances when such behaviour was anticipated were during asymmetric convergence (see section 5.3), when it was thought that the balance between the requirements of vergence and version might be struck by means of a mechanical tug-of-war between medial and lateral recti; and during movements far from the primary position, when the secondary actions of the muscles, being often synergic rather than opposed, would render reciprocal innervation inappropriate. In the latter case, Tamler et al (1959a, 1959b) found little evidence for coactivation during movements through the primary position, but movements between tertiary positions were generally associated with coactivation of all the muscle pairs except the horizontal. Asymmetric convergence was found to give rise to coactivation only if the degree of convergence was unnaturally large, that is, when the fixation stimulus approached nearer than the near point (Tamler et al, 1958; Miller, 1959). Finally, Nakayama (1975) has shown that the normally very precise reciprocal relation between firing of antagonist units is also severely disrupted during sleep.

Recording from single units gives more precise information: Reid (1949) in cats and goats, and Björk and Kugelberg (1953) in man were able to make such recordings from extraocular fibres. As would be expected from the exceptionally high fusion frequencies of the muscles, rates of discharge were also found to be very high; as Renshaw cells have sometimes been assigned the role of limiting the frequency of firing of motoneurons, it is interesting that they are not found in the oculomotor nuclei (Cajal, 1911). Accurate quantitative information about the relationship between muscle activation and movement have had to wait until the more recent development of methods of noise-free intracellular recording from the brainstem, and a moral climate in which recording from restrained, unanaesthetised animals was considered acceptable: although computer filtering of electromyogram signals promises to give as precise results (Trimble et al, 1974). In the last few years, a very large number of studies of this sort have appeared (Schaefer, 1965; Fuchs and Luschei, 1970; Robinson, 1970; Schiller, 1970; Fuchs and Luschei, 1971; Keller and Robinson, 1972; and many others). As there has been exceptionally good agreement between the reported results, the basic findings will be summarised without reference to specific authors.

The technique used is essentially to record discharges from neurons in or near the eye muscle nuclei while the animal is making either voluntary or reflex movements of different kinds: if these movements are simultaneously recorded, one can hope to correlate the two records to reveal the causal relation (if any!) between the two. It turns out that oculomotor neurons behave in a very satisfactory 'machine-like' way, so that such correlations are very close: all this means of course is that the mechanical properties of the muscle are uniform in time. As might be anticipated from the approximate linearity of these mechanics (taken as a whole) there is in most cases a linear relationship for tonic deviations between the rate of discharge and the angle of deviation of the eye, although different units may generate lines of different slope and position when plotted on a frequency–deviation graph (figure 8.9), and 'stiction' may in some cases produce a graph showing hysteresis (Eckmiller, 1974).

Again, bearing in mind that the dynamic properties of the eye mechanics can be approximated at low frequencies by a first-order low-pass filter (see section 7.5.4), it is no surprise to learn from these experiments that the transfer function linking frequency of discharge to eye position is of the same form, that is, $(k+\mathrm{D})^{-1}$. In practice, experimenters tend to express their results the other way round, as if the frequency of firing were a function of the eye position, rather than the opposite: this relationship is thus described as the inverse transfer function, $(k+\mathrm{D})$. In other words, the frequency of discharge is proportional both to the deviation of the eye—as we have seen—and to its rate of change of deviation, or velocity. The latter relationship can be investigated by looking at the rate of firing of the neuron when the eye is at a particular deviation, but crossing that deviation at different velocities (figure 8.9): the expected linear relation is again observed.

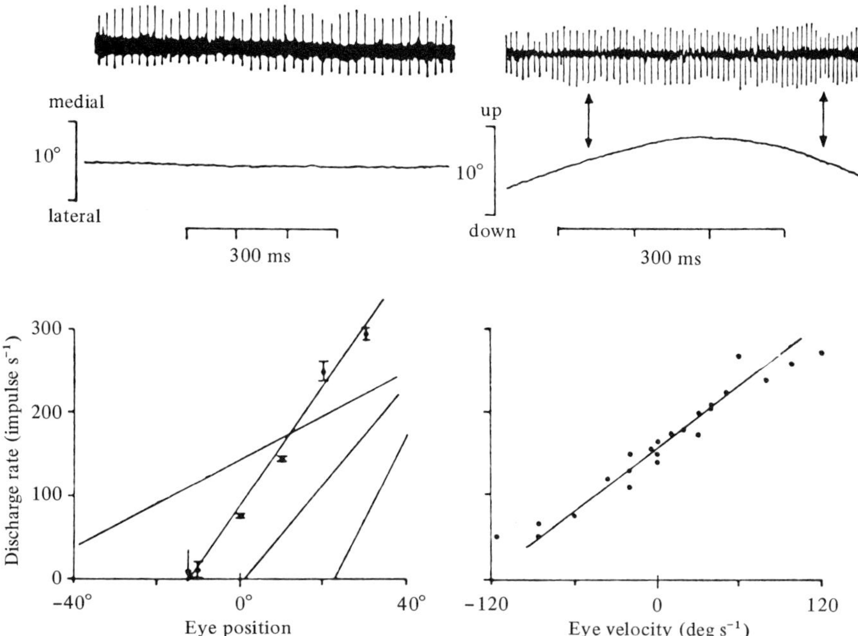

Figure 8.9. Oculomotor discharge in relation to eye movement. On the left, the steady rate of firing when the eye is stationary is shown above; and below, the relationship between this firing rate and eye position is shown for a few typical units, showing their different slopes and intercepts. On the right, the rate of firing during a slow voluntary eye movement is shown above: the arrows indicate points where the eye passes through the same position with velocity of opposite signs, and it can be seen that the associated firing rate is different in the two cases. Below, firing rate is plotted for a single unit as a function of velocity, at a particular deviation of the eye. The recordings were made in alert rhesus monkeys (Robinson and Keller, 1972).

All this simply goes to show that our analysis of the mechanics of the eye was essentially correct, although the variation of mechanical properties from fibre to fibre could not easily have been calculated in advance: it presumably reflects the morphological spectrum of fibre types noted earlier in this chapter. Thus the slope of the rate–position characteristic can vary from about one to fifteen impulses per second per degree, with a peak at about four, while the rate–velocity characteristic ranges from 0·3 to five impulses per degree, peaking at around 0·6. Collins (1975) has shown by recording simultaneously from units in different parts of extraocular muscles that the more 'phasic' units (that is, with steep rate–velocity functions) are large and globally situated, while the 'tonic' ones are small and orbital (figure 8.10).

Thresholds never exceed 25° in the direction of action, and about 16% of the units have no thresholds at all, but fire at all positions of the eye. Thus slow contractions of the muscles must be associated with increasing recruitment of fibres, presumably leading to the asynchrony of firing that can often be observed between neighbouring synergic units (Eckmiller et al, 1974). Robinson and Keller (1972) suggest that this may reflect the extra tension required to deviate the eye against increasing elastic forces from orbital tissue; but we have already seen that, because of the substantial cancellation of nonlinearities consequent on the muscles' 'push–pull' arrangement, the variations in threshold seem unnecessarily large for such a function unless they represent a strongly nonlinear relationship betwen frequency of firing and active tension. Collins and Scott (1973) have found a comparable nonlinear (power function) relation between total activity in the muscle and deviation of the eye.

The regular behaviour of these units is even more marked during saccades in the direction of action, when the roughly constant-velocity change of position is associated with a short high-frequency burst, followed by a permanent elevation of the resting discharge to a level appropriate for the new position of the eye (figure 8.11). A striking feature of the burst is

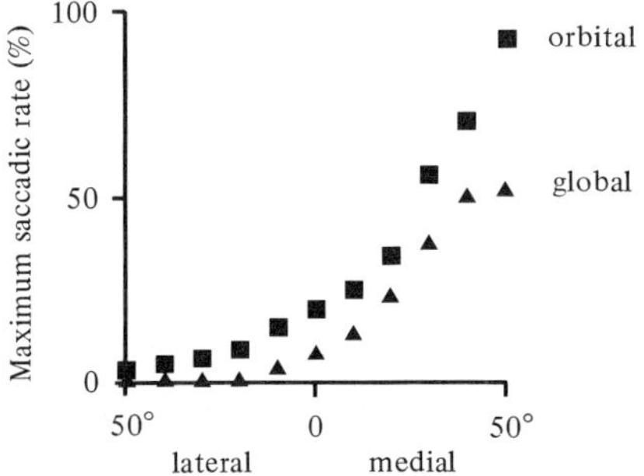

Figure 8.10. Contributions of orbital and global fibres as a percentage of their maximum saccadic activity, at different steady fixation positions (after Collins, 1975).

that its frequency does not alter with saccades of different extent: what happens is that the *duration* increases as the size of the saccade increases (figure 8.12), as was anticipated in Robinson's mechanical analysis (see section 7.5.5) (Fuchs and Luschei, 1970; Schiller, 1970). (This is not true of the *total* muscle electrical activity during saccades, which shows variable amplitude as well as duration as a function of saccade size, on

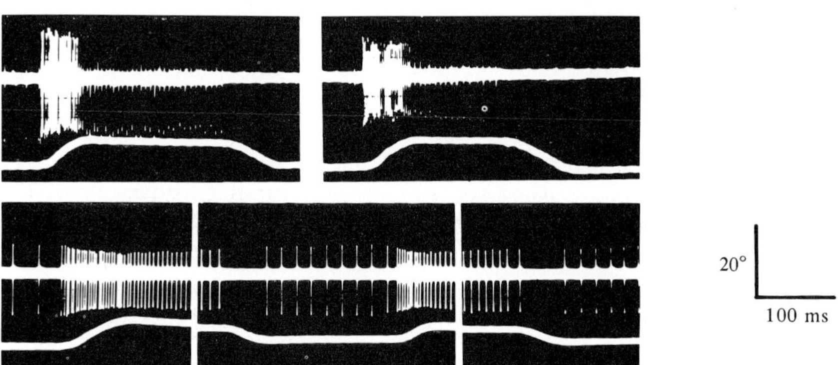

Figure 8.11. Bursts and pauses in oculomotor units during saccadic movements. The records are of spikes from two abducens units (above and below), and the lower trace indicates lateral eye position (upwards = abduction) (Fuchs and Luschei, 1970).

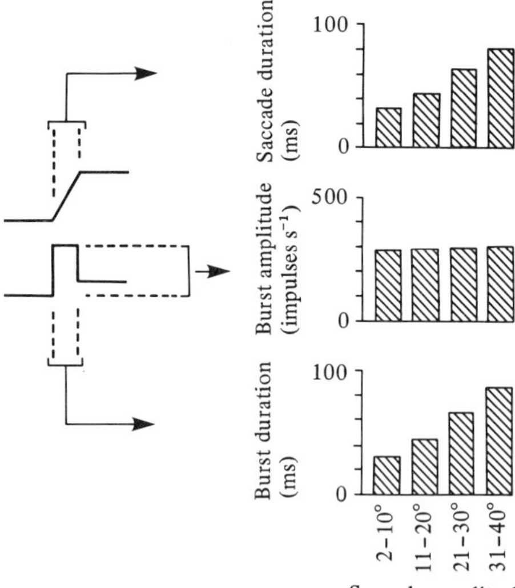

Figure 8.12. Variation of certain parameters of the oculomotor saccadic bursts as a function of saccade amplitude. On the right, from top to bottom, saccade duration, burst amplitude, and burst duration: data from alert monkey (data from Fuchs and Luschei, 1970).

account of the progressive recruitment of extra fibres at different deviations of the eye.) The behaviour of a unit during a saccade also depends to some extent on its particular position characteristic and rate characteristic. If the former is steep, the amplitude of the burst may not be constant in absolute frequency, but vary with the starting eye deviation in such a way that the *change* in frequency is roughly constant; if the velocity characteristic is steep, the burst frequency is less dependent on eye position and appears to represent a saturating value of some 600 impulses per second or more (in the monkey: Robinson, 1970). Saccades in the opposite direction are normally associated with a silent pause whose duration is dependent on the saccade size: but again, some units may not show complete inhibition at extreme deviations. There is thus a satisfactory correlation between the behaviour during tonic deviations of the eye and during fast saccades: in fact these units continue to discharge in a predictable, regular way whatever the *type* of movement taking place, whether saccade, following movement, vestibular reflex, or vergence (Keller and Robinson, 1972; Keller, 1973) (figures 8.13, 8.14).

This is obviously strong evidence against the notion (section 8.1.2) that different types of muscle fibre might be responsible for different classes of eye movement, and in particular that twitch fibres are used only in saccades and slow fibres in vergence and other slow movements. But it is clear, all the same, that the units with higher velocity sensitivity will tend to fire preferentially during fast components of movements, whatever their origin. Yamanaka and Bach-y-Rita (1968) have produced evidence for selective firing of fast and slow fibres in the quick and slow phases of vestibular nystagmus, while Henn and Cohen (1973) have shown that in the alert

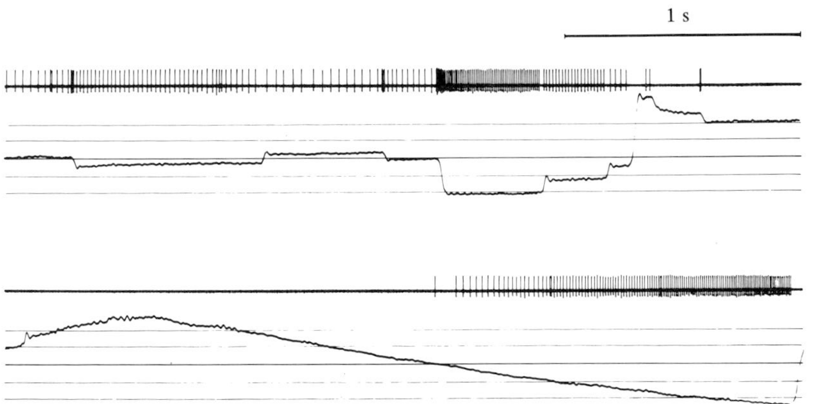

Figure 8.13. The same motor units participate in slow and fast movements. Above, firing frequency of a single unit during voluntary saccades of different sizes and directions; below, the same unit firing in a comparable manner during slow following movements (alert monkey) (Keller and Robinson, 1972).

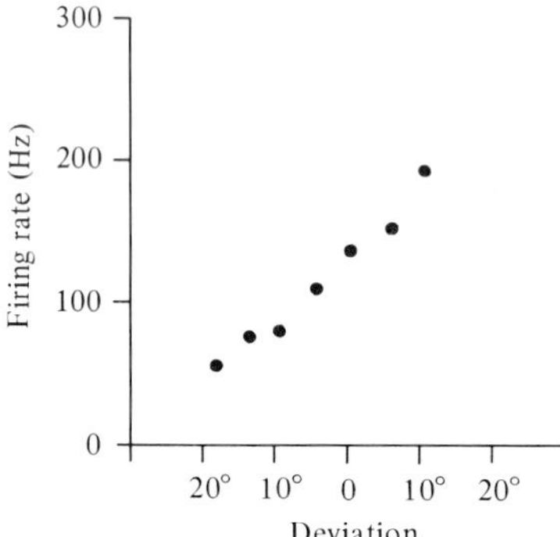

Figure 8.14. Equivalence of oculomotor unit behaviour during vergence and version. The shaded area shows one standard deviation on each side of a measurement of an abducens unit firing rate for far fixation at different deviations. The points show measurements of firing frequency as a function of deviation, when converging by 4°. No discrepancy between the two sets of data can be discerned (data from Keller and Robinson, 1971).

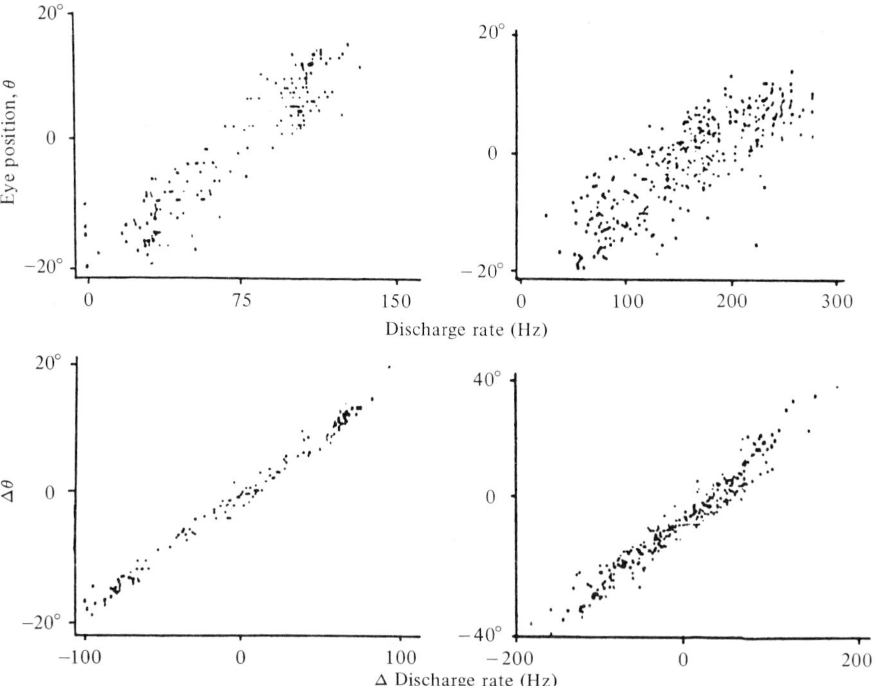

Figure 8.15. Changes of position and of firing frequency of oculomotor units correlate better than absolute values. Data from a predominantly tonic unit in abducens (left) and medial rectus (right) of alert monkeys. Above, in each case, absolute position is plotted against absolute frequency; below, the changes in the quantities are plotted against each other. The reduction in scatter is evident (after Henn and Cohen, 1973).

monkey there is generally a much better correlation between relative *change* of position and of discharge frequency (figure 8.15) than there is between absolute position and absolute frequency before and after saccades, which might well be the result of slowly altering levels of tonic activity from other, unrecorded, units. In the rabbit, Yagi (1974) finds two distinct populations of oculomotor units, one of 'regular' units that correspond with the previously described type, and lie nearer the centre of the nucleus, and a second 'burst' type nearer the periphery. Both show responses on antidromic stimulation of nIII, though the second type is of rather longer latency: a somewhat paradoxical finding since one would anticipate that the burst fibres would be the faster. The possibility that the burst units are actually associated with afferent proprioceptor fibres cannot wholly be ruled out, nor that the 'burst' unit is really a conventional unit with a very high threshold.

A similar distinction between tonic and phasic (or burst) units is seen in recordings made in the regions immediately surrounding the eye movement nuclei (Luschei and Fuchs, 1972; Fuchs and Luschei, 1972; Keller, 1974): such units were first described by Duensing and Schaefer (1957a; 1957b). Further categories described in these regions are 'burst-tonic' (having, like the oculomotor units themselves, both characteristics), and 'pause', which are silent during saccades. The time relation of their activity to the movements varies from unit to unit: some fire 20 ms or more in advance of the movement, while others are active simultaneously with it, or even slightly after. These units presumably directly or indirectly connect with the oculomotor units themselves (though see above, section 8.4.2), and thus provide the path by which the tonic and phasic elements of the motoneuron response pattern are combined from separate pathways.

One suggestive characteristic of at least some of these reticular formation units whose firing is precisely linked to eye position is that they often have preferred directions that are neither horizontal nor vertical, nor indeed correspond to the direction of action of any of the extraocular muscles (Westheimer and Blair, 1972b). In chapter 7 it was pointed out that a complicated transformation has to take place somewhere along the oculomotor final common path between the specification of a desired direction of gaze in visual space, and the set of muscle activities for each eye that are necessary to bring the eye to point in that direction. It is tempting to suppose that these reticular formation units, which fire some 20 ms before activity in the eye muscles, embody eye movement commands expressed in 'visual' coordinates (in fact, in terms of meridional angle and eccentricity, as would be expected from Listing's law: section 7.3.2), and that it is the relative effectiveness of their connections with oculomotor units that translates from this coordinate system into patterns of eye muscle innervation. This is further discussed in section 12.1.

More puzzling are the findings described by Taylor (1965a) and Melvill Jones and Sugie (1965) when recording from neurons in or near N.VI: not only are some units apparently antagonistic, firing when the muscle is relaxing (described also by Precht et al, 1969), but even more oddly, some fire in bursts during both contraction *and* relaxation; such units cannot apparently be fired by antidromic stimulation of nVI (Gogan et al, 1973). Similar 'omnidirectional' responses have also been described by Westheimer and Blair (1972a). It is very difficult to see what possible function they could have.

8.4.4 Stimulation experiments

Experimenters who have stimulated regions in and around the eye muscle nuclei have usually either been interested in purely anatomical matters like the topography of the oculomotor nucleus (already discussed in section 8.4.1), or have been more interested in the functional relation between the characteristics of the stimulus and the resultant response from the muscles. Both types of experiment are open to criticism of the type referred to earlier, but used with caution can provide useful results. Thus Bender and Shanzer (1964) were able, by electrical stimulation of the brainstem of the monkey, to delineate some of the possible pathways converging on the eye muscle nuclei: in particular, they were able to show the existence of a 'physiological' decussation at the level of N.III, in the sense that stimulation above this level tends on the whole to evoke contralateral movement, while that below gives ipsilateral.

Zuber's experiments (Zuber, 1968a; 1968b) were of the second type. He showed that stimulation of the oculomotor area at different frequencies could produce tonic deviations of the eye, with a nearly linear relationship between the two (figure 8.16). If the frequency of stimulation is itself sinusoidally modulated, sinusoidal eye movements can be recorded from which measurements of the frequency transfer function (gain and phase) can be made. His results show a roughly first-order low-pass system (figure 8.17) with a characteristic frequency of about 1–2 Hz. Further experiments (Reinhart and Zuber, 1970) have shown that the phase characteristics can also be adequately represented by a first-order model, if an added transport delay of some 12–13 ms is included: their results are then in good agreement with those expected from Robinson's mechanical model (figure 8.17). However, a delay as large as 12 ms does not accord well with the direct measurement of latencies of movements in response to electrical stimulation of the motor nerves (Robinson, 1968a), which gives values nearer 4–5 ms. The latter figure is of the order that would be expected from consideration of the various components making up the delay: Robinson estimates some 0·3 and 0·7 ms respectively for conduction and synaptic delay, and 2·2 and 1·0 ms for excitation–contraction coupling and mechanical lag. The reason for the disagreement with Zuber's measurements is not clear.

Finally, intracellular stimulation of oculomotor neurons (Barmack, 1974; Daley and Barmack, 1974) has been used to investigate their electrical membrane properties, in the hope of trying to localise the generation of the tonic and phasic components in the neurons themselves rather than in the pathways that control them. They find that the rate of discharge during applied current steps shows an adaptational decline at the beginning, just as in spinal motor neurons, and suggest that this increased firing at the beginning may represent the mechanism producing preemphasis in the saccade. We have already seen that the presence of burst and tonic units in the areas around the oculomotor nuclei makes such an idea unlikely: in any case, the adaptation in these experiments is only superficially similar to the preemphasis of the saccade. The former is of fixed time scale and variable amplitude; the latter, as we have seen, fixed in size but of variable duration.

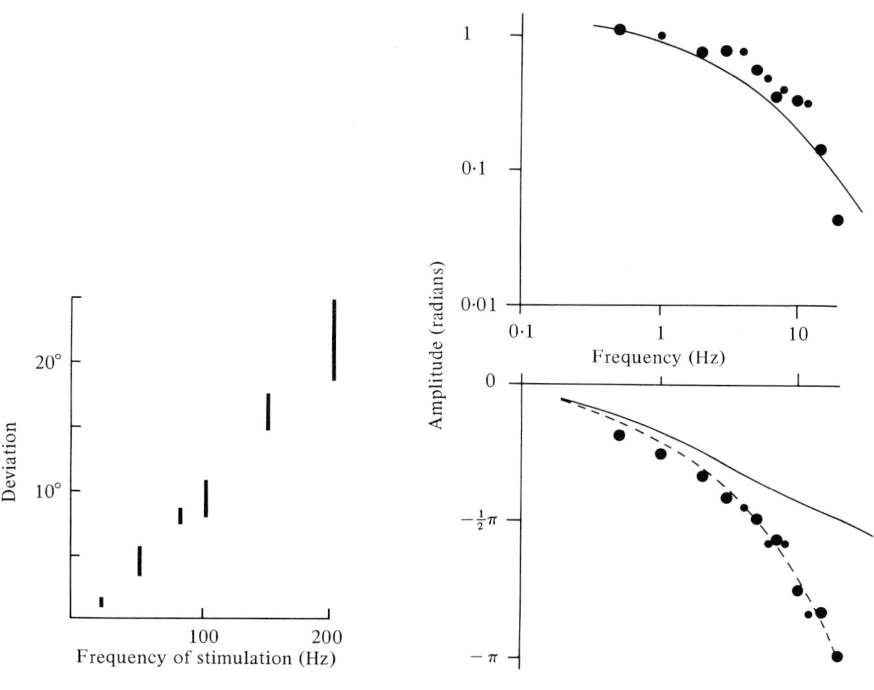

Figure 8.16. Figure 8.17.

Figure 8.16. Deviation of the eye as a function of frequency of electrical stimulation: anaesthetised cat. The third nerve was stimulated within the brainstem. The vertical bars indicate the range of the data points (data from Zuber, 1968).

Figure 8.17. Frequency transfer function for amplitude of eye movement in response to sinusoidal modulation of stimulation frequency of cat oculomotor nerve (after Zuber, 1968a). The smaller circles are single data points, the larger are means of several. The solid lines show Robinson's (1965) transfer function; the broken line is the same function with an added 13 ms delay.

9

Central eye movement pathways

"Let nothing then hinder us from acknowledging the braine to bee the most noble part of the whole body. This is that magnificent and stately turret of the soule, this is that goodly royall palace, the consecrated house of *Pallas*..."

Very many areas of the brain have been shown, at one time or another, to play some part in the control of eye movements: because of their interrelationships it is not easy to deal with them in a systematic way. In this chapter they have been assigned—rather arbitrarily—into four groups, which are examined in their apparent hierarchical order, viz: vestibular nuclei–superior colliculus–cerebellum–cerebral hemispheres. Inevitably, any such division must lead to overlap, and material is sometimes repeated where necessary to reduce the need for continual cross-referencing.

9.1 Vestibular pathways

The basic physiology of the vestibular receptors themselves has already been outlined in chapter 2. Here we will be concerned with the vestibular nuclei and their relation to the oculomotor nuclei and associated regions.

9.1.1 The primary vestibular projection

The *vestibular nuclei* are fundamentally the sensory nuclei of the vestibular nerve; together they form a compact group of cells having an elongated lemon-like shape and forming the lateral floor of the caudal half of the fourth ventricle. Not all the primary vestibular fibres terminate in these nuclei: some pass through them and continue to the cerebellum, mostly to the floccule, nodule, and uvula (Brodal and Høivik, 1964). Four main divisions of the vestibular complex are recognised: they are the *inferior* (or descending) nucleus, the *lateral* (or Deiters') nucleus, the *medial* nucleus, and the *superior* nucleus (figure 9.1). All four nuclei receive at least some primary vestibular fibres, and they differ as to the types of fibre that they receive. Information from the three canals is predominantly represented in the superior and (rostral) medial nuclei, the saccule projects primarily to the (dorsolateral) inferior nucleus, and the utricle to the medial and inferior nuclei (figure 9.2) (Stein and Carpenter, 1967; Gacek, 1969). It is clear from the pattern of vestibular projection within individual nuclei, and from cytoarchitectonic studies, that each is far from being functionally a single unit, and that further subdivisions ought certainly to be made (A Brodal, 1972a). In particular, in each nucleus there are regions—for example the dorsal part of the lateral nucleus—that do not receive a projection from primary vestibular fibres at all: and there are other accessory nuclei lying just outside the classical outline of the vestibular complex (for example the *x, y,* and *z* nuclei) which from their connections ought to be considered as part of the vestibular nuclei (Brodal and Pompeiano, 1957). Brodal (1972a) has reviewed this topic at length.

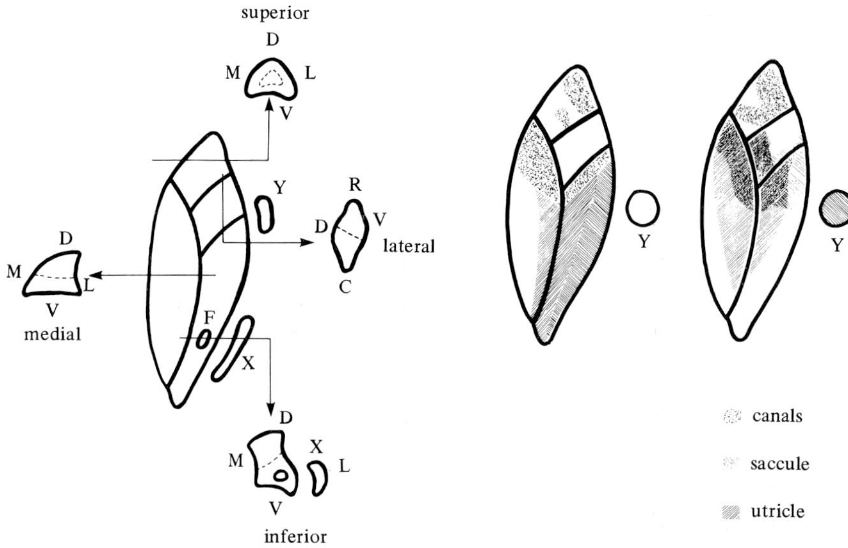

Figure 9.1. Figure 9.2

Figure 9.1. Diagrammatic representation of the main divisions of the left vestibular nucleus (ventral aspect), showing also representative cross sections of the subregions, in the directions indicated by the thin lines. The dotted lines show further subdivisions of a functional nature.

Figure 9.2. Distribution of primary vestibular fibres to the vestibular nuclei, from the sources indicated. Left: according to Stein and Carpenter (1967); right: according to Gacek (1969).

9.1.2 Other afferents to the vestibular nuclei

Apart from fibres originating in the vestibular apparatus, a large afferent contribution to the vestibular complex comes from the cerebellar cortex and the fastigial nuclei. Some fibres originate in the flocculonodular lobe—the classical 'vestibulocerebellum'—and also in the other parts of the vermis that receive primary vestibular fibres as well. The paraflocculus, though it receives primary vestibular fibres, does not project back in this manner (Angaut and Brodal, 1967) These cerebellar fibres project ipsilaterally in a pattern characteristic of their origin (figure 9.3).

The crossed fibres leaving the fastigial nucleus in the uncinate fasciculus project to the superior, (ventral) medial, (ventrolateral) lateral, and inferior nuclei; uncrossed fibres pass mainly in the juxtarestiform body to project to dorsal parts of the inferior medial and lateral nuclei (Walberg et al, 1962). The projection on the lateral nucleus is regular and orderly, reflecting the somatotopic disposition of the original cells in the vermis (figure 9.4).

Another source of afferent fibres is the contralateral vestibular complex. As shown by degeneration studies (Ladpli and Brodal, 1968) and electrical recording (described in section 9.1.3), the most prominent appear to be the mutual connections between the two inferior nuclei and between the two superior nuclei, although other comissural connections may be traced as well (figure 9.5). Such connections would be anticipated on theoretical grounds, to provide complete vestibular information on each side of the brain (because of the functional polarisation of the vestibular receptors discussed in chapter 2). Some physiological consequences of the commisural connections are mentioned in section 9.1.4 below.

It is doubtful whether the nuclei receive fibres *directly* from higher levels of the brain: it is generally proposed that descending influences on the vestibular nuclei are exerted by way of the interstitial nucleus of Cajal, along the medial longitudinal fasciculus: another possible route is

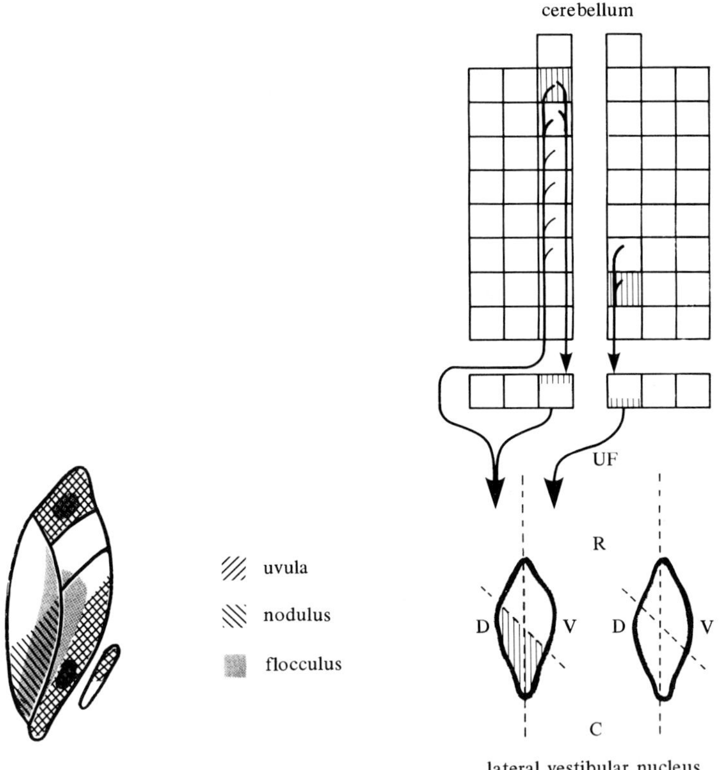

Figure 9.3. Distribution of fibres to the vestibular nuclei from the vestibulocerebellum (after Angaut and Brodal, 1967).

Figure 9.4. Cerebellar projections to the lateral vestibular nucleus (shown below in lateral projection, as in figure 9.1) showing the differential distribution of crossed and uncrossed fibres in the fastigial nuclei. UF is the uncinate fasciculus ('hook bundle'): the highly schematic representation of the cerebellum is explained in figure 9.8 (data from Brodal et al, 1962).

through neurons in the pontine and medullary reticular formation, which sends a small number of afferents to the nuclei (Pompeiano and Walberg, 1957). These latter connections have also been suggested as mediating the well-known effects of arousal level on vestibular nystagmus, and possibly also the rapid eye movements associated with certain states of sleep (Markham, 1972; Pompeiano, 1972). The fibres from the interstitial nucleus appear to project only ipsilaterally, to the dorsal and caudal medial nucleus: since one important input to the interstitial nucleus is from the superior colliculi (see below), it is possible that such projections might also be responsible for the recently demonstrated responses of vestibular neurons to visual field movement (Henn et al, 1974) and to eye movements (Miles, 1974).

One must mention finally that the vestibular nuclei also receive fibres from the spinal cord, largely from the lumbosacral region, but these presumably have little to do with eye movements: conceivably, however, proprioceptive information from the neck may influence oculomotor neurons via vestibulo-ocular paths originating in this way (Hikosaka and Maeda, 1973). These somatic endings are found most abundantly in nuclei *x* and *z*, and less so in caudal regions of the inferior, lateral, and medial nuclei.

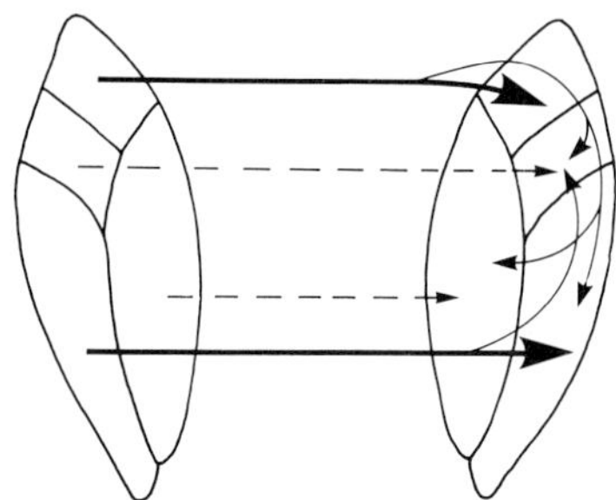

Figure 9.5. Diagrammatic representation of the main commissural connections between the vestibular nuclei on the two sides. The broken lines show connections that are less important or not fully established (after Ladpli and Brodal, 1968).

9.1.3 Efferent pathways

The vestibular nuclei provide the largest single source of fibres to the eye muscle nuclei, and it is clear from physiological (for example Highstein, 1972) and anatomical (for example McMasters et al, 1966) studies that the main projection—via the medial longitudinal fasciculus—is rather precise and orderly. Now one might expect, from a consideration of the axes of the semicircular canals in relation to the muscular axes of the eye, that in the vestibulo-ocular reflex, particular canals need only predominantly activate a small subset of the total of twelve individual extraocular muscles: and this appears to be largely true (figure 9.6: see for example Cohen et al, 1964; Ito et al, 1973a; 1973b). Szentágothai (1950) showed by stimulation of individual canals that the most direct projection of each was to only two extraocular muscles, although more indirect paths, probably not using the medial longitudinal fasciculus at all, could result in small supplementary contributions from other muscles. The latter is perhaps only to be expected from the known secondary actions of the muscles in positions away from the primary, and from inexact correspondence between canal and muscle axes, and in fact the orthodox view since Barany (1906a) has been that every canal is connected to every eye muscle. All the same, one would hope to be able to show projections from the vestibuli nuclei to the eye muscle nuclei corresponding in their pattern to the main canal–muscle relationships: but although the distributions of the projections from the various vestibular nuclei to the oculomotor nuclei are quite precise and distinctive (figure 9.7), they cannot easily be related to the functional requirements of the vestibulo-ocular system. One reason for this is that our knowledge of where *individual* canals project within the vestibular complex is very incomplete—indeed virtually nonexistent—so that for example the fibres that degenerate after destruction of a large area in the superior nucleus, and are rather widely scattered throughout

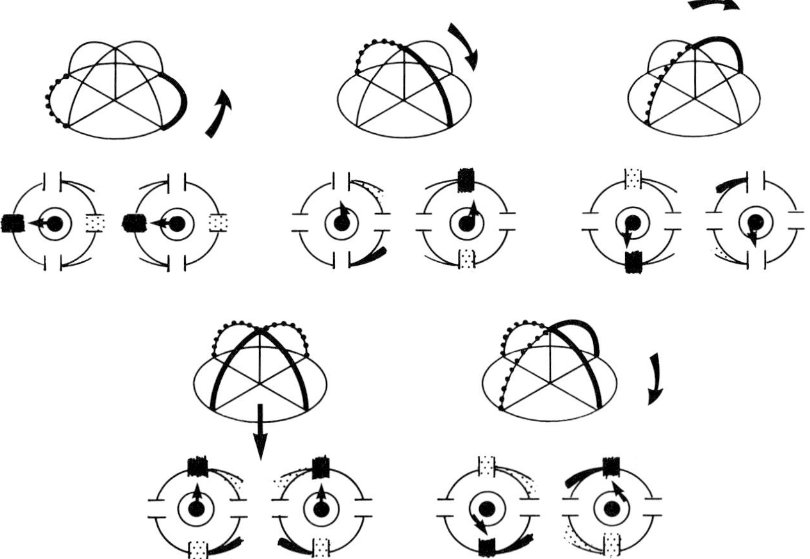

Figure 9.6. Relationships between the semicircular canals and the eye muscles. In each of the five cases, the upper diagram shows a schematic frontal representation of the six canals, the arrow showing the direction of the stimulus rotation, the thickened line the canal that is thus stimulated, and the dotted line the canal that is inhibited. Below, in each case, is a front view of the two eyes and their muscles, the active muscle being shown in black and the inhibited muscles in stipple: the small arrow near the pupil shows the resultant motion of the globe (partly after Cohen et al, 1964).

the oculomotor nuclei, are likely to have been second-order neurons of all three canals. Recent electrical recordings have been able to clarify these relationships with much more accuracy, and are discussed in the next section.

Similarly precise projections, in a rather simple scheme, have been suggested as linking the otolith organs to particular muscles (Szentágothai, 1964); although in the cat, single shocks to the utricular nerve can give almost pure torsion of the eyes, suggesting a more complex projection (Suzuki et al, 1969).

The major descending outflow from the vestibular nuclei is to the spinal cord, in the *vestibulospinal tract* (originating in the lateral nucleus, which is somatotopically arranged), and in the *medial longitudinal fasciculus* (from the medial nucleus). The former projects to all spinal levels and probably influences muscle tone and posture, while the latter projects only to cervical areas (very likely serving the vestibulocollic reflexes), and possibly sending off small collaterals en route to the medullary reticular formation [where gravity responses have recently been demonstrated (Spyer et al, 1974)], and perhaps to visceral motor nuclei.

The last main efferent system of the vestibular complex is that which projects from the (lateral and caudal) inferior and medial nuclei and nucleus X to the cerebellum, via the juxtarestiform body (figure 9.8). Fibres project ipsilaterally to the flocculus (Brodal and Torvik, 1957) and bilaterally to the nodulus and uvula, and possibly the fastigial nuclei; those to the cortex appear to end as mossy fibres (Brodal and Høivik, 1964)

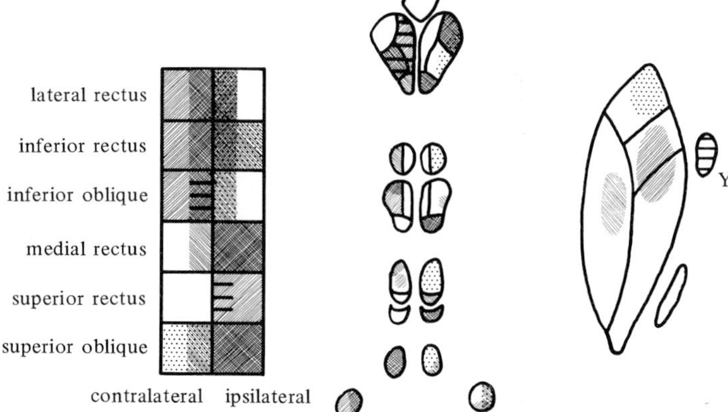

Figure 9.7. Connections between the vestibular and oculomotor nuclei. Lesions placed in the vestibular nuclei as shown on the right resulted in degeneration in the regions of the oculomotor nuclei shown in the centre (using Warwick's representation: see figure 8.8). By correlating these areas with the muscles with which they are associated, one can obtain the schema on the left, which shows the approximate correspondence between the areas of the vestibular nuclei and the eye muscles, suggested by these results. The projection from cell group Y is based on electrophysiological evidence: see also figure 9.16 (data from McMasters et al, 1966).

Brodal (1972b) emphasises that the areas of the vestibular complex that project to the cerebellum are *not* those that receive primary vestibular terminations: thus it seems that no secondary vestibular fibres go to the cerebellum. The main afferent projection to these areas of the vestibular nuclei is the spinal cord, so that it is really more correct to think of these pathways as part of a second spinocerebellar route. But it is possible that secondary vestibular fibres may reach the cerebellum

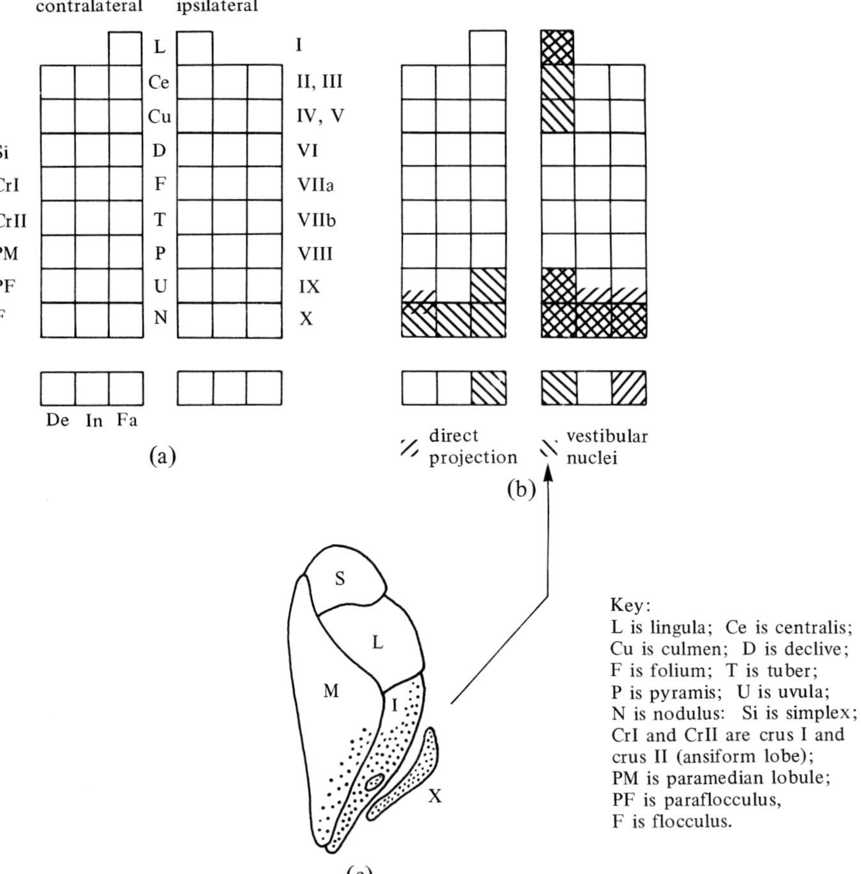

Figure 9.8. Projection from the vestibular nuclei to the cerebellum: (a) key to the highly schematic representation of the cerebellar cortex and deep nuclei (Roberts, 1967). The three columns represent respectively (from inside to outside) vermal, paravermal, and lateral regions of the cortex, divided horizontally as indicated: underneath them lie the fastigial (Fa) interpositus (In) and dentate (De) nuclei. The meanings of the other letters are given in the key. On the right, the corresponding Roman numeral nomenclature is shown. (b) distribution of direct primary vestibular fibres, and secondary fibres from the vestibular nucleus; the origins of the latter are shown stippled in (c) (data from Brodal and Torvik, 1957).

indirectly by means of relays in the reticular formation: the lateral nucleus projects ipsilaterally to the lateral reticular nucleus, and the superior and lateral nuclei both project contralaterally to the reticular tegmental pontine nucleus (figure 9.9). Both of these reticular nuclei have projections to the cerebellum, that probably are not confined to the classical vestibulocerebellum (Brodal, 1972b). Finally, the efferent fibres to the labyrinth that were mentioned in section 2.1.2 appear to originate at least in part in the lateral vestibular nucleus (Gacek, 1961; Rossi and Cortesini, 1965).

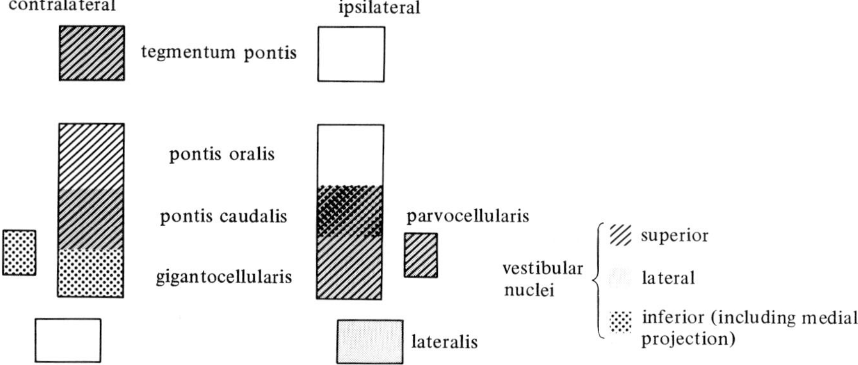

Figure 9.9. Vestibular projections to regions of the reticular formation. Crossed and uncrossed routes are shown respectively on the left and on the right (data from Ladpli and Brodal, 1968).

9 .1.4 Electrical responses from the vestibular nuclei

We saw in chapter 2 how the behaviour of primary vestibular units corresponds quite well with what would be expected from calculation of the mechanical properties of the labyrinth. It turns out that rather little modification of these responses takes place at their first synapse in the central nervous system, with secondary vestibular neurons.

The responses of the secondary units to static tilting (that is, to a stimulus intended to be effective only for the otolith organs) may be classified as monosynaptic or polysynaptic according to their latencies: the monosynaptic responses appear to exhibit no qualities that are not already demonstrable from the primary neurons, and respond oppositely to tilts in opposite directions (Duensing and Schaefer, 1959; Fujita et al, 1968; Peterson, 1970). This is not always true for the apparently polysynaptic responses, which may show an increase (or decrease) in firing rate for tilts in either direction. As would be expected from the topography of the projection of the macular areas to the vestibular nuclei, the most prominent responses of this kind are found in the lateral and inferior nuclei: their distribution within these areas has been discussed by Peterson (1972).

Secondary cells responding primarily to canal stimulation have been investigated by many workers. Shimazu and Precht (Shimazu and Precht, 1965; Precht and Shimazu, 1965) found that in decerebrate cats the units responding to stimulation of the canals could be classified into *type I* (Ewaldian) or *type II* (non-Ewaldian) according as they responded with increased firing to ipsilateral or to contralateral canal stimulation, and into *tonic* and *kinetic* classes according to whether they did or did not show spontaneous firing in the absence of stimulation. Roughly two thirds of the neurons examined were of type I, and one third of type II, while a small number (around 3%) of the cells showed increased firing with rotation in either direction, and an even smaller number showed a *decrease* in activity in either direction (respectively types III and IV). The same proportions of types I and II were found by Melvill Jones and Milsum (1970), although more recently Ryu and McCabe (1973) found, in the inferior nucleus, nearly equal numbers of each type: they also reported that around 40% of the cells in this area showed no response at all to angular acceleration. The existence of the two major types of neuron can most easily be accounted for by invoking the use of the commissural fibres that pass from one vestibular complex to its counterpart on the opposite side. Physiological evidence for a crossed inhibitory pathway comes from evoked field potentials (Shimazu and Precht, 1966) and more recently from a demonstration of ipsilateral excitatory, and contralateral inhibitory, postsynaptic potentials in neurons of the vestibular nuclei as a result of electrical stimulation of ampullary nerves (Kasahara and Uchino, 1974).

The classification of secondary units into tonic and kinetic types is more debatable. Transient stimuli are not necessarily the best way of demonstrating such properties in the presence of strong nonlinearities, because some aspects of the stimulus may exceed the linear region of the device being examined, leading a confusion between effects that are due to a genuine sensitivity to rate of change, and those that are simply the result of the nonlinearity itself. For this reason, sinusoidal stimuli have much to recommend them as they are less likely to overload the system (because of the moderate amplitudes of their higher derivatives), and the effect of varying their frequency on the amplitude and phase of the response gives a direct measure of the system's transfer function, and hence whether it is truly 'tonic' or 'phasic' in nature.

Melvill Jones and Milsum (1970; 1971) have measured the firing frequency of units in the decerebrate cat's vestibular nucleus during sinusoidal rotation in the horizontal plane. Some units—presumably equivalent to Precht and Shimazu's tonic units—fire all the time during such a stimulus, and show a roughly sinusoidal modulation of their frequency of firing in response to it: others are found to show behaviour analogous to rectification, cutting off during part of the cycle (figure 9.10).

Some of these latter cells do not fire when the head is at rest, and would presumably be called 'kinetic' by the previous investigators. But the distinction is not a clear-cut one: often a unit may show both types of behaviour, giving nearly sinusoidal responses for small input amplitudes, and rectification for large. More important, the phase relation between stimulus and response—an indicator of its tonic/kinetic classification—does *not* depend significantly on whether the unit is of the first or second type. The distribution of characteristic phases at any frequency is in fact unimodal, and roughly Gaussian; thus there is no evidence from these studies for the existence of units that are phasic and tonic in the proper sense, and the phase relations found—allowing for a 180° phase change in the type II cells—are virtually identical to those found in the primary fibres themselves (Melvill Jones and Milsum, 1971) (figure 9.11).

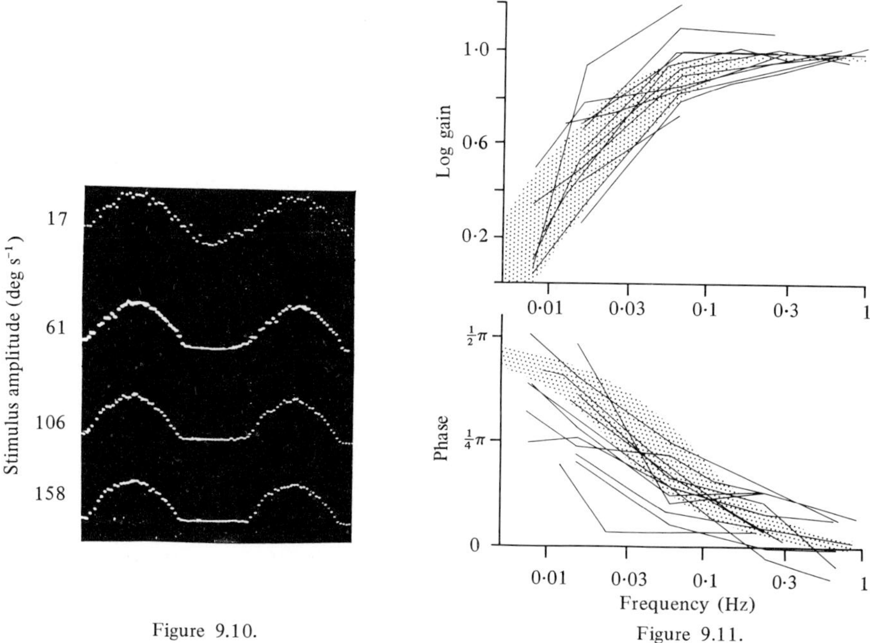

Figure 9.10. Figure 9.11.

Figure 9.10. Firing frequency of a single unit in the decerebrate cat's vestibular nucleus during sinusoidal rotation of the head and body, showing the transition from quasi-linear to rectification behaviour as the amplitude of the stimulus is increased. The frequency of the oscillation was 0·25 Hz (Melvill Jones and Milsum, 1970 (retouched).

Figure 9.11. Frequency transfer functions relating the amplitude and phase of a number of units such as that in figure 9.10 to the sinusoidal input, at different frequencies. Each line represents a separate unit: the shaded area shows what would be expected for a simple first-order system having a time constant lying between 2 and 6 s (data from Melvill Jones and Milsum, 1971).

These results have recently been fully confirmed by Shinoda and Yoshida (1974), and extended to transient behaviour: their careful analysis shows no discrepancy between sinusoidal and transient behaviour, and no suggestion of 'tonic' and 'kinetic' units, although there is some variability in the individual time constants.

Thus over the physiological range of frequencies these units fire at a rate that is—barring nonlinearities—essentially proportional to the angular velocity of the head. Indeed there are very strong reasons why we would certainly not expect to find units responding in a phasic manner to the vestibular input. If this *velocity* information is to be used to control the *position* of the eyes in the vestibulo-ocular reflex, the afferent signal must be *integrated* by the neural pathways with respect to time: exactly the converse operation to the *differentiation* implied by a phasic or adapting response. Maeda et al (1971) have shown, for example, that vestibular afferent fibres in N.VI show a steadily increasing firing rate in response to steady electrical stimulation of nVIII, that is, that these vestibular neurons —not necessarily second-order—are already showing an integrating (and certainly not differentiating) response to vestibular input. If it were true that the second-order neurons gratuitously differentiated the signal they receive, the rest of the vestibulo-ocular pathway would have to undo the damage by performing not one, but *two* integrations to achieve the same end: on the grounds of economy such a scheme seems improbable. This argument does not apply to the otolith organs, which in their function of monitoring the tilt of the head do not have built into themselves the velocity sensitivity associated with the canals. Using sinusoidal tilt, Schor (1974) has recently shown that many units responding to otolith stimulation in lateral and inferior vestibular nuclei show a response that does depend essentially on rate of tilt (figure 9.12), certainly to a much greater extent than the rather slight adaptational component that can be seen in the primary otolith fibres. This in a sense leads to a uniformity of response in the vestibular nuclei to angular *velocity*, whether signalled by otoliths or by the canals.

One further complicating feature of the response of second-order units under sinusoidal stimulation is that they seem to show an intrinsic dynamic asymmetry in addition to their rectifying properties (Milsum and Melvill Jones, 1969), such that the leading edge of the response is often sharper than the trailing edge (figure 9.13). One might suppose that this was the origin of the apparent tonic and kinetic behaviour seen by earlier workers, but it appears that this skewness is also unimodally and quasi-normally distributed, so that it could not be used as a criterion for dividing the cell population into two categories.

Some degree of convergence, and interaction between modalities, appears to take place in the labyrinthine projection to the vestibular nuclei. Markham and Curthoys (1972) found that of the type I and type II horizontal units, more than a third also responded to otolith organ stimulation, while 20% were connected to canals other than the horizontal. Obviously in these experiments one must be careful to refine one's stimulus so that only one mechanism is stimulated at a time: Wilson and Felpel (1972) found that only 6% of their units in the pigeon showed true convergence, although the figure was more than 25% if due account was not taken of this source of error. Kasahara and Uchino (1974) found very little evidence for convergence at all, although they suggest that this may in part be due to the anaesthetic they used. Apparent convergence may be due to interactions in the labyrinth itself, rather than to imprecise stimulation or actual neuronal convergence. Benson et al (1970) showed that certain patterns of linear acceleration may stimulate the *canals* even in the absence of angular movement (see section 2.1.4). Finally, convergence between visual and vestibular input has recently been demonstrated (Henn et al, 1974); units that for example respond to horizontal acceleration to the left can sometimes be found to respond also to an optokinetic stimulus moving to the right. Cooperation between the two modalities is found: at very low frequencies where the canals begin to introduce a phase advance, if an objectively stationary object is presented in the visual field, the units response shows a relative phase lag to maintain the same phase relationship as at higher frequencies.

As far as horizontal angular accelerations are concerned, the relationship between type I and type II units seems well established, and it is possible

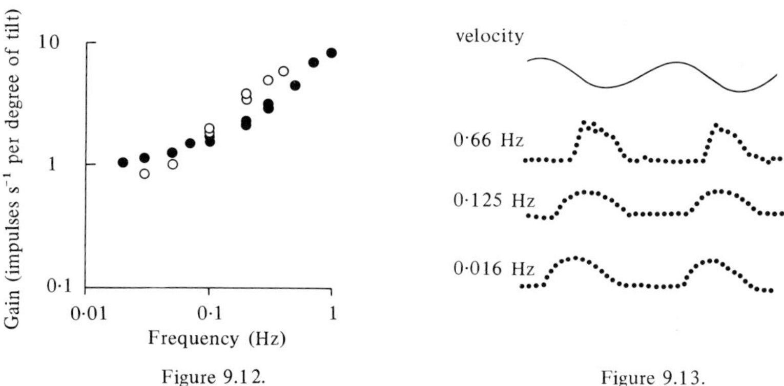

Figure 9.12. Figure 9.13.

Figure 9.12. Frequency response of cells in the vestibular nuclei of a cat during sinusoidal roll tilt: ordinate shows impulses per second per degree of tilt. Filled circles are for a unit in the lateral nucleus, open circles for a unit in the inferior nucleus. Responses of the sort are virtually unchanged if the canals are chronically plugged, and are therefore presumably primarily due to the otolith organs (data from Schor, 1974).

Figure 9.13. Asymmetry of vestibular response as a function of frequency: the three lower traces are averaged tracings of responses to sinusoidal head rotation from units of the same type as in figures 9.10 and 9.11, made at the three frequencies indicated (after Milsum and Melvill Jones, 1969).

to present a tentative scheme of connections to represent the bilateral pathways between the pairs of vestibular nuclei (figure 9.14). One advantage of such an arrangement is that it converts the essentially nonlinear (in fact, unidirectional) responses of the vestibular end organs into a signal that is more or less linear, by a process closely analogous to a push–pull output amplifier stage (figure 9.15). We saw the same arrangement occurring—for slightly different reasons—in the mechanics of the opponent eye muscles (section 7.5.3): Linearisation may perhaps be a more common feature of the bilateral organisation of the nervous system than has hitherto been suspected.

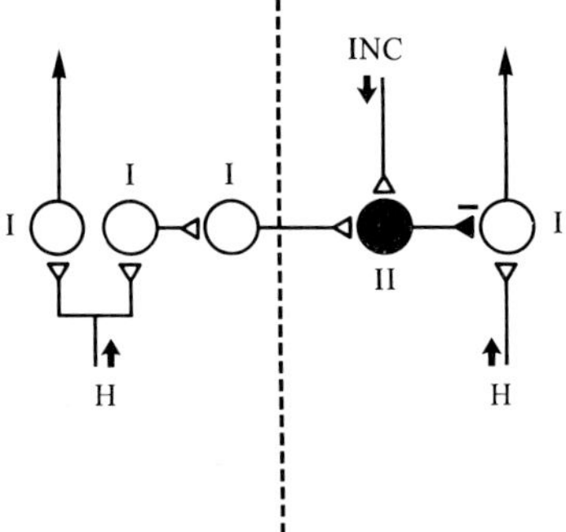

Figure 9.14. Schematic representation of bilateral relationships between cells in the vestibular nuclei driven by input from the horizontal canals (H), showing type I and type II cells, as well as descending influences from the interstitial nucleus of Cajal (INC).

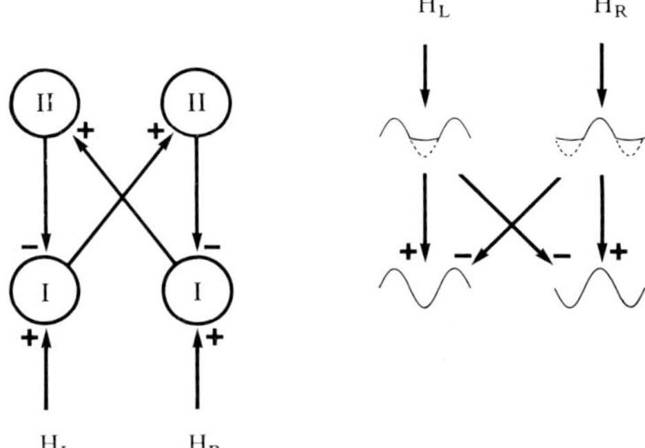

Figure 9.15. Left: simplified summary of the bilateral relationships between type I and type II cells, and their horizontal canal inputs on the left and right (H_L and H_R). On the right, showing how an arrangement of this sort can convert the essentially rectified input from the horizontal canals into a bilateral input that is much more closely linear, in an analogous manner to a 'push–pull' amplifier.

9.1.5 Physiology of the projection to the eye muscle nuclei

There are at least three routes by which the vestibular nuclei can influence the eye muscle nuclei. Signals can travel directly via the medial longitudinal fasciculus as part of the 'three-neuron arc'; through (presumably polysynaptic) paths in the reticular formation; or possibly via the cerebellum. Only experiments relating to the first two routes will be discussed here: cerebellar pathways will be discussed when the cerebellum itself is dealt with (in section 9.3.5). It is convenient to begin with the rather older observations on the effects of lesions in the pathways concerned, and then to turn to more recent electrophysiological evidence.

One of the oldest points of dispute concerned the relative importance of the medial longitudinal fasciculus and reticular pathways. Despite the simplicity and directness of the 'three-neuron arc', it is clear that it cannot represent the only vestibulo-ocular pathway, for destruction of the medial longitudinal fasciculus, although reducing the amplitude of vestibulo-ocular reflexes (especially the faster components) does not abolish them (Lorente de No, 1933). On the other hand, even localised lesions in the medial longitudinal fasciculus can have profound effects specifically on voluntary lateral deviations of the eyes, suggesting either that the pathways for such movements include neurons in the vestibular nuclei, or possibly that they use fibres entering the medial longitudinal fasciculus other than vestibular ones. The effects of such lesions depends on the level at which they are made. Experimental studies in the monkey (Carpenter and McMasters, 1963; Carpenter and Strominger, 1965; and others) showed that lesions rostral to the abducens nucleus produce an unyoking of lateral movements (the clinical 'anterior internuclear ophthalmoplegia') presumably due to a severance of the pathways responsible for the coordination of medial and lateral rectus, while large bilateral lesions at the level of the abducens nucleus produce paresis of lateral gaze in both directions, with convergence and vertical movements unaffected.

Since unilateral lesions of the medial longitudinal fasciculus produce degenerative changes only in the area of the oculomotor complex corresponding to the ipsilateral medial rectus (Carpenter, 1971), it would appear that vestibular fibres to the eye muscle nuclei for planes of rotation other than horizontal must pass in some other route. Pasik et al (1969a; 1969b) found that lesions in the pretectal area, especially in the region of the accessory oculomotor nuclei, could produce specific disturbances of vertical movements, without affecting horizontal, and there is evidence now that neurons in the paramedian pontine reticular formation may send ascending fibres either in the medial longitudinal fasciculus or near it, that project to the eye muscle nuclei (reviewed in Cohen, 1971). Monosynaptic afferent inhibitory and excitatory connections from units in the pontine reticular formation to the oculomotor nucleus have recently been demonstrated by Highstein et al (1974). Indeed it was the observation that extensive lesions in this area—sparing the medial longitudinal fasciculus—had a profound effect on vestibular and other eye movements that led Lorente de No (1933) to doubt the all-suffiency of the three-neuron arc; although his findings were criticised at the time (Spiegel and Price, 1939), recent work has confirmed them fully (Bender and Shanzer, 1964; McCabe, 1965).

Some of the disagreement may partly have been due to the rather coarse descriptions of eye movements that were—and indeed often still are—used to characterise the result of a particular experimental procedure. Now that we know a little more about the neural activity associated with fast movements such as saccades—in particular the existence of separate fast and slow components—it is evident that it is simply not good enough merely to observe that saccades are or are not present. If for example a particular lesion were to result in the abolition of the initial bursts in saccades, whilst the tonic component remained, casual observation might well not notice anything amiss, since the eyes would still execute movements of the same amplitude as before, and one might conclude that the lesion had no effect. In fact a comparison of the effects of lesions in the mesencephalic reticular formation on the quick and slow phases of nystagmus shows that these more subtle differences do in fact occur (McCabe, 1965; Harris et al, 1967): quick phases and slow phases of nystagmus are strongly differentially affected ipsilaterally and contralaterally by such lesions. Evidence supporting the idea that the paramedian pontine reticular formation may be especially concerned with the slower components comes from electrical stimulation (Bender and Shanzer, 1964; Cohen, Komatsuzaki, and Harris, 1967): whereas stimulation of the medial longitudinal fasciculus typically results in a steady deviation of the eye lasting much the same period as the stimulus, stimulation in this region results in a constant *velocity* of deviation, as if integration of the signal were being performed peripherally to the point of stimulation (Cohen and Komatsuzaki, 1972). The fidelity of integration is greater than would be expected from a consideration of the mechanical properties of the eye, implying that the function is not pure integration, but of the 'proportional plus integral' form noted previously in the generation of saccades (Keller, 1974).

Another recent finding lending support to the idea of separate pathways for slow and fast components of eye movements is Westheimer and Blair's (1973a) observation that low-level electrical stimulation near the midline in pretectal dorsal areas and pontine areas ventral to the medial longitudinal fasciculus can produce selective inhibition of saccades and nystagmus quick phases, but not of on-going slow movements. However, Sparks and Travis (1971), Cohen and Henn (1972) and Sparks and Sides (1974), recording from pontine reticular formation units near the abducens nucleus, find on the contrary that at least some units respond only to fast movements, showing either a burst or a pause, in the manner described earlier for other cells in and around the eye movement nuclei (see above, section 8.4.3). No doubt the truth is that both types of response are represented in separate intermingled populations in the reticular formation, and that it is misleading to think of it as a single structure, or even as a series of homogeneous subregions. Our knowledge of reticular mechanisms is at present rather scanty, partly because workers have preferred to concentrate on the more easily defined—but not necessarily more important—route through the medial longitudinal fasciculus.

Microelectrode recording from the abducens nucleus during vestibular stimulation has clarified some of the synaptic relations involved (Baker et al, 1969; Maeda et al, 1972; Schwindt et al, 1973). Single shocks of the ipsilateral vestibular nerve produce inhibitory postsynaptic potentials, while during repetitive stimulation the abducens neurons show periodic electrical phenomena in step with the resultant horizontal nystagmus. During this nystagmus it is possible to show that the slow phase is associated with a slowly increasing inhibitory current and a subsidiary slow decrease in excitatory current, while the quick phase is predominantly due to a sudden increase in the excitatory drive. Almost symmetrically inverted responses can be simultaneously recorded from contralateral abducens neurons: excitatory and inhibitory effects both seem to be disynaptic. By similar methods (Precht, 1972; Highstein, 1972; Baker et al, 1973; Baker and Berthoz, 1974) it can be shown that neurons in the trochlear nucleus receive ipsilateral inhibitory connections from neurons in the superior vestibular nucleus, and excitatory ones from neurons in the

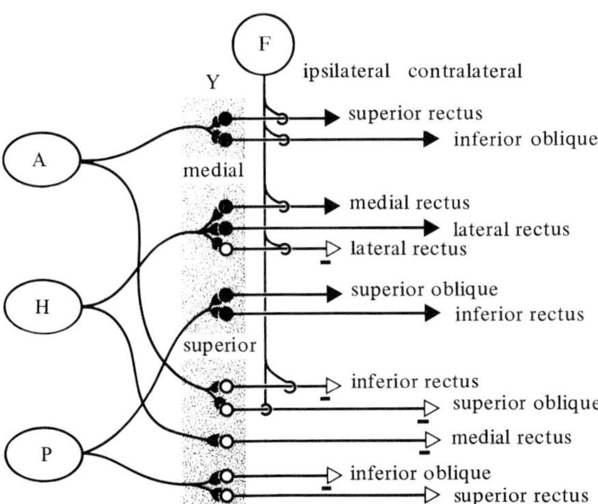

Figure 9.16. Postulated scheme of connections between primary vestibular fibres from the three semicircular canals (A, H, and P) with secondary units in the vestibular nuclei, and their projection in turn to the eye muscles: the inhibitory influence of the flocculus (F) on some parts of the latter are shown by encircling loops. Filled arrows show excitatory projections; open arrows, inhibitory (data from Ito et al, 1973c).

contralateral (rostral) medial vestibular nucleus: pathways for other muscles have been worked out by comparable means (for example Berthoz et al, 1973; Ito et al, 1973a; 1973b) (figure 9.16), and at least some of them are influenced by proprioceptors in the neck (Hikosaka and Maeda, 1973).

Finally, some evidence is beginning to accumulate that ordinary chemical synapses are not the only means by which information can be transmitted from the primary vestibular fibres to the medial longitudinal fasciculus. Extremely short latency responses (around 0·4–0·5 ms) can be recorded in the fasciculus following electrical stimulation of the labyrinth (Wilson and Wylie, 1970; Horcholle-Bossavit and Tyc-Dumont, 1971; Grey and Barnes, 1973), and it seems possible to rule out stimulus spread, antidromic invasion of efferents to the labyrinth, and the existence of primary vestibular fibres in the medial longitudinal fasciculus. Studies of antidromic graded depolarisations suggest that the synapse in the vestibular nucleus may indeed be partly electrical in nature (Korn et al, 1973), possibly involving the 'tight junctions' observed in the lateral vestibular nucleus (Sotelo and Palay, 1967), though it is perhaps too early to give full acceptance to such an unexpected conclusion.

9.1.6 The interstitial nucleus of Cajal

This is a convenient point to mention recent work on the synaptic articulations of the interstitial nucleus, on account of its involvement both with the oculomotor nuclei and with certain parts of the vestibular complex. This nucleus projects bilaterally to all parts of the third nerve nucleus except the region corresponding to the medial recti (Carpenter, 1971): and in fact the results of electrical stimulation suggest that it is concerned only with vertical movements of the head and eyes (Szentágothai, 1943; Hyde and Toczek, 1962; Hassler, 1972; and others). Schwindt et al (1974) have recorded excitatory and inhibitory postsynaptic potentials from neurons in N.IV and N.III, arising apparently monosynaptically from stimulation of the interstitial nucleus: no responses could be evoked in the abducens nucleus. Matsunami (1972) has recorded from neurons in and around this area, and found units that discharge during saccades in the dark, some 2–12 ms before the beginning of the movement: this latency is very similar to that found in the eye muscle nuclei.

It also projects ipsilaterally to the (caudal) medial vestibular nucleus (Pompeiano and Walberg, 1957), and electrophysiological studies (Markham et al, 1966; Markham, 1968) show that stimulation of the interstitial nucleus can produce, on the ipsilateral side, both inhibition of type I neurons in the vestibular nucleus, and excitation of type II neurons (figure 9.14). These effects are probably mediated by the medial longitudinal fasciculus: after section, Markham et al (1966) found that some of these effects were reversed, and suggested a secondary route through the reticular formation, having opposed effects. One slightly puzzling feature is that the inhibition is most marked on type I cells corresponding to the *horizontal* canals (Markham, 1968—precisely the plane of rotation which the interstitial nucleus was thought not to be interested in. It is difficult to see how antagonism between rotatory responses in orthogonal planes would serve any purpose.

Possible roles for the interstitial nucleus of Cajal in mediating signals from the superior colliculi and from the cerebral hemispheres are discussed in subsequent sections of this chapter.

9.2 Superior colliculus

9.2.1 Structure and fibre connections

The two pairs of colliculi—inferior and superior—form the tectum or roof of the mesencephalon (figure 8.7). The superior colliculus is homologous with the relatively larger optic tectum of submammalian vertebrates, but with the increasing consequence of cortical visual areas as one proceeds through mammals to man, the importance and size of the superior colliculus has declined. In man it appears to have little to do with the elaboration of visual sensations and is primarily concerned in the automatic control of eye movements in relation to visual stimuli, and of other simple visual reactions. The *inferior* colliculus is primarily auditory in function, but may form part of the mechanism by which saccades can be evoked by localised sounds: eye movements can be elicited by electrical stimulation of the inferior colliculus (Syka et al, 1973), but the area has been largely neglected by oculomotor physiologists.

The superior colliculus is conventionally divided into four layers: starting from the inside, they are the *stratum lemnisci,* the *stratum opticum,* the *stratum cinereum* and the *stratum zonale* (figure 9.17). The stratum lemnisci, which may be further divided into gray and white layers, has many large and medium sized cells whose axons form the main output of the colliculus: these fibres project bilaterally into the pontine and medullary reticular formation [to the same regions that receive fibres from the cerebellum, cerebral cortex, and vestibular nuclei (Kawamura et al, 1974)], and to the interstitial nucleus of Cajal and the nucleus of Darkschewitsch (Altman and Carpenter, 1961; Graybiel and Hartweig, 1974). There is thought to be no direct projection to the oculomotor nuclei themselves (Szentágothai, 1950). Afferent fibres from the frontal eye fields seem to terminate mostly in the stratum leminisci (Astruc, 1971). Other efferents project to the tectospinal tract, to parts of the lateral and medial geniculate bodies, the pulvinar of the thalamus, the pretectum, and to dorsolateral pontine nuclei (Altman and Carpenter, 1961). This last-mentioned tectopontine tract may also be a route by which visual information can reach the cerebellum, although direct projections from the (ventral) lateral geniculate to the pons have also recently been demonstrated (Edwards et al, 1974). It is interesting to note that there is a disynaptic route to cervical motoneurons, via the tectospinal and tectoreticular tracts (Abrahams et al, 1975).

The stratum opticum consists largely of afferent visual fibres from the retina and lateral geniculate, terminating mostly in the stratum cinereum, and in deeper layers, where responses to extraocular stretch have also been reported (Cooper et al, 1955). The stratum cinereum is composed of radial bipolar cells, conducting inwards; they also receive afferents from the occipital cortex, which form the fibres of the stratum zonale: small horizontal cells are also found in this latter layer. In the cat, several areas of the cortex project in characteristic patterns to different layers of the colliculus (Sprague, 1963). Finally, afferent fibres from the reticular formation can be demonstrated (Scheibel and Scheibel, 1958; Nauta and Kuypers, 1958) which might provide a possible route by which vestibular information could reach the superior colliculus: some such arrangement is required to explain the visuovestibular responses described by Bisti et al (1974). Auditory responses, particularly to moving sounds, and responses to touching the skin have also been described (Gordon, 1973).

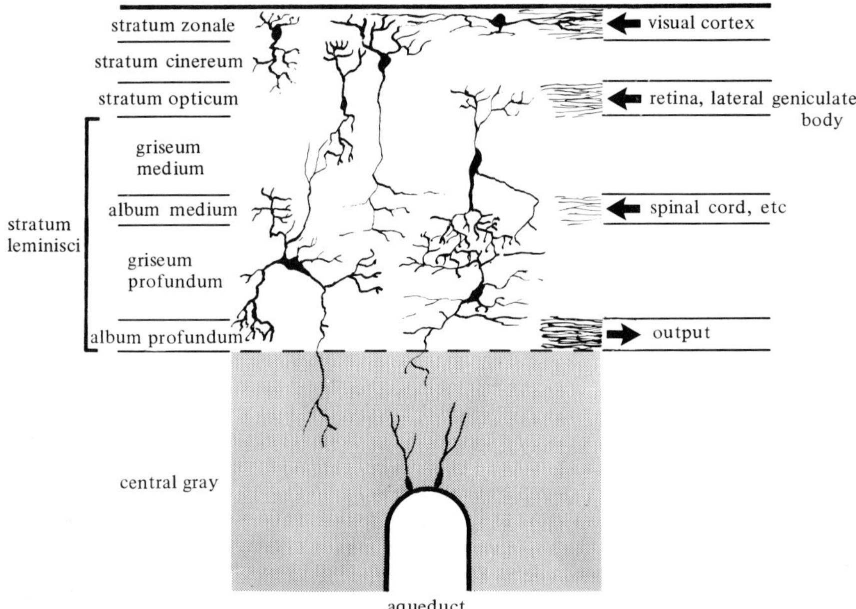

Figure 9.17. Schematic cross section of the layers of the superior colliculus, showing typical cell types (in the centre), and fibre connections (on the right).

9.2.2 Electrical responses to visual stimulation

Species differences in the types of visual response that can be recorded from the superior colliculus are less marked than one might expect, considering its changing role in the evolution of the vertebrate visual system, perhaps because corticotectal fibres can send back to the colliculus the results of some of the kinds of elaboration of visual information that the colliculus used to do for itself, and have now been taken over by the cortex. Thus, after ablation of the visual cortex of the cat, the directional sensitivity of collicular units is lost (Wickelgren and Sterling, 1969; Richard et al, 1973). In all species studied, units can be found that respond to the movement of visual objects (Cronly-Dillon, 1964; Straschill and Hoffmann, 1970; Masland et al, 1971; Straschill and Rieger, 1972) and to stationary spots (Grüsser-Cornehls et al, 1963; Schaefer, 1972): only about half typically respond to diffuse illumination. The organisation is retinotopic, and may be either contralaterally or bilaterally organised, depending on the species (Lane et al, 1973). The projections from the striate cortex are such as to preserve retinotopicity (Crosby and Henderson, 1948; McIlwain and Fields, 1971; McIlwain, 1973), although it is not always true that cells that are close together in the colliculus receive fibres from cells close together in the visual cortex. The cells seem to be arranged in columns, with moving- and stationary-stimulus cells being found at opposite ends (Michael, 1970): the former type may be innervated by complex cells in the visual cortex (Palmer and Rosenquist, 1974).

In the cat (but not in the monkey: Schiller, 1972; Wurtz and Goldberg, 1972a) the preferred directions of collicular units appear to be arranged in a highly systematic way that has some significance in relation to the structure's optomotor function: the preferred direction for a particular cell is highly correlated with its position in the visual field, in such a way that it responds best to objects moving away from the point of fixation (Straschill and Rieger, 1972; 1973). Such an arrangement would provide automatically for convergence of information about both the displacement of an object from the point of fixation, and the rate at which this displacement is increasing, and might thus form the neural mechanism underlying the elegantly coordinated responses to ramp-step stimuli that were described in section 4.2.2.

9.2.3 Modification of visual responses by other afferent information

A certain amount of evidence is accumulating that can be interpreted as meaning that some collicular units are able to distinguish between movements of images over the retina that are due to actual movement of an object in space, and those that are merely due to eye movement. Such a discrimination demands either proprioceptive information from eye muscles, or knowledge, derived from the centres that initiate the eye movements, that an eye movement is about to occur ('corollary discharge' or 'efference copy'). The difficulty with the latter idea is that, if—as appears to be the case—the superior colliculus is *itself* in some sense a centre of this kind that can initiate eye movements, it is difficult to see how one would set about demonstrating 'efference copy', or even what meaning—if any—could be attached to the notion. All the same, it is clear that discharges related to eye movements in a manner independent of visual stimulation can be recorded (Johnstone and Mark, 1969; Straschill and Hoffmann, 1970; Hermann, 1971; Wurtz and Goldberg, 1972b).

Straschill and Hoffmann found that in the cat's superior colliculus some 10% of the cells studied fired when the eyes moved, irrespective of whether or not there was any simultaneous visual stimulation; of the rest, half responded to eye movements only in the presence of stationary visual objects, and about a fifth responded only to 'real' shifts of objects in space, and not to shifts caused by eye movements. This last class of cell might therefore form the basis of an 'objective' map of the visual world in the superior colliculus, rather than a strictly retinotopic 'subjective' map. But it is very difficult to see how both maps could exist in an intermingled fashion amongst the neurons of the superior colliculus: one could conceive of an entirely subjective organisation, or just possibly of an entirely objective one, but to have *both* seems something of an *embarras de richesse.* The idea of an objective map introduces enormous difficulties in itself: to be useful, it would presumably also have to take account of head movements, and even displacements of the whole body. Evidently such a map is potentially infinite in extent: in any case, collicular neurons do not in fact respond to head movements in this kind of way, even when the head movement is such as to alter—through the vestibulo-ocular reflex—an on-going eye movement (Robinson and Jarvis, 1974). A further difficulty lies in the relative timing of the visual and eye-movement discharges. Although visual responses typically show a latency of some 50–100 ms, the responses associated with saccades actually occur *before* the eye movement (Schiller and Koerner, 1971). While this is only to be expected if the eye movement responses represent essentially *motor* discharges, it clearly limits their usefulness as corollary information.

A different type of modification of visual response by eye movements has been described by Wurtz and Mohler (1974), who find the visual sensitivity of a collicular unit rises just before the animal makes a saccade to the equivalent region; saccades to other regions do not have the same effect. Possibly this represents a shift of attention or awareness prior to the eye movement. Other, more complex, effects are described by Hayashi et al (1974). A related observation is that visual responses can apparently be reduced when other, 'newer', visual stimuli are introduced into the visual field (Rizzolatti et al, 1973; Camarda et al, 1974). Such a process may represent a mechanism for directing attention to interesting visual objects, and a competitive arrangement of this type is only to be expected in the release of visually evoked saccades. Clearly, if two visual objects appear suddenly in the visual field, a foveating saccade must be directed at either one or the other of them: any kind of compromise—for example, fixation of a spot somewhere in between them—is useless. Simultaneous electrical stimulation of two parts of the colliculus (Robinson, 1972) does produce a movement virtually equivalent to the vector sum of those obtainable from each point separately, however; although if the two stimuli are separated in time a refractory period is observed after the first stimulus, after which the second can evoke its own characteristic movement.

9.2.4 Optomotor functions

The superior colliculus was one of the first areas from which eye movements were obtained by electrical stimulation, over a hundred years ago (Adamück, 1870), yet the importance of the colliculus in the control of eye movements was underestimated for a long time on account of the very slight effects that lesions here often have on eye movements in animals (see Pasik and Pasik, 1964), and the lack of a *direct* projection to the oculomotor nuclei. But as we have seen, collicular fibres certainly terminate in the interstitial nucleus of Cajal and in the nucleus of Darkschewitsch, and a large number of investigators over recent years have revealed a highly organised representation of ocular movements in the superior colliculi. All the same, one should not jump to conclusions: not everything that moves the eyes on stimulation is necessarily oculomotor, except in the most trivial sense, and it may be that the animal that makes saccades when his colliculus is stimulated is merely deciding to look at an interesting visual phosphene. The point is argued more forcibly in connection with the cerebral cortex (section 9.4.3), where it is perhaps more relevant still.

The first evidence for a close correlation between visual responses and oculomotor responses in the colliculus was provided by Apter (1946): he showed that if strychnine was applied to a small area of it, and a flash of light presented to the eye, the eye moved to roughly the same part of the visual field as that from which a spot of light evoked the greatest electrical response in the region of strychninisation, thus demonstrating a rough equivalence between the two kinds of map. Recent work has fully confirmed and elaborated his findings (Robinson, 1972; Schiller, 1972; Schiller and Stryker, 1972; Wurtz and Goldberg, 1972b; Straschill and Rieger, 1972). Electrical stimulation, especially in the deeper layers, produces natural-looking saccades of a direction and amplitude such that, if the eye starts in the primary position, it finishes up looking at the part of the visual field corresponding to the receptive field for visual responses from the same area (figure 9.18). This response is very little related to any parameter describing the stimulus except its position on the surface of the colliculus: even depth of penetration has little influence (Robinson, 1972). There is not, unfortunately, total agreement about what happens if the eye starts in some position other than the primary. Robinson, Schiller, and Wurtz and Goldberg all agree that the resultant saccade has a direction and an amplitude that are *not* influenced by the initial position of the eye: in particular, prolonged repetitive stimulation over the course of a second or so results in a series of saccades—a staircase—each of which is of roughly the same size and direction, despite the movement of the eye across the field (figure 9.19).

Straschill and Rieger (1972; 1973), on the other hand, are equally positive that the direction and amplitude are profoundly influenced by the initial position, and that indeed the evoked saccades are *goal-directed,* bringing the eye to a point fixed in *space* rather than one having a fixed relation to the initial position of the *eye* (figure 9.20) see also Hyde and Eason (1959). They have suggested that a possible reason for the discrepancy may lie in the rather lower stimulation currents that they have used, compared with those of other workers (Straschill and Rieger, 1973). All the same, the obvious theoretical difficulties associated with a space-fixed oculomotor map are so great that at present the other findings must inevitably carry greater weight. It seems inconceivable, if the superior colliculus is really an important oculomotor region, that it should first laboriously convert the retina's subjective visual map into a

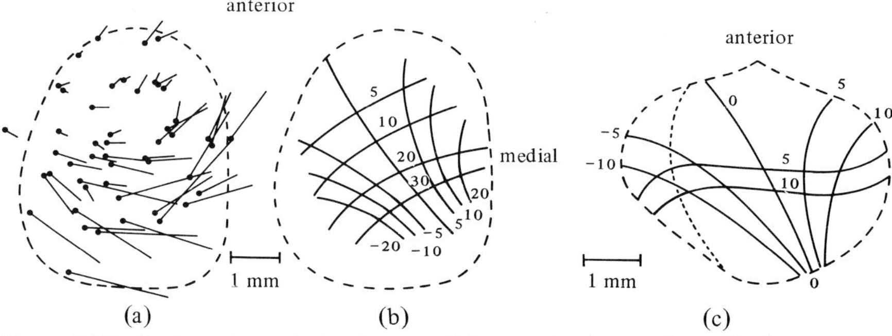

Figure 9.18. Oculomotor and visual maps of the monkey's superior colliculus: (a) outline plan of left colliculus, showing points of stimulation, with the resultant eye movements indicated by the amplitude and direction of associated lines; (b) approximate oculomotor map derived from observations like those on the left, the amplitudes and direction in degrees being shown by the horizontal and vertical coordinates; (c) visual map obtained by electrical recording and plotted in a corresponding fashion: the general accordance between the two maps is evident (data from Robinson, 1972; Cynader and Berman, 1972).

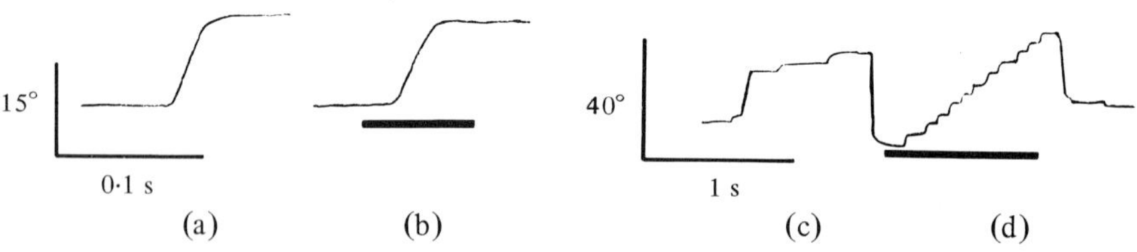

Figure 9.19. Saccade-like movements from electrical stimulation of the monkey's superior colliculus: (a) a normal voluntary saccade; (b) a saccade obtained by electrical stimulation of the colliculus for the time shown by the bar: the 'realistic' appearance of the saccade is obvious: (c) a sequence of spontaneous saccades, followed by (d) a saccade staircase obtained by prolonged electrical stimulation, as indicated (after Robinson, 1972).

collicular objective map before calculating the necessary eye movements: particularly as an objective oculomotor map would then have to be reconverted back into subjective form before it could be made use of by the peripheral oculomotor apparatus! The staircase effect with repeated stimulation is particularly strong—surely incontrovertible—evidence in favour of a subjective map: and it is noteworthy that Apter (1946), in the very first experiments of this type and using a stimulus in a sense more 'physiological' than even Straschill and Rieger's tiny currents, described exactly the same staircase phenomenon with repeated flashes of light.

Of course, the more closely matched we find the visual and oculomotor maps to be, and the more independent the evoked eye movements are of the nature of the stimulus, the more our suspicions must grow that this region is not really any more essentially oculomotor than any other part of the visual system. Certainly the fact remains that lesions in it have strikingly little effect on visually evoked saccades. Wurtz and Goldberg (1972a; 1972c) have shown that if small lesions are made in the superior colliculi of monkeys, and visually evoked saccades to the corresponding area are compared with those to other parts of the field, *no* significant differences can be observed in the velocity, amplitude, or accuracy with which they are made. The only apparent difference is that they are delayed relative

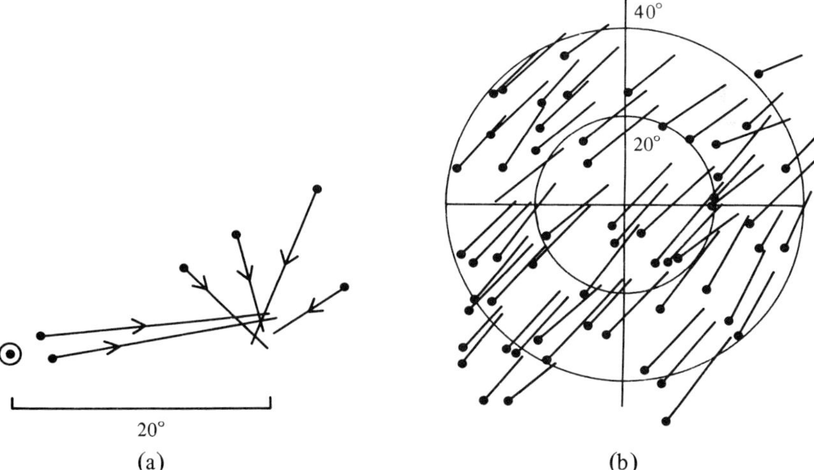

Figure 9.20. The difference between goal-directed and position-independent evoked saccades. (a) Goal-directed movements: electrical stimulation when the eye started in the positions shown by the dots resulted in movements that were clearly dependent on the initial position, and directed approximately to a goal situated at some 20° from the primary position (circled dot). (b) Quite different findings in another preparation: here the direction and amplitude are hardly affected by the initial position, even when it is more than 40° from the primary position, and the movements are certainly not goal-directed (after Straschill and Rieger, 1972; Schiller, 1972).

to normal saccades by some 150 to 300 ms. Similarly, latencies are increased for contralateral eye movements after hemicolliculectomy in man: but even this effect is lost with the passage of time (Heywood and Ratcliff, 1975). It seems therefore that whatever the function of the superior colliculus in eye movements may be, it is one that is also carried out—though with less despatch—by some other part of the brain: a possible candidate for this role is the visual cortex, whose rise to prominence in the phylogenetic tree has coincided with the eclipse of the optic tectum.

9.3 The cerebellum

9.3.1 Structure

The situation and external appearance of the cerebellum are too well known to need description here; but it may be helpful to indicate the nomenclature of its various divisions, and describe briefly what is known of its neuronal connections: these aspects are excellently reviewed in Eccles et al (1967) which may be consulted for further details.

The primary division of cerebellar neurons is between those whose cell bodies lie in the *cortex* and those in the four pairs of intrinsic *nuclei.* These four nuclei—globose, emboliform, dentate, and fastigial—to a large extent act as relay stations for the efferent fibres from the cerebellar cortex, although some of these fibres pass directly to the brainstem without relaying. The cerebellar cortex can be divided vertically into a narrow medial *vermis* with lateral *hemispheres* on each side (figure 9.21); horizontally, a deep cleft, the *primary fissure,* divides the surface into an *anterior* and a *posterior lobe.* These lobes are further subdivided by secondary fissures into *lobules*, which are named differently in the vermal and hemispheric divisions. One particular grouping of the lobules has an important functional and developmental significance, namely the division into the *archicerebellum* (consisting of the flocculonodular lobe), the *paleocerebellum* (effectively synonymous with the anterior lobe), and the *neocerebellum* (all the rest). The archicerebellum is the oldest part and is primarily concerned with the vestibular system; the paleocerebellum is more recent, and is concerned more with proprioceptive information from the spinal cord; and the neocerebellum is the most recent of all, having developed roughly in parallel with the cerebral cortex, with which it is associated. Despite the functional importance of these horizontal divisions, the efferent pathways via the intrinsic nuclei seem to be vertically organised. Anterior and posterior parts of the vermis project to the fastigial nuclei, paravermal regions to the globose and emboliform nuclei, and lateral regions mainly to the dentate.

Curiously enough, this almost grid-like arrangement of horizontal planes of input and vertical planes of output is also reflected in the microstructure of the cortex. The only efferent cells are the large *Purkinje* cells, which have elaborately branched flat dendritic structures, oriented in the sagittal direction: their axons are wholly inhibitory in action (Ito et al, 1964).

Afferent *mossy fibres* synapse with *granule* cells whose axons ascend to the surface layer and bifurcate to form *parallel fibres* running in a horizontal direction and piercing the planes of the Purkinje cells at right angles (figure 9.22). Contact between the two is made by synapses on dendritic spines on the Purkinje dendritic tree. A second afferent system, thought not to originate primarily from sensory pathways but mostly from the contralateral olivary complex (Szentágothai and Rajkovits, 1959), is formed by the *climbing fibres*: these ascend to the Purkinje dendritic tree, whose branches they intertwine like ivy creeping up an oak. The climbing fibres are excitatory, and thanks to their intimate entanglement have an overriding all-or-nothing excitatory effect on the Purkinje cells. Their tight functional connection with the efferent cerebellar pathways is reflected in the fact that climbing fibres—like Purkinje cells but unlike mossy fibres—seem to be functionally arranged in vertical (parasagittal) planes (Oscarsson, 1969).

Other interneurons are found in the cerebellar cortex. *Basket* cells appear to receive an input from the parallel fibres, and send off a single axon in the same direction as the planes of the Purkinje cells: branches of this axon envelope each of a row of Purkinje cells with inhibitory endings.

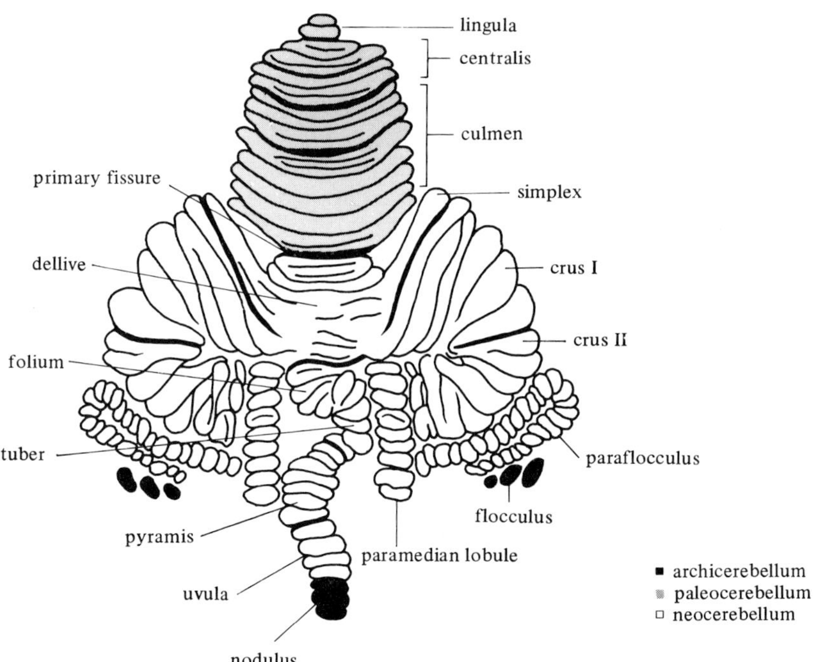

Figure 9.21. Schematic view of 'unrolled' cat's cerebellum, showing the names of the main divisions and lobules (after Roberts, 1967).

Other interneurons include *Golgi* cells, that appear to send information from the outer layers back to the inner in such a way as to modify the transmission of afferent information from mossy fibres to granule cells, and *stellate* cells. The synaptic relations between these various neurons are comparatively well understood; yet despite this knowledge, and the beautifully systematic way in which the various parts of the cerebellum seem to be arranged, the functioning of this 'neuronal machine' is still largely a matter for speculation.

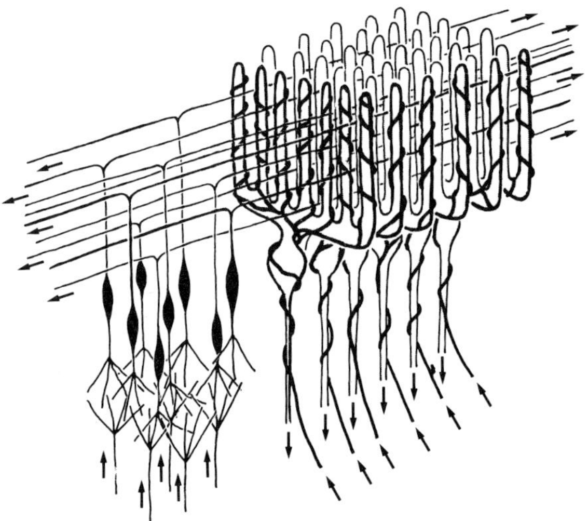

Figure 9.22. Schematic representation of the connections between mossy afferents (bottom left), granule cells and parallel fibres (left), Purkinje cells and climbing fibres (right).

9.3.2 Afferent fibre systems

The source of the climbing fibres has already been mentioned: the inferior olivary complex in turn receives projections from the cerebral cortex, the red nucleus, and the periaqueductal gray of the mesencephalon (Walberg, 1956). Thus the climbing fibres form in effect a route for descending control of cerebellar activity from higher levels of the brain; the deep nuclei receive some fibres from the same source. Recently it has been shown that visual information also projects via the inferior olive to climbing fibres in the flocculus (Maekawa and Simpson, 1971; 1973), a point which may have considerable significance in theories of cerebellar control of eye movements (see chapter 12). It is possible that the ultimate origin of this visual information is from the geniculate and collicular projections to the pontine reticular formation (Kawamura and Brodal, 1973; Graybiel, 1974).

The mossy fibres have different origins in different areas of the cerebellum. Primary vestibular fibres, and fibres from the inferior, and parts of the medial, vestibular nuclei, and nucleus *x*, project mostly ipsilaterally to the archicerebellum, paraflocculus and uvula, which together can be called the 'vestibulocerebellum' (A Brodal, 1967; Precht and Llinas, 1969): in the frog, a part of this projection is in fact via climbing fibres. Purkinje cells in the flocculus can be found that respond to vestibular stimulation either by excitation or by inhibition; their patterns of discharge are not very different from those of second-order neurons in the vestibular nuclei (Llinas et al, 1971). Some of the fibres from the vestibular nuclei pass to the contralateral vestibulocerebellum, and to the fastigial nuclei (Brodal and Torvik, 1957; Carpenter et al, 1959).

Tactile and proprioceptive information from the spinal cord is carried in the anterior and posterior spinocerebellar tracts and cuneocerebellar fibres: they terminate in the anterior lobe and parts of the pyramis and paramedian lobule; among them are afferents from joint receptors in the neck (Berthoz and Llinas, 1974). Fibres also enter the cerebellum from the reticular formation. The lateral reticular nucleus projects ipsilaterally to the paramedian lobule and the anterior lobe, while the paramedian reticular nuclei send fibres—mostly ipsilaterally—to parts of the vermis: both of these reticular areas probably project also in part to the fastigial nuclei. We have already seen that the lateral reticular nucleus in particular receives a number of fibres from the ipsilateral vestibular nucleus, and therefore might provide a path for secondary vestibular fibres to send information to the cerebellum: the direct paths from vestibular nuclear regions to the cerebellum are probably not composed of secondary vestibular fibres (A Brodal, 1972b). Afferent fibres from the fifth nerve nuclear complex are of interest here because of their likely involvement in conveying proprioceptive information from the eye muscles. Secondary fibres from the mesencephalic nucleus appear to pass to the emboliform and dentate nuclei (Pearson, 1949a; 1949b), and electrical responses to extraocular stretch can be recorded from cerebellar cortex, mainly from the central vermis and the superior cerebellar penduncle (Cooper et al, 1953b; Fuchs and Kornhuber, 1969; Azzena et al, 1970; Batini et al, 1974; but see Rahn and Zuber, 1971, for an experiment conflicting with this view). They probably influence Purkinje cells as both mossy and climbing fibres (Batini et al, 1974).

Finally, a second projection from higher levels descends through relays in the pons. Since these pontocerebellar fibres terminate in the same manner as the simple sensory afferents—as mossy fibres—it is probable that they also represent a sensory input of similar function, but presumably elaborated and refined by cortical processing. The main cortical projection to the pontine nuclei is from the frontal and temporal lobes, and especially the sensorimotor cortex; the latter projects in highly specific somatotopic maps which coincide with the maps obtained by direct stimulation of mechanoreceptors in the periphery (Snider, 1950). Projections from all parts of the visual cortex to rostral pontine areas have been described (P Brodal, 1972a; 1972b; Glickstein et al, 1972). It is probable that the superior colliculus also projects to the cerebellum via pontine relays (Altman and Carpenter, 1961), providing another route apart from climbing fibres by which the electrical responses to visual stimuli that can be recorded from the cerebellum might be mediated (Snider and Stowell, 1944). In the cat, the visual input is mostly—and in the pigeon, entirely—through mossy fibres rather than through climbing fibres (Clarke, 1974; Buchtel et al, 1972).

Figure 9.23 shows, in schematic form, the different projection areas discussed in this section.

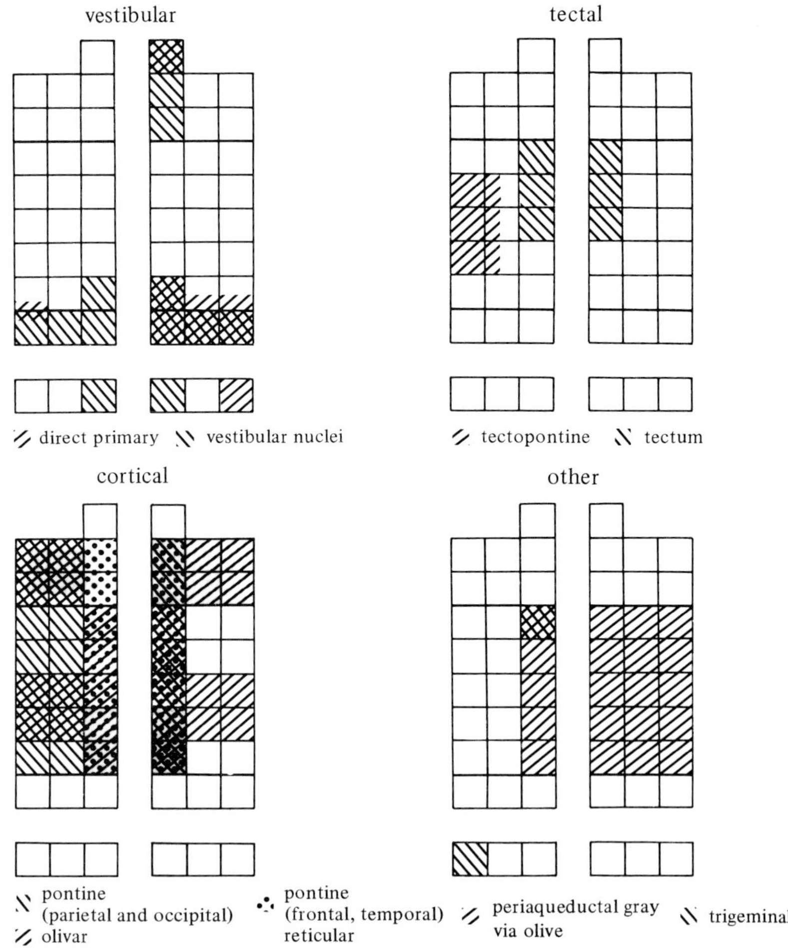

Figure 9.23. The approximate cerebellar distribution of certain afferent systems, with the use of the diagrammatic representation explained in figure 9.8 (after Roberts, 1967).

9.3.3 Efferent pathways

We have seen that nearly all the Purkinje cell axons pass down to the intrinsic nuclei, and it is from these, consequently, that the bulk of the cerebellar outflow ultimately issues. Efferent fibres from the dentate, emboliform, and globose nuclei form the *superior cerebellar peduncle:* all cross to the contralateral side, and project mainly to the red nucleus (mostly globose and emboliform fibres) and to the ventrolateral nucleus of the thalamus (mostly dentate). Of particular interest here is a small projection from the dentate nucleus, which crosses the midline and terminates in the oculomotor nucleus, preferentially in the regions corresponding to the vertical recti (Carpenter and Strominger, 1964); and a further group of fibres passing contralaterally and caudally to end in the paramedian reticular formation (Carpenter and Nova, 1960), an area we have seen to be implicated in vestibulo-ocular connections. The projection to the oculomotor nucleus seems to be the only example of cerebellar fibres ending directly on motor neurons.

Fibres from the fastigial nuclei take a different course, through the *uncinate fasciculus* and *juxtarestiform* body. Crossed fibres in the former pass from the fastigial nuclei to parts of the superior vestibular nucleus, and to ventral and lateral portions of the other three nuclei of the vestibular complex, while the uncrossed fibres in the fasciculus and in the juxtarestiform body end in dorsal parts of the medial inferior and lateral vestibular nuclei, so that the projections hardly overlap (Walberg et al, 1962) (figure 9.4). We saw earlier, in section 9.1.2, that the vestibular complex also receives fibres *directly* from the cerebellar cortex, not relaying in the intrinsic nuclei (Angaut and Brodal, 1967). The nodulus and uvulus project to peripheral parts of the superior nucleus, the (caudal) inferior nucleus, and group x, while the nodulus also projects to caudal and medial parts of the medial nucleus: the flocculus sends fibres to selected parts of all the main vestibular nuclei (figure 9.3).

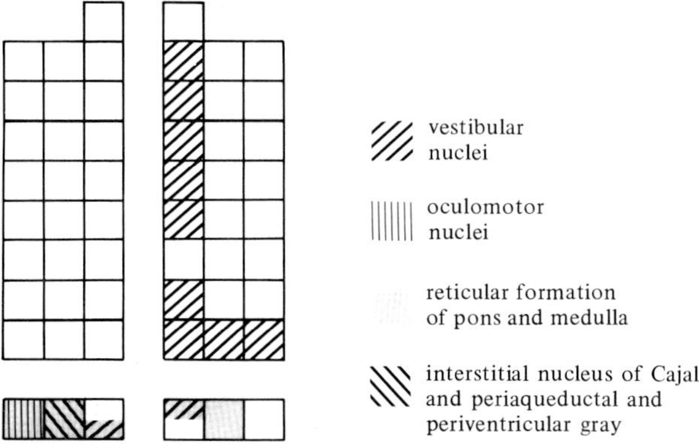

Figure 9.24. Cerebellar origins of certain efferent systems, with the use of the same representation as in figure 9.23 (after Roberts, 1967).

Other fastigial projections include those to the dorsomedial regions of the pontine and medullary reticular formation, and certain higher regions that probably do not concern us here: figure 9.24 summarises the cerebellar topography of the efferents mentioned in this section.

9.3.4 Electrical cerebellar activity related to eye movements
Hitzig (1874) seems to have been the first to note that stimulation of the cerebellum could provoke eye movements: the early history of such observations has been reviewed by Dow and Manni (1964), and more recent work by Precht (1975). Horizontal movements are the most commonly evoked (see, for example, Magoun et al's (1937) account of an extremely thorough electrical exploration of the cerebellum), and often over a very wide area. Since the only direct cerebello-oculomotor pathways that have yet been demonstrated are exclusively for vertical movements, it seems likely that these electrically evoked movements are mediated by much longer pathways, very likely through vestibular neurons, or the pontine reticular formation. Much of the earlier work is of rather little interest now, because experimenters on the whole did not appreciate the importance of describing the exact form of the eye movements that they observed, being content with simple characterisations such as 'deviation' or 'nystagmus'. For this reason it is probably more helpful to proceed immediately to the most recent findings.

Two separate problems have been receiving attention in recent years: the first is the classical one of the nature of the eye movements evoked by cerebellar stimulation, while the other is the question of what influence cerebellar activity may have on coexisting eye movements evoked by *other* means, for example by vestibular stimulation. The vestibulo-ocular reflex is of particular interest here because of the close relationship between the cerebellum and the vestibular system, and the likelihood of vestibulo-ocular paths that actually pass through the cerebellum, of which several are possible (figure 9.25). Our knowledge of these relationships is still very limited: we know a little about the electrophysiology of the projection to the vestibular complex itself, but virtually nothing about its influence either directly on the oculomotor nuclei, or on the pathways that pass through the reticular formation.

Extracellular electrical stimulation is a crude procedure at best, and perhaps particularly so in the cerebellum with its tightly packed neurons and their closely knit excitatory and inhibitory effects. It can never be wholly certain whether the stimulating current is acting directly on Purkinje cells, or on the afferent fibre systems, or on interneurons, or on all of these simultaneously: and the synchronous activation of many elements over a wide area is likely to be a grossly unphysiological situation. Perhaps, then, it is not surprising that some of the results obtained by electrical stimulation have been contradictory and mutually confused, even among more recent workers who have been at pains to give useful descriptions of the movements obtained. Thus whereas Fernandez and Frederickson (1963) could not demonstrate eye movements at all on stimulation of the vestibulocerebellum, and found in fact that stimulation in this area seemed to inhibit on-going vestibular nystagmus (leaving the slow component intact), Ron and Robinson (1973) found that stimulation in this region had exactly the opposite effect, namely that it evoked a nystagmus of natural appearance [also observed by Nashold et al (1969) in man]. One is reminded of the old analogy, that such experiments are like trying to see how a computer works by sticking into it a crowbar connected to the mains, to see what happens! At the very least, one must be particularly on one's guard against jumping to premature conclusions on the basis of such evidence.

Some of the details of the cerebellar involvement in the control of vestibulo-ocular reflexes have recently been clarified by recording from the vestibular nuclei and from the neurons in the eye muscle nuclei to which they project (for example Shimo-oku, 1970; Shimazu and Smith, 1971; Fukuda et al, 1972; Baker et al, 1972; Baker et al, 1973). After a single shock to the vestibular nerve, electrical responses can be obtained from the trochlear nucleus, consisting of an IPSP followed by a more complex pattern of depolarisation and hyperpolarisation. If the cerebellum is ablated, this second component appears to be lost: since the equilibrium potential is identical for the original IPSP and the delayed components, it is probable that whatever the cerebellar influence on this pathway is, it is

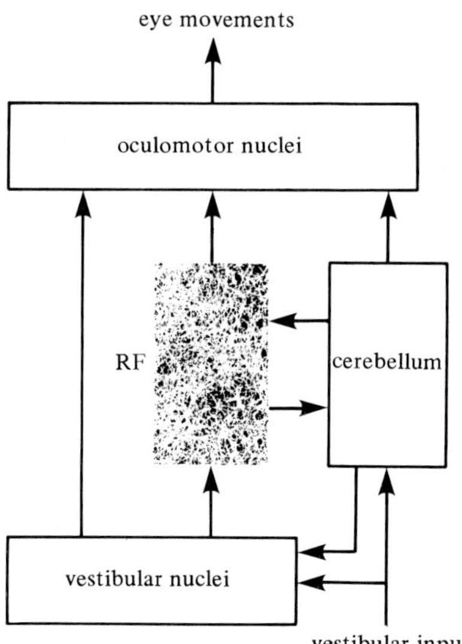

Figure 9.25. Possible routes by which vestibular information can reach the eye muscle nuclei: apart from the direct projection from vestibular nuclei via the medial longitudinal fasciculus (left), other possibilities include routes through the reticular formation of the brainstem (centre) or the cerebellum (right) or a combination of both.

exerted at the level of the second-order neurons rather than by convergence on the trochlear neuron. They suggest that Purkinje axons synaptically inhibit the second-order vestibular neurons and thus 'control' the vestibulo-ocular reflex in some way. This would of course fit in with Fernandez and Frederickson's (1963) observation on the inhibiting effect of cerebellar stimulation on the reflex [and Precht and Llinas's (1969) converse observation of prolongation of vestibular nystagmus after lesions of the vestibulo-cerebellum], and possibly even with Ron and Robinson's (1973) apparently contradictory observations: with the existence of reciprocally inhibitory connections across the midline, it is not beyond the bounds of possiblity that a sufficiently strong inhibitory signal on one side might, as it were, drive the reflex in the opposite direction and thus provoke a nystagmus. It is perhaps significant that the nystagmus thus evoked starts with the slow phase, as does vestibular nystagmus (figure 9.26): although here again there is an unfortunate conflict of observation, since Cohen et al (1965) found that nystagmus evoked in this way in spinal cats actually began with the quick phase. Clearly the electrophysiology of cerebellar influences on the vestibuloocular reflex arc needs further study, perhaps especially in relation to the reticular paths, since it is evident from recent work by Ito et al (1973c) that not all of the classical medial longitudinal fasciculus pathways receive these influences (figure 9.16).

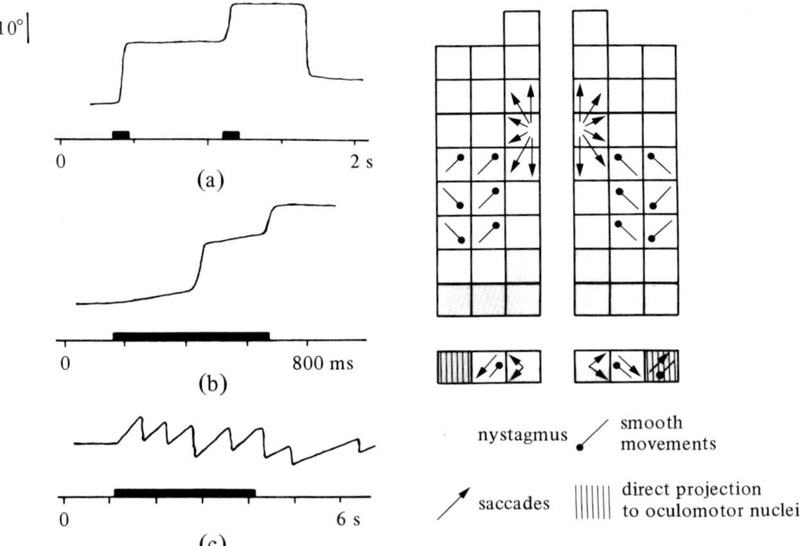

Figure 9.26. Eye movements resulting from stimulation of an alert monkey's cerebellum: (a) realistic saccades; (b) a slow movement with superimposed saccades; (c) nystagmus (Ron and Robinson, 1973)

Figure 9.27. Cerebellar areas from which eye movements can be obtained on stimulation. The direction of the evoked movements is indicated by the direction of the lines or arrows (data of Ron and Robinson, 1973).

Apart from observing evoked nystagmus from the vestibulocerebellum, Ron and Robinson (1973) were able to obtain eye movements by electrical stimulation of a number of other cerebellar areas, though not in lobes I–IV, the paramedian lobe, or the paraflocculus (figure 9.27). These negative results for certain regions are in conflict with several previous investigators (see Magoun et al, 1937), and, although their records of eye movements are rather more complete than those of other investigators, even with simpler methods of description one can hardly be mistaken about the *existence* of some kind of movement. The most likely explanation for these discrepancies is that some of the positive results were due to current spread. Thus Dow (1935) found that it sometimes made no difference to the movements obtained by stimulation of the rabbit cerebellum whether the dura was intact or not, and the currents necessary were often so great as to cause evident stimulation of cranial motor nerve nuclei. As a result, he concluded that although it was indeed possible to obtain eye movements from large areas of the cerebellum, including the paraflocculus, most of these effects were entirely due to spread of current. The observations of Ron and Robinson (1973) are less open to this criticism, since they took care to limit their currents to such a level (about a milliamp) that no excitation was probable at distances of more than a few millimetres from the electrode. Both slow movements and realistic saccades could be evoked in this way (figure 9.26), and the sites where the two kinds of movement were obtained were found to be arranged in an orderly way on the surface of the cerebellum (figure 9.27). Simultaneous stimulation of two points apparently results in vectorial summation of responses (Cohen et al, 1965).

Unlike the saccades obtained by collicular stimulation, most (78%) cerebellar saccades are not of fixed amplitude, but vary with the current density used (figure 9.28): if the eye is in the primary position, the direction of the saccade is fixed for a particular site of stimulation, and

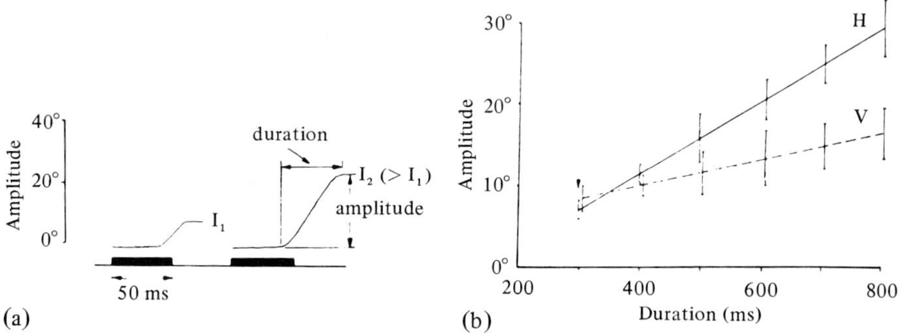

Figure 9.28. (a) Saccade duration (and hence size) increases with increased current of stimulation; (b) the relationship between duration and amplitude for the horizontal (H) and vertical (V) components of a number of evoked saccades of this type (alert monkey cerebellum) (Ron and Robinson, 1973).

both direction and amplitude are independent of the pulse width or repetition frequency of the stimulus, so long as the train used exceeds some 100 ms in length. Shorter trains produce smaller saccades, while longer ones provoke a series of saccades (a staircase) separated in time by between 100 and 200 ms. Cerebellar saccades appear to be unaffected by the nature of the visual field, whether textured, blank, or dark. On the other hand, in 90% of cases the starting position somewhat modified the size and direction of the evoked saccade (figure 9.29) in a way that might be described as goal-directed; but the goal was usually found to lie outside the oculomotor range of the eye, so that saccades were simply observed to get smaller in the direction of their action. This is very far from providing evidence for the kind of 'objective' map that has been suggested in the superior colliculus: since the saccades grossly fail to reach their goal, and are so little modified by their starting position, it may be that these observations represent a quite different mechanism, possibly one that—under natural circumstances—allows for the changing mechanical actions of the muscles at different positions of the globe. At all events, it is likely that the extraocular muscle proprioceptors that project to the same region of the cerebellum provide the information about eye position that causes the modifications.

The same quasi-goal-directed behaviour was seen with evoked slow movements (figure 9.26), whose velocities also generally depended on eye position, as well as linearly on the current strength and on the pulse width and frequency of stimulation: velocities as high as $150° s^{-1}$ could be obtained in this way. Unlike the saccades, the slow movements were very strongly inhibited by the presence of a textured visual scene, so that larger currents were necessary to invoke them. Presumably this was due to opposition from the smooth pursuit system. If stimulation was attempted during optokinetic nystagmus, with a sufficiently great stimulus the evoked slow movement would replace (rather than add to) the previous nystagmus. Similar slow movements, saccades and nystagmus could be recorded from stimulation of the deep nuclei of the cerebellum, generally with rather shorter latencies (up to 30 ms). Some sites giving vertical movements in the dentate nucleus showed extremely short

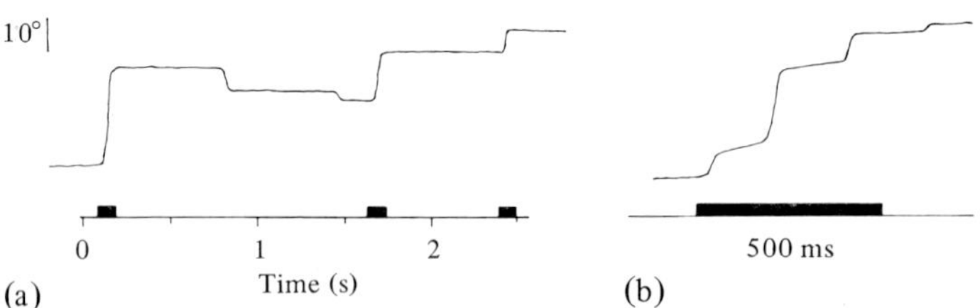

Figure 9.29. Position dependency of saccades evoked by cerebellar stimulation: (a) saccade size varies with deviation of eye and is quasi- 'goal-directed'; (b) continuous stimulation evokes a staircase of diminishing step size (Ron and Robinson, 1973).

latencies—down to 9 ms—and a time course of the evoked movement very similar to that seen after stimulation of oculomotor neurons. These responses are almost certainly due to the direct pathway mentioned earlier from the dentate to the oculomotor nuclei, and concerned with vertical movements (Carpenter and Strominger, 1964).

The fact that cerebellar movements depend more strongly than collicular movements on the nature of the stimulus that provokes them suggests that it is further down the oculomotor system, and that the movements obtained are not merely the reflex effects of stimulation of an essentially sensory mechanism. This is suggested also by Wolfe's (1971) observation that cerebellar potentials that *precede* spontaneous eye movements by some 30 ms can be recorded from unanaesthetized cats: similarly, Purkinje cell activity starts to build up some 25 ms before a saccade (Llinas, 1974) (rather oddly the activity appears to vary inversely with the amplitude of the saccade). On the other hand, the fact that the movements obtained by stimulating the deep nuclei are so similar to those obtained from stimulating the cortex suggests that in both cases it is essentially the *output* of the cerebellum that is being activated (although the fact that deep-nuclei responses are not of opposite sign to cortical responses raises doubts as to whether it is only the Purkinje cells, with their inhibitory output, that are being stimulated in the cortex). This implies that the observed relationship between the stimulus and the response—for example, the integration that converts a steady stimulus current into a constant-velocity smooth movement, or the pulse generator that produces the saccades—is not wholly the work of the cerebellum and must be generated by structures further down the neural pathways: but it does not exclude, for example, the possibility that the cerebellum forms part of a feedback circuit performing these functions.

9.3.5 Cerebellar lesions and eye movements

One might think that the use of lesions or ablations was an even cruder technique of investigating functional neuroanatomy than electrical stimulation: but this is not necessarily so. If a particular function is completely unaffected by removal of a particular part of the brain, even immediately after the operation, then it is as certain as anything can be in neurophysiology that the part of the brain removed plays no role in the execution of the function. The converse can never be argued with equal conviction, because of the possibility of unintentional damage or disturbance to structures other than the one in question. However, in the first case the onus is on the experimenter to show that the function really is *completely* unaffected: this demands some precise and quantitative way of recording the system's performance under a variety of natural conditions. Unfortunately, as we have seen, many early experimenters were not sufficiently aware of the importance of recording the *form* of eye movements as well as their mere existence, and the value of their observations as to the effects of such procedures as cerebellectomy is correspondingly reduced. Consequently there is a great deal of confusion and contradiction in the literature describing the effects of cerebellar lesions on eye movements, which is only just beginning to be resolved. Added to this difficulty is the probability—in chronic preparations—that other structures may begin to take over the function of the damaged part (see for example Westheimer and Blair, 1974), and the results obtained from such preparations are not as useful as they might otherwise be. For all these reasons, no attempt is made here to review early work in any detail, and readers who are interested may find the necessary information in Dow and Manni (1964). A brief review of clinical signs of cerebellar damage is given by Dichgans and Jung (1975).

One of the more constantly observed effects of cerebellar lesions is a spontaneous nystagmus, especially on trying to deviate the eyes (Holmes, 1917; Ferraro and Barrera, 1938; Cogan, 1956; Dow and Manni, 1964; Kommerell, 1975). A possible explanation for this phenomenon is suggested by recent observations of the effects of cerebellar lesions on the time-course of saccades. In the chronic rabbit (Collewijn, 1970a), monkey (Aschoff and Cohen, 1971; 1972; Westheimer and Blair, 1973b) and in the cat (Robinson, 1974; 1975b) a constant finding is that, although the initial part of the saccade or nystagmus quick phase is more or less of normal speed speed and amplitude, the gaze cannot be maintained in deviation, but drifts back to a 'neutral' position in a roughly exponential manner (figure 9.30). The position of this neutral zone tends to wander about, resulting in slow random wandering of the eyes in the dark. Unilateral cerebellar ablation results in a continuous drift in the dark away from the side of the lesion (Westheimer and Blair, 1974).

It is not difficult to see how such an inability to hold a deviation of gaze could result in nystagmus on trying to look to one side. After the first attempted saccade the eye will tend to drift back and the line of sight will be seen not to coincide with the desired object; a second corrective saccade will occur, with the same effect as the first: then a third, and a fourth, and so on—resulting in a nystagmus whose quick phases are directed towards the object of interest, and in which the slow phases are exponential in shape: this is precisely what is clinically observed (for example Kommerell, 1975). The further the desired position of the eye from the neutral zone, the faster the rate of drift and hence the higher the expected frequency of the nystagmus: again, this is the clinical finding [Alexander's Law: see for example Dix and Hallpike (1966); similar effects can be induced by barbiturates (Bergmann et al, 1952)]. Hood et al (1973) recently observed that in a series of patients with chronic cerebellar disease deviation nystagmus of this kind showed both a slow adaptation during long attempted deviations, and a corresponding 'rebound' on trying to regain the primary position: it may be that in such circumstances the neutral point slowly catches up with the desired point of regard (possibly by a process of parametric feedback: see section 10.3.3), with a time lag that results in a reversed, rebound nystagmus when the subject stops trying to deviate his gaze.

A simple explanation for this defect in gaze holding comes to mind if one considers the two separate components of the signal sent to the eye muscles during a normal saccade: the pulse that drives the eye quickly to its new position, and the step that holds it there. If for some reason the pulse occurred without the step, the effect would be very much what is observed in these cases: the eye would move with normal velocity to the correct place, but drift back afterwards because of the absence of the tension needed to hold it in place. In fact, a loss of gain for 'slow' components of movement seems characteristic of cerebellar damage. In the monkey, smooth pursuit movements are greatly reduced (Westheimer and Blair, 1974) although in *chronic* rabbits Collewijn (1970a) found little defect in the slow phase of optokinetic nystagmus: but, as has been repeatedly emphasised, closed-loop measurements of optokinetic nystagmus minimise any functional differences that may be present. In the acutely decerebrate cat, Carpenter (1972a) found a large decrease in the low-

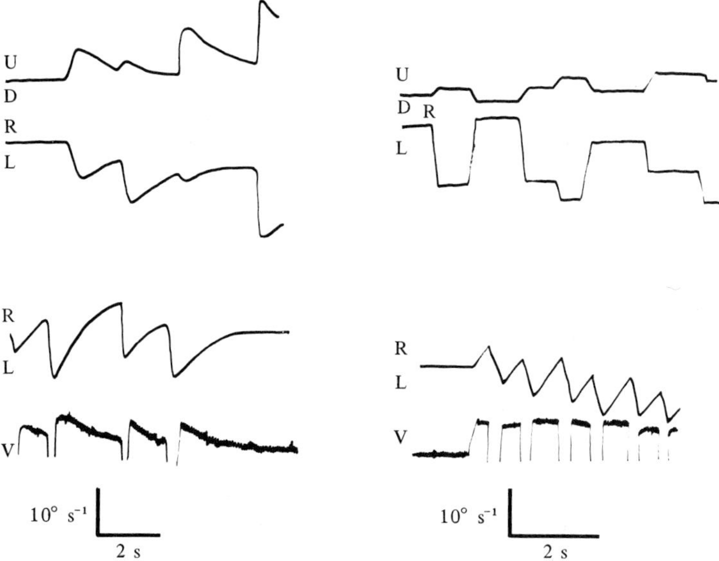

Figure 9.30. Eye movements after ablation of the cat's cerebellum. On the right, vertical and horizontal components of spontaneous saccades made by a normal animal (above), and of normal horizontal vestibular nystagmus: the lower trace of the nystagmus (V) shows the instantaneous velocity, which can be seen to be virtually constant during the slow phases. On the left, similar records after ablation of the cerebellum: velocities of saccades are comparable, but the deviation cannot be maintained and the eye drifts back to the midline. During vestibular nystagmus (below) the slow phase shows a similar exponential decline of velocity (after Robinson, 1974).

frequency gain of the vestibulo-ocular reflex after cerebellectomy or local surface cooling (figure 9.31), a drop which could be accounted for very well by supposing that cerebellectomy had the effect of disabling a neural integrator in parallel with other paths in the vestibuloocular reflex. The high-frequency gain is only slightly affected (Carpenter, 1972a; Westheimer and Blair, 1974), and unilateral cerebellar damage produces asymmetric defects in vestibular response. The same lack of an integrator can be deduced from the report of Precht et al (1969) on abducens discharges during vestibular stimulation in the decerebrate, decerebellate, cat; but the significance of their findings in this respect was not realised at the time. The location and properties of the integrator are further pursued in chapter 12.

The older notion, that the cerebellum had no role in the vestibuloocular reflex—because nystagmus could still be obtained after total cerebellectomy (see for example Dow and Manni, 1964)—came about because experimenters could only conceive of two possibilities: nystagmus, or no nystagmus. Just as saccades are modified, but not abolished, by cerebellar lesions, so the removal of the parallel integrator will modify, but not abolish, vestibulo-ocular reflexes. In practice, the quick phases are substantially unaffected (figure 9.30), while the slow phases, instead of being of roughly

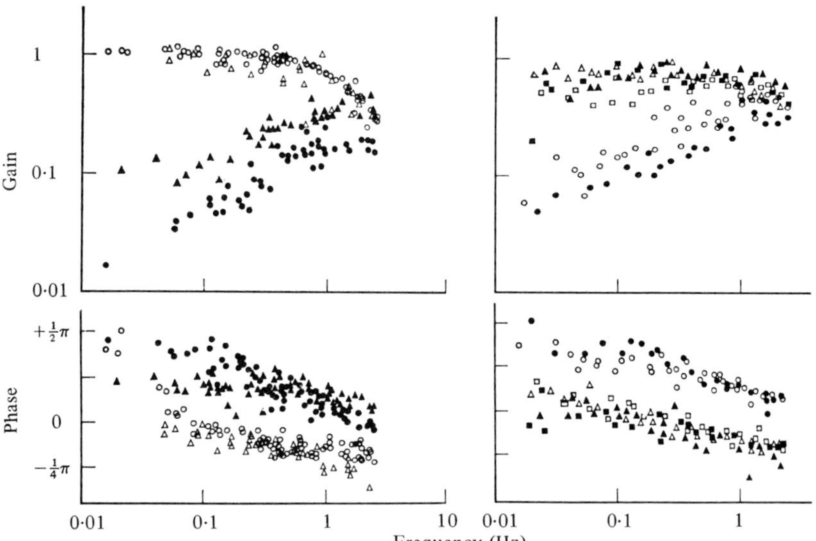

Figure 9.31. Frequency transfer functions of the vestibulo-ocular reflex in a number of decerebrate cats, before and after cerebellectomy, and during and after local cooling of the cerebellum. Left (open symbols) before and (closed symbols) after cerebellectomy in two cats: right, triangles and squares respectively before and after local cooling, and circles during cooling, in two cats (filled and open symbols). In each case, interference with the cerebellum results in a loss of low-frequency gain, and in an increase in phase lead or decrease in lag (Carpenter, 1972a).

constant velocity, show the same exponential drift towards the neutral zone as in the case of saccades. In the same way, little defect would be expected in the slow phases of sinusoidal vestibular nystagmus, if the frequency is sufficiently high.

The relation between the effects of lesions and the electrophysiological findings outlined earlier is more obscure. Two points have to be borne in mind: first, that the electrophysiological studies have as yet only been made on the classical medial longitudinal fasciculus pathway, whereas, as we have seen, it is the other, parallel, pathways that are likely to be concerned with the slower integrated components; and second, that although electrical stimulation of the cerebellar cortex leads exclusively to inhibitory responses, this should not be taken to mean that the function of the cerebellum is to *depress* the vestibulo-ocular reflexes. It is important to make a clear distinction between inhibition as the opposite of excitation, and inhibition as a reduction in gain. In the first case, the inhibition is simply the manifestation of a signal that happens to have a sign opposite to the one the experimenter considers to be the primary input: and if—as was the case for half the neural pathways examined by Fukuda et al (1972) and Ito et al (1973c)—this primary input itself happens to be 'inhibitory' in this sense, then it is evidently a matter of taste as to which input is excitatory and which inhibitory as far as the functioning of the whole reflex is concerned. In a bipolar, bilateral system like that of the vestibulo-ocular reflex such distinctions are largely meaningless: only reductions in gain (as might be produced, for example, by presynaptic inhibition) can usefully be considered to be functionally inhibitory. In this sense, there is no electrophysiological evidence that the cerebellum's role in the vestibulo-ocular reflex is primarily inhibitory: only that it provides an added signal to the classical three-neuron reflex arc that in half the cases is of the same sign as the vestibular input, and in half the cases of opposite sign.

This is a field of active exploration, and it is likely that the next few years will show a greater clarification of these mechanisms than is possible now. In particular, recent work has suggested that an important role for the cerebellum may be in coordinating visual and vestibular information in the control of eye movements, especially in the suppression or even reversal of vestibulo-ocular responses that may occur under artificial visual conditions (Ito et al, 1974; Lisberger and Fuchs, 1974; Takemori and Cohen, 1974b; Robinson, 1975b; see also sections 2.3.3, 10.3.3 and 12.3). It is precisely under these circumstances of mismatch between visual and vestibular stimulation that motion sickness commonly occurs, and it is interesting that lesions in the vestibulocerebellum are also reported to reduce motion sickness (Wang and Chinn, 1956). In chapter 12 an attempt is made to bring together some of these ideas about the cerebellum and its function in the control both of eye movements, and of the motor system in general.

9.4 Telencephalic oculomotor areas

9.4.1 Basal ganglia

The basal ganglia form a complex conglomerate with diffuse and largely controversial connections with many levels of the central nervous system. Experimenters have not yet become particularly interested in any possible oculomotor role they might have, and so such little information as there is derives almost exclusively from clinical material. It is probably not worth while to attempt to outline even sketchily the anatomy of these regions: many standard textbooks of neuroanatomy (for example Truex and Carpenter, 1969; A Brodal, 1969) present as clear expositions of the general topography and connections of the basal ganglia as can be expected. Astruc (1971) has recently described projections of the frontal eye fields of the monkey to parts of the basal ganglia (caudate nucleus, putamen and subthalamic nuclei).

A further difficulty is that is not yet possible to correlate particular pathological states associated with damage to the basal ganglia (for example, paralysis agitans, or Huntington's chorea) with lesions in particular structures: indeed the picture is more often one of multiple diffuse degeneration, involving both brain stem and cerebral cortex. Thus oculomotor defects found in such patients may not be primarily the result of the damage to the basal ganglia. Lesions of the basal ganglia of experimental animals do not mimic naturally occurring pathological states, except to the extent that ballistic and choreiform movements can be produced by lesions in the subthalamic nuclei (discussed in Truex and Carpenter, 1969).

A general finding with Parkinson's disease is that movements are infrequent (akinesia), too small in amplitude for the task (hypokinesia), and slower than normal (bradykinesia): more obvious positive phenomena such as tremor and rigidity are also found (see for example Martin, 1967). The eye movements of these patients can often show the same general negative characteristics, sometimes also with erratic bursts of coactivation of antagonists (Slatt et al, 1966; de Jong and Melvill Jones, 1971; Melvill Jones and de Jong, 1971; Chaco, 1971). There is an increased latency for visually triggered saccades, which are reduced in amplitude: sometimes, especially in the vertical plane, paralysis of the gaze may be complete (Cogan, 1964; 1974). The velocites of saccades are not markedly reduced, however, and their amplitude–duration curves are essentially normal (Melvill Jones and de Jong, 1971): but because of the reduction in saccade size, a large movement is split up into a series of small steps (in a manner analogous to the 'cogwheel rigidity' classically associated with Parkinsonism) so that the total time for executing a given movement is increased (figure 9.32: de Jong and Melvill Jones, 1971; Yamazaki and Ishikawa, 1972). This suggests a defect in initiation and specification of the eye movement rather than in its execution.

A rather different kind of defect was noted by Starr (1967) in a patient with Huntington's chorea: here the patient could produce neither saccades nor the quick phase of vestibular nystagmus. Smooth pursuit appeared to be unimpaired, and voluntary deviations of the eyes could only be executed by means of long slow movements. It seemed to be the visual surroundings that were slowing the eyes in this case, for a much quicker movement could be made if the subject blinked.

In the absence of precise information linking defects of this kind to lesions in specific structures there is little point in attempting to incorporate the basal ganglia into any general scheme of the oculomotor control system, although it is worth noting that here again we find evidence for differential effects on slow and fast components of eye movements.

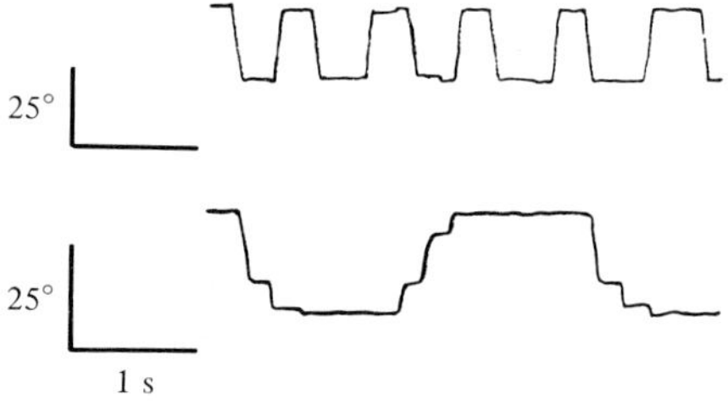

Figure 9.32. Decomposition of saccades in Parkinsonianism. Above, normal voluntary saccades of 25° amplitude; below, the same task as performed by a Parkinsonian patient, showing decomposition of the saccades into a number of small components (after de Jong and Melvill Jones, 1971).

9.4.2 Cerebral cortex: anatomy

Just like the cerebellar cortex, the cerebral cortex can be divided into three parts, of different degrees of antiquity: *archicortex* (hippocampus), *paleocortex* (pyriform cortex), and *neocortex*. Only the last division has been shown to play a direct part in the control of eye movements: in mammals it is by far the largest division, and with its increasing area as the phylogenetic tree is climbed it has become enormously furrowed and convoluted into the familiar pattern of sulci and gyri. In many cases the pattern of gyri reflects underlying functional differentiations, and associated patterns of cytoarchitectonics, and they are useful as landmarks for specifying particular areas of cortex. Two regions are mainly associated with eye movements: they are the *frontal eye fields* lying bilaterally in the posterior half of the middle frontal and inferior frontal gyri, and the *occipital eye fields* situated in an area extending bilaterally from the occipital pole roughly to the intraparietal fissure: the boundaries of both areas are somewhat diffuse (figure 9.33). Electrical stimulation in either region can elicit eye movements, but only the frontal eye fields are likely to be *primarily* concerned with oculomotor control: the occipital region from which eye movements can be obtained on stimulation also happens to be the region from which electrical responses to visual stimulation can be obtained most easily, and which includes the primary projection area for the optic radiation from the lateral geniculate body. Although there are slight architectonic differences between the two areas, and between regions within each area, the general arrangement of neurons and fibres is roughly similar in each (figure 9.34).

The efferent fibres of the cortex arise from large or medium-sized pyramidal cells, occupying two distinct layers in the cortex. Those in the more superficial layer tend to project to other parts of the cortex—providing 'association' fibres—while those in the deeper layer project mainly to subcortical regions and thus form the true efferents of the cortex: both cells have long dendrites extending sideways and also upwards to the very top of the cortical substance. Two groups of association fibres have been found which presumably have an oculomotor function, linking the occipital and frontal eye fields (possibly in both directions: Larmande, 1973). Afferent fibres can similarly be divided into the associational afferents from other parts of the cortex, and the true afferents from subcortical structures: both show an essentially vertical distribution of connections, and in fact electrophysiological

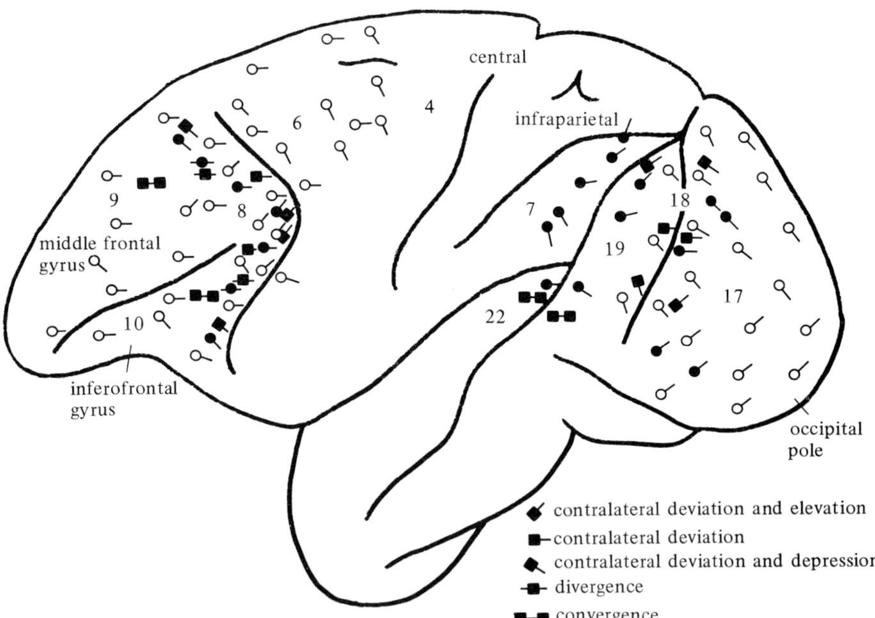

Figure 9.33. Oculomotor areas of the monkey cerebral cortex, showing the numbers and names of some of the principal surface features, and an indication of the direction of the movements that can be obtained on stimulation, according to the various authors mentioned: ● Crosby and Henderson (1948), Crosby et al (1962), ○ Wagman et al [1958; 1961 (summary)], ■ Jampel (1960).

evidence both in the visual and in the somatosensory areas suggests that the normal functional organisation of the cerebral cortex is in *columns* (Mountcastle, 1957; Hubel and Wiesel, 1962; 1968). In the cat's striate visual cortex, some columns correspond to constant directions in space, while others correspond to regions of constant binocular disparity (Barlow et al, 1967; Blakemore, 1970); these two types of column may well be concerned in the initiation of version and vergence movements respectively. Jampel (1960) has observed convergence and divergence responses—amongst others—to stimulation of parts of the monkey's visual cortex. Although the frontal eye fields do not receive direct visual fibres, they do receive a projection from the pulvinar of the thalamus, which in turn receives fibres from the cortical visual areas (Trojanowski and Jacobson, 1974). Apart from the main afferent and efferent fibre systems, the cerebral cortex has a wealth of interneurons of different types, that may convey information from column to column and from layer to layer (figure 9.34) (Lorente de No, 1949). The main difference between the cytoarchitectonics of the frontal and occipital eye fields is the greatest number and size of pyramidal cells in the former, and of interneurons (particularly granule cells) in the latter (von Economo, 1929).

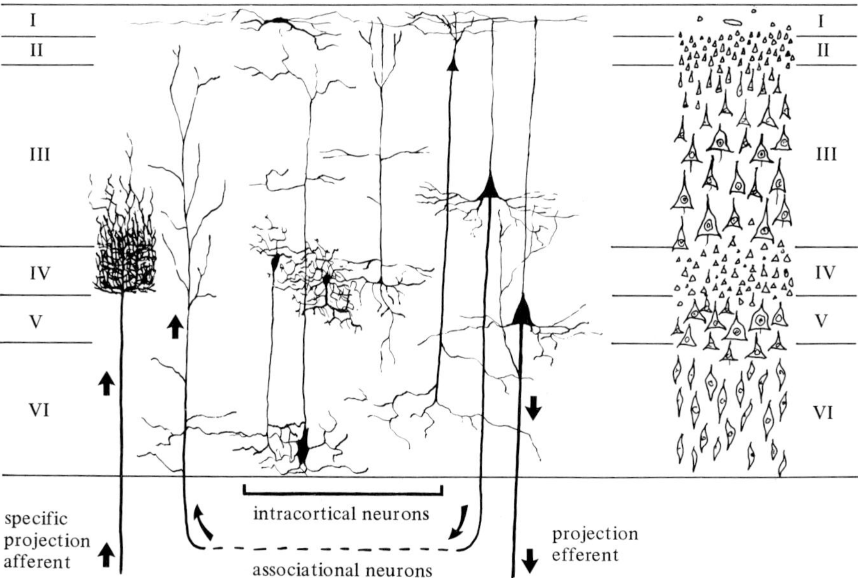

Figure 9.34. Diagrammatic representation of the neuron types in the cerebral cortex, and their principal connections. On the left, afferent systems; in the middle, intracortical neurons; and on the right, efferent systems. On the far right, the general histological appearance of the different layers is indicated.

Apart from the corticospinal pyramidal tract, which does not concern us here, corticofugal fibres project mainly to the pontine nuclei, the reticular formation, the thalamus, and other nuclei in the basal ganglia and midbrain. Corticopontine fibres project mainly to the medial pontine nuclei, passing from the frontal eye fields in the frontopontine tract (bundle of Arnold) and providing a means by which the frontal eye fields can influence the cerebellum. The occipital pontine tract is much smaller, and projects to lateral and dorsolateral rostral pontine areas (P Brodal, 1972a, 1972b). Many more fibres project from the frontal than from the occipital eye fields to the reticular formation: they terminate bilaterally, mostly in the pontine reticular formation and in the region of the nucleus reticularis gigantocellularis of the medulla, areas which project both to the spinal cord and to the midbrain. Other cortical efferents terminate in such areas as the lateral reticular nucleus, the medullary paramedian nuclei, and the tegmental reticular nucleus: we have seen that parts of these regions are associated with the vestibular nuclei, cerebellum, and possibly reticular vestibulo-ocular transmission. Of the other possible terminations of corticofugal fibres, the most relevant is of course the possibility of fibres ending directly on oculomotor neurons, in a manner analogous to the corticospinal tract fibres in certain species. In the cat, no cortifugal fibres terminate in any cranial motor nerve nucleus (for example Lloyd, 1941), and although in primates and in man a direct projection may exist to some of the cranial nerve nuclei, none have been demonstrated going to the eye muscle nuclei (Kuypers, 1958; Astruc, 1971).

Thus it seems that cortical influences on eye movements must be exerted either—most directly—via the reticular formation, or possibly through the thalamus, cerebellum, superior colliculus [to which both eye fields send an important projection (Kuypers and Lawrence, 1967; Astruc, 1971)], interstitial nucleus of Cajal, and nucleus of Darkschewitsch (Szentágothai and Rajkovits, 1958; Kuypers and Lawrence, 1967; but see Pompeiano and Walberg, 1957), or the vestibular nuclei (Spiegel, 1933; Markham, 1972). But in the latter case, Pompeiano and Walberg (1957) again have evidence that no direct projection exists: the observations that the effects of frontal eye-field stimulation are profoundly modified by lesions in the vestibular nuclei (Spiegel, 1933; Spiegel and Aronson, 1934), and conversely that vestibular nystagmus is influenced by cortical lesions (Dusser de Barenne and de Kleijn, 1923), are presumably due to a cortical oculomotor route that projects only indirectly through the vestibular pathways, perhaps reaching them via the interstitial nucleus of Cajal, which we saw in section 9.1.4 to have direct connections with inhibitory neurons in the vestibular complex. Lesions of the vestibular nuclei disrupt optokinetic nystagmus of both 'cortical' (that is, 'look') and noncortical kinds (Scala and Spiegel, 1938).

9.4.3 Cortical eye movements: experimental studies

There is a difficulty that attends the experimental study of regions like the cerebral cortex which lie in the hinterland between the sensory and motor systems, that the dividing line between what is an interesting motor effect, and what is merely a trivial sensory effect, becomes hard to draw. No one would be particularly excited to learn that section of the optic nerve results in a loss of visually evoked eye movements: but what is to be our reaction to the effect of lesions in the occipital eye fields? The answer is, no doubt, that distinctions between 'sensory' and 'motor' mechanisms at this level have rather little meaning: one is only too inclined to assume that the cerebral cortex represents the highest level of the nervous system, in the sense that its afferent paths are sensory and its efferent ones motor. Behind this notion is the unspoken assumption that the cerebral cortex in some sense represents the interface between the nervous system and the 'ghost in the machine' which provides the ultimate distinction between sensory and motor mechanisms. Without wishing to labour the point, one should perhaps be particularly on one's guard against assuming that, because stimulation of a particular cortical area results in a movement, that the area is therefore essentially a motor area. There is really no evidence that any part of the neocortex is concerned with anything except the elaboration of sensory information: even the outflow from the motor cortex may only represent the tapping-off of integrated sensory information to activate a sophisticated type of reflex (see for example Brooks and Stoney, 1971). Thus one must be more than usually cautious in one's interpretation of experiments on cortical eye fields.

The early history of this topic has an enormous literature, which starts with the discovery of the frontal eye fields by Fritsch and Hitzig (1870), and of oculomotor responses from the occipital cortex by Schäfer (1888), but which for similar reasons as in the case of the cerebellum is not of very great interest today. It has been well reviewed by Mettler (1964).

Electrical stimulation of the frontal eye fields generally results in conjugate deviations of the eyes to the opposite side, although other types of movement with an upward or downward component added may also be represented, possibly in twin regions on each side in an orderly sequence (figure 9.33) (Crosby et al, 1952; Lemmen et al, 1959; Wagman et al, 1961; Jampel, 1960). Jampel (1960) has also reported convergence and divergence movements from the frontal eye fields. In the occipital region, conjugate eye movements can be evoked by stimulation over a wide area: currents required are on the whole greater than for the frontal eye fields, and the resultant movements are slower and have a greater latency. The direction of the occipital movements is roughly what would be expected from the retinotopic projection, if the eyes have to look in the direction corresponding to the part of the cortex being stimulated: but for the parastriate areas there is more disagreement about the topographical arrangement (Crosby and Henderson, 1948; Jampel, 1960; Wagman et al, 1958; see discussion by Mettler, 1964). Jampel (1960) again finds that disjunctive movements can be elicited, from the lower half of area 19 and area 22.

Unilateral ablation of the striate cortex in monkeys leads to an oculomotor and visual neglect of the impaired visual field: lesions in the frontal eye fields have a similar effect, the visual neglect apparently representing a true hemi-amblyopia (G Clark and Lashley, 1947; Latto and Cowey, 1971a; 1971b; similar effects have been reported in man by Silberpfennig, 1941). Recently, Mohler et al (1973) have shown that nearly half the units in the frontal eye fields have visual input, with large, undiscriminating fields quite unlike those of either the occipital visual cortex or the superior colliculus. Yet bilateral ablation of the frontal eye fields has rather little effect on either optokinetic nystagmus, slow pursuit, or saccades (Henderson and Crosby, 1952; Pasik et al, 1959; Pasik and Pasik, 1964): in man, such bilateral lesions are said to lead to a difficulty in making voluntary shifts of fixation (Holmes, 1938; Larmande, 1973), and a reduction or abolition of the quick phase of certain kinds of nystagmus (Jeannerod et al, 1968). With unilateral lesions of cortical areas, vestibular nystagmus may actually be enhanced to the side of the lesion (Bauer and Leidler, 1911; Dusser de Barenne and de Kleijn, 1923; Carmichael et al, 1954). Bilateral lesions of the occipital regions abolish optokinetic nystagmus in primates, though not in other mammals (Smith, 1937; Pasik et al, 1959; Wood et al, 1973): apart from this, it appears only to be fast movements (saccades, or quick phases of nystagmus) that are affected by cortical lesions, and on the whole electrical stimulation also results in fast movements.

The exceptions to this are Jampel's disjunctive movements, and Robinson and Fuch's (1969) finding that barbiturate and possibly other kinds of anaesthesia convert fast movements from electrical stimulation of the frontal eye fields into slow ones. Otherwise, these authors find that stimulation of the frontal fields results in realistic saccades having the same amplitude-duration characteristics as normal voluntary saccades, and whose amplitude and direction are substantially independent both of the initial eye position and of the parameters of the pulse train used to evoke them, except in so far as pairs of stimuli delivered to the same side show a refractory period (figure 9.35). Similar pairs delivered to opposite hemispheres do not show a similar refractoriness for horizontal movements, but do for their *vertical* components. The latency for these saccades is quite short, of the order of 15 ms, and thus less than the 20 ms minimum latency reported by Robinson (1972) in the superior colliculus.

Thus, although the findings in the frontal eye fields are so strongly reminiscent of those in the colliculus, and despite the demonstration by Guitton and Mandl (1973) of a functional pathway from frontal eye fields to the superior colliculus (in the cat), it is clear that the frontal eye field responses cannot be due to indirect activation of collicular mechanisms: *possibly* the frontotectal route is a pathway for 'corollary discharge', although we saw earlier that the idea of an objectively stabilised map in the colliculus is not an attractive one. A possibility is that the pathway from the frontal lobes includes the thalamic internal medullary lamina, where lesions abolish the eye movements evoked by frontal lobe stimulation in cats. Units in this area can be found that fire in close association with eye movements, leading activity in the sixth nerve by some 12–14 ms, even in the dark (Orem and Schlag, 1971; Schlag et al, 1974). Electrical stimulation of the same regions can evoke conjugate saccadic movements to the opposite side: since this region also receives the main concentration of projections from neurons in the reticular formation, it has been suggested that these eye movements are perhaps the result of stimulation of collaterals of reticular neurons also projecting to oculomotor nuclei, and hence embodying some kind of corollary discharge (Schlag and Schlag-Rey, 1971). There is an analogy here perhaps with the projection of somatic motor areas such as the cerebellum and basal ganglia to other thalamic nuclei.

Bizzi (1968; also Bizzi and Schiller, 1970) has examined discharges in single units in the frontal eye fields of unanaesthetised monkeys during movements of the head and eyes, and finds two types of units that are

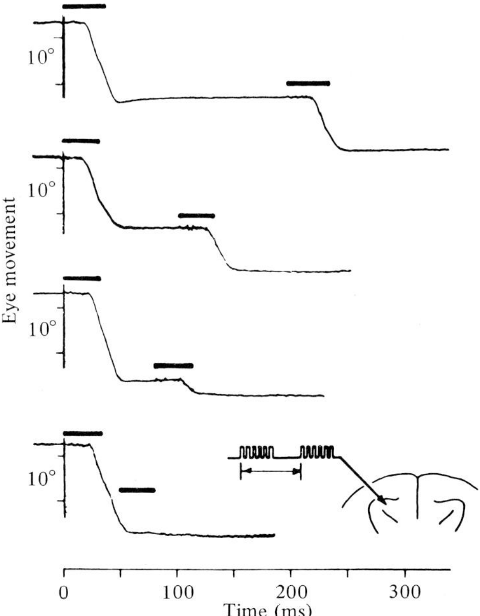

Figure 9.35. Stimulation of frontal lobe of alert monkey with pairs of pulse trains, showing realistic evoked saccades, and the refractoriness (as shown by the diminution in size of the second saccade) seen when both stimuli are applied to the same hemisphere (Robinson and Fuchs, 1969).

linked with eye movements. The first is associated with saccades and with the quick phase of nystagmus, and in accordance with Robinson and Fuchs's findings fires in a manner which is independent of the initial eye position. The second type fires preferentially during smooth pursuit and other slow movements: neither cell type is influenced by the position of the head. A third cell type can be found—rather less frequently—that responds only during movements of the head and not in any particular association with eye movements. But it is quite clear that none of these units can have much to do with the *initiation* of eye movements, since they consistently fire after the beginning of the movement. One must conclude that they are essentially sensory, and respond either to visual, proprioceptive, or 'corollary discharge' information about the movement of the eyes. More recently, Straschill and Schick (1974) have shown

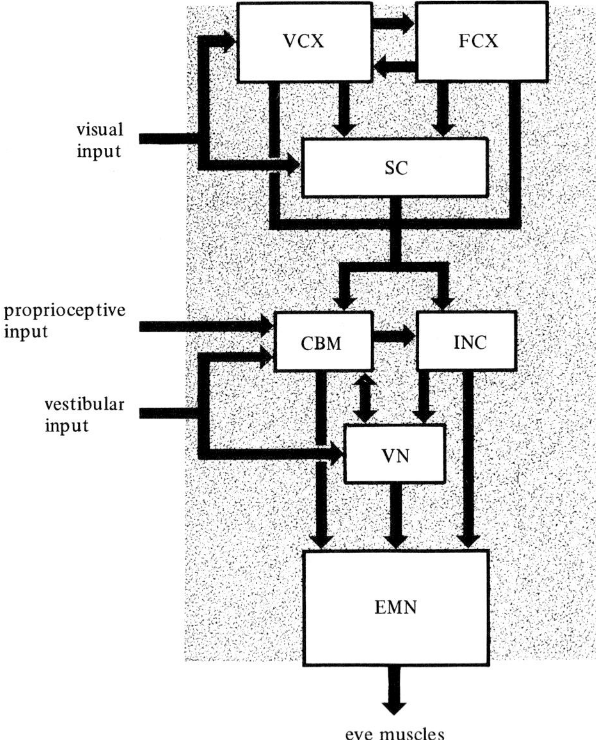

Figure 9.36. Highly schematic representation of the *principal* pathways that may subserve oculomotor function. The grey background represents the reticular formation of the pons and medulla, parts of which can be shown to connect with all the other structures named: no attempt is made to distinguish subdivisions of larger units such as the vestibular nucleus. VCX is visual cortex; FCX is frontal cortex; SC is superior colliculus; CBM is cerebellum; INC is interstitial nucleus of Cajal; VN is vestibular nuclei; EMN is oculomotor nuclei.

patterns of firing associated with eye movements in the parietal lobe of the cat, an area not hitherto associated with eye movements. More than three quarters of the units there that respond to visual stimulation also fire in association with saccades: their responses are weakened (but not wholly abolished) in the dark. The important point about these units is that they fire during or even *before* the saccade takes place, and so *may* represent a link in the causal chain that leads to a voluntary saccade being made. But as far as the *frontal* eye fields are concerned, there is nothing to show that they are not essentially sensory, and that the eye movements that they can evoke are anything more than a high-level reflex.

9.5 Summary of central oculomotor pathways

It may perhaps be helpful to draw together some of the anatomical pathways presented in this chapter, by means of a greatly simplified scheme of connections (figure 9.36). There is a danger in accounts of this sort of hiding the wood with trees, and of giving the impression that everything is connected to everything else. But if one is willing to ignore paths that are not well-established or of substantial size, and not too careful in distinguishing the subgroups of regions such as the reticular formation or vestibular complex, one can achieve a representation which, if nothing else, can serve as a tangible target for criticism. Of course, a tract that is insignificant in size may nevertheless play a crucial role in the system: and of course the observations themselves are biased by preconceptions about what the pathways are likely to be, because that is where one first looks for them. But taken in the right spirit, such diagrams can often be a stimulus to the imagination when trying to discern the larger-scale aspects of the organisation of complicated neural systems. More specific speculations about the functional anatomy are presented in chapter 12.

Part 3

The system as a whole

10

The propriceptive input

"... the proofe wherof may easily be had, if with thy finger thou force the one of thine eyes either higher or lower than the other."

We saw in part 2 that sensory receptors sensitive to stretch—and in some cases, at least, with some degree of gamma control—are an almost universal feature of eye muscles, and that the patterns of impulses they produce in response to mechanical stimulation differ very little from those of ordinary spindles in skeletal muscle. Nothing without a cause: yet the fact remains that after a diligent search by physiologists over a period of rather more than a century we have really no idea at all what these receptors are actually for. It is easy to think of all kinds of functions they *might* serve: for example, by analogy with skeletal stretch receptors one might suppose that they were involved in a rather peripheral mechanism of feedback regulation, similar in its effects to the classical stretch reflex. Attempts to demonstrate such a reflex in extraocular muscle have led to often contradictory results, though it is evident that the contribution of any such mechanism to normal eye muscle tone must be very slight indeed, and not at all comparable with the gross effects observed in the limbs. One possibility is that they may give us conscious sense of the position of our eyes, as Sherrington (1918) thought. But a great weight of evidence makes it clear that this is not the case, or at best that such sensations are so feeble that they can only be perceived by highly trained subjects under conditions of extreme sensory deprivation, and even then give only crude and unreliable indications (Skavenski, 1972).

If, then, the receptors are not sensory in the strict sense, if they have any function at all it must be one of some kind of feedback into the visual or eye muscle control system, even if it is not a classical stretch reflex. Ordinary skeletal muscles send a large projection to the cerebellum, as well as participating in spinal mechanisms like the stretch reflex, and it is perhaps significant that similar cerebellar projections have been demonstrated for the extraocular stretch receptors (Fuchs and Kornhuber, 1969; Azzena et al, 1970, Batini et al, 1974). There are essentially two uses to which such information might be put: one might be described as immediate, the other long-term. Many *immediate* uses for knowledge of the position of the eye have been suggested: for example, stretch of the eye muscles beyond a certain point might inititate the quick phase of nystagmus. Evidence concerning this and other possible short-term functions is considered in section 10.3. In the *long term,* information from stretch receptors could be used by the control system to check that the eye movements actually being made correspond with the commands being issued, and thus to keep a watch for drift or other kinds of deterioration of performance by the muscles, or indeed by the neural circuits that control them. One might imagine parametric feedback of this sort exerted over a rather long time scale in response to repeated discrepancies between the actual and the desired performance, by which the gain and dynamic characteristics of the control system were under continual and gradual adjustment: we have already seen in part 1, the remarkable extent to which the eye movement control system is able to alter its performance to suit unnatural conditions imposed on it from outside. These possibilities are discussed in section 10.3.3.

A thoughtful discussion of earlier ideas on possible roles for eye muscle proprioception may be found in Irvine and Ludvigh (1936).

10.1 Stretch reflexes

10.1.1 General considerations

Figure 10.1 shows an idealised representation of a simple monosynaptic reflex pathway of the type embodying a spinal stretch reflex. The afferent fibres from the stretch receptor synapse excitatorily with motor neurons innervating the main muscle fibres in parallel with the spindle. It is evident

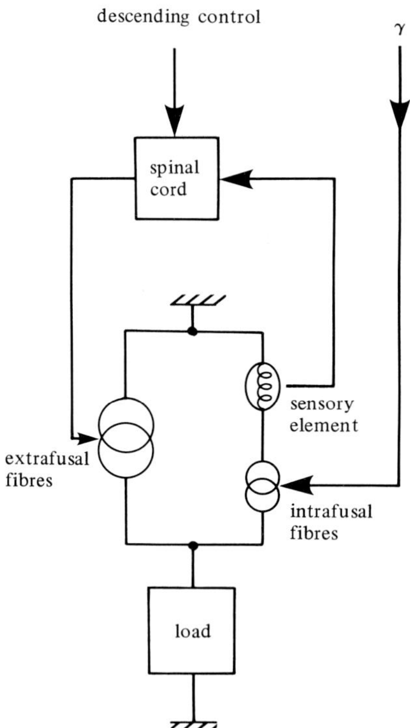

Figure 10.1. Highly schematic representation of the mechanical and control elements of the notional muscle servoloop. The contractile elements are shown by the overlapping circles.

that, if the muscle is stretched, the receptor will initiate a reflex contraction of the muscle fibres, with the result that extra tension is developed in opposition to the stretch. From the point of view of the experimenter who is pulling on the muscle, the effect of the reflex is to make the muscle appear to be stiffer than would be expected from its intrinsic passive mechanical properties alone: and indeed the only way to distinguish a stretch reflex from an ordinary mechanical response is either by accurate measurement of latencies, or by opening the feedback loop by severing the afferent nerve. It is no good separating the muscle altogether from the nervous system, because any drop in stiffness that is then observed may simply be due to loss of tonic activation of the main fibres. In the spinal cord the afferent and efferent fibres are conveniently sorted out into the dorsal and ventral roots, so that opening the loop is a simple matter: but the sensory and motor fibres associated with the eye muscles are not clearly differentiated in this way (section 8.3.2), and the equivalent experiment is not easy to perform with certainty of what one is actually doing.

Two further features must be introduced to bring this simple picture nearer reality. The first is the presence of intrafusal fibres with their small innervating γ efferents. The effect of stimulating these fibres is to stretch the receptors beyond what they experience as a result of changes in length of the muscle as a whole. One would therefore expect that excitation of the fibres would lead to a reflex contraction of the whole muscle, and indeed it has been suggested that in the limbs these fibres form the input of a follow-up length servo (Merton, 1951) controlling the length of skeletal muscles in a way which is relatively independent of any external loads that may be applied to them (figure 10.2). If such a load stretches the muscle beyond the 'desired length' signalled by the γ fibres, the stretch reflex will induce an extra opposing force, tending to restore the *status quo*. The usefulness

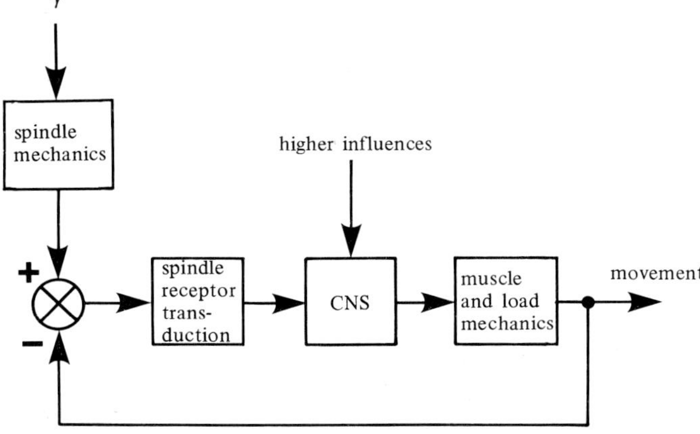

Figure 10.2. A block diagram of the servosystem of figure 10.1, showing the different individual stages of signal transfer that make up the control system.

of such a mechanism in the limbs, with their continually changing loads resulting from the work they have to do against gravity and in accelerating external objects is obvious: but it is not so obvious that such a mechanism would be of much use in the eye. The centre of gravity of the eye is very near its centre of rotation, so that changes in the loading of the extraocular muscles as a result of changes in the attitude of the head must be very slight indeed. In normal use the eye is not loaded with external masses, and so its moment of inertia is constant; the same is true of the elastic and frictional forces with which it has to contend. There is thus no necessity for a length servo, because a particular pattern of firing will always—at least, in the short term—be associated with precisely the same position and velocity of the globe.

The second modification of the simple model of the stretch reflex comes from a consideration of the cooperation between antagonist muscles. Skeletal and eye muscles both exhibit reciprocal innervation of antagonists: contraction of one muscle of a pair is normally associated with relaxation of the other, by a mechanism that in the spinal cord involves in part a crossed inhibitory influence from stretch receptors. An afferent fibre from a stretch receptor in the agonist muscle synapses excitatorily with an interneuron, which in turn inhibits a motor neuron of the antagonist muscle (figure 10.3). Thus the effect of stretching the agonist is to cause both reflex contraction of the same muscle, and reflex relaxation of its antagonist. In the case of the eye, one *might* suppose that such a crossed relation could in principle exist even in the absence of the simple monosynaptic stretch reflex: but it is difficult to see what use it would be.

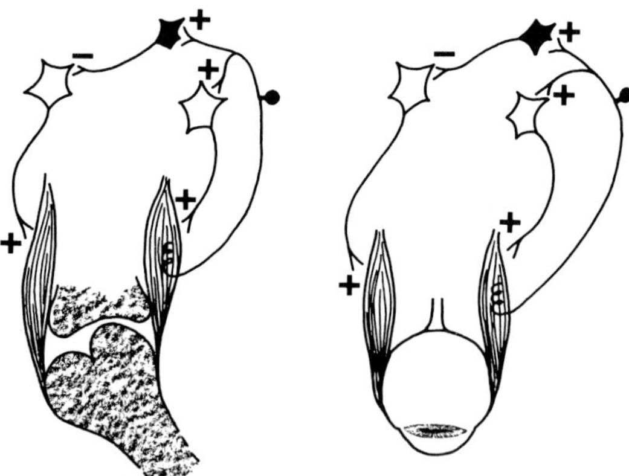

Figure 10.3. Comparison of cooperation between antagonists in a typical skeletal joint (left) and cooperation in the eye (right). In the first case, crossed stretch reflexes as shown tend to produce relaxation of one muscle when the other is contracted; the equivalent arrangement in the eye is only hypothetical and has not been clearly demonstrated.

Another kind of muscular cooperation that is more necessary in the eye perhaps than in most skeletal joints is that between the pairs of muscles that move the eye in different rotational planes. We saw in chapter 7 how changes in length of any one muscle inevitably modify the action of all the others: by a simple extension of the idea of the crossed stretch reflex, one could well imagine cross-linked stretch reflexes between all six muscles of the eyes, that would automatically take care of the complications that these secondary actions introduce in the computation of the oculomotor commands (Kornhuber, 1971). By a further extension, one might imagine that similar cross-links between the muscles of the two eyes might be of assistance in the coordination of conjugate movements. However, we saw in section 5.3 that the yoking of the eyes in binocular movements is not the rigid phenomenon that might be expected if it were the consequence of a peripheral reflex mechanism, and is no longer observed if one of the eyes is occluded: it seems more likely that binocular coordination is achieved by means of visual feedback. Reinecke and Simons (1975) have suggested that *phoria*—latent squint revealed by excluding visual feedback—may be the result of imbalance in a proprioceptive mechanism of this kind.

Finally, there are a number of reasons why a stretch reflex, though present, might not be as simple to demonstrate as in the case of skeletal muscles. One could imagine, for example, that the mechanism might be switched on for some kinds of movements but not for others, the switching effectively being performed by activation of the γ fibres. For example, the vestibular system might exert its control of eye position by means of a length servo, while visually evoked eye movements might use visual rather than proprioceptive feedback (being intrinsically closed-loop anyway). The retina is well adapted to giving accurate information about relative movements of the eye (in stable surroundings), and its messages are more closely related to the needs of the oculomotor system, whose ultimate function, after all, is to *look* rather than to point the eye. In the words of Sherrington (1918): "The spatial endowment of the retinal sense itself is of such pre-eminent and exquisite degree that it has seemed... a sufficient source in itself for almost every spatial attribute of vision." Secondly, the stretch reflex may exhibit gross nonlinearities, and be brought into action only with extreme deviations, or conceivably only during the high *rates* of stretch experienced during saccades: although it is true that the receptors themselves do not exhibit this sort of behaviour, one can easily imagine filtering of their information by the neural structures to which they project. Lastly, it might be that the stretch reflexes influence only the slow fibres in the muscle, generating slow sustained changes in tone that might well be overlooked in ordinary investigations (Baichenko et al, 1968).

10.1.2 Mechanical studies

We saw in chapter 7 that the nonlinearities in the passive properties of the eye muscles, combined with the passive elastic elements linking the globe to the orbit, together result in a net elastic force that tends to restore the eye roughly to the primary position after displacement. This fundamental fact means that we must do more to demonstrate an extraocular stretch reflex than simply show that there is a tendency for the globe to resist external displacements from its position of rest. Thus Skavenski's (1971) observation that the miniature eye movements made in the dark are more often corrective than not does not by itself imply the presence of a proprioceptive mechanism. He showed that there was a significant negative correlation between the error in the direction of gaze (with respect to the mean position measured over a longer period) at any instant, and the size and direction of the movement made in the succeeding half second. But this is exactly what would be expected if there were a purely passive tonic process tending to centre the eye, with random microperturbations superimposed, whose size and direction are not related to the position of the eye at all: the same would be observed if, for example, one were to drop a marble into a bowl and then shake the latter about in a random fashion.

The only wholly satisfactory experiments must involve opening the hypothetical feedback loop. As we have seen, this is not nearly such a simple matter as in the spinal cord. The drastic procedure of cutting the *whole* nerve supply to the muscles is unsatisfactory because they will then lose any tone they may derive from sources other than stretch reflexes, for example from tonic vestibular reflexes. McCouch and Adler (1932) tried to get round this problem by first sectioning the vestibular nerves: under these circumstances they found that the tension associated with a particular degree of stretch was not reduced after cutting the muscle nerve, implying that no stretch reflex component was present. But the conditions they used were clearly highly artificial. De Kleijn (1921a) attempted to open the loop by partial anaesthesia of the nerve endings with novocaine: but it is impossible with this procedure to be sure that there is a level of dosage for which the sensory nerve endings are significantly depressed, while the motor ones are not affected at all. Sherrington (1893) cut the insertion of the inferior oblique on the globe, and found that pulling on it sometimes resulted in reflex movements of the other muscles, suggesting a stretch-reflex-type cooperation between the muscles of the globe along the lines proposed in section 10.1.1 above. But the movements were small and sometimes altogether absent, and also associated with quite unrelated movements such as twitching of the ears, which suggests that he may simply have been causing pain.

All these mechanical methods were eventually superceded by electrical methods of analysis, which offer a greater measure of certainty of interpretation. But it is perhaps worth mentioning one other aspect of the mechanical properties of the extraocular muscle which at first sight appears to support the notion of a tonic stretch reflex, namely the shapes of the length–tension curves under different degrees of innervation (section 7.5.3). Figure 10.4 shows a set of curves of this type from a human subject attempting to fixate at different angles to the left and right. Now if the effect of different degrees of voluntary effort were merely to add different extra tensions to the passive tension exerted by the elastic elements of the globe and muscles, whether or not a stretch reflex were present, one would expect the various curves to be superimposable by simple vertical sliding. But in fact, the curves are much better described by *horizontal* displacements, as if the effect of different acts of volition were to change the 'desired length' of the muscle—via the γ efferent mechanism—and thus only indirectly causing contractions of the muscle through the stretch reflex. In other words, the fact that the different curves can be generated by sliding along the length rather than the tension axis is *prima facie* evidence for a length servo (Granit, 1971). The argument rests on the assumption that the mechanical properties of the muscle fibres should be unaffected by changes in length or activation: but as we have seen, the known nonlinearities of the mechanics demonstrate exactly the reverse. In the cat, there is clear evidence that the approximate superimposability of the curves under lateral displacement is merely an internal property of the muscle, and not the result of an external feedback loop (Collins, 1971): precisely the same relationship is found for different rates of stimulation of the muscle nerve (figure 10.5), even when its

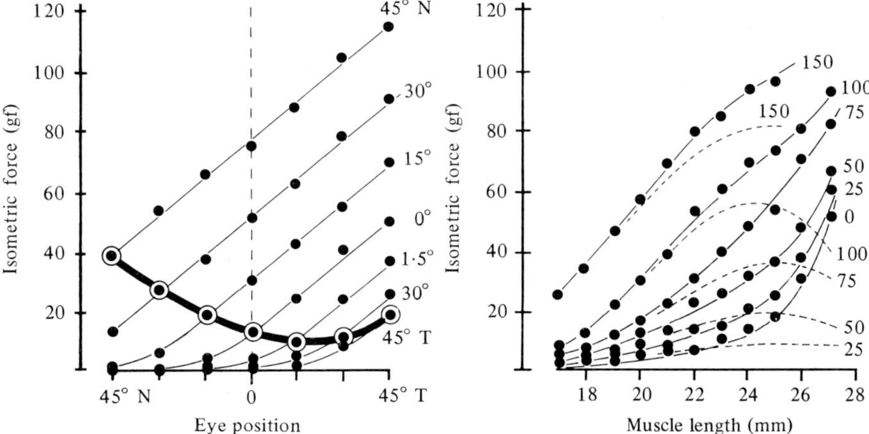

Figure 10.4. Length–tension relationships for human rectus muscles, when the subject attempts to fixate an object at different eccentricities: see figure 7.28.

Figure 10.5. Length–tension curves for cat lateral rectus, when the nerve is stimulated at the different frequencies shown; the central connections of the muscle are severed, therefore conventional stretch reflexes can play no part in determining the shape of the curves.

central connections have been severed. It is quite clear then that the shape of the length–tension curves, suggestive though it is, does not provide evidence for a stretch reflex of any kind.

10.1.3 Electrical recordings

The confusion between responses that are simply the result of essentially passive properties of muscle, and those due to a stretch reflex, is avoided if electrical responses either in the muscle or in the motor neurons that supply it are taken as a measure of the active contribution of the muscle to movement. If a simple monosynaptic stretch reflex exists, then pulling on the muscle should result in an increase in its electrical activity. Crossed inhibitory influences should show up as a change in the electrical activity of the antagonist or of the other muscles. Unfortunately, few experimenters have been able to demonstrate such clear unequivocal results, and different workers have reached quite contradictory conclusions. Thus McIntyre (1939) showed that the tonic rate of discharge of the abducens nerve was unaltered when it was severed from the muscle itself and thus permitted to relax completely; conversely, Perryman and Breinin (1971) could observe no increase in the extraocular EMG on pulling on the muscles. Breinin (1957), Maruo (1964) and Jampolsky (1970) all find, on the contrary, that there is a simple excitatory stretch reflex component, though only for stretches lying between full relaxation and the primary position, with no effect on any of the other muscles. Sears et al (1959), under what appear to be identical conditions, find no evidence at all for stretch reflexes when the eye is near the primary position, nor any changes in a muscle's tonic activity when either it or its antagonist is disinserted. The only effect reported is the quite unexpected one that extreme stretch causes a *decrease* in the electromyogram of both agonist and antagonist. This is of course the exact opposite of what would be expected from a stretch reflex, and it is possible that the inhibition is due to stimulation of tendon organs, rather than true stretch receptors, by analogy with the clasp-knife reflex of ordinary skeletal muscle. Jampolsky (1970) reports a lack of graded cross-innervation—that is, of normal reciprocal firing—after cutting the muscle insertions: but since this was only exhibited when it was the operated eye that attempted the fixation (the relation being normal when the other eye was used), it is likely that this was simply due to the effective opening of the visual feedback loop on the affected side, with resultant very high gains.

Recordings from oculomotor nerves in experimental animals are perhaps less prone to error through lack of knowledge in the human case of how the subject may be perturbing the results by the intrusion of semivoluntary influences, and results have shown a good measure of consistency in denying the existence of stretch reflexes. [An exception is Bach-y-Rita's (1972) finding of very slight increases in the discharge rates of selected oculomotor units when a distal branch of the abducens nerve is stimulated: but as the muscle was isometrically clamped, the results are difficult of interpretation].

McIntyre's (1939) completely negative finding has already been mentioned and has been fully confirmed recently in a very thorough series of experiments by Keller and Robinson (1971) in the alert monkey. Recording from single units in the abducens nucleus, they found a total absence of any sign of a stretch reflex either for lengthening or for shortening of the muscle, at any position of the globe (figure 10.6). Nor could any differences in the discharge pattern during a saccade be found between trials where the eye was allowed to move freely, and when it was suddenly clamped (figure 10.7). This effectively rules out the possibility

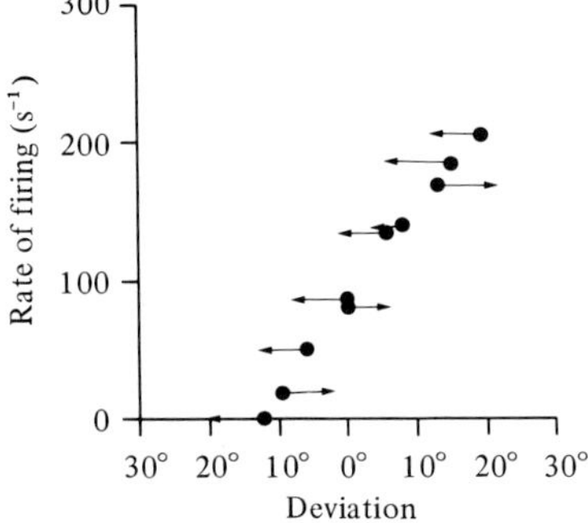

Figure 10.6. Absence of a tonic stretch reflex in extraocular muscle. Data points show unimpeded deviation-frequency relationship for a single monkey abducens unit; arrows indicate the (lack of) effect of stretching and shortening externally applied upon the firing rate at different deviations (data of Keller and Robinson, 1971).

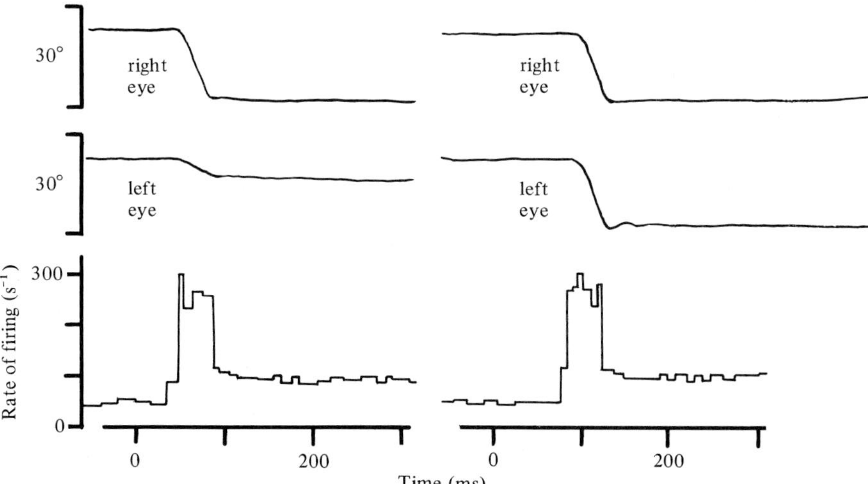

Figure 10.7. Lack of stretch reflex during fast movements. Left, the left eye was impeded whilst a conjugate saccade was attempted by the monkey (upper traces); the time course of firing frequency of one of the abducens units is shown below. On the right, for comparison, the behaviour of the same unit during a normal, unimpeded, saccade (after Keller and Robinson, 1971).

suggested in section 10.1 that feedback might only operate in fast movements, since these are the fastest movements that the eye can make. Keller and Robinson admit that their results do not rule out the possibility of stretch reflexes involving only slow fibres, whose neurons might not be accessible to ordinary microelectrode recording, but otherwise the force of their conclusion that there is no stretch reflex in monkey extraocular muscles can hardly be disputed.

Further evidence that the primary mode of controlling eye muscles is not by means of a length servo activated by γ fibres comes from observations of the relative timing of discharges in the γ fibres and in the main motor fibres—the α fibres— in the goat (Whitteridge, 1958). If such a servo-mechanism provided the prime activation of the contraction, one would expect that the γ fibres would fire first, followed by an increase in the frequency of firing of the afferent fibres from the stretch receptors, and followed in turn by increased firing in the α fibres and contraction of the muscle. The observed sequence of events in vestibularly evoked eye movements is quite different: the α fibres fire before the γ, and the response of the afferent fibres consists of an initial *decrease* in firing rate, followed sometimes by an increase. It is clear that, although there may be length-servo component to the response, it is dominated by a more direct system of activation via the α fibres.

10.1.4 The possibility of an intrinsic stretch reflex

Although the evidence presented so far has been to some extent conflicting, and although this is an area where there are marked species differences in structure, and no doubt also in function, it is probably fair to say that studies on the firing rates of the nerves and nuclei have been virtually unanimous in denying the existence of a stretch reflex, while on the other hand those that have studied the electromyogram have on the whole supported the notion, at least under particular conditions. At the same time, we have seen that the intrinsic properties of the muscles, as exhibited in the length-tension curves, are very much what would be expected from a length servo, although there is irrefutable evidence that they cannot be the result of an ordinary stretch reflex loop.

One possible way in which these various observations might be reconciled is to postulate the existence of a stretch reflex that is entirely *intrinsic* to the muscle: for example, one could endow some of the muscle fibres with the property that, when stretched, they respond with electrical activity and contraction. Such a response would not of course show up in recordings made from the muscle nerve or nuclei. Now we have seen that the extraocular fibres contain a high proportion of 'slow' fibres, fibres that lie somewhere in the middle of the continuum of muscle types that runs from striated twitch fibres on the one hand to classical smooth muscle fibres—as found for example in the uterus—on the other. A well-established feature of smooth muscle is precisely the property that we are postulating here for some of the extraocular fibres: stretching such fibres induces an increase in their electrical activity, which in turn results in a 'reflex' contraction (for example Bülbring, 1955). It is perhaps not too farfetched an idea to suppose that some of the many types of slow fibre in eye muscle, whose function we have seen to be something of a mystery, may in fact serve to generate an intrinsic stretch reflex of this type. It is even possible that the small nerve fibres that innervate them might play an analogous role to the γ fibres of skeletal spindles, and specify a 'desired length', though Bülbring's (1955) observation that in smooth muscle it is the tension rather than the degree of stretch that determines the rate of firing perhaps makes this unlikely. Even if they do not participate in a length servomechanism, such fibres could well contribute to the control and regularisation of the overall mechanical properties of the muscle, which we have seen to be so well adapted to its function: However, this idea is wholly speculative, and one must bear in mind that extremely similar length–tension curves are shown by the *retractor bulbi* muscle of the cat, whose fibres are wholly of the twitch variety (Lennerstrand, 1974).

10.2 Sensation

The fixity of the relationship between the degree of activation of the eye muscles and the resultant movement of the globe, which we have seen to be a strong argument against the need for extraocular stretch reflexes, argues just as strongly against the need for proprioceptors to tell us where we are looking. As Helmholtz (1909) pointed out, we need only monitor the signals that are *sent* to the eye muscles to have perfect knowledge of the position of the eyes; for, as Merton (1961) puts it: "there is no reason why we should not be able to judge the size of motor volleys leaving the brain as accurately as we can judge the size of sensory volleys arriving". The idea seems first to have been suggested by Sir Charles Bell (1823), who called it the 'sense of voluntary exertion': nowadays it is usually referred as the 'outflow theory', in contrast with the 'inflow theory' that supposes, as Sherrington (1918) did, that such information is derived only from proprioceptors in the muscles.

The signal that is imagined to be tapped off from the motor pathway and used as a basis for sensation is sometimes called a *corollary discharge* (Sperry, 1950) or *efference copy* (figure 10.8). Different people mean different things by 'sensation', and it is important to emphasise that, although a subject might be able, for example, to use information from stretch receptors to point his eyes in a determined direction in the dark, it does not follow from this that the receptors give him conscious sensation of eye position, for the proprioceptive information may be used only at an unconscious level of integration, to ensure that the commands sent out are actually obeyed (Merton, 1961). In this example, although proprioception is essential if the sensation derived from outflow is to correspond with reality, it does not directly provide the sensation. The same distinction applies to the role that is often suggested for extraocular muscle receptors, of informing the visual system whether a shift of the retinal image is due to an actual movement in the outside world, or merely to an eye movement. Common experience tells us that, when we move our eyes, the world around us does not appear to move in the opposite direction but remains apparently stationary. Even if it were true that this is because stretch receptors in the eye muscles have in some way cancelled the shift of the retinal image at some level of the visual system, this certainly does not imply that they give conscious sensation of eye movement. These three kinds of sensation are discussed separately in the three ensuing sections. Thoughtful discussions of earlier arguments about the role of inflow and outflow may be found in Merton (1964) and Festinger and Canon (1965).

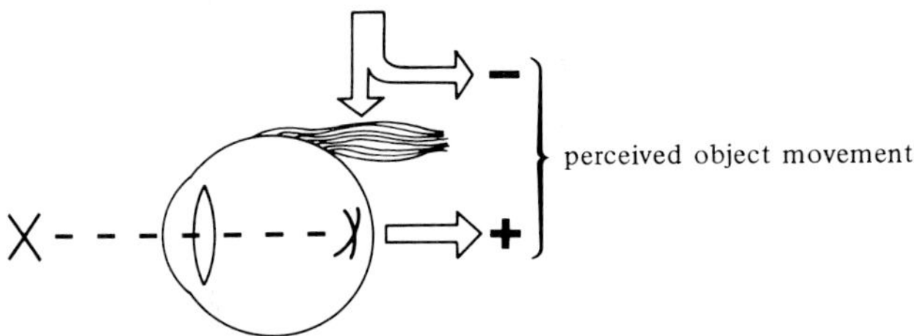

Figure 10.8. Schematic representation of the notion of 'efference copy' or 'corollary discharge'. Two sources of information are proposed for perceiving object movement and distinguishing it from eye movement: they are retinal image movement (below, right) and knowledge of the signal sent to the eye muscles (above, right). They are imagined to be subtracted one from the other in some central mechanism to cancel out the effects of eye movements (after von Holst, 1957).

10.2.1 Conscious sensation

It is clear from experiments that proprioceptors in the orbit contribute very little, if anything at all, to conscious sensation. Both Irvine and Ludvigh (1936) and Brindley and Merton (1960) found that a subject could not tell if an experimenter was deviating his occluded eye to one side or the other by means of forceps, so long as the surface of the eye was anaesthetised with cocaine, and care was taken not to disturb the eyelids. Nor could subjects tell whether an intended eye movement had actually taken place, or had in fact been held back by the experimenter. Such a negative finding carries very much more weight than a positive one, because in the latter case one cannot ever be sure that *all* possible sources of information other than stretch receptors have been eliminated.

Skavenski (1972) applied external forces to a subject's eye by means of a tightly fitting contact lens with a stalk attached, and found that highly trained subjects could, in the dark, name the direction in which their eye had been pulled correctly in about 70%–80% of the trials. But the onus is on the experimenter here to show conclusively that, for example, differences in pressure on the two sides of the contact lens may not have been unconsciously sensed by the subject and used as clues to the direction of pull. At all events, the significant finding is perhaps that even under conditions designed to be as free from distracting stimuli as possible, and with experienced and practised subjects, the supposed mechanism is so feeble that in something like half the trials the subject cannot be sure of naming even the direction of the pull correctly, and has to guess. It is difficult to believe, even if these results do in fact represent a sensory function for the proprioceptors, that such a function could be of any great utility in normal life.

That any such signal is swamped by visual information is clearly shown in an experiment by Ludvigh (1952a; 1952b), who arranged for a subject to fixate a stationary point of light situated behind a half-silvered mirror that filled his (restricted) visual field and reflected the surrounding room. If, while the mirror was moved back and forth about a vertical axis, the subject tried to maintain fixation on the point of light, he had the sensation that the visual field was stationary and that it was the light that was moving around; and also that he was making large corrective eye movements to follow it, when in fact his eyes were not moving at all.

10.2.2 Cancellation of the visual effects of eye movements

There is an abundance of evidence that the apparent stability of the visual world when we move our eyes is not the result of information from our eye muscles. The simplest, though not perhaps the most convincing, demonstration that this is so is that if the eye is moved by an external force—for example, by pressing on the eyelid with a finger—the visual scene appears to move in the opposite direction (Helmholtz, 1909). One could well argue that this results in unnatural mechanical stimulation of the muscles, and possibly also affects the optics of the eye; and also that the other eye, being stationary, may possibly override any sensory effects from the manipulated one. Finally one cannot be sure that the apparent motion of the image is the same as the amplitude of the motion of the eye, in other words that there is not *some* degree of cancellation induced by stretch of the muscles. Experiments that demonstrate the contribution of outflow signals are perhaps more convincing (figure 10.9). Mach (1886) partially immobilised his eyes, and found that the visual world moved when he tried to make eye movements: Brindley and Merton (1960) observed exactly the same thing when the subject tried to move his eyes, when both were forcibly held by the experimenter. Hughlings Jackson and Paton (1909) showed that a patient with unilateral weakness of the eye muscles, when asked to point at a visual object (his hand being screened from his own sight) invariably pointed too far in the direction of the paresis. A similar experiment is to paralyse, or at least weaken, the eyes by pharmacological means: Kornmüller (1931), using novocaine, and Hammond et al (1956), who used tubocurarine, both reported apparent movement on trying to move the eyes.

Further evidence comes from patients with a pathologically immobile eye (for example Helmholtz, 1909; Hughlings Jackson, 1932), who observe exactly the same phenomenon: these findings have, however, been criticised on the grounds mentioned earlier, that some account ought to be taken of the unaffected eye and its possible contribution (Sherrington, 1900; James, 1950). A more disturbing consideration is that if the eye is *completely* immobilised (Siebeck, 1954; Stevens et al, 1976; Brindley et al, 1976) *no* movement of the visual world on attempting to move the eye is observed. Thus it seems that *some* retinal image movement is a prerequisite for the sensation of movement of the visual world: but if this retinal slip can be accounted for by a concomitant eye movement, it is ignored. The observations with completely paralysed eyes are therefore not as devastating for the outflow theory as they perhaps seem at first,

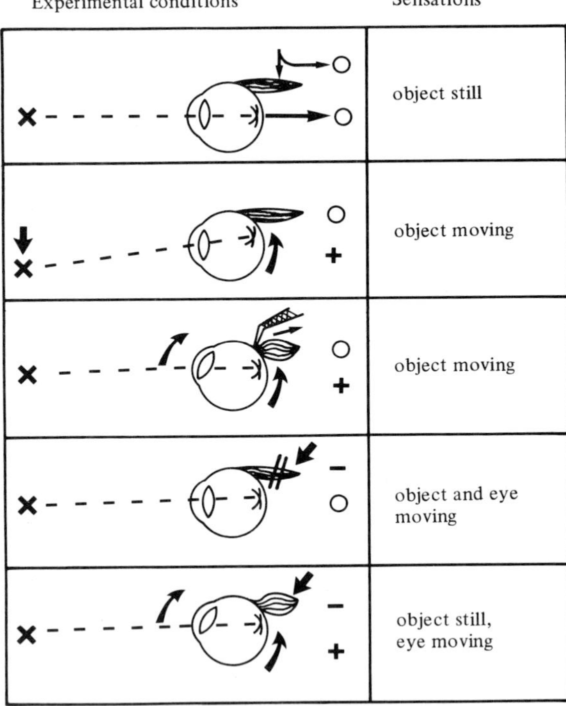

Figure 10.9. Perceived object motion under a number of different experimental conditions, predicted from the efference copy mechanism. From top to bottom, they are: eye and object at rest; object moves with eye still; object still, eye is moved independently of the will of the subject; object still, subject wills an eye movement but eye is paralysed; and normal movement of eye with object still. The symbols just to the right of the eye in each case indicate the relative contribution of the efference copy and retinal sources of information, and the right-hand column lists the subject's sensations in each case.

although they rule out a simple model in which perceived external movement is under all circumstances equal to the difference between retinal image movement and desired eye movement.

Afterimages—necessarily fixed relative to the retina—in some cases provide a more critical test of the outflow theory. The behaviour of the afterimage is the exact opposite of that of images of the real world in experiments like those described above. Thus afterimages do *not* move if the eye is pushed (Bell, 1823; Helmholtz, 1909; Karrer and Stevens, 1930; but see also Oppel, 1959), but *do* move when voluntary eye movements are made, even when the muscles are detached from the globe (Jampolsky, 1970). But a recent report (Brindley et al, 1976) claims that under complete curarisation an afterimage in the paralysed eye does not move (though one in the other eye *does*). The question of whether the afterimage moves during involuntary movements has never been decisively settled. Bell (1823) thought that it did not, at any rate for some kinds of involuntary movement; Mack and Bachant (1969) on the other hand found a good correlation during semiautomatic tasks like afterimage 'tracking' between eye position and apparent afterimage position: true smooth pursuit cannot of course be examined under stabilised-image conditions. It is not clear what happens during vestibular nystagmus: as the reader can easily verify for himself by forming an afterimage from a light bulb and then moving his head appropriately, the slow component of the vestibuloocular reflex causes an apparent movement, while nothing corresponding to the quick phase can be seen at all. Karrer and Stevens (1930) suggest that this is because the afterimage actually disappears during the quick phase: but it is difficult to see why this should also suppress the perception of the consequent displacement of the image, since equivalent fast displacements produced by voluntary saccades are perfectly easily seen. It seems more likely that the quick phase does not in fact contribute to afterimage movement, though the observations are difficult to make with confidence.

During a vergence movement, the images in the two eyes move—under natural conditions—in opposite directions: no mechanism exists for compensating for each eye's movement separately, and under these conditions the world appears to move. This can most clearly be demonstrated by making a convergence movement on to an object with one eye covered: preferably an asymmetric convergence such that the uncovered eye does not need to move at all (figure 10.10) (Helmholtz, 1909). The object will then appear to move in a direction opposite to the motion of the eye. The equivalent afterimage experiment is to perform an afterimage version of an ordinary phoria test, one eye viewing the afterimage of a scale, and the other of a pointer on it. Voluntary convergence and divergence do not result in *tonic* displacement of the scale relative to the pointer, although there may be a transient impression of relative movement between them even though one can see throughout the course of the whole

loaded or hindered in some way by external forces, so as to upset the normal relation between efferent activity and eye position. Such an experiment has been reported by Skavenski (1972). By means of a lever attached to a tightly fitting contact lens, Skavenski arranged for various displacing forces to be applied to a subject's eye while—in total darkness—he was endeavouring to maintain a fixed direction of regard. He found that subjects could still maintain roughly constant gaze, with a standard deviation of between 1 and 3°.

The interpretation of this finding is complicated by our ignorance of what part may be played by the eye that is *not* subjected to the disturbing forces, and it is unfortunate that records were not made of its movements in the experiment. Either the eyes move conjugately, in which case the correction for the disturbed eye is inappropriate for the other; or only the disturbed eye is corrected, and the other remains stationary. Neither alternative is very satisfactory. Why, if they move conjugately, should one eye be corrected at the expense of the other? If on the other hand the eyes are corrected independently, why is it that if the undisturbed eye is allowed to fixate a small target, *no* corrections are made by the (occluded) manipulated eye? These considerations make it hard to accept Skavenski's conclusions, and it is possible that in this experiment too the well-practised subjects were unconsciously using faint sensations from the cornea in response to the loads being applied to the contact lens. There is good evidence that such apparently unconnected sensations can be used to improve the accuracy with which the eye can be held stationary in the dark (McLaughlin et al, 1968). If an auditory signal is given to the subject whenever the deviation of the eye exceeds some bound (say 1° from the desired direction), there is a significant increase in the accuracy of his stabilisation. Even greater effects are observed if the auditory clue is directional, and related to the direction of the error. Thus it is clear that the task of directing the eye in the dark is susceptible to influences at a high level of integration in the brain.

10.3 Other possible functions

10.3.1 The quick phase of nystagmus

Since the effect of the quick phase of nystagmus is to reset the position of the eye when the steadily increasing deviation of the slow phase would otherwise bring it to the limit of its rotation, it is natural to assume, as Bartels (1911) did, that it would be appropriate for stretch receptors in the extraocular muscles to initiate this function. Experiments soon showed that this was not the case. De Kleijn (1921a) injected novocaine into the muscles during caloric nystagmus in the hope of paralysing the proprioceptive endings before paralysing the motor endings, and observed that the effect was a sudden cessation of all movement. If the proprioceptors were responsible for the quick phase, one would have anticipated a period during which the slow, but not the quick, phase was produced. The weakness of this argument is of course that one cannot be sure that the proprioceptors really were knocked out first. Better evidence was provided by McCouch and Adler (1932), who showed that the rhythm of caloric nystagmus was unaltered by pulling on the muscles, and by McIntyre's (1939) knockdown demonstration that a normal nystagmic rhythm could be recorded from oculomotor nerves even if the eye and all its muscles were entirely removed from the orbit! There can be no question, then, that the stretch receptors have very little to do with the generation of the quick phase.

10.3.2 Velocity feedback

We have already seen that the characteristics of all three types of slow movement suggest the presence of a neural integrator in the final common path of the oculomotor system, and we shall see in chapter 12 that such an integrator is probably used in the saccadic system as well. Now to say that the deviation of the eye at any moment is proportional to the time integral of a particular signal is simply another way of saying that the velocity of the eye is always proportional to the same signal. This in turn suggests the possibility that the integration might be performed by a feedback mechanism, in which stretch receptors measure the velocity of the eye, which is then compared with the input signal, and the error between the two is used to accelerate the eye and reduce the discrepancy (figure 10.11). Taylor (1965b) recorded from the abducens nucleus of an anaesthetised cat before and after curarisation of the eye muscles: if there were a loop, this would open it. He found, in fact, no significant changes in the phase of the discharge pattern in response to sinusoidal rotation, although there was a slight reduction in amplitude. In a similar experiment in which a decerebrate rather than an anaesthetised preparation was used, Carpenter (1972a) compared the pattern of the electromyogram from the lateral rectus during sinusoidal vestibular stimulation, either with the eye

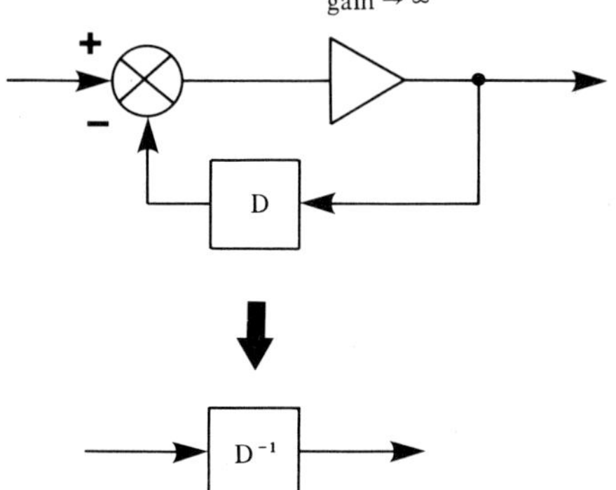

Figure 10.11. Feedback of the differential of the output, when the forward gain is very high, is equivalent to integration.

free to move, or with it held fixed relative to the head. Again, no significant difference in the pattern of firing could be observed in the two conditions. It thus seems fairly certain that any role for stretch receptors in the vestibuloocular reflex must be a slight one, and certainly not of the fundamental type implied if the integration is achieved by velocity feedback. The results of Keller and Robinson (1971) mentioned earlier make it clear that the same is true of the integration that may be required in the case of smooth pursuit, vergence and saccades.

10.3.3 Long-term parametric feedback

The arguments set out in the preceding sections against the utility of feedback from the eye muscles lose their strength as soon as one considers the long-term control of eye movements. There are many reasons why the relationship between efferent activity and eye position, though constant over periods of minutes, might not be so from day to day and from year to year. During early life the eye and its muscles are growing, while even in the mature organism pathologic or metabolic processes—or the insidious changes of age—may significantly alter their mechanical properties. Eye muscles are also subject to fatigue. All these circumstances would pass unnoticed by a system that never checked to see if its orders were being carried out, and relied entirely on outflow rather than inflow as a source of information. Indeed it is difficult to see how such a blindly autocratic system would even deal successfully with stable idiosyncrasies present from birth, since the neural model of the eye mechanics that must exist for corollary discharges to be translated back into positional terms would presumably have to be genetically specified.

A more satisfactory hypothesis is that the various parameters of the eye control system are *learnt*, by a process in which outflow signals are continually compared with proprioceptive feedback, and any long-standing errors automatically induce changes in the control system, by a process of *parametric feedback* (figure 10.12). Here the γ innervation is imagined to convey the 'desired position' to the spindle, which then acts as the

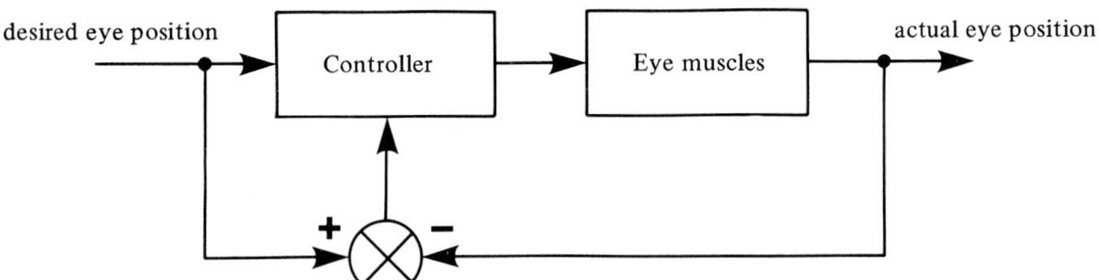

Figure 10.12. Possible role of parametric feedback in control of eye position. Actual eye position is compared with the desired eye position that forms the input to the whole system; the error signal does not *directly* cause an output response, but rather modifies the behaviour of the open-loop controller in such a way as to minimise such errors in the long run.

comparator: in normal operation the γ and α routes will be activated simultaneously, and the spindle response will indicate errors of performance. The difference between this and the servo theory is that here these spindle discharges cannot *directly* induce contractions. [In section 10.1.3 we saw that γ discharge if anything lags behind the α discharge (Whitteridge, 1958)]. The same learning mechanism could serve equally well not only for setting the system up in the first place, but also for keeping it in step with changes in the mechanical characteristics of the eye (Ludvigh, 1952b; von Holst, 1954). In particular—by an extension of the notion presented in section 10.1.1 that cross-linked stretch reflexes might help in the mutual coordination of the twelve eye muscles—it is natural to suggest that this function might be easier to learn than to specify genetically. An old observation, confirmed in 1941 but apparently not reexamined since, is that transposition of pairs of eye muscles is followed by a remarkably rapid process of recovery of functional coordination (Marina, 1915; Olmstead et al, 1936; Leinfelder and Black, 1941). The latter authors found (in the monkey) that simultaneous transposition of medial and inferior recti, and lateral and superior, led to a return of proper cooperation after only eight days, even when the animals had been maintained in the dark; while Olmstead et al (1936) found recovery of coordination after transposition of superior and lateral recti, although the eye in question was blind! It is difficult to imagine what mechanism apart from muscle proprioception could be responsible for such a recovery; but there are obvious logical difficulties, even so.

A mechanism for which this argument for parametric feedback seems particularly compelling is that which generates the pulse-step profile of excitation during a saccade. The relation of the height of the pulse and that of the step is an extremely critical one, in relation to the mechanical properties of the eye. If the pulse is too big, the eye will overshoot: if too small, it will creep only slowly to its final position (for example Easter, 1973; Bahill et al, 1975b). As we have seen, although some subjects do produce undershoots and overshoots (figure 4.4), they are both small in relation to the size of the saccades themselves—showing how well the relative size of pulse and step are matched to the mechanics—and also, perhaps significantly in this context, subject to slow variations of extent from day to day. In particular, it has been clearly shown that fatigue in the saccadic system is a potent generator of mismatch between the slow and fast components (Bahill and Stark, 1975). If we think of the pulse-step combination as being generated by an integrator in parallel with a pure gain component (see chapter 12), then this matching process amounts to an adjustment of the relative gains of the two paths. We shall see later that the same two paths probably also compute the vestibular eye movements from afferent semicircular canal signals, and that there are good reasons for believing that the direct path is embodied in the medial longitudinal fasciculus, while the indirect path involves the neurons of the pontine reticular formation and possibly the cerebellum. It is thus perhaps significant that one of the few central electrophysiological effects ever reported as a result of stimulation of extraocular stretch receptors was a depression of the response of such cells to vestibular nerve stimulation (Gernandt, 1968). Many people are coming to believe that a major function of the cerebellum is in the learning of new motor skills, and we have already seen that there is some evidence that the cerebellum is involved in long-term adaptation to unnatural relationships between head movement and movement of the visual scene (section 9.3.5). Like skeletal muscle spindles, extraocular stretch receptors have a prominent cerebellar projection, and the simultaneous convergence of visual, vestibular, and proprioceptive pathways in the cerebellum (see section 9.3.2), combined with its known involvement both in vestibular and in saccadic eye movements makes it highly probable that it is the seat of the kinds of adaptive processes that have been suggested in this section: this discussion is pursued further in the two following chapters.

Perhaps, then, the apparent uselessness of eye muscle receptors is due to experimenters' natural reluctance to perform long experiments: and perhaps it is significant that the only recent report that has even hinted at a possible proprioceptive function (Skavenski, 1972) used subjects who were highly trained in the task that was required.

11

Eye movements and vision

"The third thing which I have to testifie the excellencie of the sight, is the certaintie of the function. For it is out of all doubt that this is the most infallible sence, and that which least deceiveth: according to that which men are wont to say, when they wil assuredly avouch any thing, namely, that they see it with their owne eyes."

It is only too easy, in contemplating the elegant precision of eye movements, and in enthusiastic examination of the *minutiae* of the neuronal mechanisms that bring them about, to forget that the whole eye movement control system, impressive as it is, is after all a mere adjunct to the sense of sight. Perhaps now it is time to look at the eye movement control system as it were through the eyes of the visual system. In part 1 of this book, in describing the characteristics of the various kinds of movement, we examined the extent of the visual system's control over eye movements. This chapter will consider the reciprocal aspect of this relationship, namely the ways in which the visual system is itself influenced by movements of the eyes.

The first two topics to be discussed are at first sight paradoxical: they concern the observations that on the one hand the sense of sight is partially incapacitated during voluntary eye movements, and on the other, that unless *some* movement takes place one cannot see at all. The third topic is the very extensive one of the relation between eye movements and spatial sense: that is, of our knowledge of the distance, direction, and motion of the visual objects round us. Spatial sense is largely the province of experimental psychologists, and it is probably inappropriate to do more than touch on some of the ways in which movements of the eyes impinge on it: a more complete discussion of these matters may, for example, be found in Ogle (1962).

11.1 Saccadic suppression

11.1.1 Basic observations

We have seen that the velocity of the eyes in executing a saccade is very great, and it is not surprising to find that vision during saccades is impaired. What *is* surprising is both the degree of impairment, and the fact that it is quite unperceived, even by subjects who are intellectually aware of its existence and try hard to experience it directly (see for example Dodge, 1905). This may be simply demonstrated by means of a mirror: however closely and attentively one looks at the reflections of one's eyes whilst making voluntary eye movements, they appear perfectly stationary (Dodge, 1900). A refinement of this experiment is to arrange to record the eye movements electrically, and use the signal to deflect a trace on an oscilloscope (Ditchburn, 1973). Again, the subject is unable to see the result of his own movement, although he may do so if the brightness of the trace is substantially increased (Ebbers, 1965). In fact it is easy to show that this suppression is not absolute: if for example we have a disc with a number of holes arranged near its edge, through which a brightly lit background can be seen, and rotate it with constant velocity, there will come a point where the holes cannot be individually perceived, but fuse to form a continuous band of light. If now a saccade is made, then in that part of the disc that is moving in the same direction as the saccade, the holes suddenly spring to view and appear as bright and clear as if the disc were stationary. For this to occur, the speed of the holes must of course be adjusted to be equal to the eye's velocity in the middle of the saccade, so that their retinal images are stationary on the retina for a substantial period of time (Dodge, 1900). The observation can be made most easily by looking down from a railway carriage window: at speed, it happens that the apparent angular velocity of the sleepers is close to that of a saccade, and during voluntary eye movements made in a direction opposite to that of the train the details of the track can be seen quite clearly. Or again, if the reader happens to have a pocket calculator at hand, and moves his gaze from one side to the other of the numbers (intermittently) displayed, he will see a number of clear repetitive images of the figures, separated from each other by a distance which is given by the ratio of the velocity of the eye to the display frequency.

These observations all suggest that perhaps the impairment of vision during saccades is merely the result of what is often misleadingly called 'retinal blur' (I would prefer *velocity* blur), in which—although the optical image may be perfectly sharp—the changes in light intensity signalled by any particular receptor are too fast to be resolved by the receptor mechanism and the neural pathways of the visual system: the difficulty is one of *temporal*, not spatial, resolution. Although this factor undoubtedly plays a part in saccadic suppression (Mitrani, Mateef and Yakimoff, 1970), the fact that suppression can be observed with very brief stimulus flashes (for example Holt, 1903) shows that it cannot be the whole explanation (the flash must be sufficiently dim that no afterimage is perceived). Besides, measurements of the timing of the suppression relative to the movement itself show that some suppression occurs *before* the saccade starts. Volkmann (1962), Latour (1962), Zuber and Stark (1966), Volkmann et al (1969), Lederberg (1970), and others have measured the time course of saccadic suppression (figure 11.1), and agree that the threshold for seeing a brief flash of light is significantly elevated even some 30–40 ms before the beginning of the saccade, and does not reach its normal level again until some 100–120 ms later; there may be differences in the time courses for saccades in different directions (Volkmann et al, 1969). Similar time courses of suppression are observed as a result of the quick phase of nystagmus, and the microsaccades of fixation (Zuber et al, 1964a; 1964b; Ebbers, 1965; Zuber and Stark, 1966; Beeler, 1967), although in the latter case Krauskopf et al (1966) could observe no suppression at all: certainly the degree of suppression increases with the saccade amplitude (Mitrani, Yakimoff, and Mateef, 1970). Objective correlates of subjective suppression can be measured; for example, saccadic suppression of the pupillary light reflex (Zuber et al, 1966) and of visually evoked potentials from small pattern shifts (Gross et al, 1967; Chase and Kalil, 1972): evoked potentials from small incremental flashes suffer rather less suppression, but if stabilised relative to the retina, show a suppression time course remarkably similar to that obtained subjectively (Duffy and Lombroso, 1968).

Further evidence that velocity blur is not the only origin of saccadic suppression comes from entoptic retinal stimulation: both afterimages (Fiorentini and Mazzintini, 1965; Kennard et al, 1970) and electrical phosphenes (Riggs et al, 1974) exhibit behaviour similar to saccadic suppression, although in the case of afterimages the time course of the effect is very much prolonged: observations on afterimages are difficult to quantify, because even very slight changes in background luminance that may result from eye movements can greatly influence their visibility (Carpenter, 1972b). Of course, velocity blur might easily affect electrical retinal phosphenes as much as retinal images, if it were the neural pathways rather than the receptors themselves that cause the temporal blur: this interpretation is strongly supported by the fact that beats can be obtained between flickering light and alternating currents applied to the eye at frequencies far beyond the flicker-fusion frequency (Brindley, 1962).

Finally it is certain that velocity blur during saccades does not prevent the appreciation of the relative direction of visual objects during saccades. Hallett and Lightstone (1973; 1976a) found that if a target is moved to a new position during a saccade, and extinguished before the saccade has finished (figure 11.2), the next corrective saccade is made accurately to the new position. However, we saw in section 10.2.2 that in the absence of

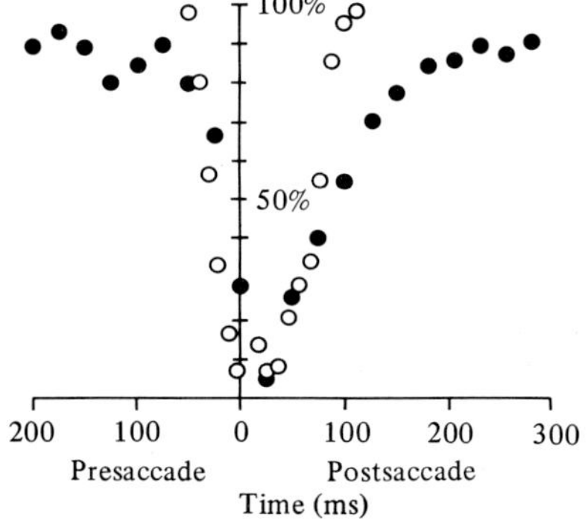

Figure 11.1. Saccadic suppression. Visibility of a test flash at various times before and after the beginning of a saccade; filled circles show the data of Latour (1962), open circles that of Volkman et al (1969).

other visual cues, the necessary allowance that has to be made for the motion of the eye itself appears to have an overprolonged time course, resulting in substantial errors of perceived direction (Matin et al, 1969; Orban et al, 1973). Matin (1974) has recently reviewed this and other phenomena of saccadic suppression.

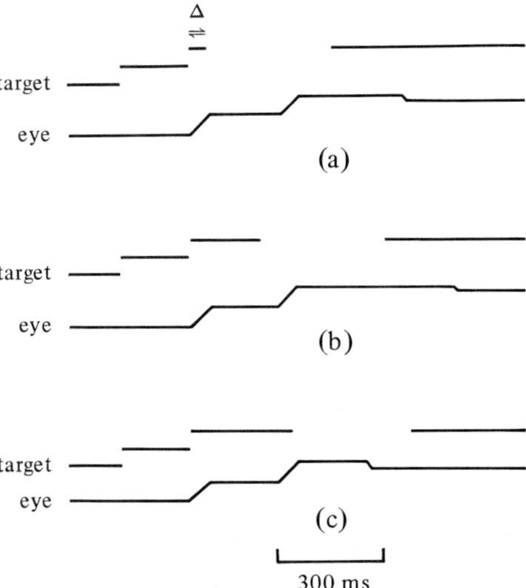

Figure 11.2. Schematic representation of Hallett and Lightstone's (1973) experimental paradigm. In each case, initial target movement evokes a saccade, and this in turn triggers a further movement of the target, which is then—after a delay Δ—extinguished for a period of 350 ms. (a) If Δ is less than the first saccade's duration, the corrective saccade is nevertheless accurate, though made in the dark. (b) If Δ is increased (~300 ms), the first two saccades are effectively unchanged, though the last correction saccade is relatively delayed because it must wait for the reappearance of the target. (c) Finally, if Δ extends into the period of the second saccade, the last correction saccade is made only one intersaccadic interval after the second, showing that information is again available for making corrective saccades *during* the preceding saccade.

11.1.2 Possible mechanisms

Many different theories of saccadic suppression have been put forward. There are essentially two possibilities: suppression may be the consequence either of the saccade itself, or alternatively of the *intention* to make the saccade. Of the former class of theory, one can distinguish those ascribing suppression to the rapid motion of the retinal image from those suggesting that it is caused by the motion of the eye itself.

Of these theories, the idea that suppression is a result of the intention to move the eyes—attractive because of its obvious parallel with the mechanism for visual-movement cancellation, discussed in the previous chapter—has received the least attention, and indeed does not appear ever to have been explicitly stated. In principle, it could be tested by seeing if suppression still occurred when the eyes were immobilised, or with accurately stabilised retinal images: but both these procedures are technically difficult in that one cannot be sure that the retinal image is truly stationary during the attempted movement. The best evidence for an outflow component of saccadic suppression comes from electrical recordings of responses in the lateral geniculate nucleus during saccades, discussed in section 11.1.3; but interesting and suggestive as these results are, it remains to be shown that such responses are accompanied by corresponding reductions in visual sensation. It is at any rate certain that outflow is not the *only* factor causing saccadic suppression: apart from experiments described below that show that suppression can be observed with rapid movements of the visual field even when the eye is stationary, Richards (1968a) has shown that it can also be produced by passive movements of the globe, for example by tapping it near the external canthus.

The possibility that saccadic suppression may be due in part merely to motion of the retinal image, rather than to eye movements *per se* has been established by MacKay (1970a; though Woodworth described a qualitative version of the experiment in 1906). A small test stimulus is briefly presented against a 10° background field: at different times relative to the test flash, the background is displaced through a few degrees with a velocity comparable to that of a voluntary saccade. Although no eye movement response occurs until well after the observation interval, 'saccadic' suppression is still observed, and its time course is broadly similar to that found during voluntary eye movements (figure 11.3), particularly with respect to the component of suppression that occurs

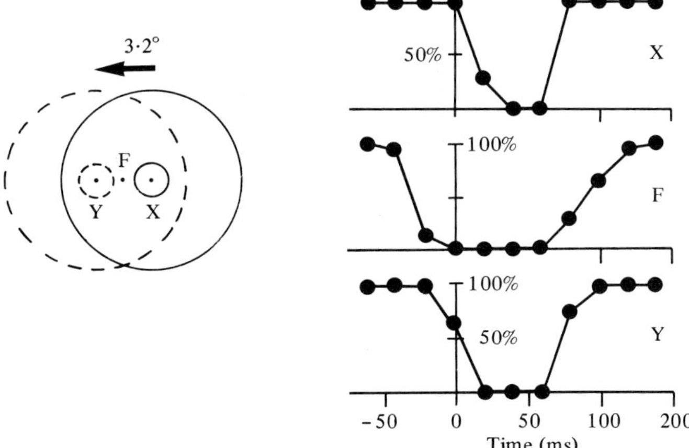

Figure 11.3. 'Saccadic' suppression without eye movements. Left, the stimulus arrangement: the large circle represents the adapting field, with the flashed target (small circle) fixed at its centre and moving with it. In the experiment, the subject fixates one of the points X, F, or Y, the complete stimulus is suddenly moved in a saccade-like manner from X to Y, and the target is flashed at some instant before or after the onset of movement. Its visibility for different moments of presentation under the three conditions are shown in the three curves at the right.

before the movement of the image. It might seem at first that such a result confounds causality by presenting an effect before its cause: but this is not so, if we suppose that the time taken for the suppressive signal to reach the point in the visual system where suppression occurs is less than the time taken by the visual signal itself. An analogous asynchronicity of perception of simultaneous events under similar conditions was noted in the previous chapter (section 10.2.2) (MacKay, 1970b). The importance of the background in saccadic suppression has been emphasised by Richards (1968b; 1969), who showed that the suppression was greatest when the colour of the test stimulus was closest to that of the background; suppression is increased when the background has a detailed texture (Mitrani et al, 1971). These observations suggest strongly that suppression is due, not to reduced retinal activity, but to *increased* activity, which results in the test stimulus being momentarily masked by the background. Such an increase would be anticipated from the preferential sensitivity of most retinal ganglion cells to changing, rather than steady, levels of illumination (for example Noda and Ross Adey, 1974), resulting in a reduction in effective figure-ground contrast: evidence for suppression of electrical responses to light flashes during displacement of a background has recently been demonstrated by Brooks and Holden (1973).

Finally, there is the possibility that suppression is caused by the mechanical results of rapid motion of the eyeball. Since the vitreous is to a certain extent left behind during rapid eye movements, and settles only relatively slowly into its final position (Hilding, 1954), it is possible that a degree of shearing movement occurs in the retina during saccades. It is not difficult to imagine that such shearing might temporarily incommode the receptors, and might even generate electrical potentials that could disturb the transmission of information (Richards, 1968a). A simpler explanation invokes the Stiles-Crawford effect, that light stimulating cones at an oblique angle is less effective than light directed along their axes. If the receptor layer undergoes shear, a depression in visual sensitivity could arise simply because of deviation of the preferred axis of the receptors: Richards (1969) has reported that the direction of peak sensitivity is indeed shifted in the expected direction during a saccade. All the same, it is clear that such *direct* effects of rotation cannot be a primary cause of saccadic suppression, because suppression starts before the movement gets under way: for the same reason, retinal shear cannot be used to explain the mislocation of objects during saccades in the dark (section 10.2.2). One cannot rule out the possibility of an *indirect* effect of movement of the globe—for example stretch-receptor discharge—which might neurally suppress the visual by a more rapid path, nor indeed of a direct mechanical effect on visual elements in the eye (for example on ganglion cells) whose latencies are sufficiently long that when the saccade occurs, they are processing information from an image received many milliseconds before.

If all the observations described here are correct, it is difficult to avoid the conclusion that all the methods by which saccadic suppression might conceivably occur do in fact contribute to it, insofar as they have been tested at all. Such a conclusion is not as improbable as might at first sight appear, since the mechanisms suggested, with the exception of the outflow theory which has no very strong evidence in its favour anyway, are all in some sense secondary consequences either of the structure of the eye (as for example in the case of retinal shear) or of the basic principles of sensory processing (in the case of masking by enhanced background activity), rather than being 'deliberate' specialisations of function. Indeed it is difficult to argue convincingly that there is any particular virtue in suppressing vision during saccades, since even blurred and degraded vision is better than nothing. But it might be argued that visual suppression is a necessary adjunct to the mechanism discussed in the previous chapter, by which the visual world appears to remain stationary when the eye moves. We have seen that, although compensation is good for the final position of the eye, it is not so good during the course of the saccade. The visual system might then prefer to have no input at all during the saccade than information that was actually misleading as to the direction of external objects: it is suggestive that the time course of mislocation is also drawn out relative to the saccade, and precedes it in time in a comparable manner. But it is quite easy to show that the correct *relative* objective positions of visual stimuli can be perceived perfectly well even if they are only visible during a saccade, and so under natural conditions there is no reason to suppose that the visual signals are any more misleading than at other times, since, as we shall see, it is the position of objects relative to their backgrounds that dominates their perceived position in space.

Almost as striking as the suppression itself is the subject's total unawareness of its occurrence. Comparable interruptions—around 100 ms—of the sight by means of a shutter are readily perceived, although it is significant that natural blinks, which last for the order of 300 ms (Miles, 1931) are not. This particular aspect of saccadic suppression seems to have received little attention. It is also interesting to note that in chickens the nictitating membrane closes briefly during each quick phase of the head nystagmus occurring during walking—possibly yet another mechanism of saccadic suppression! (Dunlap and Mowrer, 1931).

11.1.3 The possible role of the lateral geniculate nucleus

The position of the lateral geniculate nucleus as a relay on the pathway from the eye to the brain, and the arrangement of the inhibitory synapses within it, suggest strongly that it might serve to gate the flow of visual information to the central visual system, particularly during eye movements. The suggestion is even sometimes made (for example Jeannerod, 1972) that this nucleus might be the seat of the mechanism whereby movements of objects in the outside world are distinguished from movements of the eyes, though such a view is difficult to maintain in the face of the well-established indifference of the visual cortex to such a distinction (section 10.2.2). Many experimenters have demonstrated electrical responses that seem to be associated with fast eye movements in or near this nucleus (Cohen, 1966; Feldman and Bender, 1966; Feldman and Cohen, 1968; Jeannerod and Putkonen, 1971; Büttner and Fuchs, 1973), or in the geniculate projection to the visual cortex (Corazza and Lombroso, 1971). These potentials are accompanied by depolarisation of the afferent fibres of the optic tract, and so may well be related to a mechanism of presynaptic inhibition (Bizzi, 1966; Kawamura and Marchiafava, 1968). They behave as if they were generated by outflow rather than by inflow information: if the eyes are immobilised, stimulation of the semicircular canals still evokes geniculate responses, while passive movements of the eye do not (Feldman and Bender, 1966; Papaioannou, 1973). Responses can be observed within 5 ms of the start of a saccade, in other words before the eye has really got under way (Cohen, 1966), and are usually very little affected if the recordings are made in complete darkness. However, Büttner and Fuchs find that the percentage of cells within the nucleus behaving in this way is very small: only in the pregeniculate nucleus could clear responses to eye movements in the dark be consistently recorded; in contradiction to Cohen, they find latencies in the region of 80 ms after the start of the saccade, with a peak latency of some 100–200 ms. They consider that these potentials are too long delayed to be associated with any mechanism of saccadic suppression or compensation. Recently it has been shown that a large percentage of cells in the lateral geniculate are also sensitive to vestibular stimulation, possibly through vestibulo-ocular pathways (Putkonen et al, 1973; Magnin et al, 1974); and another thalamic area (the internal medullary lamina) has also been shown to be active in association with eye movements (Schlag et al, 1974).

The relevance of all these observations to saccadic suppression is far from established: particularly in the case of vestibular stimulation, it is difficult to be sure that the potentials observed are not the result of a rather diffuse and unspecific projection, or even of arousal; this was essentially the conclusion of Feldman and Cohen (1968), who obtained similar potentials by somaesthetic stimulation. What one would hope to show is that electrical responses to visual stimulation of optic nerve fibres are reduced when they are associated with a saccade or saccadic intention, and by no other stimulus. The observations that come nearest to doing this are those of Noda (1975a; 1975b). Most relay cells in the lateral geniculate nucleus can be assigned to one of two groups on the basis of their responses to shifts of the retinal image produced by spontaneous eye movements in the light: *S*-cells give a sustained discharge that is related to instantaneous eye position, whereas *T*-cells fire only transiently, during saccades. Neither response is observed in the dark, so it is clear that they are the direct result of the movement of the retinal image, rather than of a corollary discharge. If their excitability is measured (by electrical stimulation of the optic chiasm) during spontaneous saccades, it is found that both *S*-cells and *T*-cells show a depression of excitability that lasts for some 150–200 ms after the beginning of the saccade (itself lasting some 50 ms). Again, this depression is only seen during saccades in the light, or when the visual scene is suddenly shifted in a saccade-like manner. The existence of these two types of response from the two populations of cells in the lateral geniculate helps to explain the otherwise puzzling earlier observations (Ross Adey and Noda, 1973; Singer and Bedworth, 1974) that, whereas geniculate responses to stimulation of the chiasm are on the whole reduced in amplitude during saccades [though Cohen et al (1969) could see no difference], those from the visual cortex are actually increased: presumably the latter response is dominated by the *T*-cells, whose transient burst in response to the saccade may perhaps cause some kind of overriding facilitation. At all events, it seems that recordings from the lateral geniculate simply reflect the process of masking by increased background activity during saccades, already suggested earlier, rather than any extraretinal 'gating' input, whether 'inflow' or 'outflow' in nature, except insofar as the latter may—in common with other kinds of stimulation—cause an increase in alertness (Cohen et al, 1969), possibly through a mechanism involving the pontine and mesencephalic reticular formation (Cohen and Feldman, 1968).

11.2 Miniature eye movements and vision

11.2.1 Methods of stabilising retinal images

We saw in chapter 6 that even when fixating a stationary object, a normal observer makes small eye movements of a few minutes of arc in extent, of which he is generally unconscious. In the fovea of the retina, the centres of neighbouring receptors are probably less than half a minute of arc apart, so these movements can hardly pass unnoticed by the visual system. In fact, it turns out that the sense of sight is totally dependent on the small-scale irregular motion of the retinal image that results from these miniature eye movements, and that in their absence, vision ceases. Many workers have devised methods of preventing these small eye movements from moving the retinal image over the receptors, thus achieving a stabilised retinal image. One of the earliest methods (Riggs and Ratliff, 1952; Ditchburn and Ginsborg, 1952; Riggs et al, 1953) used a mirror mounted on a contact lens to reflect a target image on a screen: it is necessary to double the length of the line of sight relative to the reflected beam, since for any angle α moved through by the eye, the beam moves through an angle 2α (figure 11.4). With further refinements (Ditchburn and Fender, 1955; Ditchburn, 1963) it is possible to compensate for small movements in horizontal and vertical planes (with an accuracy of about a third of a minute of arc), but not for torsional movements: if the image is small and centred near the fovea the effect of torsional movements will be slight.

The method is incapable of dealing with translational movements, and so the head must be firmly fixed. Other authors have devised particular modifications of the method for particular circumstances: Ditchburn (1973) has recently reviewed some of the possibilities.

A fundamentally different procedure is to mount the target directly on a contact lens attached to the eye (Ditchburn and Pritchard, 1956; Yarbus, 1957b; Barlow, 1963; Evans, 1965). In principle, if the attachment accurately follows the motion of the eye, such a method provides stabilisation against all eye movements (including torsion) as well as against head movements. Yarbus (1967) has described various devices of this type with much practical detail: a specimen is shown in figure 11.5. The necessity for a small but powerful lens to focus the target tends to reduce the quality of the retinal image that can be obtained in this way, while both the foregoing methods of stabilisation suffer from the fact that contact lenses can never be made to follow the eye movements with very great precision, though it appears all the same that if the subject refrains from voluntary movements, the standard deviation of the error of stabilisation may not exceed some 40″ of arc in a minute (Riggs and Schick, 1968).

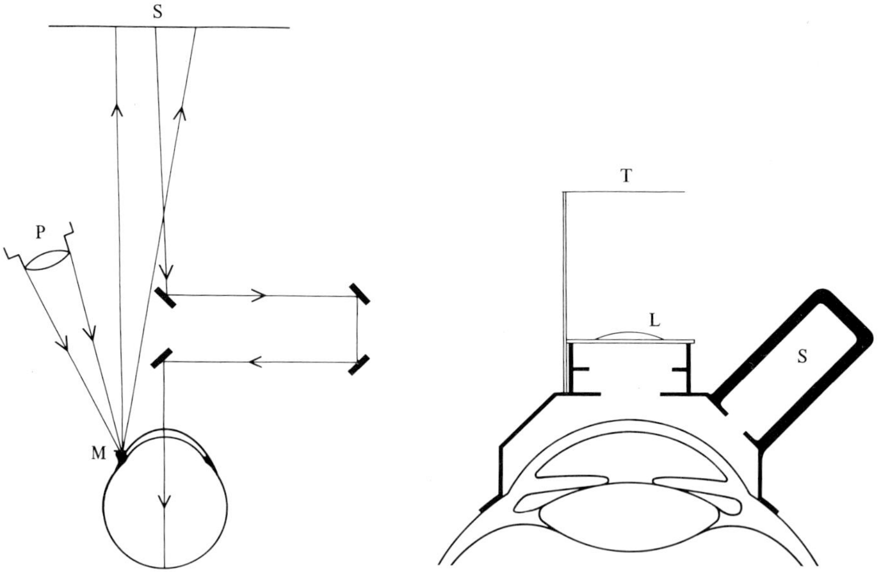

Figure 11.4. Figure 11.5.

Figure 11.4. Reflection method for generating stabilised images. The projector P reflects its beam off the corneal mirror M to form an image on the screen at S. The subject views this image through the set of path-lengthening mirrors shown on the right, which are such that they exactly double the apparent optical distance of the screen.

Figure 11.5. Stabilisation of the retinal image with a contact lens assembly. The target T is viewed through the powerful lens L mounted on the corneal contact assembly attached firmly to the eye with the aid of the sucker S.

Other methods of producing stabilised images have been suggested from time to time, including images generated within the eye [as shadows of retinal blood vessels (Campbell and Robson, 1961; Sharpe, 1972) or by auto-ophthalmoscopy (Cornsweet, 1962), or from such phenomena as Haidinger's brushes]. The advantage of this approach is that such images are stabilised not only against all kinds of head and eye movements, but also against movements of the lens, of the type discussed in section 7.2.1, which cannot of course be allowed for by methods using corneal attachments. The same advantage is shared by a novel mechanism devised by Kelly et al (1969), which was based on Cornsweet's method (1958) of measuring eye movements by tracking the position of retinal blood vessels. The fundus of the eye is scanned with a photocell, and the resulting signal is processed by a small computer to calculate the position of the retina: this information is then used in a feedback loop that stabilises the target image on the retina, to within some half a minute of arc.

11.2.2 The appearance of stabilised images

The whole subject of the appearance of stabilised images, and the performance of the visual system in general under stabilised conditions, has recently been reviewed with admirable thoroughness by Ditchburn (1973), and it is unnecessary here to do more than describe the most basic phenomena of stabilised vision, on which there is good agreement between authors.

Stabilised images are essentially fugitive. When first presented, they are clearly seen—probably as clearly as under normal vision—but in the course of a few seconds they fade away to leave a virtually uniform blank field. This disappearance is probably permanent, so long as care is taken to maintain accurate stabilisation and constant illumination of the field. A sufficiently large or rapid change in illumination results in the reappearance of the image, as do eye movements that are large enough to overpower the stabilisation apparatus. After fading, some features of the image may remain visible in a very low-contrast and blurred form, with perhaps some of the colouring of the original. For some subjects, however, the appearance after fading is of a completely black field, with no trace remaining of the target image: this appearance is more often seen when the degree of stabilisation is most accurate, and when the original image contains little detail of high contrast.

Some of these effects can be observed to a lesser extent without special stabilisation apparatus, simply by careful fixation (Troxler, 1804; Clarke, 1957): the best results are obtained by subjects who are able to exercise control over their microsaccades (section 6.1.3). After a short period of steady fixation, one finds that vision in the periphery of the field begins to blur and mist over, and that after a time this appearance begins to invade the fovea. The amplitude of tremor—and possibly also of drift—remains unchanged, and so one may conclude that it is not the loss of this component alone that produces the loss of vision associated with stabilisation.

11.2.3 The effect of imposing movements on stabilised images

To try to understand why these small movements have such a dramatic effect on vision, it is helpful to examine the efficiency of the visual system under more controlled conditions than are possible during the complex and unpredictable motions of normal fixation. There is a danger, however, with the use of oversimple and particularly with repetitive stimuli—as we have already seen in trying to investigate the smooth pursuit system with sinusoidal inputs—that the system may change its normal pattern of behaviour. Thus Sharpe (1972) found that regular oscillation of an otherwise stabilised image did *not* prevent it from fading, and that this kind of fading was specific for certain classes of visual attribute such as orientation and width: this is clearly a comparatively high-level phenomenon. In the same way, Coren and Porac (1974) conclude that fading is not just a function of the kind of retinal movement, but depends also on whether this movement is generated by the subject's own oculomotor system, or by an outside agency: in their own words, fading occurs "because the observer's interaction with the stimulus leads the higher centres to conclude that the image is not part of the behaviourally relevant environment". So one must clearly not be too simpleminded in one's interpretation of experiments involving the imposition of small movements from outside the oculomotor system.

Once we have an arrangement for producing stabilised images, it is a relatively simple matter to arrange for the original target to be moved about in a systematic way, and many experimenters have investigated the relation between the parameters of imposed image motion of this kind, and the eye's visual performance (for example Yarbus, 1957b; Gerrits et al, 1966). The experiments which are of most interest here are those in which the experimenter has tried to make the imposed motion simulate some aspect of the miniature fixation movements (for example Krauskopf, 1957; Ditchburn et al, 1959; Butler et al, 1976). If the target is moved sinusoidally at a frequency similar to the mean intersaccadic interval, and with an amplitude of some 5–30′ of arc, the characteristics of the image motion are similar in many respects to the drift component of the miniature movements under natural conditions. It is found that the visibility of a thin black line moved in this way does indeed increase with increasing amplitudes of movement, up to a peak-to-peak amplitude of about a degree; but at amplitudes equivalent to those of ordinary drift movements (for which the median is nearer 10′ of arc) only a slight improvement in visibility can be observed (figure 11.6). This suggests that the rather slow motions of drift contribute relatively little to natural visibility. On the other hand, fast movements of small amplitude—comparable in their effect to microsaccades—result in a much greater improvement (figure 11.7). Here the duration of the movement is rather shorter than in a normal saccade, being of the order of a millisecond, and maximal visibility is attained even with displacements as small as 2·5′. This is considerably smaller than median estimates of saccade amplitudes in natural fixation, and suggests that saccades play a much more important part in maintaining visibility than do drift movements.

Finally, sinusoidal movement of the target with a very small amplitude (less than a minute of arc) and at rather higher frequencies, simulating tremor, can also cause an improvement in visibility under certain conditions (Krauskopf, 1957; Ditchburn et al, 1959). The results here are rather more complex than in the case of simulated saccades and drift, and it appears that rapid vibration at amplitudes less than about a third of a minute of arc actually decreases the visibility of a thin black line. It is difficult to see why this should be so: the effect is greatest for amplitudes in the region of 0·2′ of arc, and any velocity blur introduced by the vibration is clearly less than the optical blur inevitably present: in any case, the detection of thin black lines is not essentially a test of acuity (see for example Hartridge, 1922). Besides, there is no significant difference between the visibilities of stabilised and unstabilised lines viewed for short periods (figure 11.8) (Riggs et al, 1953; Keesey, 1960)—although there must, of course, be a difference over longer periods—nor does *stereoscopic* acuity improve if the target is stabilised (Shortess and Krauskopf, 1961). The results tend to show reduced effects with increasing frequency, and it seems by extrapolation that at the frequencies associated with natural

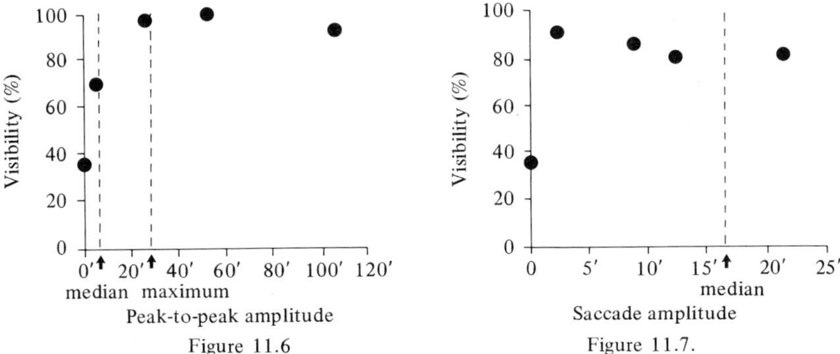

Figure 11.6. Visibility under artificial movements of the target, simulating drift. The target was moved relative to stabilisation with a 0·55 Hz sine motion, whose peak-to-peak amplitudes are indicated on the abscissa. The data points show the visibility of the target (a fine black line) at different amplitudes: the arrows show median and maximum drift amplitudes for the same subject under natural conditions (after Ditchburn et al, 1959).

Figure 11.7. Visibility with simulated saccades of different sizes. The black line target was moved in a saccadic manner with different amplitudes: as in figure 11.6, visibility is plotted as a function of this amplitude, and a median saccade amplitude for the same subject under natural conditions is also shown (after Ditchburn et al, 1959).

tremor its contribution to the maintenance of visibility may not be very great: 50 Hz movements of larger amplitude (up to 4′ of arc: Krauskopf, 1957) cause a marked *reduction* in visibility. Ratliff (1952) tried to correlate periods of greater or less tremor with performance at a visual acuity task, and found that, in general, increased tremor was associated with reduced acuity, confirming the previous results under more natural conditions. He also found that periods of large drift rate were associated with poor performance, and that on the whole the larger the drift the worse the visual acuity: this is quite the reverse of what would have been expected from the effects of the slow artificial sinusoidal drifts in figure 11.6. Possibly detection and acuity tasks are affected differently by different kinds of movement: the theoretical implications of small image movements for the visibility of different kinds of target have been examined by Bryngdahl (1961).

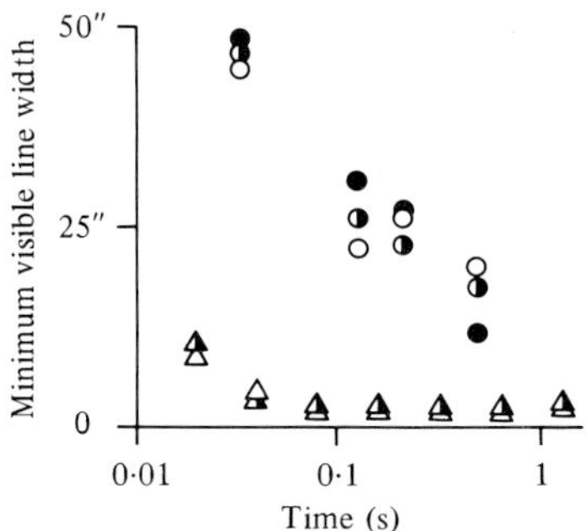

Figure 11.8. Exposure time and visibility under different conditions of stabilisation. The data points show minimum visible line width as a function of exposure under stabilisation (empty symbols), normal conditions (bisected symbols), and exaggerated eye movement (solid symbols). The circles show the results of Riggs et al (1953); the triangles, those of Keesey (1960). The difference between the two sets of results is difficult to explain: but it is clear from both curves that the presence or absence of stabilisation is of little importance in this range of exposure times.

11.2.4 Teleology

Searching for origins is not always considered to be a respectable occupation for biologists: but in this case a consideration of the purpose —if any—of the small movements of fixation may help to indicate the kind of underlying mechanism that generates them. The relationship between the fading of stabilised images and miniature eye movements is not unlike that between the chicken and the egg, and perhaps invites teleological speculation. Two possibilities exist: one might suppose that the fading of stabilised images is an accidental result of some adaptation that is particularly beneficial to the visual system, and that the miniature eye movements have had to be evolved to counteract it; or alternatively one might suppose that the miniature movements are simply the expression of unavoidable random noise in the eye movement control system, and have enabled the visual system to develop certain properties that it would not otherwise have developed. The only evidence that is relevant to this question concerns the extent to which the kinetics of the small eye movements are adapted to the needs of the visual system: consideration of the utility of the visual mechanism underlying the fading of stabilised images is neither here nor there, since both theories suppose that the visual system evolves to its best advantage. On the second theory, the visual process is merely enabled to develop an attribute that would not be possible if the eyes were truly stationary in fixation: and many authors have argued convincingly that this mechanism—which is fundamentally one of sensitivity to *change* of illumination rather than to steady levels—is indeed an advantageous one (for example Attneave, 1954; Barlow, 1959). Furthermore, if we find that the miniature eye movements *are* well-adapted to prevent fading we shall still be none the wiser, for we shall have no way of telling whether it is the visual system that has adapted to the oculomotor system, or vice versa. Thus the only finding that can be of any interest is if it turns out that the miniature eye movements are ill-adapted to this function.

The results presented in the last section on the kinds of movement that are best able to prevent fading suggested that, of the three components of the miniature movements, only the microsaccades contribute much to the maintenance of vision. The velocities of drift movements are too low, and under natural conditions probably degrade rather than enhance visual performance, while the frequency and amplitude of tremor are both such as to make it more detrimental than otherwise. One way of determining whether or not these movements, taken as a whole, are well-adjusted to the task of overcoming fading and improving vision in general is to arrange for intermediate degrees of stabilisation between complete cancellation and the natural state, by altering the degree of external feedback between eye movement and image movement: by an extension of the same method one can arrange to exaggerate rather than reduce the effect of the miniature movements. If the movements were well-adapted in their characteristics, one would expect that either an increase or a decrease of their natural size would lead to a degradation in performance. In fact, there is excellent agreement among experimenters that there is a steady improvement in vision as stabilisation is reduced, and that this improvement continues past the natural condition, so that exaggerated miniature movements generally lead to better vision than normal (Riggs et al, 1953; Riggs and Tulunay, 1959; Clowes, 1961) (figure 11.9).

The essentially random nature of the miniature movements also suggests that they are not deliberate adaptations: it is difficult to believe that a mechanism designed to prevent fading of the retinal image by moving it over the receptors would not do it in a more regular and periodic way. Although it is true, as is often pointed out (for example Gaarder, 1967; 1970), that the small movements, in conjunction with fading, can greatly assist in the preliminary visual analysis by emphasising such features as the edges of solid objects, it could clearly provide very much more help of this sort if the small movements were of constant velocity and more systematic in their scanning: arbitrary scanning patterns are likely only to increase the uncertainty of signals from the retina. This is particularly true of tremor, which is not even coordinated between the two eyes (Riggs and Ratliff, 1951). It seems unlikely, then, that we need look any further for the origin of drift and tremor than the inevitable noise and variability that is present in all neural systems, or in the case of microsaccades, further than the ordinary saccadic mechanism for bringing visual targets to the fovea.

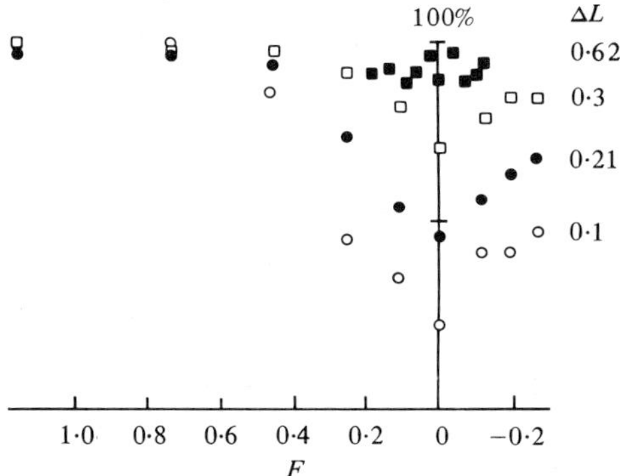

Figure 11.9. Visibility of a difference in luminance in a bipartite field as a function of the degree of stabilisation, at different luminance levels: the figures to the right of the four sets of points show the luminance differences used (in log units). $F = 1$ implies normal vision: $F = 0$ implies complete stabilisation (after Riggs and Tulunay, 1959).

11.3 Eye movements and spatial sense

11.3.1 The sense of direction and distance

Some aspects of this topic have already been covered in chapter 10, so far as they relate to proprioception from eye muscles. We concluded there that information about the position of the eyes is essentially derived from knowledge of the commands that are sent to the eyes rather than from sensory information from the muscles themselves: in Merton's (1961) words, "A subject is only conscious of his intention to move his eye and does not know whether the movement has in fact taken place or not." While one cannot rule out the possibility that proprioceptors may provide a very small contribution to this sense, it must be generally agreed that this source of information is too slight to be of practical use under natural conditions. In section 10.3.3 a rather different role for the proprioceptive input was put forward, namely that it might serve as a monitor of the proper functioning of the oculomotor system, by checking that the commands sent out do indeed result in the intended movements being correctly executed: any long-term discrepancies might then bring about a readjustment of the properties of the control pathways, by a process of parametric feedback.

Now of course proprioceptors are not the only way in which the oculomotor system can find out whether its commands are being obeyed. The retina itself provides the same information, and is in fact rather better adapted to its task than are the stretch receptors: it is not only considerably more sensitive to small movements, but also more appropriate for the task. The purpose of eye movements is after all not to move the eye, but to move the retinal image, and retinal feedback provides the ultimate test of the adequacy of the control system. In natural circumstances movements of the eye and image are closely similar. But it is a simple matter in the laboratory to upset this relationship, either with lenses that change the amplitude of retinal movements relative to eye movements, or with prisms that change their direction, and experiments of this type have greatly increased our understanding of the monitoring process in movements both of the eye and of other parts of the motor system.

To see how visual monitoring of this sort might work, it may perhaps help to begin with the simple case of parametric feedback from proprioceptors (figure 11.10). Here a command signal specifying the desired position of the eye is converted by a controller (A) into a suitable pattern of firing in the oculomotor nerves. After modification by the mechanical properties of the eye (B), this results in an eye movement and stimulation of the stretch receptors: their signal is returned to the central nervous system, where it is compared with the desired position of the eye. The resultant error signal, averaged over a comparatively long period, is used to modify the characteristics of the controller. To add visual monitoring to this arrangement we need only surround the existing feedback loop with another one of very much the same type (figure 11.11). The initial command input is now not the desired position of the *eye*, but the desired position of the retinal image of some part of an object. This is transformed by a process C into the desired eye position, which forms the input of the

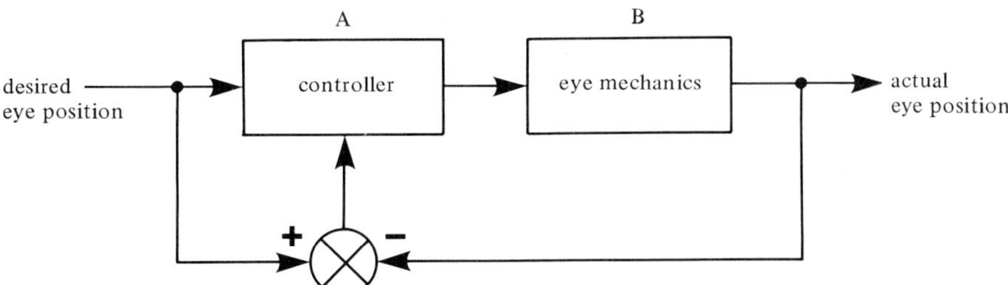

Figure 11.10. Elementary parametric feedback system in which the error signal obtained by comparison of the desired and actual positions of the eyes is used to modify the properties of the control system, in such a way as to optimise the long-term behaviour of the system.

loop already considered. The output of this subsystem—the resultant eye movement—plus any motion that the object itself may contribute, together give the retinal image movement by the usual process of intrinsic visual feedback. Any error between this and the desired retinal image movement, averaged over a period of time, is used to modify the action of controller, C.

Such an arrangement would account very adequately for the adaptive properties of the vestibuloocular reflex described in section 2.3.3, where optical devices fitted to the eyes, making ordinary reflex movements to turning of the head inappropriate in size or direction, were found to lead quite quickly to large modifications of the reflex such as to produce the best possible compensation. In this case the 'desired retinal image movement' is the input from the vestibular system: the effect of the prisms or lenses worn by the subject is to add an extra apparent object motion to the signal, corresponding to actual retinal image movement. The resultant repeated discrepancies between desire and performance will then lead to the appropriate changes in process C: since one of the modifications found was that of complete reversal of the reflex when the retinal image is reversed, one must suppose that the parametric control of process C is radical enough to include the possibility of changing the sign of its gain.

Such an arrangement is not only useful in cases where there is some sort of fault in the subject's visual or oculomotor system: it will also serve to optimise performance under conditions where one is trying to track a moving target. We have already seen that both the smooth pursuit and the

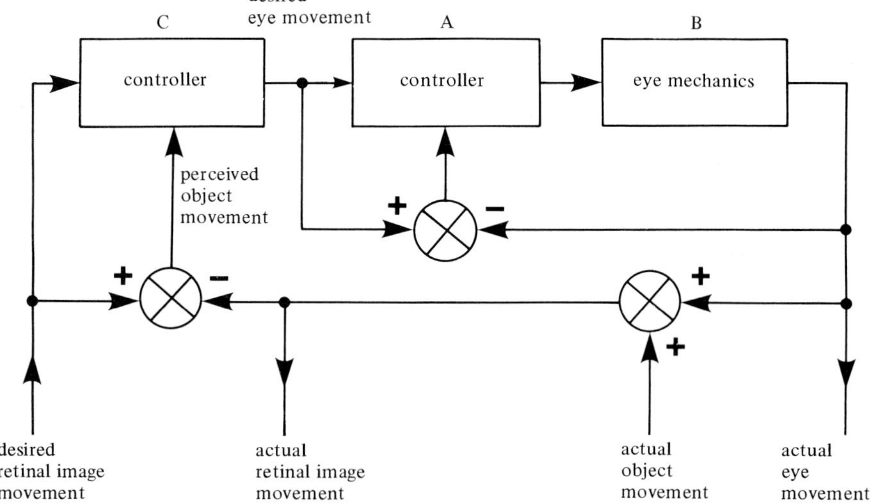

Figure 11.11. Modification of the system of figure 11.10 to include parametric feedback both from eye muscle receptors (inner loop) and from comparison of desired and actual retinal image movements: the same comparison may also generate the perception of object movement.

saccade systems are able to make use of regularities in the motion of the object being tracked to provide a better performance—in the sense of smaller mean absolute error—than is possible if the motion is unpredictable. A scheme like that of figure 11.11 is certainly capable of doing the same, provided that the nature of the parametric feedback is such that particular error patterns lead to the appropriate modifications of process C: there is no theoretical difficulty in designing such a mechanism, and devices able to modify their behaviour in this sort of way have actually been built (for example Donaldson, 1964).

But what has all this to do with the perception of visual direction? The answer comes from a consideration of the visual cancellation associated with eye movements, by which stationary objects still appear stationary despite voluntary movements of the eye. In section 10.2.2 we saw that there are overwhelming reasons for believing that this cancellation is the result of outflow rather than inflow signals. But with a system of double parametric feedback like that in figure 11.11, it is evident that there are many possible outflow signals: which is the one that is used? The answer comes from observations of what happens to the sense of visual direction when the system is forced to make parametric changes as a result of wearing distorting prisms or lenses. For, if the outflow signal is tapped off the efferent pathway at a point *after* the process C, it is clear that no parametric modification of C can alter the relationship between retinal image movement and the outflow signal and thus give rise to changes in the perception of object movement. In other words, the outflow that is used to cancel retinal image motion due to eye movements must derive from a point central to all processes whose modification leads to changes in the sense of visual direction. A specific example may make this clearer: the most complete studies of changes of this kind have been done on the eye-hand coordination mechanism, and although it is not strictly relevant to the control of eye movements, it may help to clarify the relation between parametric feedback and spatial perception.

The effect of wearing prisms that deviate the retinal image has been particularly well studied (for example Helmholtz, 1909; Held, 1961; Held and Bossom, 1961; Harris, 1963; Held and Freedman, 1963). At first, when a subject tries to point at an object—both the object and his finger being seen through the prisms—he points to one side of it: but with practice he adapts to the prisms and learns to point accurately. When the prisms are removed, he at first makes pointing errors in the opposite direction, but soon readapts to the normal situation. Similar effects can be demonstrated in trained monkeys [and appear to require an intact cerebellum (Baizer and Glickstein, 1974)], and the whole process can easily be explained as the result of parametric changes resulting from discrepancies between the desired and seen positions of the arm. It is significant that the adaptation only occurs if the subject actually tries to move his arm: observations of passive arm movements through the prisms are ineffective, presumably because there is no 'desired position' for comparison. One might therefore tentatively suggest a scheme for the control of hand position in these experiments that is rather similar to that for eye position already presented—in which the desired position of the image of the finger on the retina is the ultimate input, and a comparison of this with the actual retinal position leads to parametric changes in the process converting this input signal into finger position (figure 11.12). In this model, the adaptation is supposed to occur in the control system for hand position rather than in either the visual or the oculomotor systems: support for this assumption comes from the observation that after adaptation to prisms, the subject will point to one side of localised *auditory* stimuli (Harris, 1963): clearly such a response cannot be explained by adaptational changes confined to the visual or oculomotor systems.

It is pertinent to ask at this point what happens to the subject's perception of the direction in which he is pointing. If this percept were derived primarily from proprioceptors in the hand and arm, he would feel a permanent discrepancy even when fully adapted between this sense and the direction indicated to him by his eyes: if on the other hand his sense of direction were mainly dependent on the efferent signals entering the system of figure 11.12, in the course of adaptation a discrepancy would develop between the actual position of his hand and its felt position, such that the latter would gradually come to correspond with that perceived through sight. In fact it is the latter that is observed: the subject does

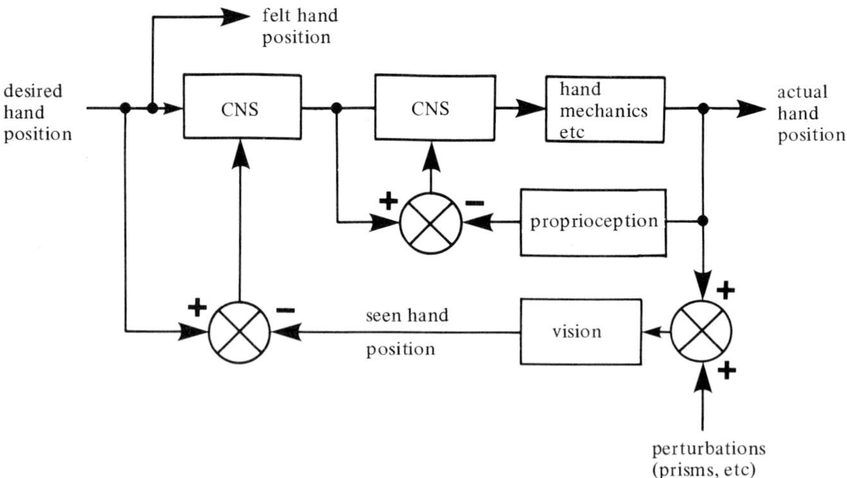

Figure 11.12. Further modification of the parametric feedback system of figure 11.11, to encompass the control of hand position. In the inner system, proprioceptors continuously monitor the error between desired hand position and actual hand position, while an outer loop supervises the inner one by comparing the desired hand position with the *seen* hand position: it is the latter system that is affected by wearing prisms and other similar devices.

not—when fully adapted—sense any discrepancy between the seen and the felt positions of the hand, and if asked to use his hand in a task that does not require vision (for example, pointing in the sagittal plane with the eyes shut) he points to one side (Harris, 1963).

To summarise, it seems first that it is the efferent signals that largely determine the sense of direction of the arm, and that adaptation is the result of a discrepancy between these signals and those derived from vision; conclusions that probably apply with equal force to the control of and to the perception of the direction of the eye. A direct demonstration of such a parallel has been given by Hay (1968) in the case of the vestibulo-ocular reflex. Hay arranged for the vertical movements of a subject's head to cause a visual target on an oscilloscope to move by a proportional amount in the *horizontal* direction, so that the desired vertical movements of the eye signalled by the vestibular system were in fact accompanied by horizontal retinal image movements: from our model, we would expect this to lead to parametric changes such that vertical head movements would generate a compensatory horizontal component in the eye response. In fact, after a short training period in the apparatus, subjects find, when the artificial feedback is turned off, that vertical head movements are accompanied by a sensation of horizontal movement of the (stationary) target, and that this only happens if they have actively tried to track the spot during the training period. Corresponding experiments do not yet seem to have been tried for other kinds of eye movements.

There are good reasons for anticipating that saccades are more likely to show marked effects of this kind than are smooth pursuit movements: whereas a system like that of figure 11.11 will do quite well for the generation of saccades, in the case of smooth pursuit there is an added complication that results from the feedback that is an intrinsic part of their control. The effect of this feedback will be in effect to reduce any discrepancies between the desired and the actual eye movement, in that the input to the system is already modified by the actual retinal position of the target. One might thus anticipate that adaptation would be faster and more complete with saccadic viewing: this has been confirmed to some extent by Slotnick (1969) with prism contact lenses. Conceivably a similar mechanism underlies Burnham's (1968) observations on the eye movements made when one is looking at the Müller–Lyer illusion: if a subject is asked to move his eyes back and forth from one end of the centre line of the illusion figure to the other, the amplitude of the movements show a gradual change, being at first comparable with the illusory length of the line, and later nearer in size to the actual length (see for example Judd, 1905: Yarbus, 1967). Burnham found that this change occurs more rapidly if saccadic rather than slow movements are made. [This does not mean, of course, that the illusion is *due* to the eye movements: geometrical illusions of this type can be perceived just as well as stabilised images (Pritchard, 1958).] The reader will find useful discussions of this and related topics in Festinger and Canon (1965), Festinger et al (1967), and Festinger (1971).

Oculomotor aspects of the sense of distance have been rather less thoroughly investigated than that of direction. Of the many sources of information about the distance of visual objects that can be shown to be used (see Ogle, 1962), only those that demand binocular vision need concern us here: they are binocular retinal disparity, and the degree of convergence. Now disparity only gives information about the depth of objects *relative* to the plane (strictly, Vieth–Müller surface) of fixation: absolute notions of depth can be derived from disparity information only if the degree of convergence of the eyes is also known, either from inflow or from outflow information. By analogy with direction perception, the latter seems more probable: but the matter does not ever seem to have been experimentally tested.

Wundt showed in 1862 that the use of two eyes rather than one increased the accuracy of depth perception from about 7% to nearer 2%. His results have more recently been extended by Gogel (1962), who found that convergence information was of little use for objects more than about a metre away: but at shorter distances convergence can certainly be used, and indeed takes precedence over information derived from accommodation where this conflicts with it (Richards and Miller, 1969). The miniature fixation eye movements appear to improve the accuracy with which depth discriminations can be made (Shortess and Krauskopf, 1961), but this may be simply because of a generalised improvement in visual performance.

11.3.2 The sense of motion

One might expect that the sense of motion would involve much the same mechanisms as those considered in the last section. Certainly there is good evidence that parametric feedback may be used to match eye velocity to target velocity (McLaughlin and Kelly, 1968). If a modification is made of Westheimer's (1954b) original experiment in which a ramp stimulus was used, such that the saccade response of the eye triggers a sudden change in the velocity of the target (figure 11.13: see also section 4.2.2), at first

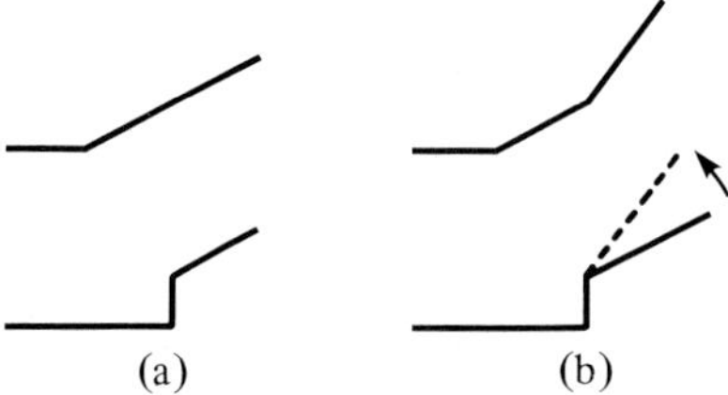

Figure 11.13. Schematic representation of McLaughlin and Kelly's experiment (1968). (a) The normal response to a target ramp; (b) the experimenter arranges for an increase in target velocity at the moment of the saccade: the response is initially the same as before, that is, appropriate for the former velocity, but with practice the eye velocity approaches the final velocity of the target.

the velocity of the eye immediately after the saccade corresponds to the velocity of the target immediately before it. With practice, however, it is found that the velocity of the eye after the saccade, begins to approach, and ultimately matches, the new stimulus velocity, long before there is any time for short-term feedback information about its magnitude. Parametric feedback offers a simple explanation of this phenomenon if we suppose that the actual velocity of the retinal image at any moment is compared with the desired velocity (presumably zero), and the recurrence of the same pattern of error at each test led to an increase in the smooth pursuit gain. It would be interesting to know what happens one reaction time after the saccade, although this is not reported: if the parametric modification of the gain of the smooth pursuit mechanism was indiscriminate in its application, one would expect an exaggerated velocity response to the final velocity of the target. Otherwise one would have to imagine a rather complex mechanism of time-dependent changes in the parameters, such that the gain is increased for a short period after the saccade, and thereafter reverts to its normal value: perhaps an implausible hypothesis. There does not, however, appear to be any evidence relating parametric changes to changed perceptions of velocity, as opposed to position: it is not self-evident that the two percepts are derived from the same system, and there are many circumstances—like the aftereffects of seen motion discussed below—where they may conflict.

A consideration of the sense of motion also brings in two factors that are all its own: the contribution of the semicircular canals, and the aftereffects caused by adaptation to visual movement. A question that will particularly concern us is how we know whether a movement of the whole visual field—such as might be experienced when one is sitting still inside a large cylinder rotating about a vertical axis—is due to *actual* rotation of the outside scene (objective, or egocentric, rotation), or due to rotation of one's own head and eyes (subjective, or exocentric, rotation). Only three sources of information can be useful here: vision, sense of ocular direction, and the semicircular canals. Of these, the first two cannot of themselves decide whether a particular apparent movement is objective or subjective; and it is an elementary property of the canals (see chapter 2) that they give no information about rotations of constant velocity. It comes as no surprise, then, to learn that a subject seated on a rotatable chair in a rotatable drum is unable, while drum or chair, or both, are revolving at constant velocity, to say whether it is the drum or the chair that moves (Mach, 1875; Dichgans and Brandt, 1972). We would, however, expect to find a difference between the two cases during the period of acceleration that leads up to the constant velocity from rest, for during this period the semicircular canals will be active in the case of chair rotation, but not in the case of drum rotation. In the first case, the subject at first feels a very strong sense of subjective rotation, which gradually subsides over the course of some 15 s to a more or less steady level: in the case of drum rotation, the subject at once senses that it is the drum that is moving, but again over the course of some 15 s this conviction is gradually replaced by a feeling that the drum is after all stationary, and that it is the chair that is going round: at this point the sensations in the two cases are identical (Brandt et al, 1973).

Now this time course is very similar to that of the return of the cupula in the canals, and suggests that the subjective sensation of rotation depends in part on the magnitude of the vestibular signal. But it is clear that it cannot depend *entirely* on this signal, since in both cases there is a strong sensation of self-rotation in the absence of any signal from the canals. A model that accounts very satisfactorily for these findings can be derived by a simple extension of the system suggested earlier (figure 11.11), in which movements of objects in the outside world (objective movement) is sensed by the difference between the outflow signal and the amount of retinal slip. All we need do is suppose that the sense of subjective rotation is simply proportional to the outflow signal itself (figure 11.14): in the experiments just described, this signal is partly the result of signals from the vestibular system, and partly the result of the action of the smooth pursuit system. Figure 11.15 shows the expected time courses of the subjective and objective components of sensation from this model, for different combinations of chair and drum rotation: in each case a good prediction is made of what is actually felt in practice.

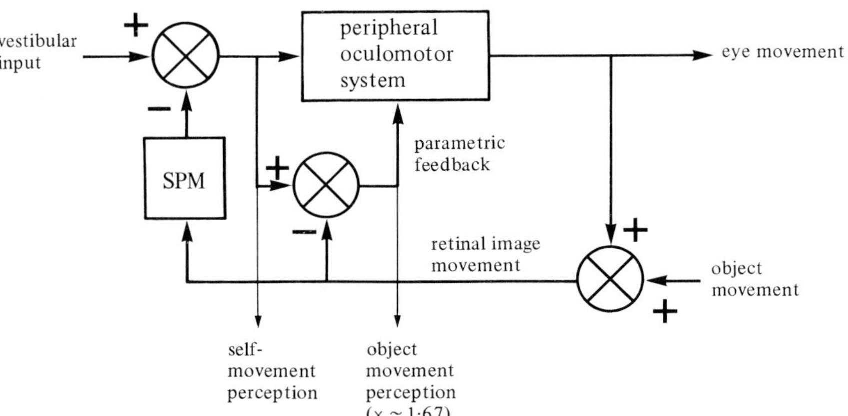

Figure 11.14. A model of possible mechanisms generating the percepts of subjective and objective movement. It is suggested that the ultimate input to the oculomotor system—the 'desired retinal image movement'—also generates the percept of self-movement, while the difference between this signal and the actual retinal image movement, magnified by a factor of around 1·67, gives rise to sensations of object movement (as well as to parametric feedback, as in figure 11.11). Retinal image movement also of course generates eye movements, through the smooth pursuit mechanism (SPM).

The model would also lead us to predict that circumstances in which the smooth pursuit system cannot accurately follow the target would also be associated with an increase in the objective component of sensation. We saw in section 3.1 that this happens when the drum speed exceeds 100° s^{-1}, and the subject's sensations are precisely in accord with this expectation (Brandt et al, 1973): as the velocity is increased beyond about 120° s^{-1}, the subjective sensation levels off while the objective component starts to increase steadily (figure 11.16). In the same way, reduction of the area of optokinetic stimulation—resulting in greater

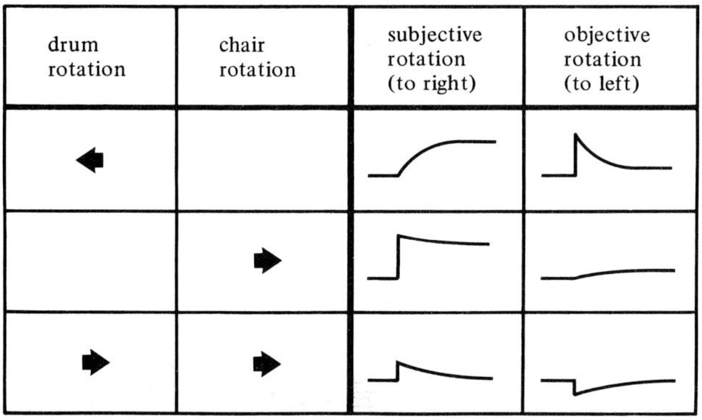

drum rotation	chair rotation	subjective rotation (to right)	objective rotation (to left)
←			
	→		
→	→		

Figure 11.15. On the right, the time courses of the subjective and objective components of sensation of rotation predicted from the model of figure 11.14 for three different combinations of drum and chair rotation: drum moving left; chair moving right; drum *and* chair moving right, with equal angular velocity.

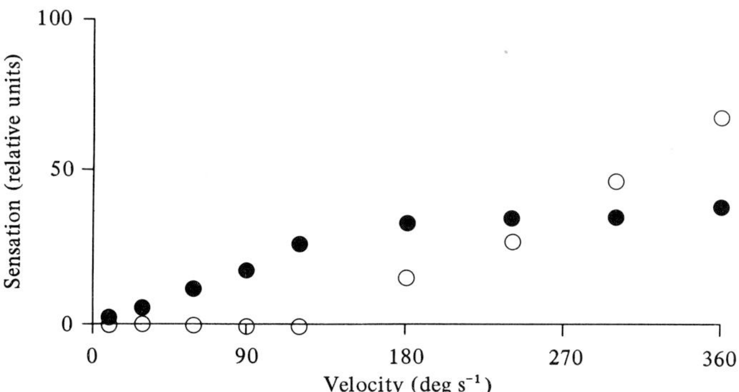

Figure 11.16. Subjective and objective sensations of rotation during prolonged drum movement at the different velocities indicated: sensations are shown as magnitude estimates. Filled circles show the magnitude of the subjective senation (that is, of self-rotation), and open circles show objective sensation (derived as the difference between total perceived relative velocity of the drum and perceived subjective velocity. Standard deviations of each data point are of the order of a third of value of the mean (data from Brandt et al, 1973).

retinal slip—also decreases the sense of subjective rotation (Brandt et al, 1973). Fixation of a point that is fixed relative to the chair usually causes a decrease in subjective sensation, as would be expected: but this observation is complicated by the fact that under these circumstances of comparatively large retinal slip in the periphery, the total perceived velocity—that is, subjective plus objective—is considerably increased and may lead the subject to think that it is the subjective velocity that has changed (see for example Hood and Leech, 1974). The reason for this seems to be that equal velocities signalled by the outflow and retinal slip pathways of figure 11.14 do not give rise to equal magnitudes of sensation, the objective (retinal slip) pathway being about 1·6 times more powerful (Dichgans, Körner, and Voight, 1969): thus, if the reader holds a finger up before his eyes and moves it slowly from side to side, its apparent velocity seems greater if the background behind it is fixated than if the finger itself is followed [the Exner–Fleischl paradox (Exner, 1875); see also Filehne's (1922) useful discussion].

When some parts of the visual field are moving and some are stationary, the question of which areas are perceived to be in motion and which stationary becomes a complex one. On a cloudy night the moon appears to sail through the clouds: in general, the larger of the areas—whether moving or not—appears to be the one that is fixed (for example Duncker, 1938; Ludvigh, 1952b). But expectation also enters into the sensation—as for example in the familiar illusion when one is sitting in a train at a station and the train next door starts to move—as does attention to one part of the field or another (for example Ter Braak, 1972): eye movements presumably play no special part in these high-level effects.

A phenomenon that may be mentioned here is that of the *autokinetic effect,* first described by von Humboldt in the 18th century (Guilford and Dallenbach, 1928): if in the dark one is looking at a small luminous object like a star, it appears to undergo small wandering movements in a more or less random manner. The size of these movements is considerably increased after muscular strain on the eyes, and after the eyes are strained in a particular meridian there is a tendency for the movement to occur mainly in the same meridian, in the opposite direction (Carr, 1910; Gregory and Zangwill, 1963). A possible explanation for the phenomenon comes from a consideration of a parametric feedback system like that of figure 11.11. During a period of strain to the right, fatigue will result in a mismatch between desire and performance, and consequently in a change in the parameters of the process C such as to increase the rightward innervation of the muscles. On reverting to central gaze, this change will no longer be appropriate: initially the eye will be directed to the right of the target: this results in the sensation that the target is to the left, while subsequent visual corrections to fixate it will give a further sensation of leftward movement. This is by no means the only possible explanation, of course (one might suggest, for example, that after the strain the eye reverts to a position to the *left* of the target because of muscular imbalance, and its gradual drift back to the centre is interpreted as a leftward movement of the target), but a clarification of the mechanism awaits precise measurements of the small eye movements made during the autokinetic sensation: although large movements can be excluded as a possible source of the phenomenon (Guilford and Dallenbach, 1928; Gregory, 1959) the accuracy of the measurements that have been made so far—some $0 \cdot 5°$ of arc—do not permit one to exclude micromovements, and indeed partial stabilisation of the retinal image reduces the autokinetic effect (Matin and MacKinnon, 1964). Theories of the autokinetic effect have been reviewed by Levy (1972).

Finally, to return to the question of the differences in the sensations derived from rotating drums and rotating chairs, a wily subject who was familiar with the dynamics of spinning bodies might try to differentiate one from the other by tilting his head to one side. If it is the chair that is rotating, such a change in the axes of the semicircular canals relative to the axis of rotation should induce rotational accelerations in their endolymph which will be felt as a rotation about some new axis (by the operation of imaginary 'Coriolis forces': see Melvill Jones, 1970). Yet there seems to be a conspiracy on the part of nature to prevent us from cheating in this way: for it turns out that precisely similar sensations are felt on tilting the head on one side, whether it is the chair or the drum that moves! (Brandt et al, 1971).

Now, it has been argued (Brandt et al, 1971) that this mimicry by the visual system of what is essentially a fault in the vestibular system implies that visual information about rotation is processed by the older pathways which serve the same function for vestibular information. This argument does not seem very compelling: if the implication is that the vestibular system has evolved neural pathways that in some way compensate for Coriolis effects, and that the same compensation is applied to visual input, then the Coriolis effects ought to be opposite in sign (for head tilt in a given direction) for drum rotation and for chair rotation, which is not what is observed. A simpler explanation comes from a consideration of the adaptational properties of the movement-detecting mechanisms of the visual system. Physical systems involving accelerations are not the only ones to show phenomena identical in their effects to Coriolis forces: *any* system that shows a degree of adaptation to constant angular velocities will behave in precisely the same way.

It has long been known that the visual system shows a tendency to adapt to continued constant movement: as in the case of the semicircular canals, this adaptation is best perceived as an aftereffect of seen motion. After gazing for a period at a scene that is in continuous motion in one direction, for example at a waterfall, on looking at a stationary field the observer may appear to see the objects in it moving in the opposite direction: this 'waterfall effect' was much studied by early physiologists (for example Purkinje, 1825, page 60), and this early work has been well reviewed by Wohlgemuth (1911). Helmholtz (1909) suggested that the effect might be due to a persistence of optokinetic nystagmus after cessation of the original motion (see section 3.3.2), since the aftereffect appeared considerably reduced if the eye attempted steady fixation during the adapting period. But this observation has often been questioned, and indeed Brindley (1970, page 146) finds exactly the opposite, namely that, if the moving stimulus is tracked as carefully as possible with the eye, no trace of aftereffect can be detected.

It is now generally accepted that the waterfall effect is mainly due to adaptation of visual motion detectors; this adaptation results in imbalance in the signals from adapted and unadapted detectors when the stationary field is viewed, which is interpreted as motion in the opposite sense (Barlow and Hill, 1963). The strongest evidence that eye movements are not the primary factor comes from observations of the aftereffects of viewing rotating figures like the spiral of figure 11.17, if such a spiral is rotated in a clockwise direction, the observer has an impression of continual expansion of the figure; on stopping the motion, the aftereffect is perceived as apparent contraction. It is difficult to imagine any kind of eye movement response that could explain such an effect. Direct evidence supporting the idea of adaptation of motion detectors has been reported by Sekuler and Ganz (1963), who adapted to a pattern of moving stripes under stabilised vision: subsequently the threshold for perceiving motion in the same direction was increased relative to that for motion in the opposite direction.

Consider now what the effect of such an adaptation would be on the perception of a continuously moving vertical grating pattern, if the head is suddenly tilted to one side. For simplicity, let us assume that the

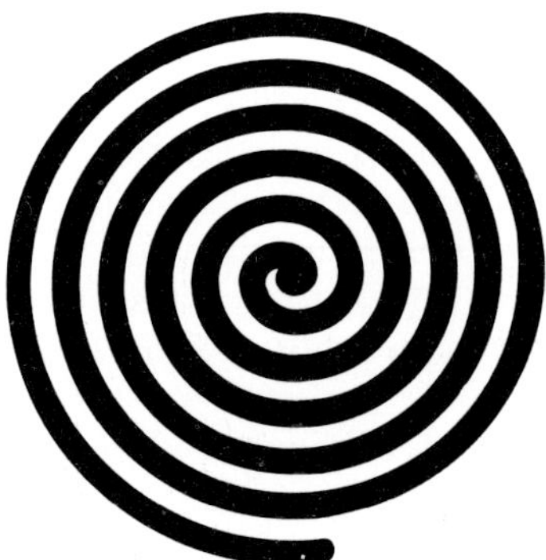

Figure 11.17. Rotating spiral to show that movement aftereffects are not the result of eye movements. If the spiral is rotated clockwise while its centre is fixated, it will appear to expand continually: the corresponding aftereffect on cessation of motion is of contraction in all directions. Clearly no eye movement could account for such a sensation.

perceived direction and amplitude of motion of such a stimulus is formed of something like the vectorial sum of the signals from motion detectors in different directions, and that orientational specificity is rather sharp: neither assumption is absolutely necessary to the argument, although some early observations (Borschke and Hescheles, 1902) suggest that motion aftereffects do indeed add vectorially. The sequence of events before and after tilting the head is illustrated diagrammatically in figure 11.18, together with the parallel case of true Coriolis (vestibular) stimulation. During the viewing period before the head tilt, the perceived velocity is gradually reduced as a result of adaptation (a and b). On tilting the head (c), the aftereffect in the original meridian will result in an apparent horizontal component of motion perception in the backwards direction, added to which will be a component from the new set of motion detectors stimulated by the new direction of motion. The resultant of these two

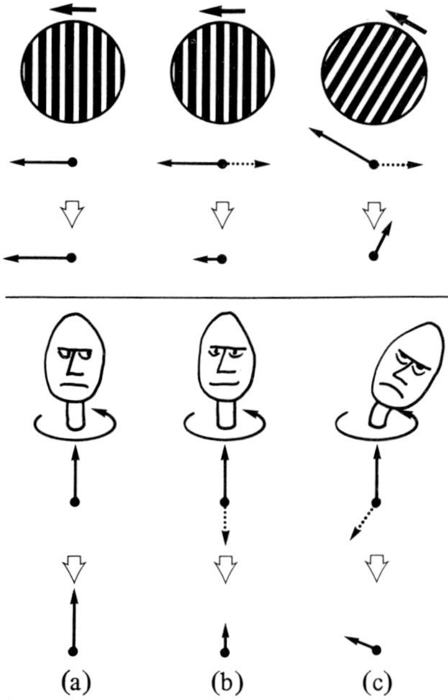

Figure 11.18. Adaptation to velocity inevitably produces Coriolis-like effects. Above, the effect of head tilt when the subject is sitting stationary with moving visual field. The upper figures represent schematically the visual field relative to the head. (a) The initial sensation is of the movement that actually occurs (vector arrows below show perceived direction and magnitude of movement). After a time (b), adaptation (dotted arrow) reduces the magnitude of the sensation. On tilting the head to the left (c), the new movement vector combines with the adaptational effect of the old to produce a sensation of movement that is different in direction from either. Below, precisely analogous effects under conditions of head rotation, when the head is tilted. Again, the new vector (c) combines with the adaptational component to generate a sensation in a totally different direction.

components will be an apparent direction of motion that is quite different from either: the visual field will appear to be moving predominantly upward. After a period of continued viewing in the tilted position, the original aftereffect will wear off, and the apparent direction of motion will veer round to coincide with the true direction. Such an effect of head tilt is thus closely similar to the 'pseudo-Coriolis effect' described by Brandt et al (1971), but does not require the postulation of any particular relationship between the visual and vestibular systems. It may, however, be that visual signals of this type are used in some way to offset the vestibular ones, a process which results in the reduction in true Coriolis effects that is observed when the visual and vestibular stimuli bear their natural relation to one another. For such a compensation to be effective, it is of course necessary for the time constant of the adaptation to seen motion to be similar to that of the semicircular canals: in view of the differences between the time constants of the different canals in man (see section 2.1.3) it would be interesting to know whether similar differences in adapting to motion in different directions is observed.

12

An attempted synthesis

"... yet the case so standeth, that in respect of the diversitie of his actions, of the difference of his instruments wherewith it serveth it selfe, and of the varietie of objects set before it: that it may seeme and appeare to the common people (after a certaine maner) to consist of divers parts."

'Divide and rule' is no less applicable to scientific study: and the intention in the previous chapters has been to make as many distinct compartments of the subject matter as seemed possible: dividing structure from function, catching from holding, large movements from small, and so on. Such an approach may perhaps seem to emphasise too much the differences between the different types of movement, and postpone too long the disagreeable task of binding our airy speculations about function to the chill rock of anatomical fact. This final chapter begins by bringing together for comparison the various functional subunits of the oculomotor system—vestibular, saccadic, etc—and attempts some condensation by looking for mechanisms that seem to be held in common. Then, having formed some idea of the irreducible kernel of the functional system, I attempt to identify its neural embodiment.

12.1 Common functional mechanisms

12.1.1 The idea of the final common path

In looking for common ground amongst the various oculomotor systems it is natural to start at the output end and work backwards. There are many sensory routes by which an eye movement can be initiated: but all ultimately lead to contractions of muscles in the orbit. We have seen that all six muscles are in general involved in any movement of the eye, so it is clear that all the subsystems must project to each muscle. Working back along the muscle's insertion in the globe—clearly the common transmitter of the forces generated by the various systems—we come to the first stumbling block: the diversity of muscle types. We saw in chapter 8 that eye muscles seem to be composed of at least five distinct types of muscle fibre, differing greatly in their mechanical and electrical properties. Numbers have a kind of magic even for the twentieth-century scientist: setting about it the right way, one can calculate that there are exactly five classes of eye movement, and five types of clinical condition resulting from lesions in the oculomotor system. For some, this is a cogent reason to believe that each type of fibre is concerned exclusively with one type of movement, and involved in one type of disorder. It is true, as we have seen in chapter 8, that, if one records directly and simultaneously from different types of fibre within the muscle, one finds that certain kinds of fibre are relatively more active in some kinds of movement than others: but this differential activity is correlated solely with the speed of the eye movement, and *not* with type of activation—vestibular, saccadic, etc—which evoked it. Of course, saccadic movements will cause a predominance of activity in the faster fibres, and vergence movements in the slower fibres: but these associations are not exclusive, and the very same fibres that were active during a vergence movement can be shown (by direct recording from the motor neurons) to be used to hold the eye at its new deviation at the end of a saccade. One can think of the fibres of any one muscle as being like the members of an orchestra: specialised in their output, made different use of by different composers, but not owing them exclusive allegiances in the sense that the trombones are only for Berlioz, or the strings for Mozart. The firing of an oculomotor neuron is essentially a function of the desired position and velocity of the eye, and of nothing else.

Now if this function was in every case a *linear* one, one might picture the various sources of eye movement commands as simply summing at the input to each neuron in the pool, to produce the summation of effects that we have seen to be characteristic (on the whole) of interactions between the different modes of stimulation. But there are several reasons why this simple model will not do. In the first place, the functions are *not* linear, in that each neuron has a threshold eye position or velocity, below which it is inactive: we have seen that it is the graded recruitment of units resulting from these various thresholds that helps to counteract the intrinsic nonlinearity of the eye's intrinsic mechanics. A saccadic command to abduct by 5° will evoke very much more extra abducens activity when the eye is already in abduction than when it is pointing straight ahead. There are two alternative modifications of the model that get round this difficulty. One possibility is to make the firing of the neuron an appropriate nonlinear (threshold) function of the summated input; alternatively, we could arrange for a signal representing the position of the eye at any moment to be sent to each neuron to modify its behaviour in the desired way. This hypothetical signal cannot literally be from the eye itself, for we know that the firing patterns associated with particular desired eye positions are not in fact modified if the eye is interfered with in such a way as to prevent these positions being attained (chapter 10). But it could be synthesised—by a process of efference copy—from the efferent activity of the neuron pool. Although the former scheme (a nonlinearity at the neuron input) is preferable on grounds of simplicity, it cannot account for the further complications introduced by the action of the other five muscles. The incremental activity for unit displacement of the eye is not only a function of the deviation of the eye in the same direction: it is equally a function of the rotation of the eye at any moment about the other two axes, and hence of the activity in each of the other muscles. The simple process of linear summation followed by a nonlinearity can no longer cope: to achieve cooperative relationships like those illustrated in figure 7.22, commands corresponding to rotations of the eye about each axis must be sent to *every* neuron, and they must be allowed to interact and modify each other before the stage at which they sum together. Only in this way can the effective 'weight' of each synapse be modified according to the position of the eye, as in figure 7.23. Bearing in mind that a command may be to move the eye about any one of an indefinitely large number of axes in Fick's plane, one can see that the number of individual synapses on each motor neuron will be very large indeed. The use of efference copy rather than an intrinsic nonlinearity in the motor neuron helps only slightly.

Now there is nothing improbable in a model that supposes a very large number of synapses on a neuron: what does begin to seem implausible is the idea that such a swarm of synaptic endings over the motor neuron's surface would be capable of anything more sophisticated than a simple summation of total weighted input. But the scheme as it stands so far requires interactions not only between the presynaptic terminals and the postsynaptic membrane, but *between the terminals themselves.* Since each terminal has to be able to reach each other terminal and influence it in a highly specific way, it is evident that the number of such connections—of the order of the factorial of the number of afferent fibres—will soon become quite unmanageable. One is forced to conclude that the linear parts of this computation—as for example the resolution of movements along oblique meridians into a common system of coordinates—must precede the nonlinear processes finally needed to match the process of neuronal recruitment: this of course also implies that the final common path for commands of different origin must also lie at least one stage further back in the oculomotor system. A possible scheme of this type is shown in figure 12.1. Here a large number of afferent fibres, corresponding to different meridians and different origins, converge onto two neurons (or more plausibly, neuronal pools) whose activity represents desired rotation about the two nontorsional axes. Although the number of afferents is just as large as in the former model, the important difference is that, since trigonometrical resolution of this kind is a linear process, the interactions *between* the terminals that proved fatal to the previous scheme are avoided. The outputs of these two channels—containing complete information about the desired movement of the eye—are then sent to each of the final motor neurons: as before, one has to postulate nonlinear interactions between them, as well as the inevitable nonlinearity in the motor neuron itself. But the number of terminals is now so reduced that this is no longer an embarrassment. Listing's Law can be taken care of by choosing appropriate synaptic weightings, and if other torsional movements are to be included, one need only postulate a third channel at level 2 working in the same manner as the other two. If figure 12.1 resembles a diagram of part of a cross-bar telephone exchange, this only reflects the fact that the same principle—that of concentration of signals through common intermediate links—guides the design of both (see Atkinson, 1950).

The complexity could of course be still further reduced if the sensory systems from which the oculomotor commands originate were already organised in a coordinate system. The obvious example that comes to mind is the vestibular system, where the transformation from the axes of the semicirucular canals to those of the hypothetical channels of level 2 would be relatively straightforward. But there is no direct evidence for an analogous process in the visual system, and nothing in the arrangement of nerve cells (with the possible exception of the cerebellum) to lend support to such an idea. In any case, as was seen in section 8.4.3, one can indeed find units in the reticular formation of the brain stem, whose properties are exactly what would be expected of units of level 3, firing in proportion to movement of the eye in a preferred direction that is neither horizontal nor vertical, nor related in an obvious way to any of the muscles. There seems little doubt that the units of level 2 are also to be found somewhere in the brain stem, but they have not been sought in precisely these terms. One might in fact think of the suggested arrangement of levels 2 and 3 as being essentially part of the visual system, condensing the afferent information until it is in a form in which it can be mixed with signals passing along the much older vestibulo-ocular system. Since the choice of the three coordinate directions of level 2 is essentially arbitrary—it makes no difference to the principle of operation of the whole network—we might go on to suppose that this mingling of visual and vestibular signals would be still more facilitated if the coordinates used at level 2 were simply those of the semicircular canals themselves.

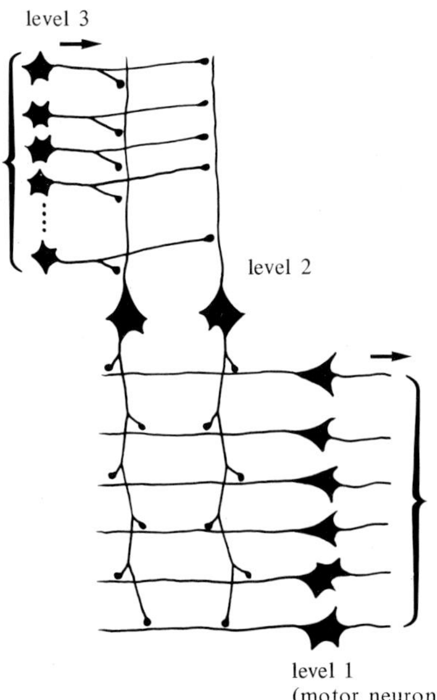

Figure 12.1. Hypothetical arrangement of final levels of the oculomotor system.

For the vestibulo-ocular reflex, level 2 must of course be identified with the vestibular nuclei (and its output with the medial longitudinal fasciculus), and it is natural to make one more speculative leap and suggest that the visual input is also funneled through the same vestibular second-order neurons. But there is no logical compulsion whatever in the scheme as it stands for level 2 to be common both to visual and to vestibular commands: the degree of synaptic complexity at level 1 is not increased very greatly if there are in fact two separate sets of level 2 inputs. All the same, as we have seen, some experimental evidence favours the idea of the medial longitudinal fasciculus as a common path for at least part of the visual input as well as the vestibular: this point is discussed again in section 12.1.7.

This difficulty, of deciding whether level 2 has separate mechanisms for visual and for vestibular inputs, is typical of what tends to happen when one tries to look for common mechanisms without detailed and anatomically related neurophysiological results as a foundation. Occam's Razor—that entities should not be needlessly multiplied—is sound advice in constructing logical systems for one's own use: but when the aim is to make deductions about the *actual* construction of a system that already exists it has no more force than any other argument based on estimates of the likely course of evolutionary development. In the next four sections the four main classes of eye movement are compared to see what functional components might be common to them all (apart, that is, from the peripheral mechanisms already discussed, the deduction of which did not need the use of the Razor). In doing so, it is convenient to use the common mathematical language of systems analysis to describe their behaviour: but it has the disadvantage that the very fact of its providing a common means of expression implies that it may indicate similarities where none in fact exist. The low-pass filter, $1/(\mathrm{D}+a)$, is a simple functional building block: by writing it as $[\mathrm{D}/(\mathrm{D}+a)]\mathrm{D}^{-1}$ (a first-order high-pass filter followed by a stage of integration) we can, if we feel inclined, pretend that it shares a common mechanism with some other system, $b\mathrm{D}^{-1}$, that really *is* an integrator. Such an interpretation could only be justified by further experiment, that is, by breaking into their respective 'black boxes'. If actions that destroy the integrator in one of the systems always, without exception, destroy the integrator in the other system, then by the ordinary standards of scientific inductive proof one can justifiably conclude that the integrator is held in common. (A more direct test would of course be to trace the neuronal connections of the two systems: but this is not generally a practicable approach.)

12.1.2 Vestibular eye movements

We saw in chapter 2 that the gain of the vestibulo-ocular reflex as a function of frequency is virtually flat from about 0·02 to 4 Hz. This finding seems to vary surprisingly little in different species and preparations; the phase response is apparently more variable, and strongly dependent on such factors as the presence or absence of quick phases: some of these difficulties may be essentially problems of measurement. At all events, measurements of amplitude are more reliable, and will be used in preference to phase measurements (where possible) in what follows; this also avoids the difficulty of estimating the distributed delays of the system.

Now it is clear that the vestibulo-ocular reflex consists of three distinct processes in series: first the transducer process of the canals, in which movements of the head are converted into firing frequencies of eighth nerve fibres; second, the neural processes by which these frequencies are converted into firing frequencies of oculomotor nerves; and third, the transduction of these frequencies into eye deviation (figure 12.2). If we confine ourselves to a physiological range of frequency—for the sake of argument, that over which the gain is constant—we can predict from previous experimental data how the two transducers (canals and eye) will contribute to the overall transfer function. Consider first the canals: the range of frequencies we are interested in is well above that in which low-frequency adaptation (see section 2.1.3) makes itself felt, and well below that in which we need to consider the inertial time constant of the canals. (This may not be true if we are interested in accurate measurements of phase, which shows a wider spread of effects on a frequency scale than does gain: even at one-tenth of the characteristic frequency of a first-order low-pass filter, a phase lag of nearly 6° is introduced, while the gain is less than 0·5% down.) We can probably also ignore the high-frequency adaptational component found by Fernandez and Goldberg (1971) in the squirrel monkey, which (for the horizontal canal) had a characteristic frequency of about 11 Hz. The canals can then be described by the transfer function (linking head position to frequency of firing): $D^2/(\lambda+D)$, where λ has a value somewhere in the range 0·06–0·16 s^{-1}, depending on the species. Similarly, the mechanics of the eye can be broadly treated as a first-order low-pass filter of characteristic frequency around 1–2 Hz (section 8.4.4). We can write this as $1/(k+D)$, where k is around 10 s^{-1}. We now know the transfer function of two of the three processes that make up the vestibulo-ocular reflex, as well as the transfer function of the whole thing: by subtraction, it is a straightforward matter to calculate the transfer function of the neural pathways that make up the missing stage.

It is convenient to begin by subtracting the effect of the semicircular canals (*a*, figure 12.3). Since the canals essentially signal head velocity, a single stage of integration is needed if the brain is to convert this *velocity* information into an eye *position*: so it is no surprise to find that a Bode

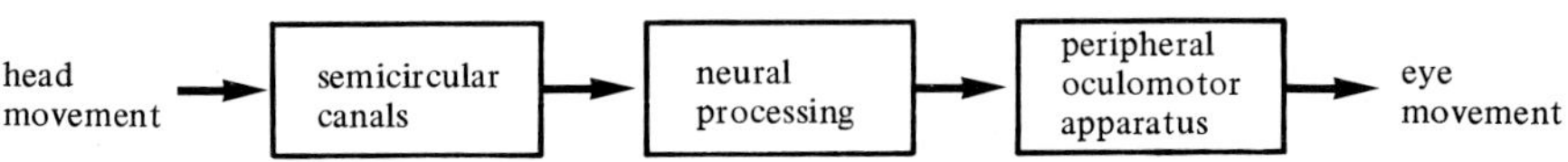

Figure 12.2. The three series elements of the vestibulo-ocular reflex.

plot of the gain of the remainder of the reflex has the slope of -1 that is characteristic of an integrator. If we now proceed to subtract the effect of the eye mechanics, so as to leave the transfer function of the neural pathways on their own (*b*, figure 12.3), we find that this function, though looking like an integrator at low frequencies, begins to level off at around 1 Hz in order to compensate for the falloff in gain occasioned by the poor high-frequency gain of the eye mechanics. Algebraically, we can represent the neural transfer function by the expression $(1 + k\mathrm{D}^{-1})$, where k has the same value as before. If we combine this expression with the transfer function representing the eye mechanics, we obtain $(1 + k\mathrm{D}^{-1})/(k + \mathrm{D})$, which simplifies to D^{-1}—as it should. In effect, the neural part of the reflex is acting to make the whole system a much better integrator of the velocity signal coming from the canals than one would expect from the sluggishness of the eye itself, by allowing a little of the velocity signal to bypass the integrator and feed directly on to the oculomotor neurons (figure 12.4). It is tempting to identify this direct bypass that is designed

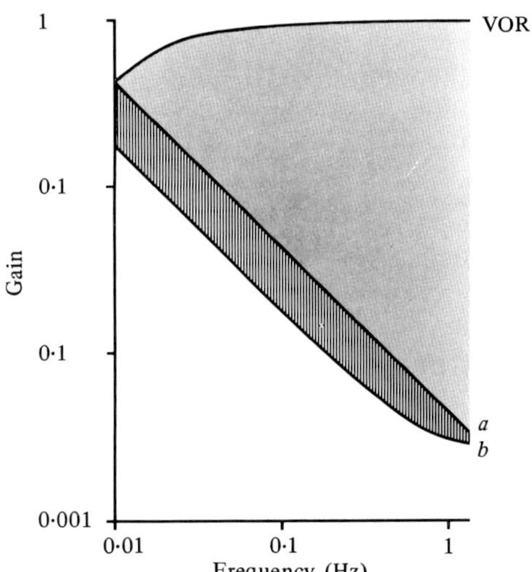

Figure 12.3. VOR = gain of vestibulo-ocular reflex as a function of frequency; a = VOR minus gain of semicircular canals; $b = a$ minus gain of peripheral oculomotor apparatus. Thus b is the transfer function of the 'neural processing' element of figure 12.2.

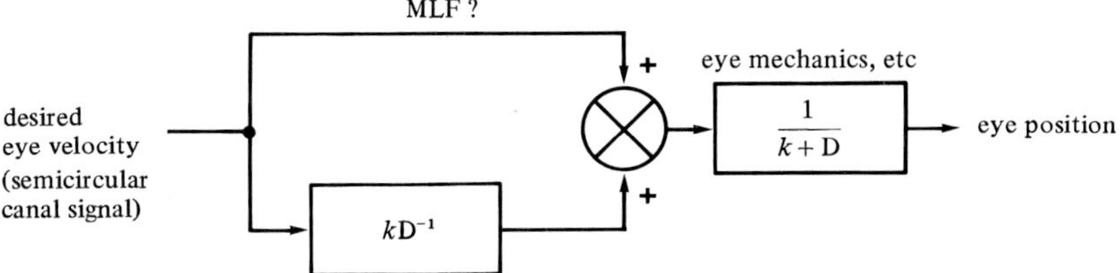

Figure 12.4. Hypothetical scheme of the conversion from the signal from the semicircular canals to deviation of the eye. (MLF is medial longitudinal fasciculus).

to speed up the vestibular response with the fibres of the medial longitudinal fasciculus (MLF), that are specialised for fast conduction and provide a direct projection from vestibular nuclei to motor neurons, and the integrator with the alternative pathways in parallel with the MLF, through the cerebellum or reticular formation. These possibilities are discussed in section 12.1.7.

12.1.3 Vergence

Like all the visual mechanisms for moving the eye, control of vergence by perceived disparity is essentially closed-loop in nature. In section 5.2.2 we saw how it was possible to open this loop by arranging an external feedback circuit that cancelled the effect of disjunctive eye movements. The open-loop transfer function linking disparity to vergence can then be measured by means of sinusoidal variation of the input. It turned out that the gain of the system under these circumstances, plotted in Bode form, showed the -1 slope characteristic of an integrator at moderate frequencies (figure 5.12): as in the case of the vestibulo-ocular reflex, the phase response is more variable, and shows inconsistencies from subject to subject. The response to steps of disparity—constant-velocity vergence movements whose velocity is proportional to the applied disparity—confirms the essentially integrating nature of the system, whose transfer function might be written as $k\mathrm{D}^{-1}$, where k has a value of around 5 s^{-1} in man.

One would hope at this point to be able to proceed as in the case of the vestibulo-ocular reflex and calculate the transfer function of the neural parts of the disparity vergence system. Certainly there is no reason in principle why we should not do this at the output stage, by subtracting the known mechanics of the eye: but it is only at frequencies above about 1 Hz that the mechanics have noticeable effects on gain, and it is precisely in this region that reliable data are missing. It is just not possible to say whether the integrator is simply of the form D^{-1}, or whether, as in the case of the vestibular movements, it is bypassed by a pathway of constant gain, to compensate for the degradation introduced by the eye mechanics. On the input side, the problem is more serious. Whereas in the vestibular system one can think of a single channel of information leading from each canal and carrying a signal whose instantaneous value is a linear function of one single dimension of the physical stimulus, the visual system, as has been repeatedly emphasised, consists of a very large number of parallel channels in which the *pattern* of activity considered over the whole ensemble (rather than the *degree* of activity in any one channel) carries the information we need. Our knowledge of visual processes is simply not sufficient at present to disentangle the spatial and temporal aspects of the processing of this information.

To take a fundamental question of obvious relevance to the control of vergence, what is the nature of the 160 ms delay? It is very unlikely that more than about 12 ms of this is due to delays in the final common oculomotor pathways, and in good photopic conditions the delay in the retina is perhaps 50 ms or so at most. What is happening in the missing 100 ms? If this delay were simply a transport delay due to neuronal conduction and synaptic transmission, there would be plenty of time for transmission through a hundred consecutive neuronal elements: but current visual neurophysiology has scarcely penetrated beyond the third. It is inconceivable that such a series of transfers would not be attended by some frequency-dependent degradation of the signal being carried, at least in its temporal aspect: its spatial properties might well be accurately preserved. Since somewhere along the line from retina to oculomotor nuclei such spatial aspects of the visual stimulus as disparity must be converted into a time-varying signal in, effectively, a single channel, the amount of temporal filtering suffered by this signal will depend on where in the chain of neurons this conversion takes place—at present a completely unknown factor. Another possibility, in some ways more attractive and plausible, is that the large delays associated with the processing of visual information are the result of some intrinsic timing mechanism that forces the system to integrate its information over a certain period of time before finally releasing its conclusions to the oculomotor pathways. One advantage of this conception from the investigator's point of view is that, by allowing the visual information as it were to gather itself together at the entrance gate to the oculomotor system (like horses under starter's orders at the beginning of a race), irregularities of phase can be eliminated, and the whole visual system treated (for purposes of analysis) as if it were simply a lumped transport delay introducing no phase distortion. In the absence of experimental evidence on either one side or the other, this is the expedient that will be adopted here when considering transfer functions of visually evoked eye movements: we have already seen in chapter 4 that similar assumptions of an intermittent gating process in the visual system account quite satisfactorily for many aspects of the generation of saccades (see also section 12.2 below).

For disparity vergence, then, this leads to the simple conclusion that the neural pathways are acting as an integrator (which may or may not have a direct bypass) when presented with simple stimuli such as sinusoids or steps of disparity (figure 12.5). More complicated stimuli can lead to

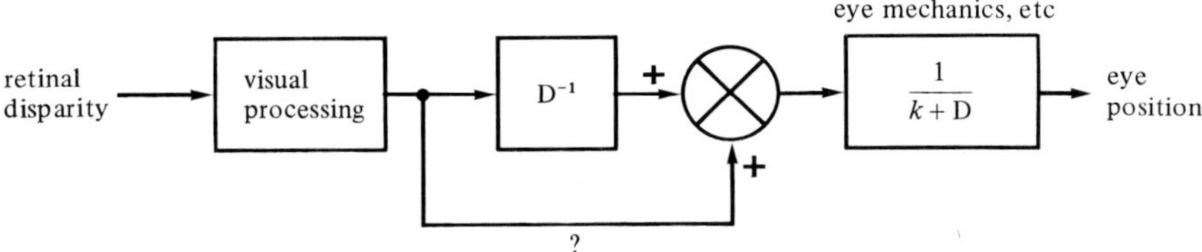

Figure 12.5. Hypothetical scheme of the vergence system.

anomalous responses showing short-term prediction: it is possible that these are the result of processing by the visual system (that is, that portion of the whole pathway that lies in front of the hypothetical 'gate' that immediately precedes the integrator). A further property noted in section 5.2 is that under natural closed-loop conditions the system may learn to improve its performance over a longer time scale when presented with stimuli that are repetitive or otherwise predictable.

12.1.4 Smooth pursuit

Measurements of the transfer function of the smooth pursuit system—with the use of sinusoidal and step inputs under either open- or closed-loop conditions—were examined in section 3.3. A fundamental difficulty in the analysis of pursuit movements that was noted there is the lack of correspondence between responses to changes of *position* and responses to *velocity*, a distinction whose ultimate origin lies in the fact that the visual system is a 'which' system, while linear systems analysis can only usefully be applied to 'how much' systems. However, it seems possible to model the smooth pursuit system quite adequately by ignoring smooth responses to positional information altogether and placing a differentiating element D at the input end of the system (Collewijn, 1972). The same policy will be adopted here, though at the end of the section an attempt will be made to incorporate a positional input as well.

We saw that the earliest studies of optokinetic nystagmus indicated that in the rabbit the transfer function of the whole system was that of an integrator (kD^{-1}), and that the value of k was around 1 s^{-1}. Ignoring the filtering effect of eye mechanics for the moment, and adding the element D at the input as mentioned above (which of course necessitates an extra compensating stage of integration at the other end) we have the basis of a model of the rabbit's optokinetic system. By adding a saturating nonlinearity after the velocity detector, and bypassing one of the integrators to improve the high-frequency phase response, we can accurately simulate a rabbit's smooth pursuit movements under a wide variety of stimulus conditions (figure 12.6) (Collewijn, 1972). The gain a of the bypassed integrator in this model happens to be of the same order of magnitude of those envisaged for the vestibular and vergence systems (about 5–6 s^{-1}): but this is really coincidental, as allowance has yet to be made in Collewijn's model for the effect of eye mechanics, whose compensation (if indeed they *are* compensated for in the same way as in the vestibulo-ocular reflex)

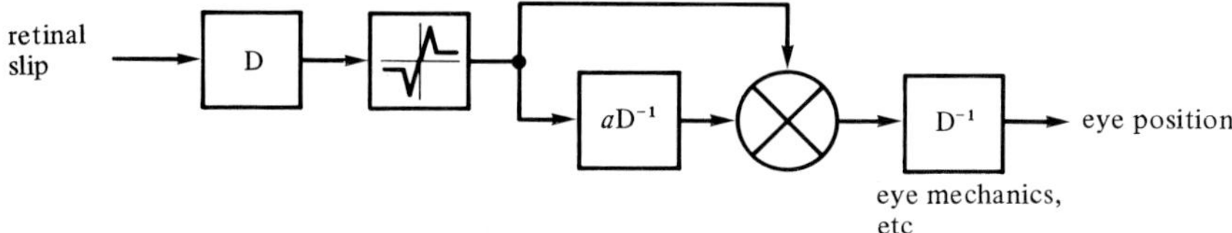

Figure 12.6. Model of rabbit's smooth pursuit system; modified after Collewijn (1972).

would require the second integrator also to have a bypass route, *this* being the integrator analogous to those in the vestibular and vergence systems.

For various reasons (examined in section 3.3.1) equivalent measurements in man do not seem to be amenable to as quantitative a treatment as those in the rabbit, because of the difficulty of making high-quality recordings under truly open-loop conditions. The positional input to the smooth pursuit mechanism in man, mentioned earlier, has also not been measured with great precision. We saw that the open-loop response to a step of position is a movement of constant acceleration whose magnitude is rather unaffected by the size of the input: linear analysis is therefore not strictly applicable, but one can easily see that such a step might simply cause a constant signal to be sent to the pair of integrators used for the smooth movements. A possible scheme for the complete system is shown in figure 12.7: as was explained in the case of vergence movements in the previous section, it is convenient to lump transport delays together in the 'visual processing' box. St Cyr and Fender (1969c) suggest that the improvement in closed-loop phase response that results from practice in following repetitive stimuli can be described as reductions in the delay associated with this element: if one imagines that the rate at which it can deal with incoming information has an upper bound, then redundancies in the stimulus, reducing the inflow of information, will enable the processing to be completed more quickly and the hypothetical 'gate' into the smooth pursuit system to be raised sooner. In addition to this stimulus-dependent delay, which may vary from nearly 40 ms for a sine wave to nearly 250 ms for a Gaussian input, there is an irreducible delay of about 70 ms due presumably to neural conduction and other immutable factors. It is not easy to see how a neural network could be devised that embodies these stimulus-dependent delays in this way.

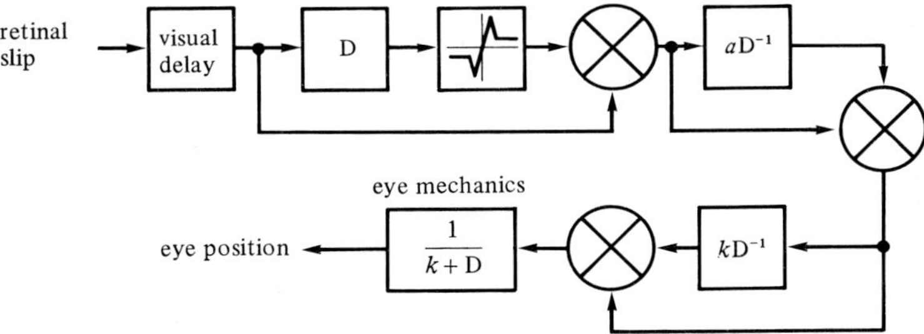

Figure 12.7. Improved version of figure 12.6.

12.1.5 Saccades

The difficulties of devising a scheme of visual processing that will explain the observed properties of visually evoked saccades are even greater than in the case either of vergence or of smooth pursuits movements, and discussion of this question is given a section of its own (12.3). Here we shall be concerned with only the final stage of saccade production, in which the signal sent to the oculomotor nuclei is elaborated from knowledge of the desired size and direction of the movement.

As we saw in section 7.5.5, there is overwhelming evidence that at some stage preceding the oculomotor nuclei, the desired amplitude of a saccade is coded by the *duration* of a brief pulse of roughly constant neural activity in a set of neurons (the desired direction is presumably coded by *which* set it is). We also saw that by the time this signal reaches the motor neurons it has been transformed from a pulse of activity into a pulse step—the sum of a pulse and its integral. The purpose of this transformation is exactly the same as in the case of the vestibulo-ocular reflex: to ensure that, despite the sluggishness of the eye's mechanics, the movement of the globe is a smart flick from one position to another—the precise integral of the original pulse. It is clear that the neural circuit required to do this is exactly the same as in the vestibular case, namely an integrator bypassed by a direct pathway: and to achieve correct compensation for the eye mechanics (as is the case) the gain of the integrator should again be of the order of 10 s^{-1} (figure 12.8).

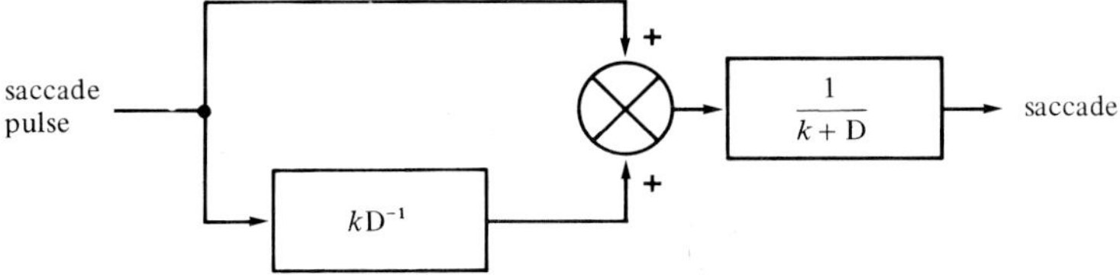

Figure 12.8. The same general arrangement as in figures 12.4 and 12.5 will also serve for generating saccades.

12.1.6 Possible mechanisms of neural integration

We have now established the necessity for an integrator in the output of each class of large eye movement (with a bypass in the case of saccades and vestibular eye movement, and very likely in the other two types as well). As far as small eye movements are concerned, microsaccades can presumably be treated as members of the same class as saccades, while tremor probably merely represents random noise in the motor neurons and muscle fibres. The 'random walk' properties of drift (section 6.1.2) suggest a model consisting of a noise source followed by a single integrator This makes five integrators in all (leaving aside for the moment the question as to whether one or more of these integrators are held in common): before considering where in the brain they might be located, we ought to consider how integration might in principle be achieved by neural circuitry, so we have some idea what we are looking for.

Broadly speaking, two approaches seem possible. On the one hand, one might try to imagine some novel property of the synaptic junction, which would act as an integrator; or on the other, one might try to

devise some kind of neural network that would perform the same function, but invoking only well-established synaptic mechanisms.
The first solution sounds quite simple: all we have to do is to invent a transmitter substance that lingers indefinitely at the postsynaptic membrane, instead of disappearing within a few milliseconds as is normally the case. This is by no means implausible, and is indeed precisely what happens under conditions when the enzyme whose function is to remove the transmitter when it has done its work is inactivated by an appropriate drug, for example eserine in the case of the transmitter acetyl choline. But there is a fundamental difficulty with such a concept. The signals that flow from black box to black box in a system analyst's model can take on positive or negative values, just as he chooses: but real neurons are not like that. Their signals are conveyed by the frequency of firing of their axons; and this frequency can be zero, or positive, but never negative. In the same way, a synapse can only add to the amount of transmitter present at the postsynaptic membrane: there is no known way in which it can reduce it. In many kinds of neuronal signal processing, the first difficulty can be obviating by arranging neurons in complementary pairs, as in the 'push-pull' scheme of figure 12.9: we have already met examples of this arrangement in the oculomotor system, with the pairs of neurons on opposite sides of the midline, and seen that it can also serve to get rid of particular kinds of nonlinearity (sections 7.5.3, 9.1.4). But the second difficulty—that of removing the long-lasting transmitter once it is there—is more serious. During sinusoidal rotation of the head in a decerebrate preparation, for example, in each half-cycle a constant amount of transmitter would presumably be released at the integrating synapse: it is inconceivable that the resulting steady buildup of transmitter would not sooner or later lead to saturation of the postsynaptic receptor mechanism, yet one can go on stimulating such a preparation in this way for periods of hours at a time without observing any kind of decrement in response. (The absence of nystagmus in such a preparation excludes the otherwise attractive hypothesis that the quick phase is the result of a sudden removal of the accumulated transmitter, perhaps by the release of an appropriate enzyme by a separate set of nerve terminals.) In the absence of direct experimental evidence for integrating transmitters, the hypothesis must be abandoned.

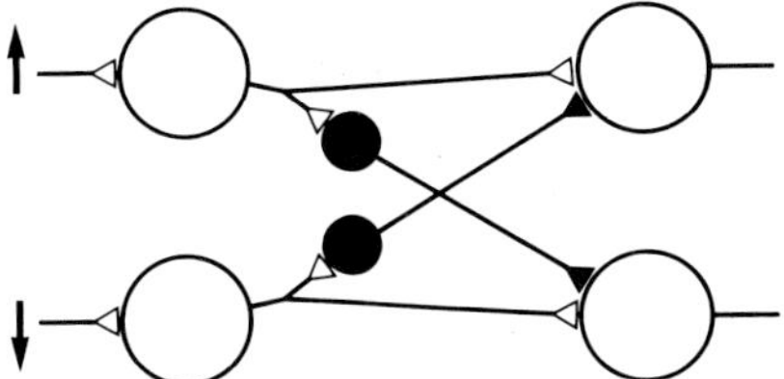

Figure 12.9. Neurons in 'push-pull' arrangement. The black neurons are inhibitory.

All integrators demand some way of storing the afferent information: the neural network hypothesis generally does this by making use of the delays inherent in transferring information from one neuron to another. In the scheme shown in figure 12.10, the input signal is sent down a long chain of interneurons arranged in series: each neuron also sends an axon to a common summating neuron, whose activity is taken to be proportional to the total activity in all the neurons of the chain. So long as the signal does not suffer distortion as it travels down the chain (this can be guaranteed so long as each cell gives exactly one output spike for each input spike) the output of the whole arrangement will be equal to the integral of the input over a finite period that is proportional to the length of the chain. The problem with this model is that we know from the vestibulo-ocular reflex that the integrator is capable of integrating over periods of 15 s at the least, so that if we allow a 1 ms delay per neuron (a rather generous estimate), we shall require a total chain length of fifteen thousand. This seems entirely implausible.

A more elegant solution is to make our chain into a loop (figure 12.11), thus making it effectively of infinite length: there is then no need for the summing element. So long as the gain round the loop is exactly unity, the transfer function of the whole arrangement (ignoring high-frequency effects due to the fact that the signals are pulse-frequency modulated) is given by $k\mathrm{D}^{-1}$, where k is the reciprocal of the delay round the loop. The system will of course misbehave when a pulse coming round the loop coincides with one coming via the input, but if there are a sufficient number of these units in parallel, with slightly different characteristic delays, such disturbances will be smoothed out. Unlike the synaptic integrator, this one will be able to vary its output both up and down (though it cannot of course produce negative values) if we add inhibitory synapses that can cancel the circulating impulses. We know

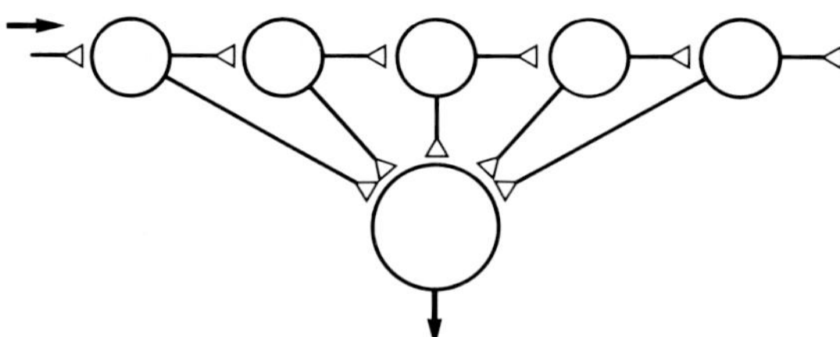

Figure 12.10. Interneurons arranged in series to form an integrator.

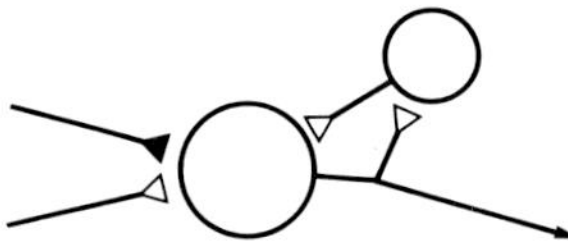

Figure 12.11. The chain of figure 12.10 made into a loop.

from the response time of the oculomotor integrators that the loop delay cannot be more than some 10 ms; but it cannot be much less than that either, from consideration of the maximum firing frequency of the neuron. This implies an extemely limited dynamic range, a major fault in the model, but one that can be corrected by imagining a population of such units with a wide spectrum of different loop delays, so that some are quick-acting but soon saturate, while others are slower but have a wide dynamic range. One attractive feature of the model is that its transfer function can be considerably altered by changes in the transmission round the loop. We have already seen that the gain depends on the loop delay: *attenuation* of the signal round the loop—which might be achieved by inhibitory endings that randomly cancel a fixed proportion of the total impulse traffic—converts the system from a pure integrator to a leaky integrator $1/(D+a)$, whose time constant depends on the degree of attenuation. This might be a convenient way of implementing some kinds of parametric feedback.

A slightly different kind of neural integrator has been proposed by Rosen (1972 figure 12.12). Here the necessary storage of information is carried out by a set of cells, each of which is at any moment either inactive, or firing at maximum frequency; each cell has positive feedback from its input to its output, and the resultant hysteresis constitutes the memory. Each has a different threshold, and receives a signal proportional to the total activity of the whole ensemble: thus, when a constant input is applied simultaneously to all, they switch on one after another at a rate proportional to the input. The sum of their activities is then approximately the integral of the input. The main criticism of this model is perhaps that it is rather uneconomical of neurons: the total information stored by 1000 of them arranged in this way is only rather less than eleven bits!

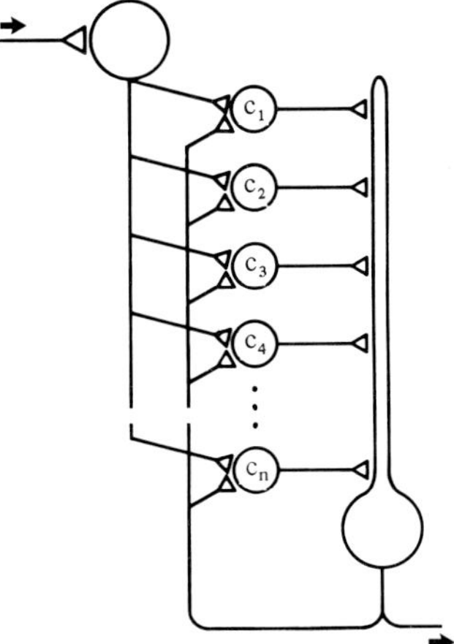

Figure 12.12. A possible neural integrator: the cells c_1–c_n have graded thresholds. Modified from Rosen (1972).

This scheme is compatible with the anatomy, as far as it is known, and also with the results of neurophysiological experiments. The PPRF tonic and burst cells are of course the tonic and burst cells described by Keller and others. Cerebellar ablations destroy the integrator but spare the fast components of saccades and vestibular nystagmus: PPRF lesions on the other hand abolish the fast and the slow components. The funnelling of the entire output of the system back through the vestibular neuron is suggested both by the effect of MLF lesions in causing complete abolition of all types of version (though perhaps not vergence) and by the fact that the discharges of MLF units are in every way extremely similar to those of the motor neurons themselves (see Robinson, 1975b, for an excellent discussion of this point): we also saw in section 9.1.4 that many vestibular units are also sensitive to optokinetic stimulation. Furthermore, it agrees with the conclusion reached in section 12.1.1 from quite different considerations, that the vestibular nucleus forms level 2 of the final common path. The scheme presented here is in some ways quite similar to that suggested by Robinson (1975b), though fundamentally different in two respects: it explicitly incorporates a reasonably plausible mechanism for the integration process, and by including cerebellar pathways it is better able to explain the known involvement of the cerebellum in this process. It is of course greatly oversimplified in many ways, particularly in its omission of the pathways of reciprocal inhibition necessary to deal with the problem of integrator saturation and the bilateral, 'push-pull' nature of the input and output. For example, 'pause' units in the PPRF, which show a brief suppression of activity during saccades, are presumably the inhibitory analogue of the burst units; and there are many well-established features of the bilateral connections of the vestibular nucleus neurons (section 9.1.4) which have been ignored.

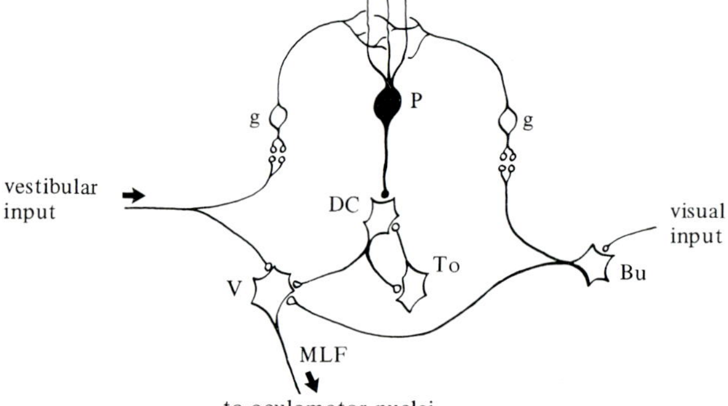

Figure 12.13. Possible vestibular and visual integrator. P is Purkinje cell; DC is deep cerebellar nucleus cell; V is vestibular nucleus cell; g is granule cell; Bu, To are burst and tonic cells of pontine reticular formation; MLF is medial longitudinal fasciculus. For simplicity, To is shown synapsing directly with DC; a more likely route is via the cerebellar cortex.

12.2 The saccadic pulse generator

In section 4.2 we examined different theories about the way in which various kinds of visual information (such as position, velocity, etc) are combined to produce a single saccadic command. In that section, we deliberately avoided consideration of exactly how this command—which we know to be in the form of a pulse of variable duration signifying the desired saccade amplitude—comes to be elaborated from the complex spatiotemporal patterns of firing in the visual system. It is a difficult conceptual problem, which most writers have been content to steer clear of; in this section, some possible models of the pulse generator will be examined in relation to their likely anatomical substrate.

One approach to this problem, that has produced a plausible solution, derives from considering precisely the opposite question: what kind of system is capable of converting temporal duration into spatial extent? One such device is the *delay line* (figure 12.14a), which converts temporal variations at the input into a travelling wave of spatial activity. It is not difficult to imagine how a delay line might be created either out of a chain of neurons, or perhaps simply through conduction along thin dendrites. (Axons conduct too fast to be useful in this context, since the pulses we are dealing with are several tens of milliseconds in length, necessitating axons of implausible length.) Now the general procedure in systems synthesis for generating the inverse of a given function is to arrange for it to form the reverse path of a negative feedback loop with a comparator. In this case we need only arrange for the spatial pattern generated by the delay line to be compared with the spatial input, and for the result of this comparison to control the duration of the pulse that is sent along the delay line, to build a rudimentary saccadic pulse generator (figure 12.14b). Here, a brief trigger pulse turns on the unit-gain positive

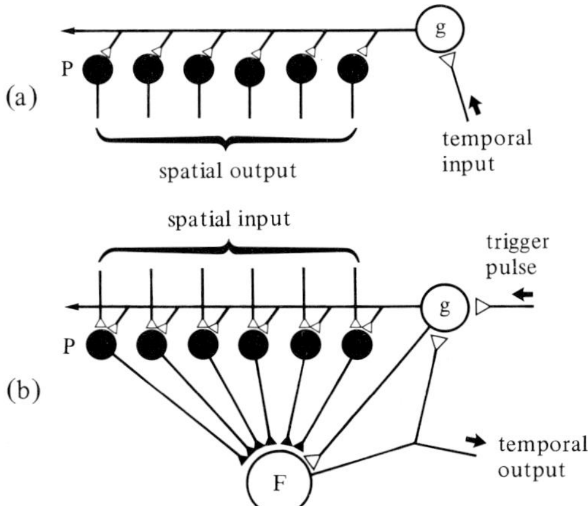

Figure 12.14. Systems capable of converting temporal duration into spatial extent: (a) delay line, (b) rudimentary saccadic pulse generator.

feedback loop formed by the two cells g and F; g is also the origin of the delay line, which projects to a sequence of cells P. Each of these cells corresponds to a different location in visual space, along the meridian defined by the relevant desired saccade direction, and has an appropriate excitatory input from the visual system. The thresholds of the P cells are such that they fire only if both the input from the delay line *and* the visual input are simultaneously active. They project back to F and inhibit it, thus terminating the sustained activity in the positive feedback loop formed by F and g. It can be seen that the output of the system, from g, will consist of a pulse of constant amplitude that is initiated by the occurrence of the trigger input, and whose duration corresponds with the desired saccade amplitude. Rosen's (1972) model, previously discussed, will clearly also behave in a similar way: instead of a delay line, the various elements (c_1 to c_n, figure 12.12) turn on in sequence because of their different thresholds. With a suitable spatial arrangement, the same mechanism can therefore generate *steps* whose height is determined by the visual input.

Now both these models have many features that strongly resemble aspects of the anatomy of the cerebellum, and it has often been suggested that the cerebellum may act as a 'tapped delay line' for the generation of duration-coded pulses, and indeed for some other kinds of spatiotemporal transformation (Braitenberg, 1961; 1967; Freeman and Nicholson, 1970; Kornhuber, 1971). The general notion is that the P cells in figure 12.14 are the Purkinje Cells, and the g cells are the granule cells, with their long straight parallel fibres running perpendicular to the plane of the dendritic trees of the Purkinje cells (see section 9.3.1). Conduction along these fibres appears to be sufficiently slow that pulses of saccade-like duration can be envisaged (Braitenberg, 1967; Freeman and Nicholson, 1970; but see also P Clarke, 1974). The visual input is presumed to enter via the climbing fibres, as is found to be the case in many species (section 9.3.2). Clarke (1974) reports that in the pigeon the visual input to folia VI to IX is crudely retinotopic, and that the parallel fibres are in effect parallel to the representation of the horizon. This is approximately the same region as that in which Ron and Robinson (1973) obtained saccadic movements from cerebellar stimulation in the monkey. It will be recalled that, with the eye starting in the primary position, the size of the evoked saccades in these stimulation studies was found to depend solely on the location of the stimulus, and not at all on its strength or duration (beyond 100 ms): this is precisely what would be expected of stimulation of the Purkinje cells that mimicked the effect of visual stimulation, although interpretation of stimulation experiments is very difficult if it is not known exactly what neural structures are affected.

If we slightly remodel the scheme of figure 12.14 to fit more closely to the actual cerebellar circuitry (figure 12.15), it is evident that the positive feedback loop needed to sustain the pulse is precisely the same as that proposed in section 12.1.7 as the final common path integrator. They cannot of course actually be identical, since the pulse generator must be *followed* by a separate common integrator to convert the pulse into a saccade: but the similarity of the circuitry perhaps makes it slightly more plausible that the cerebellum might be carrying out both functions, at first sight functions of completely different kinds. Presumably the common integrator is associated with the vestibulocerebellum, and the pulse generator with the more recent areas, around folia V to VII: one can easily imagine how in the course of evolution the pulse generator might have taken over the preexisting cerebellar integrator mechanism and developed it for its own ends.

Although the arguments for a cerebellar pulse generator seem attractive and plausible, it has to be admitted that there are experimental findings that argue against it, at least in the simple form presented here. The most obvious is that, although it is true that cerebellar damage can lead to saccades that are too slow or too small [for example in spinocerebellar degeneration (Wadia and Swami, 1971; Starkman et al, 1972; Singh et al, 1973; Zee et al, 1976) in cerebellar cortical atrophy (Kornhuber, 1971); and in experimental cerebellectomy (Collewijn, 1970b; Robinson, 1974) —though Westheimer and Blair (1973b) report no such deficits], nevertheless it is clear that rudimentary saccadic movements *are* still present. This is of course very damaging to the notion that the saccadic pulse is only generated in the cerebellum, although it might be possible to argue that these hypometric saccades are the result of the trigger pulse (T, figure 12.15) which would still feed into the oculomotor output, even if the rest of the circuit were destroyed: but on the face of it, this would only cause a saccade of a constant, minimal, size, which is not what is observed.

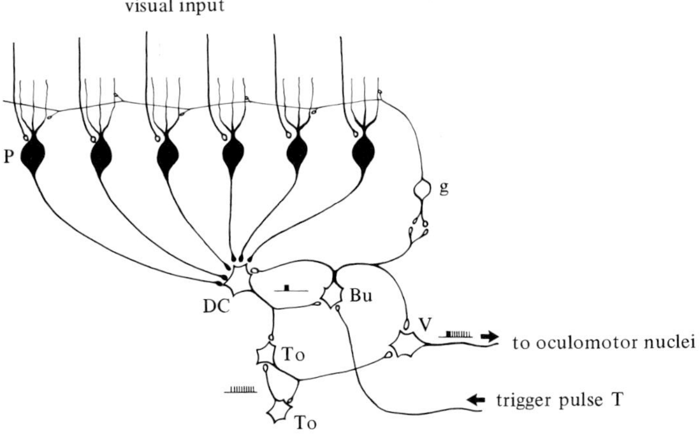

Figure 12.15. The scheme of figure 12.14 remodelled to fit more closely to the actual cerebellar circuitry.

In the absence of hard neurophysiological data, the cerebellar hypothesis must—regretfully—be put on one side. Other sites for a similar type of mechanism that might be considered are the superior colliculus and the cerebral cortex—perhaps both of them working in parallel, since damage to either alone produces rather little functional loss. But in neither case are the neuronal arrangements as perfectly suited to the task as in the case of the cerebellum.

Recently, a rather different model of the pulse generator has been suggested, prompted by observations on the slow saccades seen in spinocerebellar degeneration (Robinson, 1975b; Zee et al, 1976). This proposal does not attempt to deal with the problem of the transformation of spatial signals into temporal: rather it is intended to show how a single-channel signal representing desired saccade size by its instantaneous frequency of firing might be converted into a pulse of appropriate duration, The core of the system is shown in figure 12.16, in slightly simplified form: the *essential* difference between this and the previous model is not as great as it might seem: whereas previously the spatial input was compared with the pattern produced by the delay line and used to turn off the pulse, here the single-channel input is compared with the output of the integrator, and again used to turn off the pulse. The pulse is initiated by the trigger signal T: the 'OR' gate means that either T, or the continued existence of inequality between the input and the output of the integrator, will hold the switch shut. Either the pulse output or the step output could be used, or even the sum of both together, to generate a signal that could be sent direct to the oculomotor neurons.

The latter proposal is made by the authors, and has two important implications. First, this integrator must also be the final common path

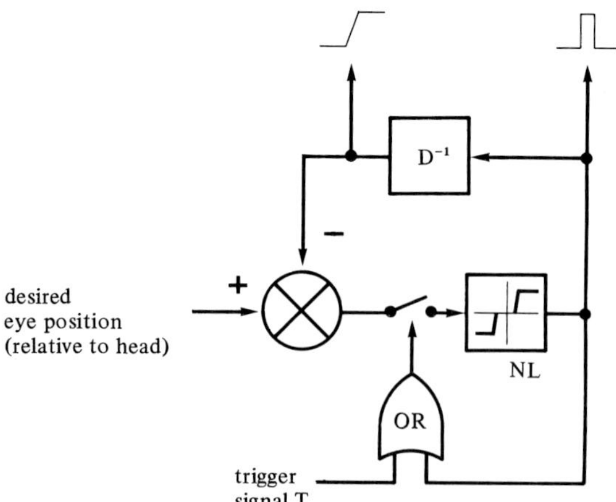

Figure 12.16. A possible saccadic pulse generator, modified from Zee et al (1976) (NL is a nonlinear unit).

integrator, and thus shared by vestibular, smooth pursuit and perhaps vergence inputs as well. These signals cannot enter at the same point as the saccadic input, because they would then only be able to act during the time that the switch is closed, that is, during saccades: they must therefore feed directly into the integrator. The consequences of this arrangement will be discussed in a moment. The second implication is that saccadic input signal is no longer retinotopic—that is, specifying a desired movement *relative* to the eye's present position—but *absolute*, specifying the actual desired position of the eye in the orbit. Since the original visual input is by definition retinotopic, the implication is that some kind of efference copy signal must be added to the visual input to produce the absolute command (which is then in effect the 'perceived object position': see section 11.3). We might as well use the output of the integrator for this purpose: the complete scheme now looks like figure 12.17. A refinement of the model is to adjust the shape of the nonlinearity NL to produce saccades of realistic appearance as far as the relation between amplitude, duration, and velocity is concerned, and by introducing a dead zone. Other simple modifications give surprisingly realistic imitation of certain pathological conditions, for example the slow saccades of spinocerebellar degeneration: (Zee et al, 1974; 1976). In particular, if the saccades and other effects are sufficiently slow relative to the time intervals between successive operations of T, the model predicts nonballistic saccades (that is, which can be modified in midflight) which are in fact a striking feature of this condition.

The consequences of having the vestibular and smooth pursuit signals feeding into this same integrator are also interesting. In the case of smooth

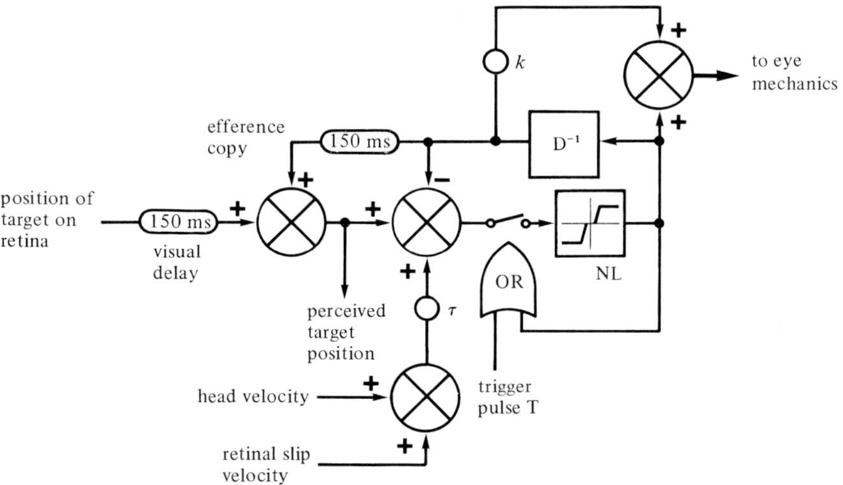

Figure 12.17. Improved version of figure 12.16. The coefficient τ is equal to the visual delay, in appropriate units.

pursuit it considerably simplifies the necessary predictive properties of the saccade size calculator—the properties seen for example in the well-known saccadic response to the sudden onset of a constant-velocity target movement (section 4.2.2). To produce a saccade of the correct size in tasks of this sort, the saccade calculator needs to estimate not only where the target is going to be by the time the saccade occurs, but also by how much the smooth pursuit mechanism will have reduced this gap in the same period. The advantage of using the common integrator as part of the saccade generator is that it obviates the necessity for the second part of the prediction: the contribution of smooth pursuit—or for that matter, of the vestibuloocular reflex—is automatically allowed for at the time the saccade is generated. This considerably simplifies the task of the saccade size calculator, since all it has to do is to predict the target position relative to the head: in practice, as we have seen, it is apparently content to use the simple linear predictor $(\mathrm{D}+k)$ for this purpose. In exactly the same way, one can immediately explain the recent observation by Jürgens and Becker (1975) that the saccades made during smooth pursuit when the target is suddenly moved by the same small amount either in the direction of the pursuit or in the opposite direction are not equal in duration in the two directions: this again follows immediately from the properties of the saccade pulse generator, since in one case the smooth pursuit signal will be assisting the saccade signal and therefore result in a shorter saccadic duration, while in the other direction it will lengthen it.

Precisely similar simplifications of the interaction between saccades and vestibular movements also accrue, although a small addition to the model is needed to make it generate the kinds of vestibularly driven saccades that are observed. Just as the intrinsic delay in the visual system can be mitigated to some extent by using a linear predictor $(\mathrm{D}+k)$ to estimate target position at the time of the saccade (the D part of this operator being presumably provided by the smooth pursuit system), so it is equally clear that an allowance for *head* movement during the same period could be made by means of a similar linear predictor, with the use of the output of the canals directly, without integration, as a head-velocity signal. Figure 12.18 may help make explain why such a mechanism is necessary.

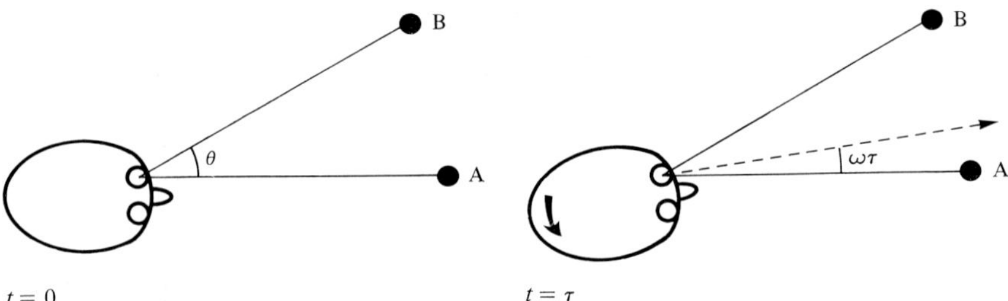

Figure 12.18. Movement of the head as well as movement of the eye must be taken into account when predicting the desired final eye position.

Imagine a subject whose head and eyes are turned toward a point A, and who suddenly decides to look at a different point, B. If he keeps his head still, there is no problem: the desired final eye position relative to the head is simply $\theta°$ from the present position, where θ is the angle subtended between A and B. But suppose, as is likely, he starts to move his head as well as his eye towards B. Then at the time τ when the saccade finally occurs, the desired final eye position is no longer θ, but $\theta - \omega\tau$, where ω is the head velocity (assumed to be constant). In other words, because the proposed saccade generator operates in coordinates defined by the head rather than in relative coordinates, it is necessary to subtract from the saccade command an estimate of where the head is going to be at the time of the execution of the saccade: the easiest way to do this is to use the value of ω provided directly by the output of the canals. The system will then, incidentally, behave in exactly the same way as the mechanism suggested by Sugie and Melvill Jones (1971) to explain the generation of the quick-phases in vestibular nystagmus, and also the anticompensatory saccades characteristic of sudden movements of the head (section 2.3.2).

There are many plausible neuronal circuits which might be devised to embody this model of the pulse generator: an example has been published by Robinson (1975b). Figure 12.19 shows another possible arrangement, derived from the cerebellopontine integrator of figure 12.13. Here, cell S elaborates the saccadic input command by adding together signals representing desired (retinotopic) position, retinal slip velocity and head velocity (for prediction), and delayed efference copy (to convert from a retinotopic to an absolute frame of reference); cell c compares this desired eye position with the efference copy signal from the integrator,

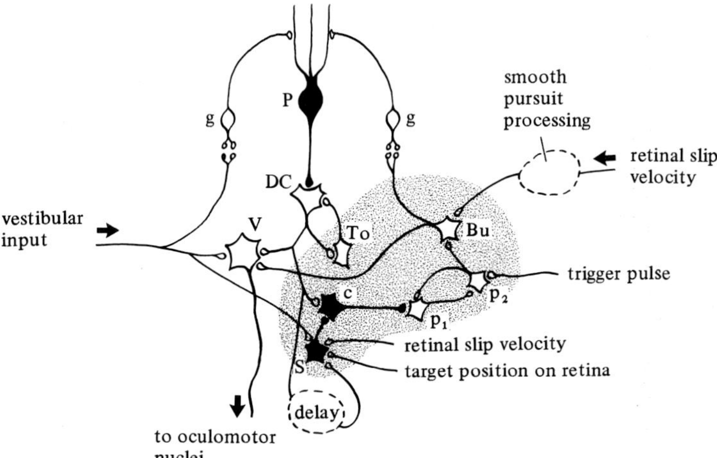

Figure 12.19. Possible neural embodiment of figure 12.17. The shaded area represents the pontine reticular formation: symbols as in figure 12.13.

and in turn controls the switch formed by p_1 and p_2. Neurons Bu, p_1, and p_2 will behave like 'burst' cells during saccades, though Bu will also fire in proportion to velocity during smooth pursuit: c will behave like a 'pause' unit, and To, as before, like a 'tonic' unit. Presumably most of these cells are to be located in the PPRF, although it seems very likely—from its anatomical connections—that the interstitial nucleus of Cajal also embodies part of this circuit. Its projection to the vestibular nuclei, its important afferent connections from superior colliculus, and its burst responses during saccades (Matsunami, 1972) suggest Bu: but it is clearly not worth trying to be very specific about a model that is largely hypothetical. As before, a parallel set of inhibitory and contralateral connections is needed to make the system work, and the fact that some of the connections shown in figure 12.19 are known to be either inhibitory or crossed or both need not be an embarrassment.

12.3 Parametric feedback and the cerebellum

The idea that the cerebellum is teachable—that it learns to modify motor responses in the light of sensory feedback during skilled actions—is rapidly gaining ground, although, it must be admitted, without a corresponding quantity of hard experimental evidence to back it up. The notion has been most carefully expressed and discussed by Marr (1969). In vastly oversimplified form, the suggestion is that any motor act takes place in a sensory 'context', some of which will be unrelated to the movement taking place, and hence different on different repetitions, and some of which will be to a certain extent *correlated* with the movement, either because it comes from proprioceptors, or because it comes from that part of the sensory environment that was responsible for initiating the movement in the first place. If we had a mechanism that could recognise a correlation between a particular pattern of sensory input and a particular motor act, and having established the correlation, then on future occasions initiate the act itself quite automatically whenever the same sensory pattern appeared, we would have a mechanism that would gradually learn to perform automatically actions that originally have to be specified in detail by conscious thought. To take a specific example, in learning to walk one has at first consciously to elaborate detailed commands for the limbs (an experience that can easily be recaptured by the adult: many cerebellar afflictions are remarkably similar to the effects of alcohol poisoning!): but with each step, exactly the same sensory feedback will be experienced from proprioceptors in the joints and muscles, and from the vestibular apparatus, which will form the context for the next step. Eventually the hypothetical mechanism will of its own accord use the sensory feedback from one fragment of the act of walking as the cue to the initiation of the next, until the whole cycle is completed with no necessity of conscious intervention beyond a general supervision of progress and reactions to unforeseen circumstances.

The cerebellum, from the arrangement of its neuronal circuits, seems ideally suited to carry out such a function. If we allow each Purkinje cell to correspond with some small fragment of motor activity—perhaps the contraction of a particular muscle—then we might think of the climbing fibres as the origin of the volitional, or in a sense hard-wired, input that is needed during the training process, and firing off the Purkinje cells in a simple one-to-one manner. The parallel fibres, conveying to each Purkinje cell's elaborate dendritic tree a wealth of information from proprioceptors, vestibular system, cutaneous receptors, and vision and hearing, provide the context to be associated with a particular action. On the simple and quite plausible assumption that the connections between parallel fibres and Purkinje cells are strengthened whenever both fire together, and otherwise tend to decay, we immediately have the makings of the kind of skill-learning mechanism we are looking for; this is the essence of Marr's hypothesis, and it still awaits experimental validation.

Now there is one area of the oculomotor system in which the evidence for some such process seems particularly strong, and that is in the relationship between the visual and the vestibular control of eye movements. We saw in section 2.3.3 and elsewhere that the behaviour of the vestibulo-ocular reflex assists the stabilisation of the retinal image in a remarkably flexible manner, and that, if the natural relationship between head movement and movement of the outside world is artifically disrupted, the reflex adjusts itself—to the extent of reversing its sign if necessary—so as to continue to be as helpful as possible. We also saw that recent evidence has shown that the integrity of the cerebellum is a prerequisite of these adjustments. It is not difficult to see how a model of the type proposed to explain cerebellar learning of skills might account for these adjustments as well [but see Ito (1972) for a slightly different conception]. If in figure 12.13 we imagine that the afferent synapses between the parallel fibres ultimately coming from the vestibular apparatus and the Purkinje cells have the property that they strengthen when there is a high correlation between their activity and that of the Purkinje cell, and weaken when there is not, then it is clear that the gain of the vestibular input to the integrator will continually adjust itself to match the activity driven by the smooth pursuit mechanism. If we allow that parallel fibres from each canal have access to all the oculomotor Purkinje cells, including those associated with antagonists, then we can explain vestibulo-ocular reversal as well as changes in gain.

Now a consequence of this model is that the alterations in the vestibulo-ocular reflex should only take place in the integrator pathway: the direct, bypass, route does not pass through the cerebellum and so is unmodifiable. This constrains the relation between phase and amplitude during vision-reversed vestibulo-ocular training: this can best be appreciated by using a vector representation of the response (figure 12.20): the reflex response is the sum of a fixed vector representing the output of the bypass, and a vector of variable length and perpendicular to it, representing the output of the integrator. The pair of vectors is tilted at an angle to the horizontal axis that represents the phase lag of the canals plus eye mechanics at the frequency in question. Gonshor and Melvill Jones (1976a; 1976b) have measured the actual form of the locus of the vestibulo-ocular response at 0·16 Hz in man under prolonged reversal of vision (figure 12.20); at this frequency the phase-lead of the periphery amounts to only a few degrees, and the contribution of the bypass is very small: the expected locus of the response during training is therefore a slow descent from a point just above the horizontal axis in the first quadrant down into the third quadrant near the horizontal axis. It can be seen that this is roughly in accord with the observations, but not very precisely: in particular, whereas the model predicts steadily increasing phase leads, in fact it is a steady increase in lag that is observed. The author's own ad hoc hypothesis—that the changes come about because the cerebellum subtracts from the output of the integrator (assumed to be elsewhere) a gradually increasing signal that slightly leads the original output (figure 12.20)—gives a better fit, but is difficult to relate to the ideas of

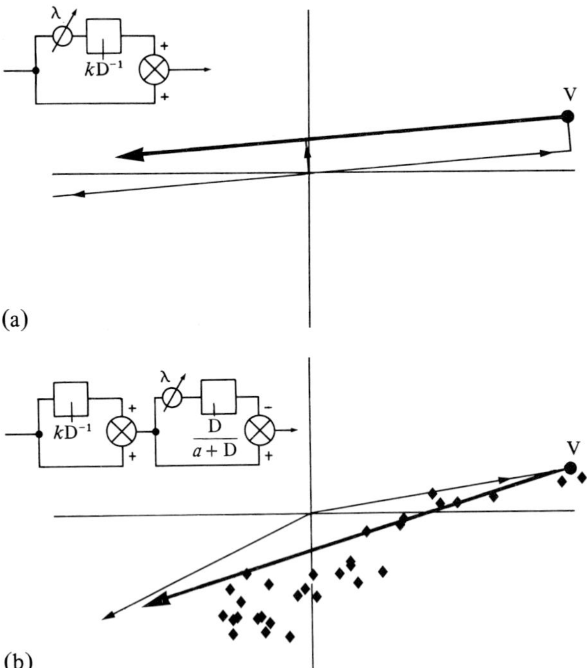

Figure 12.20. Two possible modes of parametric control in the vestibulo-ocular reflex. V represents the normal response (Nyquist plot) at 0·16 Hz, and the thick line with the arrow shows the consequence in (a) of decreasing, and in (b) of increasing, the value of λ. The lozenges in (b) show the experimental results for one of Gonshor and Melvill Jones's (1976b) subjects.

cerebellar function presented earlier in this chapter: in particular, it is difficult to reconcile with the known effects of cerebellar damage on the vestibulo-ocular integrator.

The same kind of mechanism may well cause the well-known compensation for unilateral vestibular damage noted in section 2.3.3 and due in part to a change in gain such as to restore the balance of the inputs from the opposed pairs of canals. Robinson (1975b) has argued for the importance of continual control of this balance in the maintenance of the stability of the eyes: the same mechanism of long-term parametric feedback of retinal slip modifying vestibular gain will also ensure that the small fluctuations in vestibular sensitivity that are bound to occur even in normal healthy subjects will not result in spontaneous nystagmus in the light or wandering of the eye in the dark. One of the most prominent effects of cerebellectomy in the cat is in fact the marked increase that occurs in the amplitude of such wandering movements (Robinson, 1974). Again, it was suggested in section 10.3.3 that parametric feedback from proprioceptors in the eye muscles might similarly serve to keep the peripheral oculomotor performance up to the mark despite changes in dynamic properties as a result of fatigue or aging: since the cerebellum is one of the regions that receives afferents from eye muscle spindles, it is easy to imagine how—by analogy with the visuovestibular case—this input could be used to modify the gain of the integrator in such a way as to ensure the best possible match at all times between the efference copy signal and the actual position of the eye. In each case the cerebellum is in a sense repairing—or at least covering up—deficiencies in other parts of the nervous system. The question is, whether the cerebellum is *only*—in Robinson's memorable phrase—a general repair shop, or whether it simply carries out its *own* repairs. The rapidity of developments in this field suggest that a solution to the enigma of the cerebellum may only be just around the corner.

12.4 The oculomotor system in prospect

The possibility of cerebellar circuits that, Proteus-like, change their guise as we attempt to pursue them should perhaps warn us to cut short our speculations and take stock of our position. What parts of the oculomotor system can we confidently say we understand? Where is our ignorance most glaringly evident? In what ways can our knowledge assist either the clinicians or our colleagues studying other branches of neurophysiology?

Of course, in a sense these questions are interconnected: if our models are really accurate and quantitative enough to be worth using for clinical purposes, and proved to work under conditions very different from the noise-free and highly simplified environment of the experimental laboratory, then they can surely be accepted as true representations. As far as the peripheral oculomotor apparatus is concerned, this aim has probably been achieved. Our knowledge of the kinematics and dynamics of the eye has progressed steadily since the first conceptions of such men as Fick and Helmholtz, a little over a century ago, to the point where we can now simulate the relationship between the activity in the six muscles and the resultant position of the eye with accuracy, and predict in advance what the effect will be of particular ophthalmic surgical procedures such as artificial lengthening or shortening of individual muscles to correct squint (Robinson, 1975a). Perhaps the main block to the acceptance of quantitative evaluation of such procedures is the novelty of the notion that such preoperative calculations can provide more than an approximate indication of the actual outcome.

Proceeding backwards along the oculomotor pathway, after the eye and its muscles we come to the neurons of the oculomotor nuclei. None, I think, would disagree with the notion that we have here a population of units that fire more or less linearly in proportion to eye velocity and position in an appropriate direction, with constants of proportionality and thresholds that vary from cell to cell. How they correspond to the different types of fibre found in the muscles is less clear, but from the purely functional point of view it is possible, after a few brief measurements to establish the basic parameters, to predict the frequency of firing of such a cell during virtually any kind of eye movement that one cares to evoke. But as we attempt to penetrate further back into the system, any confidence we may feel soon vanishes. Even the vestibulo-ocular reflex, the simplest and oldest of all the eye movements, shows quite unexpected complications and subtleties. There is certainly general agreement on the broader properties of the reflex—the need for an *integrator* to convert the velocity information from the canals into eye position, and the need to bypass this integrator with a direct pathway to act as a goad to the sluggish eye muscles. Yet estimates of phase in this system in different species—or for that matter in different examples of the same species—have led to wildly different results. Since we also know that the behaviour of the system is being continually modified to bring it in line with visual experience, it may well be that these otherwise inexplicable variations may be more a function of the particular subjects' visual experiences than of the hard-wired properties of their brains.

If this kind of flexibility is found even in the most archaic and straightforward of the oculomotor subsystems, what can we expect in the visual control of eye movements? Both vergence and smooth pursuit can modify their behaviour in the course of a few cycles of repetitive stimulation so as to carry out their jobs more efficiently: the mechanism of this adaptation is entirely unknown. Only under conditions when this kind of prediction is prevented are these systems amenable to techniques of systems analysis, and even so there is no more than broad agreement between investigators using different techniques and different animals: but the need for an integrator at the output stage of each is generally recognised. Our knowledge of saccades is, if anything, even less complete. It is true that we can deduce with certainty the necessity of a pulse of variable width as the primary command signal that goes to the final common path—an integrator being again implied, together with its direct bypass—but what in general triggers off the pulse, and how its width is calculated, are matters strictly for speculation. Part of the difficulty is again that under different conditions the saccadic system seems to be able to select and use whatever aspect of the stimulus enables it to perform best. In these circumstances, the 'black box' approach is unlikely to succeed. The anatomy of the oculomotor system is, however, almost as much a mystery as the details of its function. Even the arrangement of the final motor neurons is controversial: while the three most prominent areas of the brain concerned with eye movement—cerebral cortex, cerebellum, and superior colliculus—have no *established* functions whatever (though the site of much creative imagination). The pathways linking its various parts are uncertain and incomplete: after seventy years of experimentation, we still do not even know for certain where the afferents from the muscle spindles go!

A gloomy picture, but not an exaggerated one, and it may serve as a healthy antidote to the happy complacency that tends to be engendered by too much making and contemplation of *models*. Schemes like that in figure 12.19 have a kind of built-in vitality or survival power that is often only slightly connected with the correctness with which they represent the real thing. Even a cursory glance at some recent published symposia reveals rival models of one and the same process—for example the production of saccades—that are as fundamentally dissimilar in their basic form as they are detailed and even finicky in their specification. When new facts seem not to fit, it is easier to add an inhibitory synapse here, or adjust a parameter there, than to discard it altogether and sit down and think, and in this respect the present author has been as guilty as any. Model-making is a kind of playing: on the one hand it gives one practice in trying to see new similarities between apparently dissimilar things, and flexes the muscles of the imagination so that when the time is ripe it can make the speculative jump that leads to new understanding: on the other hand, it forces one to be specific and even quantitative when one would much prefer to be comfortably vague. But the important thing is not to *believe* in a model.

In fact, perhaps the most impressive result of the last ten years or so of research in this field is not so much new knowledge as such, as the demonstration of the utility of trying to examine the nervous system in a determinedly quantitative way. The widespread use of systems analysis and its vocabulary is a good example of this: as Robinson (1975b) has pointed out the use of terms such as 'integrator' and 'pulse generator' is now commonplace in this field; and from personal experience it seems that far from raising it to rarefied heights accessible only to the *cognoscenti*, such an approach is readily appreciated by students with only a minimum of mathematical training, who thereby acquire in a short space of time a feel for the oculomotor system that previously could only be assimilated by years of clinical and experimental practice.

Finally, the same techniques are now being applied with success to the investigation of other parts of the motor system—where the difficulties are considerably increased because of the much greater number of degrees of freedom, and the more prominent intrusion of volition—and, most excitingly, parallels are beginning to emerge between the control of eye movements and that of other parts of the body: not superficial similarities like that of ocular nystagmus to head nystagmus in birds or ear nystagmus in rabbits (Schaefer et al, 1971), but fundamental equivalences of modes of movement control. For example, it is clear that the notion of an integrator in the final common path is one of quite general utility in the motor system. Most parts of the body spend only a tiny fraction of the time actually in motion: the normal condition is one of sustained posture. If they are linked to the motor control system by integrators, then the brain is relieved of the burden of sending them a continual stream of commands: it need only signal to them when a *change* is required. This is in a sense the inverse argument of that which identifies the desirability of *differentiating* the sensory information entering the central nervous system by mechanisms of sensory adaptation. The fundamental consideration here is that the bandwidth of the brain is rather higher than the average rate at which interesting things happen in the outside world, so that economies in the number of computational channels can be made by reducing the amount of redundancy in the signals that are handled: this preference for dealing always in terms of *change* implies integration at the output just as much as differentiation at the input (Carpenter, 1972a).

Some of the recently discovered properties of the oculomotor system had already been deduced by Kenneth Craik in 1947 as desirable features of motor systems in general: these include such notions as intermittent ballistic control, integration, and parametric feedback as a fundamental mechanism. Amongst more recent experimental work that comes to mind is Partridge and Kim's (1969) study of a vestibulomotor reflex in the triceps, and the work of Brooks and his colleagues (Brooks, 1974; Brooks et al, 1974; Conrad and Brooks, 1974) on the control of arm movements by the monkey. Some of these findings seem to show clear parallels with saccadic eye movements: for example, the demonstration of linear amplitude-duration curves, and of control via pulse width. They have also been able to show the involvement of the cerebellum in generating the command pulse: cooling the dentate nucleus lengthens it, as would be expected if a cerebellar integrator were in use, similar to the one suggested earlier for the saccadic system. Kornhuber (1971) has also made some extrapolative generalisations along similar lines. At all events, it is clear that we now at least have an appropriate vocabulary for talking about motor processes. But perhaps the outstanding contribution of the study of the oculomotor system to neurophysiology as a whole has been —sadly—the realisation that nothing in the brain is ever as simple as it seems.

Appendices

Appendix 1. Methods of measuring eye movements

The measurement of movements of the eyes presents a nice problem in technology. An ideal system should be able to measure rotations of the globe about all three axes, yet be completely insensitive to translational movements; linear over a range of more than 90°, yet sensitive enough to record micromovements of a few seconds of arc; and have a bandwidth extending from zero to a few hundred Hz. The device must not interfere with vision—indeed ideally should not even be visible to the subject—and must not require the attachment of anything to the eyeball. It must either be unaffected by movements of the head, or light enough that the subject can wear it rigidly fixed relative to his skull.

Perhaps not surprisingly, no system has yet been devised that meets all these conditions, and the experimenter must choose the method that best suits the kind of investigation he wishes to make. In the review of methods that follows, the aim has been to emphasise the particular advantages and limitations of a large range of procedures, in the hope that it may assist experimenters in the selection of appropriate methods for particular tasks. Similar reviews have been made by Ditchburn (1973), Crickmar (1969), and L R Young (1963); and most recently, with particular emphasis on commercially available devices, by L R Young and Sheena (1975).

A1.1 Direct viewing

Simply observing a subject's eyes—without any optical aids—one can, with a little practice, probably detect movements of 1° or so without difficulty (Yarbus, 1967). This is perhaps quite adequate for preliminary clinical examination, if one is only trying to establish the presence or absence of nystagmus, gaze paresis, or other obvious signs, but cannot by itself enable more than very crudely quantitative measurements to be made. If the head can be held steady, and one is interested only in tonic movements of the eyes, then examination of the iris, or of the sclera (using blood vessels as reference marks) with a travelling microscope can provide accurate measurements. The main application for this method in man is for measuring torsional movements (difficult to measure by other means) and it has been used with success in this way by Merton (1956).

It is a relatively simple matter to fit the microscope with a cinecamera so that permanent records of eye movements can be made. Dodge and Cline (1901) arranged for an image of the subject's eye to fall on a horizontal slit, which was then photographed on a moving photographic plate: in this way they were able to make the first records of the time course of saccades, with a time resolution of about 1 ms over a range of some 40°. An improvement of the method is to increase the intensity of the photographic image by attaching a bright marker to the cornea: for example a small blob of mercury (Barlow, 1952). With the development of fast cinefilm, it became possible to photograph the whole eye at speed, and thus record rotations about all three axes simultaneously (Wendt, 1952; Melvill Jones, 1963). The main disadvantages of this procedure are first that the time resolution is necessarily limited by the speed of the emulsion and at best is unlikely to be better than some 10 ms, and second the tedium of having to measure the eye position in each individual frame of the film, and calculate the corresponding direction of the visual axis, although this task might well now be performed by a small computer: Nakayama (1974) has published matrix solutions of the relevant transformations.

A1.1.1 *Photoelectric viewing*
Because of the ease with which electrical signals can be amplified, displayed, and stored, most workers have preferred to use some sort of photoelectric cell to take the place of the eye or camera in the direct-viewing method (for example Richter, 1956; Johnson and Winter, 1958). Very often the photocell looks at the high-contrast edge between the white sclera and the darker iris at the limbus: the method is then only useful for horizontal movements, since in the vertical direction the limbus is normally covered by the lids. In animals the sclera is commonly invisible at the sides as well, and the method is then inapplicable for movements in any direction. Under these circumstances it is possible to make use of the difference in the amount of light scattered from the iris and from the pupil itself, although the consequent reduction in the total available intensity inevitably reduces the sensitivity or speed of the recording device.

In its simplest and crudest form, a spot of light can be projected on the limbus, with a nearby photoresistor arranged to pick up the scattered light (Blakemore and Carpenter, 1970). As long as care is taken that *reflected* light is not received by the transducer, the quantity of light it receives will be more or less proportional to the area of sclera lying under the spot of light (see figure A1.1a). For small movements, this will in turn be proportional to the eye's angular deviation in the horizontal plane. In practice, even a very simple device of this type will behave linearly over a range of some 10°, and with a simple bridge circuit can give some 10 mV per degree and a time resolution of about 10 ms: since it is extremely cheap to build, it is ideal for class use. With three simple modifications, the method can be used for the most exacting measurements. The first is to use infrared radiation rather than visible light (Richter and Pfaltz, 1956), to counter the criticism that the presence of an intense source of light in the subject's field of view is likely to disturb the natural form of his eye movements: it turns out that modern photodetectors are in any case often actually more sensitive to the near infrared than to the visible spectrum. The second improvement is to use not one but two spots of light, and record differentially from a pair of photocells (figure A1.1b). This both improves the linearity of the response and reduces the noise introduced by fluctuations in the illumination of the eye (see for example Stark and Sandberg, 1961). Nykiel and Torok (1963) have extended the method in a simple nystagmograph for clinical use in which the eye is diffusely illuminated with infrared, and viewed by four photodetectors disposed symmetrically round the orbit. No slits or imagining devices are used, but nevertheless differences in the quantity of scattered light received by the two pairs of detectors are approximately linearly related to eye position in the vertical and horizontal directions over a range of some $\pm 10°$. The whole assembly can be mounted on goggles worn by the subject: this eliminates problems related to head movements, but unfortunately completely obscures the subject's vision.

The third improvement is to replace the spots of light with thin bars, so that the relation between eye rotation and photocell current is both more linear and more independent of rotations in the perpendicular direction

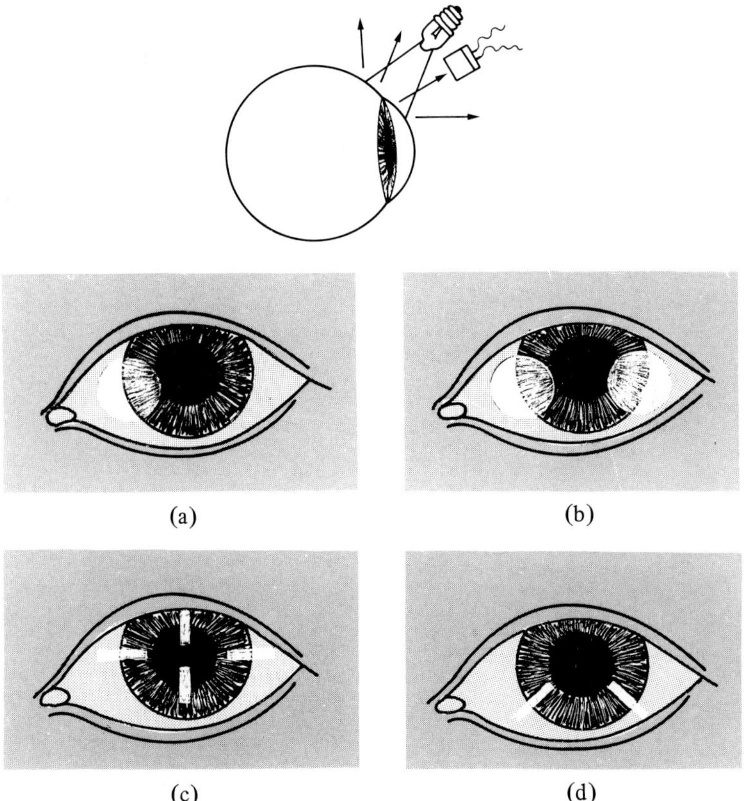

Figure A1.1. Photoelectric registration of the position of the limbus. Above, the general arrangement: a defined spot on the eye is illuminated, and a fraction of the scattered light is picked up by a photocell; the roles of the light and photocell may equally well be reversed. Below, some configurations of light spots (or photocell fields of view) that can be used. (a) The simplest arrangement; (b) a pair of spots with differential recording; (c) two pairs of slits at right angles, the vertical pair straddling the pupil rather than the limbus; (d) two slits at right angles, capable—like (c)—of measuring eye movements in the horizontal and vertical directions.

(for example Krauskopf et al, 1966). With two pairs of slits arranged as in figure A1.1c one can measure vertical and horizontal movements simultaneously: or the same result may be achieved more simply with a pair of slits set at an angle to one another (figure A1.1d) (Jones, 1973). A further refinement, which aids in the setting-up procedure (the correct placing of the slit of light on the eye being somewhat critical) is to illuminate the eye diffusely, and form an enlarged image of it on a translucent screen (Smith and Warter, 1960). Slits, with photodetectors behind them, can then be positioned in the same plane. After setting up, the translucent screen can be removed, and the illumination changed from visible to infrared. Finally, one may save light by using a fibre optics bundle flattened at one end instead of a slit, and increase sensitivity further by recording differentially with 'chopped' illumination and phase-locked amplification of the transducer signal, enormously increasing the signal-to-noise ratio (figure A1.2) (Wheeless et al, 1966). This arrangement gives a sensitivity of 3′ of arc over some 30° for horizontal movements, and 10′ over 20° for vertical movements (when the inner edge of the iris is used).

A final refinement, due to Rashbass (1960), is to image a spot of light from an oscilloscope screen on the limbus, and use the amount of scattered light picked up by a nearby photocell to shift the spot on the screen in such a way as continually to track the limbus as it moves, by means of a suitable feedback circuit (figure A1.3). A second photocell, looking directly at the oscilloscope screen, can be used as a comparison to allow for fluctuations in the spot's brightness. This method is intrinsically much more linear, as it does not rely on any particular relationship between displacements of the eye and the amount of light scattered: it is claimed to have a sensitivity of about 5′ of arc, with a resolution of some 5 ms. A major disadvantage is that surrounding illumination must be rather dim.

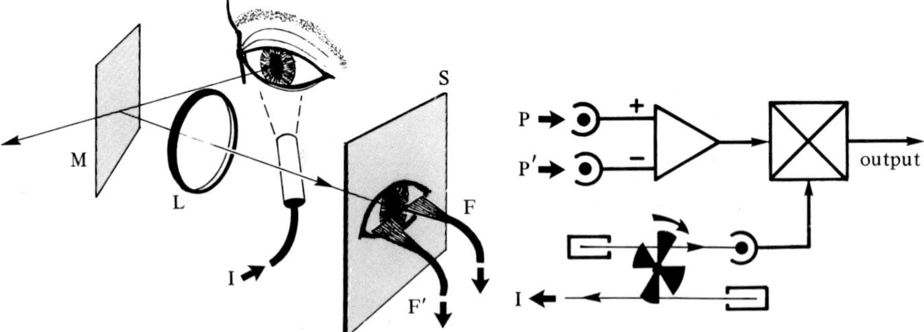

Figure A1.2. Refinement of the scattered-light method: the eye is illuminated with chopped infrared light I, and its image formed by the half-silvered mirror M and lens L on the ground-glass screen S. In setting up, the two fibre-optic slit bundles F and F′ are adjusted to the image: they are connected to photodetectors P and P′, whose differential signal is correlated with a signal from the illumination chopper to provide the output. The screen S can be removed once the system is set up.

Another method that falls in the same general category is the novel technique of Cornsweet (1958), in which the fundus is scanned through an ophthalmoscope while a photocell records the light scattered back from it. If the scan is positioned to pass over a retinal blood vessel whose course is nearly vertical (figure A1.4), the time course of the signal from

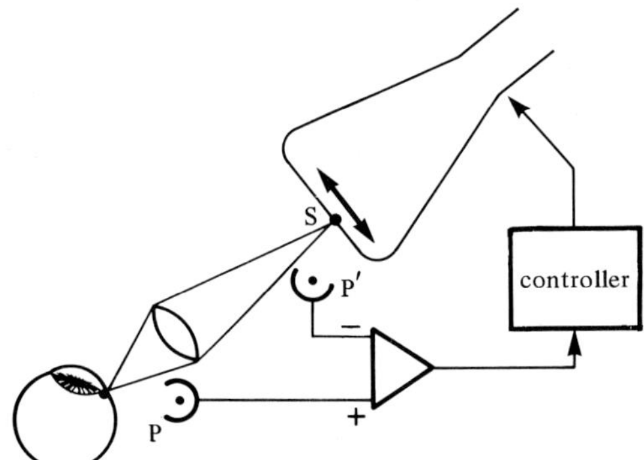

Figure A1.3. Tracking the limbus. The spot S on the oscilloscope screen is imaged on the eye, and the scattered light received from photocell P: its output is compared with that from the comparison cell P′, which views the original source, and the difference drives the oscilloscope deflection circuits in such a way as to maintain the image of the spot exactly on the limbus.

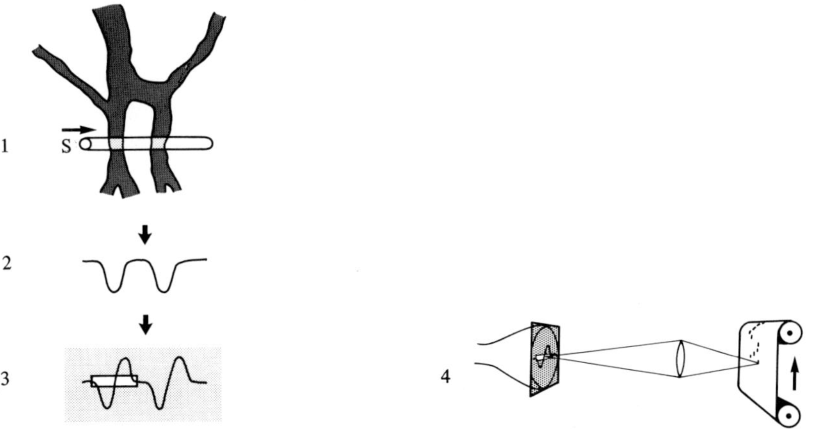

Figure A1.4. Tracking a retinal blood vessel: (1) Simplified drawing of a network of blood vessels in the retina horizontally scanned by the point of light S: the corresponding time course of the intensity of the light scattered back is shown immediately below (2). If this signal is electrically differentiated (3) and viewed through a mask so that only the point of zero crossing is visible (this corresponds with the minimum of the received light intensity), one can arrange (4) for this point to be imaged on moving photographic film and thus indicate the movement of the blood vessel as a function of time.

the photocell during the sweep will show a pronounced dip when the scanning spot meets the blood vessel, and the displacement of this point along the time axis after the beginning of the sweep will correspond with horizontal movements of the retina. In this way one can apparently resolve some 10″ of arc (that is, about 1 μ on the retina) over a range of about 4°. Unless the blood vessel chosen is absolutely vertical, there will be some interference from vertical movements, and changes in the calibre of the vessel may lead to slow artefacts. The method has more recently been developed (Kelly et al, 1969) by using a small computer to scan the retina and store an image of the fundus: by comparing successive 'frames' it can calculate the motion of the eye in all three directions, with an accuracy of some 0·5′ of arc.

These photoelectric methods are for the most part quite simple to set up, and cause no appreciable discomfort to the subject. They share a common disadvantage, that head movement relative to the transducer will be interpreted as eye rotation. If we take the rotational radius of the eye as some 13 mm (Ditchburn and Ginsborg, 1953), it is clear that a displacement of the head of only 100 μ will be misread as an angular deviation of the eye of some 26′ of arc, or nearly 0·5°. It is essential therefore either to clamp the head, or arrange like Nykiel and Torok (1963) that the transducer assembly moves with it.

A1.2 Devices using reflection

A1.2.1 *Reflection from the cornea*

The front surface of the cornea of the eye, being shiny and convex, will form an image of an external point source (the first Purkinje image) which will lie some 3·5 mm or more behind the corneal surface, depending on the distance of the source. Since the centre of rotation of the eye is not identical with the centre of curvature of the cornea, when the eye moves, the apparent position of this image will move as well. For small angles, the apparent displacement of this image will be rather less than half the displacement of the surface of the eye itself (figure A1.5b). Thus, other things being equal, a device that measures eye movements by observing this image is likely to be twice as insensitive as one that, for instance, looks at the border between the sclera and the iris. But there are two advantages of this method that make it useful in particular applications: first, that the brightness of the image and the contrast between it and the surroundings can be made very great by having a sufficiently intense source, so that faster photographic emulsions or relatively insensitive photoelectric devices such as television cameras can be used: and second, that motion in both the horizontal and the vertical plane can be recorded with equal ease. For both reasons, this method was favoured by Mackworth and Mackworth (1958) in their apparatus for determining the way in which the eye moves over natural visual scenes (figure A1.6). Here the output from a television camera viewing the corneal image is electronically mixed with the output from another camera viewing the scene that the subject is looking at: the resulting display, when the magnifications have been properly adjusted, has a bright spot at the point in the field of view which the subject is fixating at any moment. In this form, the method has an accuracy of some 1°–2° in a total range of about 20°. A head-mounted version of the same apparatus has been used successfully by Shackel (1960b), Mackworth and Thomas (1962), and others.

Considerably greater accuracy and freedom from interference from translational movements are possible if the first Purkinje image is used in conjunction with other features that move with the eye. The front surface of the cornea is of course not the only optical surface traversed by light

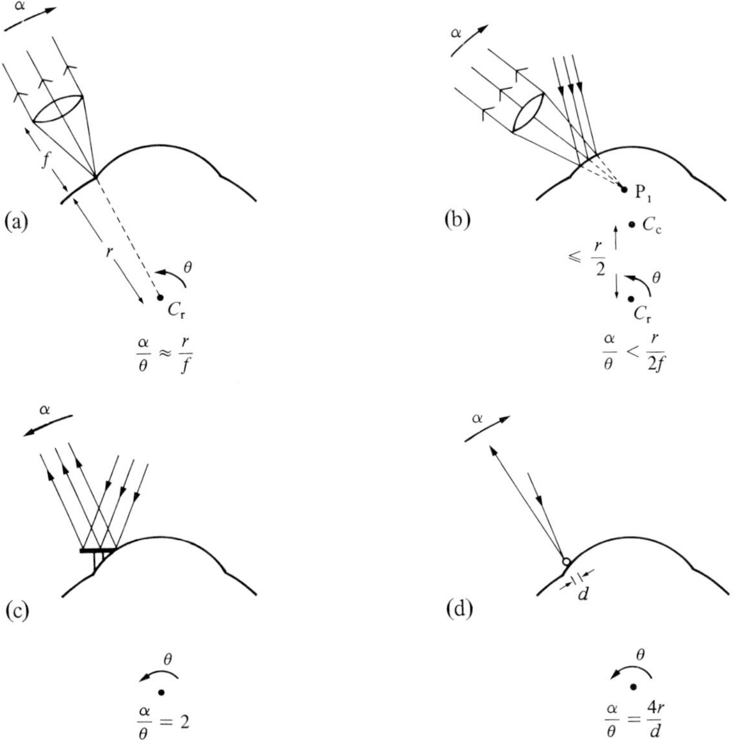

Figure A1.5. A comparison of the four basic varieties of optical eye movement recording. (a) The scattered-light method, in which the ratio of the angular displacement of the final beam α to the angle moved through by the eye θ—the figure of merit—is given by the ratio of the radius of the body of the eye r to the focal length of the objective f; (b) the method of observation of the first Purkinje image, where the figure of merit is given by about $r/2f$, because the distance between the centre of rotation of the eye C_r and the centre of curvature of the cornea C_c is approximately equal to $r/2$; (c) reflection off a plane mirror: the figure of merit is exactly 2; (d) reflection off a small sphere of diameter d: the figure of merit is roughly $4r/d$, which is potentially very large indeed.

entering the eye: and in fact secondary reflected images can be formed by the back of the cornea, and both surfaces of the lens (figure A1.7). These are called, respectively, the second, third, and fourth Purkinje images (the whole set may be referred to as P1 to P4; they are not as striking as P1, and P4 in particular is rather dim). Since P4 is formed by a concave surface, it is real and not virtual. As a result, whereas under eye *displacement* P1 and P4 move by equal amounts, under eye *rotation* they move relative to one another: this is the basis of a refined device described by Cornsweet and Crane (1973). Two four-quadrant photocells

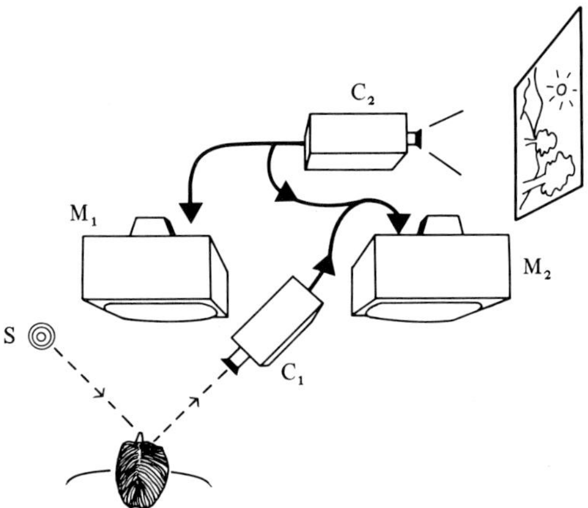

Figure A1.6. Measuring eye movements made in viewing a scene, by a reflection method. The reflected image of the source S is picked up by the television camera C_1, whose signal is added to that of the camera C_2 that views the original scene and which drives the monitor M_1 which is seen by the subject. M_2 thus displays the scene with the eye movements in superimposition.

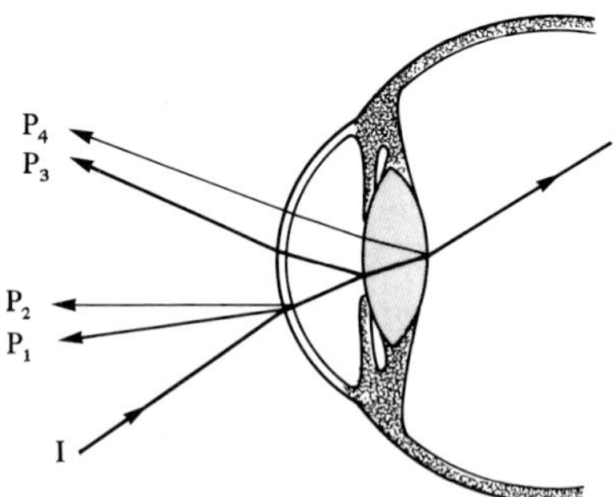

Figure A1.7. Formation of the four Purkinje images. The incident beam I is first reflected at the outer corneal surface to give rise to beams such as P1 that forms the first Purkinje image; subsequently, further reflections occur at the posterior surface of the cornea and at the anterior and posterior surfaces of the lens, to give the images P2 to P4. See also figure 7.3.

are used in a double feedback loop: the output of the first cell is used to move a mirror in such a way that an image of P1 is always centred on it, while the second cell drives an x–y positioning system that makes it track an image of P4 (reflected in the same mirror that is driven by the first photocell). Thus the movable mirror automatically cancels any translational component that may be present, while the position of the second cell is directly related to rotation of the eye. In this way a sensitivity of about 1′ of arc over a range of some 10°–20°, at up to 100 Hz may be achieved.

The same principle—that of using two separate measures of eye movement, differentially affected by rotation and translation—has been applied by Rashbass and Westheimer (1960). By recording both reflected and scattered light simultaneously, it is again possible to eliminate the interference caused by head movements (other than rotations, of course). They scan the limbus region with an image of a spot generated on the face of an oscilloscope (figure A1.8) and pick up the reflected and scattered light with a pair of photocells. The waveform from the cells during a single sweep of the oscilloscope time base shows two clearly differentiated components: one is step-like and caused by the spot crossing the limbus, the other pulse-like and generated when the reflected beam falls on the photocell. Under translation, both components are displaced equally in time relative to the start of the sweep: but if the eye rotates, they move relative to one another. The linear range of this device seems to be of the order of 8° or so.

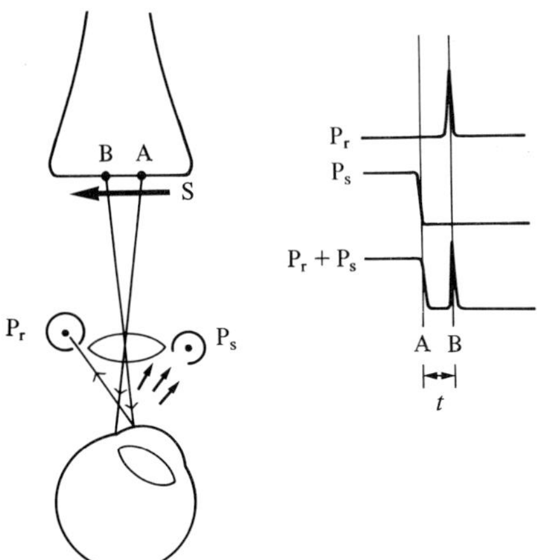

Figure A1.8. Simultaneous measurements of reflected and scattered light to record rotation independently of displacement. A scanning spot on the oscilloscope (S) is imaged at the surface of the eye: at one point A in its travel, it passes over the limbus and so there is a sudden drop in the signal from the photocell P_s that receives scattered light (see curve P_s on right). At another point, B, the light is specularly reflected in such a way as to be received by photocell P_r, whose output thus momentarily increases: the relative interval t between these two events (see right) is thus a measure of the eye's rotation, and uncontaminated by translation, which displaces each event equally.

Palmieri et al (1971) also use a method in which a spot on the face of an oscilloscope is focused on the cornea: in this case, a four-quadrant photocell receives only the reflected beam, and a feedback circuit moves the spot on the oscilloscope in such a way as to keep the beam falling always in the centre of the detector. The movements of the spot on the face of the oscilloscope thus mimic the movements of the eye, and can be superimposed on a television picture of the scene the subject is viewing. By interrupting the spot at regular intervals of time, the trace can indicate the velocity as well as the size and direction of the subject's eye movements. One of their records is shown in figure A1.9. Both this and the Mackworths' procedure suffer from extreme sensitivity to head movements: a 100μ head displacement will produce an artefact of about 1°, and unless one is willing to take Barlow's (1952) heroic measures—head resting on a stone, and clamped in an iron frame—this is probably unacceptable for laboratory use.

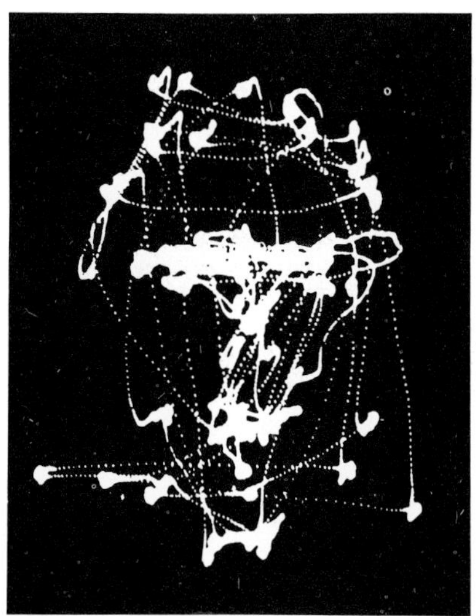

Figure A1.9. Record of eye movements in scanning a picture of a face (Palmieri et al, 1971).

A1.2.2 *Reflection from attachments to the eye*

This sensitivity to head movements arises because of the marked curvature of the cornea: if it were replaced with a plane reflecting surface, it would become essentially insensitive to small translations. In practice this means fitting the eye with a contact lens assembly that has a small plane mirror mounted on it—a technique first attempted by De La Barre in 1898 but abandoned because of inadequate recording equipment; Orschansky (1898) was more successful, and obtained the first photographic records of eye movements. With suitable optical arrangements (Fender, 1955) one can record in tnis way movements about all three axes. Torsional movements have also been measured by Davies and Merton (1958) by adding a birefringent mica filter in front of the mirror and photoelectrically measuring the transmission through a crossed analyser of an incident beam of polarised light (figure A1.10): they were able to achieve a sensitivity of some 20′ of arc.

The use of contact lenses can cause some discomfort to the subject, and is open to other objections as well. Barlow (1963) has shown that of the two main types of contact lenses, the ordinary scleral-fitting ones allow appreciable slip even when the subject is trying to hold his eye steady (with in practice some 3′ root-mean-square deviation), although the Yarbus-type lens (Yarbus, 1967)—which is held to the eye by suction—is better in this respect by a factor of four or five. When larger movements of the eyes are executed, quite large errors can develop as backlash—for example, some 6′ of lag after a 9° saccade (Byford, 1962). On the other hand, Ratliff and Riggs (1950) showed that their lens did not slip during fixation, even when the moment of inertia of the whole assembly was deliberately increased by attaching a 20 gm mass to it: it seems probable that small individual variations in the fitting and use of contact lenses produce significant differences in their adhesion to the eye. Some probable causes of slippage are discussed by Byford (1962), while Boyce and West (1968) have made a critical examination of the kinds of mechanical resonance that occur in contact lens assemblies. At all events, most workers would probably agree that contact lens methods are unsuitable for the accurate measurement of eye movements when saccades of a natural extent are permitted (see for example figure A1.11), when the inertia of the device is likely to make itself apparent.

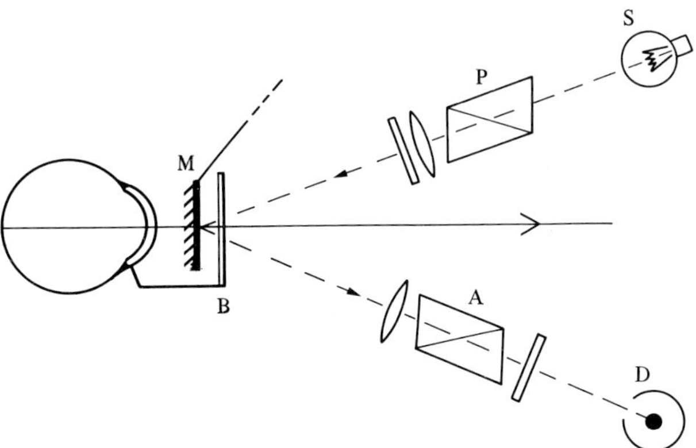

Figure A1.10. Method for measuring torsion. Light from the source S is polarised (P) and reflected from a fixed mirror M in such a way that it passes twice through a birefringent mica plate B attached to the eye. It then passes through the crossed analyser A to the photodetector D (after Davies and Merton, 1958).

If only very small movements are of interest, and the head can be adequately clamped, a possible method that potentially offers very great sensitivity is that of reflection off a small mirror having a *very* small radius of curvature, for example a droplet of mercury. Barlow's (1952) use of such a droplet was slightly different from what is envisaged here: instead of using the image (inside the drop) of an external source of light to mark the position of the eye, one could measure the angle of reflectance of an incident collimated narrow beam; a laser can now provide the kind of illumination required. Such a method would be intrinsically exquisitely sensitive (figure A1.5d), but equally, disastrously responsive to head movements.

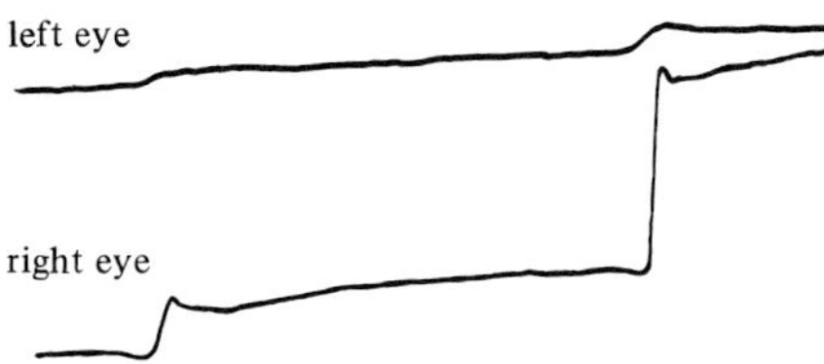

Figure A1.11. Records of movements of the two eyes during a saccade of some 40′ amplitude. The movement of the left eye was measured by direct corneal reflection, and that of the right by reflection from a plane mirror on a contact lens. It is clear that the latter method introduces overshoot artefacts that are absent in the other trace, even allowing for the fact that its gain is some eight times less (Riggs et al, 1954).

A1.3 Electro-oculography

Early in this century, when experimenters were busy recording electrical potentials from every conceivable part of the body, it was soon noticed that electrodes placed in the region of the eyes registered potentials that changed in synchrony with their movements (Schott, 1922; Meyers, 1929; Dewar had described the potentials much earlier, in 1877, without appreciating their origin). At first it was thought that these potentials were due to action potentials in eye muscles, but it is now generally believed that they are the result of a permanent potential difference between the cornea and the fundus of some 10 to 30 mV (positive at the cornea). This sets up an electrical field in the tissues surrounding the eye, which moves as the eye moves and can be recorded by electrodes anywhere on the head, but most easily by electrodes taped to the upper and lower lids (for vertical movements) or the external canthi (for horizontal). With a sufficient degree of amplification this provides a simple means of measuring eye movements and has proved attractive to countless investigators and clinicians: but the method has a number of severe drawbacks.

The fundamental difficulty is that we have really very little idea what the origin of the corneoretinal potential is. Lippold and Shaw (1971) describe electro-oculographic-like recordings from an enucleated subject, synchronised with the intention to move the (nonexistent) eyes. This casts doubt, to say the least, on the assumption that it is the corneoretinal potential that generates the electro-oculogram (EOG), or that the EOG is particularly closely related to the motion of the *globe.* At all events, it is well-known that the EOG is far from being constant in magnitude, but is influenced not only by the metabolic state of the eye [and thus by temperature, pCO_2, pO_2, etc (Marg, 1951)] but also, more seriously from the experimenter's point of view, by visual stimulation (Kris, 1958; Arden and Kelsey, 1962; Troelstra, 1972). Byford (1963) recorded eye movements simultaneously by electro-oculography and with contact lenses, concluding that "corneo-retinal potentials in no way reflect faithfully the time-course of saccadic movements". He suggests that the velocity of the eye may contribute an extra component to the EOG, causing a particularly marked distortion in fast movements (for example Boghen et al, 1974), and demonstrates also both that eye movements can occur with no corresponding EOG indication, and that changes in potential can occur when the eye is stationary (figure A1.12). Added to this noise generated by the eye itself are components produced by the contacts between the electrodes and the skin, particularly the galvanic skin response, which is liable to give sudden unexpected artefacts in subjects unaccustomed to the apparatus (Marg, 1951). These difficulties can be reduced if the outer epidermis is abraded to reduce the resistance of the contacts (Shackel, 1959). If cross-talk between horizontal and vertical channels is to be avoided, the pairs of electrodes must be carefully aligned with the eye: alternatively a suitable bridge circuit with inputs from all four electrodes can be used to balance out any residual misalignment (Rémond et al, 1958).

Finally, the generally unspoken assumption behind this method of recording eye movements is that the movement of the electrical field in the conducting tissues surrounding the eye is related in a simple way to movements of the eye itself: because of the nonuniformity of these tissues, and the shapes of the surfaces round them, this can only be an approximation to the truth. It is particularly questionable for vertical movements of the

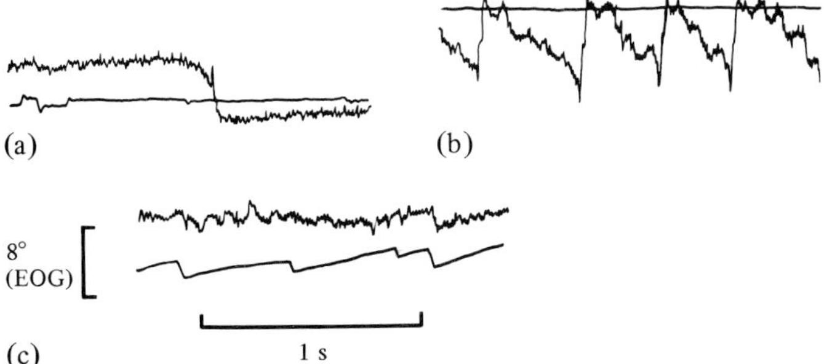

Figure A1.12. Difficulties with the EOG; in each case the smoother record is of eye movement, using a contact lens method, while the other is of EOG: (a) an EOG artefact with no eye movement; (b) rhythmical EOG artefacts: (c) clear nystagmus, undiscernible in the EOG (after Byford, 1963).

eyes because of the effects of the concomitant movements of the lids (Barry and Melvill Jones, 1965). Nevertheless, for horizontal movements, a range of some 30° is generally accepted as linear (Shackel, 1960a), with about 1° resolution. Much more could be said on the methodology of the EOG: there is a wealth of information to be found in Shackel (1967) and Crickmar (1969).

A1.4 Electromagnetic recording

To use the mutual inductance of a pair of coils, one mounted on the eye and another on the head, might seem an obvious way of recording eye movements, yet this method was not used successfully until comparatively recently (Robinson, 1963; Fuchs and Robinson, 1966). A typical arrangement is shown in figure A1.13: for simplicity, only the horizontal channel is shown, although the method may be extended to measure all three axes of rotation. A uniform alternating magnetic field (which may be generated by a coil on each side of the head, preferably in the Helmholtz configuration to improve uniformity) induces an alternating voltage in the eye coil, the amplitude of which is proportional to the sine of the angle between the plane of the eye coil and the direction of the magnetic field. This signal can be amplified and then phase-detected with respect to the magnetic field to give, after low-pass filtering, a signal that corresponds to

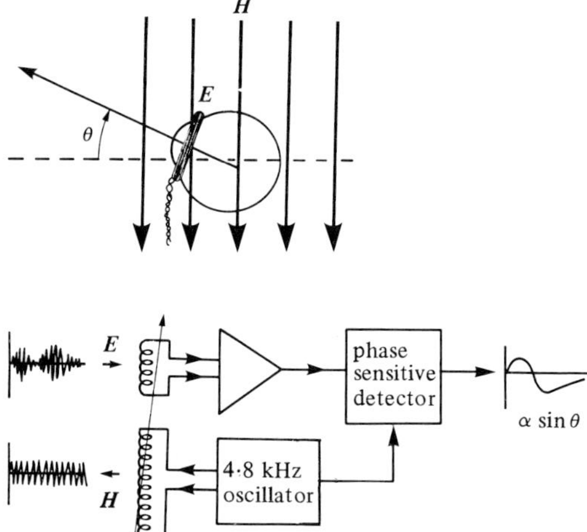

Figure A1.13. Electromagnetic eye-movement recording. Above, small coil mounted on eye: large arrows show the direction of the alternating magnetic field round the eye. Below, schematic circuit arrangements: the oscillator at the bottom drives the coils mounted on the head, that provide the alternating high-frequency magnetic field. A variable component of this—depending on eye position—is picked up by the eye coil *E*, amplified, and then phase-sensitively rectified with respect to the oscillator's own output to yield a signal which after low-pass filtering is proportional to the sine of the angle θ between the plane of the eye coil and the direction of the magnetic field.

movements of the eye in the horizontal plane. By adding a second alternating field in quadrature with the first and spatially at right angles to it, and with a second eye-coil set at an angle to the first, movements about all three axes can be resolved with appropriate detection circuitry. It is preferable to use the eye coil to generate the field, and detect it with the head coils, as then only a single eye coil is needed (if torsional movements are not of interest) and the detection circuits are considerably simpler (Carpenter, 1972a). The eye coil can either be sewn to the eye for chronic recording in animals (Fuchs and Robinson, 1966) or be attached to a contact lens (Robinson, 1963); better still, the coil may be mounted on a scleral ring, fitted in the same way as a contact lens but not subject to as many criticisms on the grounds of discomfort and inertia (Collewijn et al, 1975).

The method is capable of great sensitivity, as the noise level can be made very small indeed by choosing an appropriate value for the frequency of alternation of the magnetic field: Robinson claims some 15″ of arc. Apart from the intrinsic sine relation between the electrical signal and the deviation of the eye, which can easily be compensated for by subsequent nonlinear signal processing, the method gives regular and reproducible responses to eye movements. The method is insensitive to translation, even relative to the head, so long as the field is adequately uniform in space. The main source of error probably arises in the leads joining the eye coil to the amplifier, since they are liable to couple inductively with the magnetic field: this error can be reduced, but never entirely eliminated, by tight twisting. The entire arrangement can be made extremely light and may easily be carried on the head: this electromagnetic method is indeed perhaps the nearest one can get to an ideal eye movement measuring device for laboratory, though probably not for clinical, work.

A 1.5 Other methods

Some other methods are perhaps worth mentioning, for completeness. Mechanical methods of recording are probably only of historical interest: they seem first to have been proposed by Raehlmann (1878), and a distinctly unattractive system involving a plaster-of-Paris contact lens linked to a bristle writing on a smoked drum was used by De La Barre (1898) to show that the eye movements made while scanning illusory figures such as the Müller–Lyer figure corresponded to their illusory rather than real dimensions. Mechanical methods were subsequently developed by Buys and Coppez (1909) and by Ohm (1928), who rested a glass rod on the upper lid, attached to a mechanical lever system to magnify displacements of the cornea. More recently, Faraday (1969) used a silicon strain gauge taped to the upper lid to measure the durations of periods of rapid eye movements in sleep. A similar mechanoelectrical transducer using a probe touching the globe is described by Bengi and Thomas (1968a). They also describe a related method whereby the change in capacitance between the globe and a nearby fixed probe alters the frequency of an oscillator as the eye moves: this is a very light piece of apparatus indeed and can be attached with ease to the head of a mobile subject. Thomas (1965) has attached a piezoelectric accelerometer to a contact lens: being a transducer of acceleration rather than position, it is essentially suitable only at rather high frequencies.

Another class of methods uses subjective visual impressions to give information about eye movements. With care, quantitative information can be gained in this way with a minimum of apparatus. One of the oldest techniques is to examine the trace made by an intermittently illuminated source as the eye moves (Lamansky, 1869). From the angular extent of the interruptions along the path traced by the light one can estimate the velocity of the eye at various times in the movement, although a psychophysical assumption about the perception of direction during eye movements must first be made (see section 10.2.2). There are some advantages in using a television picture as the intermittent source! (Crookes, 1957). Alternatively, a light moving with constant velocity in the horizontal direction, viewed while the subject is simultaneously executing a vertical eye movement, will faithfully trace out the time course of the vertical displacement: a spot moving across an oscilloscope screen at some 20–50 rad s^{-1} may provide a suitable source (Thomas, 1961). Many devices [for example the Maddox rod (Maddox, 1907)] use a subjective method to measure the angular difference in the direction of the two eyes: the principle is for the subject to view a separate scene with each eye (to prevent fusion) and either to report on their relative apparent separation or to adjust their actual separation until they appear to superimpose. The latter procedure is questionable because of uncertainty regarding *central* fusion mechanisms (section 5.1.1).

Afterimages can also provide an indication to the subject of his actual direction of regard, as in Verheijen's (1961) useful demonstration of the miniature movements (figure 6.1). More quantitatively, a pair of afterimages from two flashes separated in time can indicate by their relative displacement the amount of movement that took place in the interval between the flashes. This special case of Lamansky's method was used effectively by Barlow (1952) to estimate the magnitude of errors of fixation.

If our reason for measuring eye movements is that we want to know how the retinal image moves (rather than how the eye muscles are controlled) then of course these subjective methods can provide a check that movement of the image really does correspond to movement of the globe. This is not necessarily the case: it is easy to imagine that under the rapid accelerations experienced in a saccade there could be displacement of the lens (Park and Park, 1940) or even retinal shear (Richards, 1968a), leading to displacement of the 'neural image': in any case, the fact that the centre of rotation of the globe is not identical with the (principal) nodal point means that eye rotation can never be exactly the same as the angular displacement of the retinal image. In controversial cases it is thus essential that objective measurements should be checked against subjective, as Thomas (1961) was able to do in the case of overshoots in saccades. Cornsweet's method described above (Cornsweet, 1958) shares some of these advantages, as it effectively records the position of the retina as seen through the eye's own optics, and might similarly be used to validate measurements made solely on the globe.

No account of methods of measuring eye movements would be complete without mentioning what is perhaps the most bizarre (and certainly one of the simplest) methods in the literature. Ewald Hering (1879b) discovered that it was actually possible to *hear* eye movements simply by listening to the muscles in action through a kind of miniature stethoscope. In this way he was able to distinguish two types of activity associated with attempted steady fixation: a steady background noise corresponding presumably to drift and tremor, and dull clicks occurring at intervals, associated with the microsaccades. This method potentially offers a simple way of checking the steadiness of one's fixation in visual experiments, and no doubt deserves to be revived.

in figure A2.4, the output is always by definition exactly the same as the input, whatever the nature of f may actually be. As we shall see later, an inverse to a function cannot always be found that behaves in a regular way.

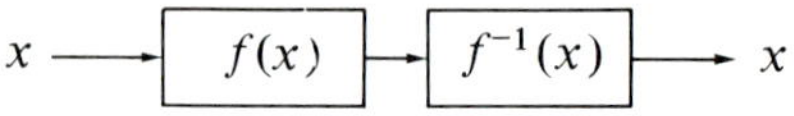

$$x \longrightarrow \boxed{f(x)} \longrightarrow \boxed{f^{-1}(x)} \longrightarrow x$$

Figure A2.4.

But neither of these first two problems has much interest for the investigative scientist. He is faced with the third case, namely the one illustrated in figure A2.5.

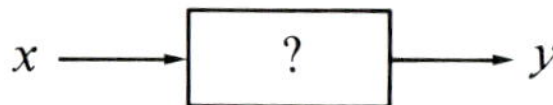

Figure A2.5.

By observing the system in which he is interested, he has obtained a list of the various inputs he has applied, and the corresponding outputs that resulted from them, and now wishes to formulate some rule that will economically describe the relation between the two. Perhaps he has measured the rate of firing of a nerve from a muscle spindle at different degrees of muscle stretch: his aim is then to provide a description of the action of the spindle that can be used to predict the rate of firing for any conceivable kind of stretching, and not just under the particular circumstances that he has actually measured. At all events, this kind of problem is clearly completely different in kind from the other two. In fact it provides the information by which they can be solved, for even in the simplest cases—like the square fields—someone must first make an analysis of observations to establish the nature of the function f from which the equations can be formulated and answers obtained. Powerful though traditional mathematical methods are for dealing with the first two cases, they are at best clumsy when applied to the third, and it is for this reason that the methods of a systems analysis were evolved. Systems analysis provides techniques for converting experimental data about how a given system responds to different inputs into an economical description of the system itself. This description can then be used either as a guide to further analysis of the components of the system, or conversely to evaluate its contribution to any larger system of which it may form a part. Finally, we shall see later that systems analysis can also tell the experimenter what *kinds* of input he should apply to obtain this information with as little experimental effort as possible.

The experimenter's job, then, is to try to guess the properties of the 'black box' of figure A2.5 by looking at how it responds to different patterns of input. To guess successfully, he clearly needs to have a good working knowledge of the kinds of black box that occur with greatest frequency in the natural world. Fortunately, it turns out that there are a rather limited number of types of function that commonly arise in physical systems—perhaps even fewer in biological ones—and that even systems that at first sight seem extremely complex can often on closer analysis be shown to be an aggregate of a number of simple functional building blocks of a standard type. Before starting on systems analysis proper, it is perhaps worth spending a little time in describing the major classes of function that are commonly met, with particular examples. Readers with a good mathematical background can probably proceed at once to section A2.4.

A2.2 Classes of function

So far we have only considered functions of a single variable, of the form $f(x)$. But there is no reason why a particular dependent variable should not be under the influence of a number of different inputs (as for example if we consider not square fields but rectangular ones, where the area depends on the length *and* the breadth).

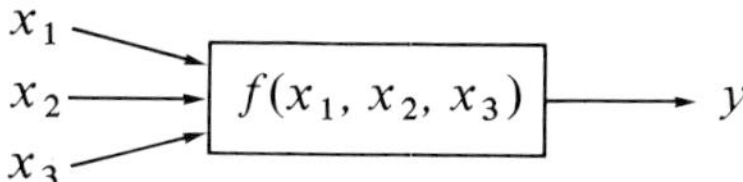

Figure A2.6.

Indeed this situation is the rule rather than the exception: for example, a stretch receptor's rate of firing is not just a function of its extension, since many other factors such as pH, pO_2, temperature, and so on will clearly affect its performance. Nevertheless, nature cooperates with the experimenter here to the extent that in living animals these extraneous variables are kept carefully within bounds, and in practice can often be ignored. In other cases this is not so—an experimenter cannot for example afford to ignore the fact that a photoreceptor's response will depend on both the intensity and the wavelength of the incident light—and it is up to the experimenter himself to design his experiment in such a way that only one thing changes at a time. In any case, no important new principles are involved in discussing functions of two or more variables rather than just one, and for simplicity we shall deal here only with the latter case.

Functions of a single variable can be represented conveniently as a graph of output versus input, and a number of the main classifications of functions are closely related to the general features of such a graph. If the graph is a straight line, and it is true that the output is zero when the input is zero, then the function is a *linear* one (figure A2.7). In fact, the only linear function of one variable is of the form $y = kx$, where k is a constant *parameter* that determines how quickly the output increases as the input increases, that is, the slope of the graph. Linear functions show additivity: the output in response to the sum of two particular inputs is equal to the sum of the outputs that would result from each applied separately. In other words, a linear function has the property that for all values of a and b,

$$f(a+b) = f(a)+f(b).$$

As a special case of additivity, it must follow that, if the input is doubled in size, the output will also double.

All other functions of a single variable are nonlinear: but there are degrees of nonlinearity. The most severe case is that of *discontinuity*: a good example is the step function that is often used as a model of threshold processes (figure A2.8). We might define the output of such a device as equal to some constant k when the input is equal to or greater than some threshold value θ, and 0 otherwise. Clearly this is not a linear function—it certainly does not obey additivity—and it is discontinuous in the sense that however closely we explore the region around θ we can never obtain an output of any intermediate value between 0 and k. Incidentally, it is also an example of a function with a very badly behaved inverse: no inverse at all can be defined for values of the output other than 0 and k, and even for these values there is evidently an infinite number of possible inputs that could have generated them.

A slightly less severe case of nonlinearity arises if the function has kinks in it: if we plot the slope of such a graph as a function of the input, these kinks become apparent as *discontinuities of slope* (figure A2.9).

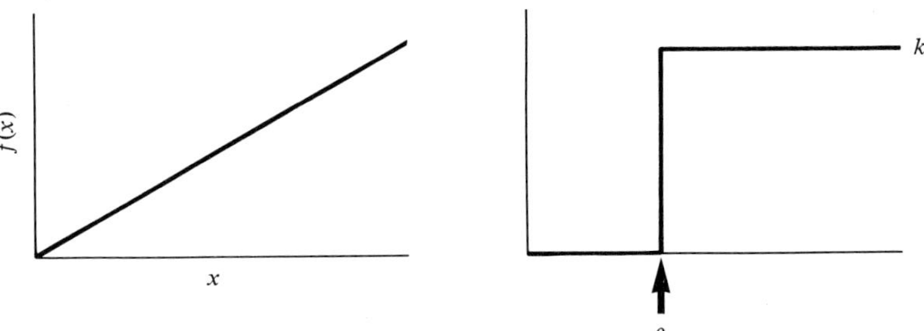

Figure A.2.7. A linear function.

Figure A2.8. A discontinuous function, the step function.

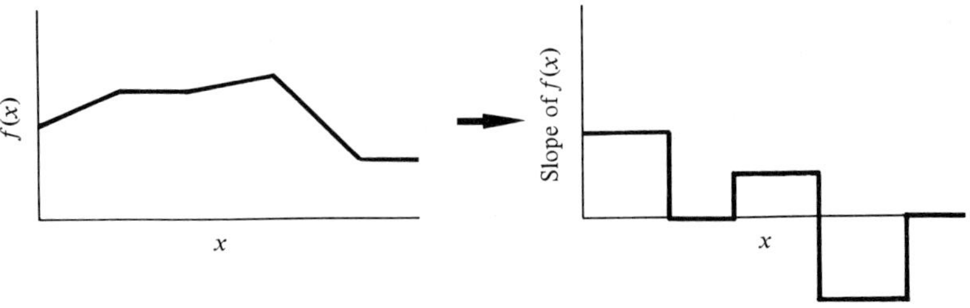

Figure A2.9. A less severe case of nonlinearity.

The mildest nonlinearities occur in those functions that neither are discontinuous nor show discontinuity of slope. An example of a smooth nonlinear function of this type is the saturating response of figure A2.10: because, ultimately, energy is not available in unlimited quantity, *all* systems show saturation of one form or another. Real systems that seem to be linear are simply those in which the initial portion of the curve does not depart significantly from a straight line for any input that can occur under 'physiological' conditions.

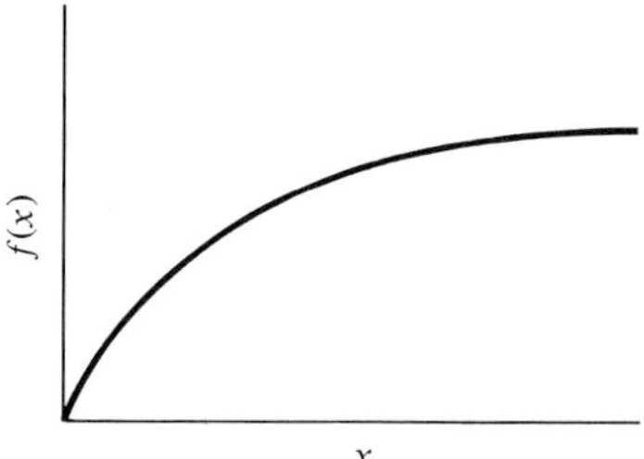

Figure A2.10. A smooth nonlinear function.

All smooth functions can be treated as linear, so long as the excursions of the input are kept within sufficient bounds, so that only a very small portion of the whole extent of the function is actually used. As the range of variation in the input is reduced, so also is the degree of departure from strict linearity: it is as if one were magnifying a small section of the complete function. Functions that are not smooth do not behave in this agreeable way: however small we make the range of input values, if it happens to include any kind of discontinuity a straight line can never be a good approximation to it (figure A2.11). For this reason, nonlinearities are sometimes divided into *essential* nonlinearities like discontinuities, that cannot be neglected by considering a sufficiently small range of input, and *inessential,* which can.

Essential nonlinearities tend to cause great difficulties in mathematical analysis, but happily do not occur in real physical systems—still less in biological ones—in their strict form. The reason for this is the all-pervading noise and uncertainty that effectively rubs the hard edges off discontinuities by preventing the observer from pin-pointing their exact position on the graph. Thus real thresholds in physiology and psychology never have the idealised form shown in figure A2.8: in practice they can only be described probablistically, so that an input near the threshold may on some occasions produce the full output and on others no output at all under conditions that are as near identical as the experimenter can achieve (figure A2.12).

In practice, then, noise turns essential nonlinearities into inessential nonlinearities, and inessential nonlinearities can in turn be treated as if they were linear if the range of inputs is sufficiently small. For this reason, linear systems analysis can often be applied with great effect to systems that the experimenter knows are not really linear at all. Useful discussions of linearising statistical processes in neurophysiology may be found in Verveen (1969) and Spekreijse and Oosting (1970).

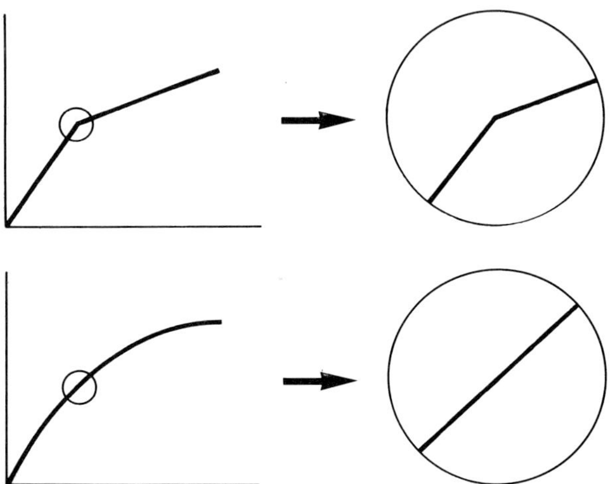

Figure A2.11. Essential and inessential nonlinearities: above, linear interpolation over a small change of input cannot always be justified if the function is essentially nonlinear; below, an inessentially nonlinear function, whose behaviour can always be treated as being linear if small enough input changes are considered.

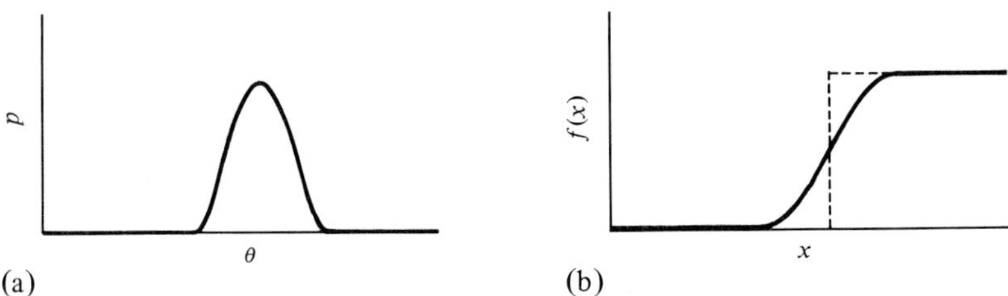

Figure A2.12. Effect of random variation in converting essential nonlinearities into inessential: (a) probability distribution of different values of the threshold value in a hypothetical threshold function; (b) effect of this variation on the observed function if averaged over a number of observations.

A2.3 Some common functions

There are three types of functional building-block that arise so frequently in an account of systems analysis that it may perhaps be useful to describe them here in brief. They comprise:

(1) power functions (of the form x^2, x^3, x^4, etc),

(2) exponential functions [$\exp x$, $\exp(-x)$],

(3) trigonometric functions (sine, cosine, etc).

Power functions

These can be written in the form $y = kx^n$, where n is a parameter that determines the shape of the graph of the function, and k is in effect a scaling factor determining its size. If $n = 0$ we have the 'function' $y = k$ for which the output is not affected by the input at all; $n = 1$ gives the elementary linear function $y = kx$ discussed previously; if $n = 2$ the graph is a parabola centred on the y-axis. The function is symmetrical about this axis (figure A2.13), since x^2 is always equal to $(-x)^2$, a property shared by all power functions having even values of n. For this reason, symmetry of this type in which the graph is unchanged after reflection about the y-axis is often called *even symmetry*, and functions made up entirely of even powers are called *even functions.* The case when $n = 3$ produces a cubic curve of which the branch corresponding to positive values of the input is similar to that for $n = 2$, but changes slope more rapidly. The negative branch is the same as the positive, but rotated through 180° round an axis perpendicular to the x- and y-axes: this is also a kind of symmetry, often called *odd* or S-*symmetry* because it is the same as that of a letter 'S'. All functions composed entirely of odd powers of x share this same kind of symmetry, and can be called *odd functions.* Higher values of n produce curves that are similar either to x^2 or to x^3, depending on whether n is even or odd, but show a progressive increase in the sharpness with which they bend into their extreme portions (figure A2.14). As n tends towards infinity, this sharpness approaches that of an actual discontinuity at the values $x = \pm 1$, since even a value of x only very slightly greater than unity can, if multiplied by itself often enough, produce an arbitrarily large result: conversely, if x is only very slightly less than unity, repeated self-multiplication can make the corresponding output vanishingly small.

These large powers of x are not commonly met by themselves, but are important as components of *power-series approximations.* The family of curves $y = kx^n$ shows such a variety of shapes within itself, as n is varied, that in fact many other functions can as it were be imitated or *synthesised* by adding suitable proportions of selected members of the family. A recipe for such a synthesis simply consists of a summed series

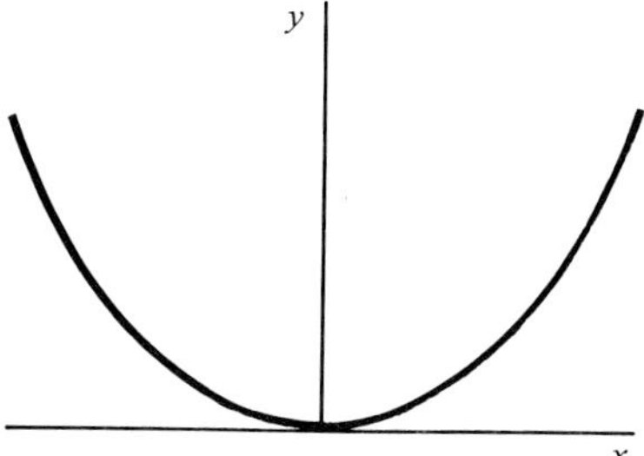

Figure A2.13. The graph of the power function, $y = kx^2$.

of terms, each of the form kx^n, for $n = 0, 1, 2, \ldots$. Normally each term will have its own associated value for k, or *coefficient,* which together specify in effect the relative proportions of each power function that must be mixed to produce the final approximation. Thus for example the function $y = 1/(1-x)$ has the particularly simple series approximation,

$$y = 1 + x + x^2 + x^3 + \ldots,$$

where all the coefficients are equal to one (figure A2.15). However, although approximations can always be made to a function in this way over a specified limited range of input values, they can often go disastrously wrong if this range is exceeded. In the example above, if x is allowed to take a value greater than one, the sum of the series will clearly get

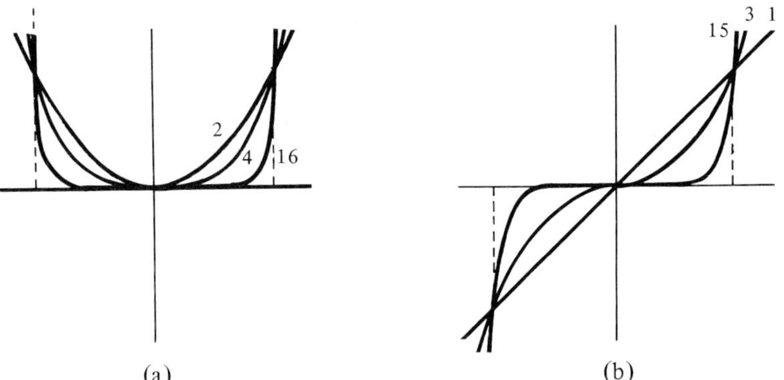

Figure A2.14. Power functions of different values of n: (a) even values of n; (b) odd values.

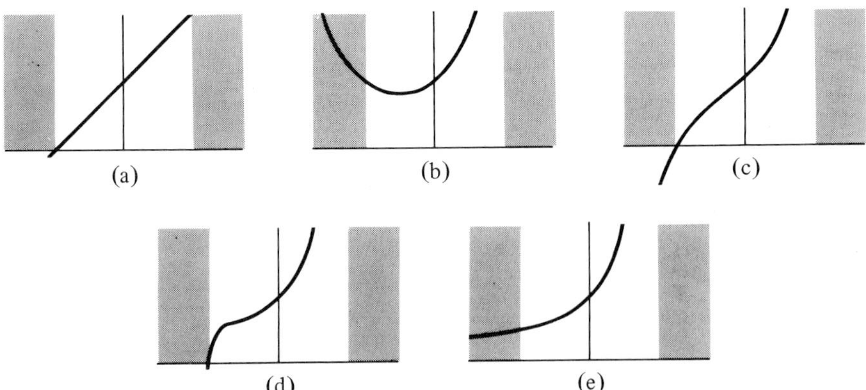

Figure A2.15. Example of a power-series approximation. The approximation is $1/(1-x) = 1+x+x^2+x^3+\ldots$; (a) shows the sum of the first two terms, (b) of the first three, (c) of the first four; (d) of the first eight, and (e) shows the function itself. The approximation is valid only in the unshaded area: outside this range it can be seen to diverge widely.

explosively larger and larger as n increases: such a series is called a divergent series. On the other hand, if x is between one and zero, the terms get smaller and smaller as one goes along, and the sum is said to converge on the correct answer [corresponding problems arise as x approaches -1 (figure A2.15)]. But as long as one takes care to ensure that a series approximation is valid for the range of inputs under consideration—and it will be seen later that some of the most important series are valid for *all* values of x—it can greatly clarify the relationships between different types of function by translating them all into a kind of *lingua franca* in which they can be compared term by term. A second useful property of series of this type is that one can use them to make linear approximations: if x is sufficiently small, so that x^2, x^3, etc are even smaller and can safely be neglected, the series can be abbreviated to its first two terms,

$$y = k_0 + k_1 x,$$

which when plotted is simply a straight line passing through a point lying a distance k_0 up the y-axis. This linear approximation is thus the exact counterpart of the process of linearisation described in the last section for the case when only small variations in the input are permitted.

Exponential functions

We have seen that a function of the form $y = kx^n$ can produce a variety of types of graph as the parameter n is allowed to assume different integer values. It is natural to ask what would happen if it were x that was held constant, and n treated as the input: or, rewriting the equation, if $y = kn^x$. Functions of this type are called *exponential* functions (x here is an exponent) and arise most frequently in biological systems as a description of growth or decay. Suppose for example that we have a cell culture that doubles its volume every hour, and that, when we first observe it, it has a volume V_0. Then after the first hour it will have a volume $2V_0$; after the

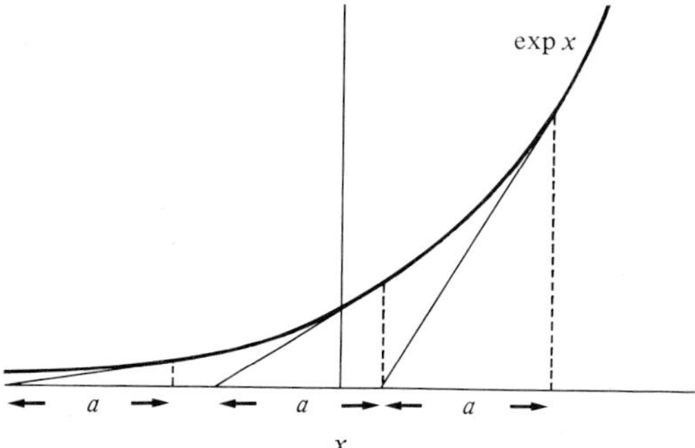

Figure A2.16. The exponential function, $\exp x$. The slope is everywhere proportional to the ordinate, so it follows that the three distances a must be equal (the thin lines are tangent to the curve).

second, $2^2 V_0$; after the third, $2^3 V_0$; and so on: thus after t hours its volume will be $2^t V_0$, which is of the same form as our original exponential expression. The graph of a growth process of this kind has an explosive appearance, because the rate at which the output increases—the slope of the graph—is at every point proportional to the output value.

An important property of exponential functions, in which they differ markedly from power functions, is that the shape (as opposed to the size or scale) of the graph is *not* affected by the value of the parameter n. For example, if our cell culture had quadrupled, instead of doubling, every hour, then the volume after t hours would be given by $4^t V_0$. We can rewrite this as $(2^2)^t V_0$, or simply as $2^{2t} V_0$. In other words, the only difference in the function is a change in the time scale, so that if the graph were plotted in units of half an hour instead of one hour, it would be indistinguishable from that of the first case. Since the actual value of n has no effect on the essential character of the function, it is usual in mathematical work to rescale exponential functions to a standard value of n—the exponential constant e (= 2·718 ...). The reason for using this rather awkward value rather than something simple like 10 or 2 is that the function e^x ($\exp x$) has a particularly simple power series expansion:

$$\exp x = 1 + x + \frac{x^2}{2!} + \frac{x^3}{3!} + \frac{x^4}{4!} + \ldots$$

(! means factorial of the number in front, that is, $2! = 2 \times 1$; $3! = 3 \times 2 \times 1$; $4! = 4 \times 3 \times 2 \times 1$; etc).

The factorial function grows so rapidly with increasing inputs that the coefficients of succeeding terms in the series diminish very rapidly indeed: consequently the series is valid for values of x that can be as large as one cares to choose. Different rates of growth can be expressed by the *time constant* of the system: this is defined as the time taken for the output to grow by a factor e, and is usually written as τ. Thus the expression describing the growth of the output of a system with time constant τ is of the form $V_0 \exp(t/\tau)$, where V_0 is again the value of the output at time zero. Decay is amenable to exactly the same kind of description as growth. If for example we have a quantity of radioisotope whose activity, initially Q_0, is *halved* every hour, then the activity after t hours is given by $Q_0(\frac{1}{2})^t$, or $Q_0/2^t$, which can be rewritten as $Q_0 2^{-t}$. Decay is thus distinguished from growth only by the negative sign of the exponent, and simple decay of this type can always be described by an expression of the form $Q_0 \exp(-t/\tau)$, where τ is again the time constant of the decay—the time taken for the output to *fall* by a factor e.

Trigonometric functions

The trigonometric functions—notably sine and cosine—are associated in elementary mathematics with essentially geometrical problems: but in systems analysis they are extremely important when dealing with sine waves and other periodic phenomena, as we shall see. A sine wave is a periodic function of time and can be expressed as

$$A \sin 2\pi\nu t$$

where ν is the *frequency* of the wave in Hz (cycles s^{-1}) and A is its *amplitude.* In mathematical work it is usual to express angles in radians rather than in degrees and minutes: 2π radians are equal to 360° or one complete turn. Thus $\sin 2\pi$ is equal to $\sin(0)$, so that the output is the same at $t = 1/\nu$ as it is at $t = 0$, and in fact the function repeats itself at regular intervals as t increases, with a period $1/\nu$. The function $\cos 2\pi\nu t$ has exactly the same shape as a sine wave, but is shifted in time—since $\sin\phi$ is always equal to $\cos(\phi - \frac{1}{2}\pi)$—and both kinds of wave are loosely referred to as 'sine waves'.

It is sometimes helpful to think of a sine wave as the projection of a point moving at constant angular velocity round a circle (figure A2.17). If the circle has a radius A, and the point moves with angular velocity ω (radians s^{-1}), the projection of the point on the x-axis is given by $A \cos\omega t$.

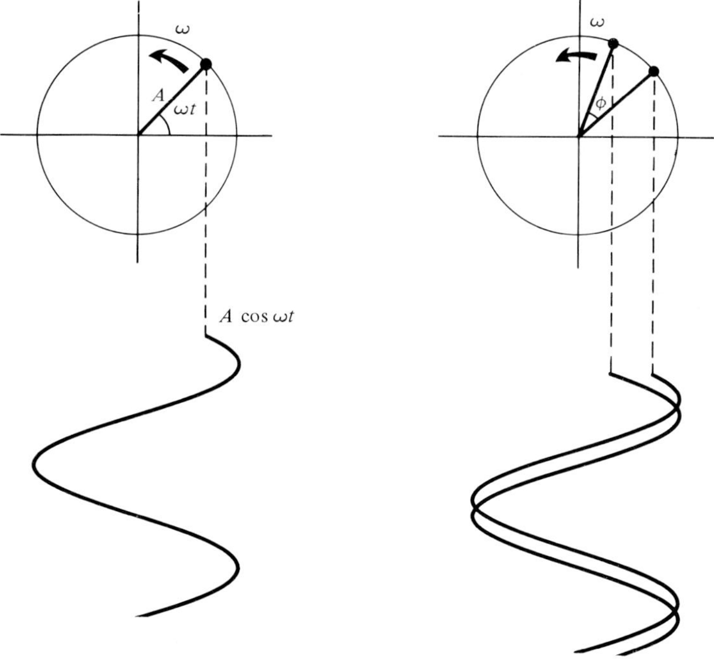

Figure A2.17. Generation of the wave $A \cos(\omega t)$ as the projection of a point moving with constant angular velocity ω round a circle of radius A.

Figure A2.18. Two points moving as in figure A2.17, but with a fixed angle ϕ between them, generate two waves with a phase difference of ϕ.

This is a 'sine' wave (actually cosine) whose frequency is $\nu = \omega/2\pi$. It is very often convenient to specify the frequency of a sine wave as the angular velocity of the generating point (ω) rather than as the reciprocal of the period of the wave (ν), and when used in this way ω is referred to as the *angular frequency*. The relation between the two is simply that $\omega = 2\pi\nu$. One could imagine two points moving round the circle with the same ω, but displaced relative to one another by a fixed angle ϕ (figure A2.18). The corresponding sine waves generated by the two points would then be displaced relative to each other by a time ϕ/ω. It is usual to refer to relative shifts of waves of the same frequency simply by the corresponding *phase* angle ϕ: thus $\phi = \pi$ (or 180°) means a phase shift of half a period, which means that the wave is in effect inverted, whereas a shift of 2π brings the two waves into coincidence again. A sine wave with a phase advance of ϕ can be written as $A\cos(\omega t + \phi)$: a phase lag is indicated by a minus sign instead of a plus sign.

Imaginary numbers

Now, to introduce sine waves efficiently and elegantly into problems of systems analysis we need to use the concepts of imaginary and complex numbers: a topic traditionally regarded as particularly abstruse and difficult for nonmathematicians. But this need not be so, and the benefits of using imaginary numbers in systems analysis are so great that it is worth getting to grips with them at an early stage.

Perhaps the simplest approach comes from considering the problem of the representation of functions of more than one variable in graphical form. Graphs of functions of *one* variable can of course easily be drawn in two dimensions, as one dimension suffices for the input axis and one for the output axis. But if there is a second input variable, a third axis and thus three dimensions are required to represent the function, which then appears not as a line on a plane, but as a surface in space (figure A2.19).

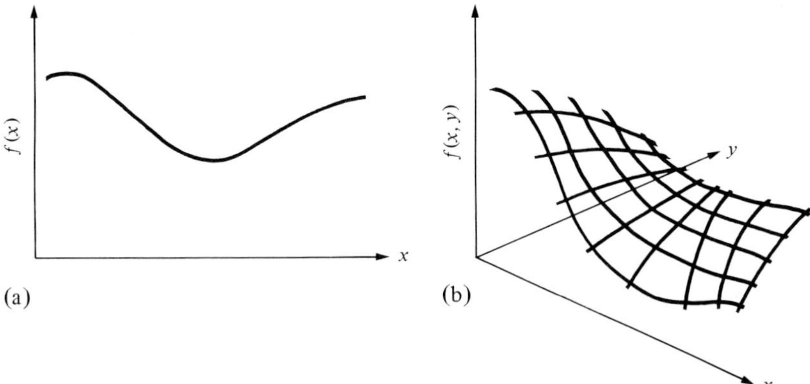

Figure A2.19. (a) A single function of one variable can be represented as a line in a plane; (b) a similar function of two variables is equivalent to a surface in space.

Just as in the one-input case the output was a function of the position of the input point on the line representing the input axis, so now the output is a function of the position of the input point on what might be called the input plane formed by the two input axes.

A common way of referring to a point on a plane defined by two axes (x- and y-axes) is as (x, y), where x and y are respectively the x- and y-coordinates of the point. Simple as such a notation is, it has one very severe drawback. To see what this is, let us return for a moment to the case of a function of one variable—say $f(x)$—and suppose that we are interested in two particular values of the input, x_1 and x_2. Apart from the outputs $f(x_1)$ and $f(x_2)$ whose meaning is obvious, we can also form expressions like $f(x_1+x_2)$ or $f(x_1-x_2)$ and so on, in which the two inputs are combined with arithmetical operators. There is no difficulty in interpreting these expressions in graphical terms, for operation like + and − are formally equivalent to operations on distances on a line like the x-axis. Thus (x_1+x_2) could be interpreted as "go along a distance x_1, *and then* go along a distance x_2". Similarly, (x_1-x_2) means in effect "go along a distance x_1, and then *turn through 180° and* go along a distance x_2". One can think of the minus sign in (x_1-x_2) as a shorthand way of writing $[x_1+(-1)x_2]$, where (-1) stands for the operation of turning through 180°, or an 'about face'. It follows that $(-1)(-1)$, two such turns in succession, has no effect at all, corresponding to the elementary arithmetical tag that 'two minuses make a plus'. At all events, it is clear that by defining algebraic operators in appropriate ways, and in particular by using (-1) to represent a 180° turn, we can use these operators to apply as easily to movements along a line as to handling numerical quantities (figure A2.20).

Returning now to the case of two input variables, it is clear that here too it would be useful if we could combine inputs by means of arithmetical operations, in other words if we could form expressions like $f[(x_1, y_1)+(x_2, y_2]$, dealing with movements around the input plane as easily as we can deal with movements along a line. The immediate difficulty that prevents us from doing so is our (x, y) notation, because the ',' has no immediate arithmetical interpretation. In geometrical terms, (x, y) means something like "go along a distance x, *then turn through 90°* and proceed a distance y", but although we have invented (-1) to represent

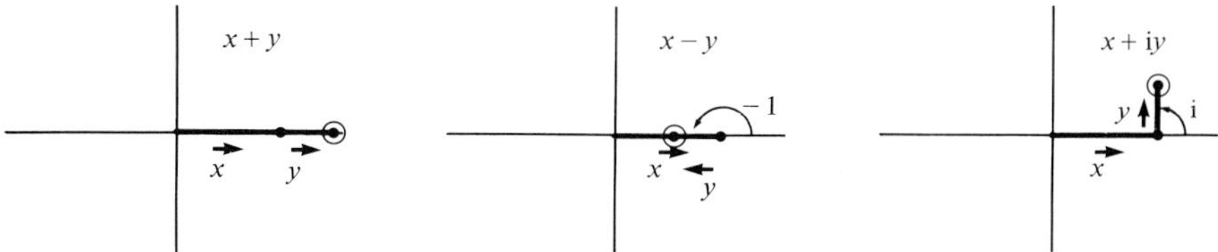

Figure A2.20. Arithmetical operations for dealing with movements along a line and within the input plane.

a turn through 180°, we do not yet have any way of incorporating a turn of 90° into our existing algebraic system.

The solution is not hard to find if one considers the analogy of (− 1). In a sense, one can almost define a turn of 180° as "what you have to do twice to get back where you started" (leaving aside the trivial case of doing nothing at all). In the same way, it is perhaps not too far-fetched to think of a 90° turn as "what you have to do twice to turn through 180°". The solution is then obvious: just as (− 1) meets the requirement for 180°, because $(-1)(-1) = 1$, so, if we use the symbol i to stand for the operator we are looking for, we can say that

$$\mathrm{i}^2 = -1, \text{ or that } \mathrm{i} = \sqrt{-1}.$$

So we can now write the point (x, y) as simply $(x + \mathrm{i}y)$, an expression in which all the terms have recognised algebraical interpretations. Operations on points on a plane now become as easy as those on a line:

$$f[(x_1 + \mathrm{i}y_1) + (x_2 + \mathrm{i}y_2)]$$

simply becomes

$$f(x_1 + \mathrm{i}y_1 + x_2 + \mathrm{i}y_2),$$

or by rearrangement,

$$f[(x_1 + x_2) + \mathrm{i}(y_1 + y_2)].$$

This latter operation of separation of the terms that do and do not contain i is called resolving into real and imaginary parts: the *real part* of the expression consists of those terms without i, and represents the x-coordinate of the whole, and the *imaginary part* similarly represents the y-coordinate. An expression of this type that consists of both real and imaginary parts is called a *complex* expression, and the corresponding plane is the *complex plane.* The fact that quantities like i are 'imaginary' in the sense that they cannot, for example, be used to represent the sizes of objects in the outside world is in a sense irrelevant: in any case, the same is equally

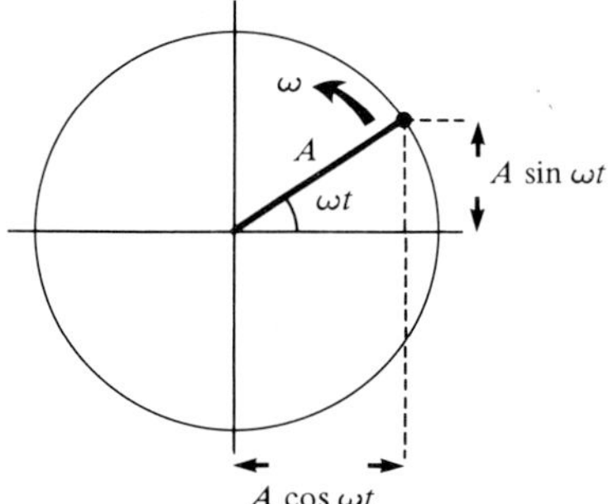

Figure A2.21. The generation of a sine wave from a circularly moving point in the complex plane.

true of negative numbers. The fact that negative apples have no existence does not stop one using '–' as an arithmetical operator *on* apples! Negative numbers only seem more real to us than 'imaginary' numbers like $\sqrt{-1}$ because we meet them much earlier in our mathematical studies, and they are more commonly used in the mathematical transactions of everyday life.

One immediate application for complex numbers is in describing the generation of sine waves from circularly moving points in the way described in the previous section. From simple trigonometry (figure A2.21) it is clear that the x-coordinate of the point at any moment is $A \cos \omega t$, and the y-coordinate is $A \sin \omega t$. Thus the point itself can be described by the complex expression $A(\cos \omega t + \mathrm{i} \sin \omega t)$. To simplify this expression, it is only necessary to look at the power series expansions for $\cos x$ and $\sin x$:

$$\cos x = 1 - \frac{x^2}{2!} + \frac{x^4}{4!} + \ldots,$$

$$\sin x = x - \frac{x^3}{3!} + \ldots,$$

so

$$\mathrm{i} \sin x = \mathrm{i}x - \mathrm{i}\frac{x^3}{3!} + \ldots,$$

and

$$\cos x + \mathrm{i} \sin x = 1 + \mathrm{i}x - \frac{x^2}{2!} - \mathrm{i}\frac{x^3}{3!} + \frac{x^4}{4!} + \ldots,$$

Now, the series for $\exp x$ was previously given as:

$$1 + x + \frac{x^2}{2!} + \frac{x^3}{3!} + \frac{x^4}{4!} + \ldots,$$

and so we can write the series for $\exp(\mathrm{i}x)$ as:

$$1 + \mathrm{i}x - \frac{x^2}{2!} - \mathrm{i}\frac{x^3}{3!} + \frac{x^4}{4!} + \ldots,$$

which is identical with what we have obtained for $\cos x + \mathrm{i} \sin x$. Thus we can write the expression describing the moving point as simply

$$A \exp(\mathrm{i}\omega t),$$

so that the corresponding cosine wave is the real part of this. In general a rotation through any angle ϕ is equivalent to a multiplication by $\exp(\mathrm{i}\phi)$: in particular we can obtain the somewhat esoteric-looking formula that relates e, i, and π:

$$\exp(\mathrm{i}\pi) = -1.$$

Phase shifts by an angle ϕ can likewise be represented by multiplication by $\exp(\mathrm{i}\phi)$, so that the expression for a phase-shifted wave becomes

$$A \exp(\mathrm{i}\,\omega t)\exp(\mathrm{i}\phi), \text{ or simply } A \exp[\mathrm{i}(\omega t + \phi)].$$

The advantages of this notation will become clearer later on.

A2.4 Operators and filters

So far we have considered functions in which the output is completely defined by the instantaneous value of the input(s) at any moment. In practice, especially in biological systems, the output depends not just on the momentary value of the input, but also to a large extent on its *past history*. Thus stretch receptors in muscle spindles typically respond not just to the stretch itself but to the *rate* of stretch; and the concentration of transmitter at a nerve ending depends not only on the immediate rate of release, but also on the amount that *has been* released. What we have in these cases is a system whose input is not a single variable, but rather is some function of time: and the output is some new function of time. Such a device is called an *operator*: just as a function transforms one variable into another, so an operator transforms one function of a variable into another function of the same variable (figure A2.22).

The physical embodiment of such a device is called a *filter,* and the input and output functions of time may be referred to as *signals.* Practically everything the nervous system does by way of information processing can be thought of as filtering of one sort or another: the vestibulo-ocular reflex, for example, with its input signal of head movement and output signal of eye movement. Complex systems like the vestibulo-ocular reflex can nearly always be broken down into a succession of individual stages of signal processing, and the nearer one gets to isolating what might be called the elementary components of such a sequence of filters, the more one tends to find that they fall into one of a very limited number of standard types. The purpose of this section is to describe the five or six most common types of linear operator, of which the first two are familiar as the operations of *differentiation* and *integration.*

Figure A2.22. (a) A *function* converts one variable into another, whereas (b) an *operator* converts one function of a variable into another function of the same variable.

Differentiation

One of the features of a function of time that may be of interest is its rate of change, the slope of its graph. As we have seen with rotations, the problem in bringing an intuitive concept like slope within the fold of conventional mathematics is often one of finding a means of describing it in terms that already exist and can be manipulated by ordinary algebra: this is what the differential calculus does for the idea of slope.

The technique is the same as that of making a linear approximation, described earlier in section A2.2. If we consider a sufficiently small change in the input t of a function $f(t)$—we can write such a small change as δt, where δ means 'a small change in'—then a straight line joining the points $[t, f(t)]$ and $[t+\delta t, f(t+\delta t)]$ can be considered to be a satisfactory linear approximation to the curve over the range δt (figure A2.23). (Difficulties will of course arise if there is an essential nonlinearity within this range; we assume that we are dealing with a function that is inessentially nonlinear.) The slope of this line is then given by the ratio of the corresponding small change in $f(t)$, $\delta f(t)$, and δt itself, or in other words by

$$\frac{\delta f(t)}{\delta t} = \frac{f(t+\delta t)-f(t)}{\delta t} .$$

The value of this expression can easily be found for a particular value of t, once we know what f is. For example, if $f(t)$ is kt^2, the slope is given by:

$$\frac{k(t+\delta t)^2 - kt^2}{\delta t} = k(2t+\delta t).$$

If δt is allowed to get vanishingly small, this expression clearly approaches a limiting value $2kt$. If the notation $\mathrm{d}t$ is used for a vanishingly small increment in t, then we can write the slope in the limit as $\mathrm{d}[f(t)]/\mathrm{d}t$, or even as $\mathrm{d}f/\mathrm{d}t$. So we can write

$$\frac{\mathrm{d}}{\mathrm{d}t}(kt^2) = 2kt,$$

and the slopes of other functions can often be found by similar methods without much difficulty. Since we have started with one function of t and ended up with another one, differentiation is evidently an 'operation' in the sense defined earlier. It is a *linear* operation, because the change in the sum of two functions is the sum of their individual changes: this

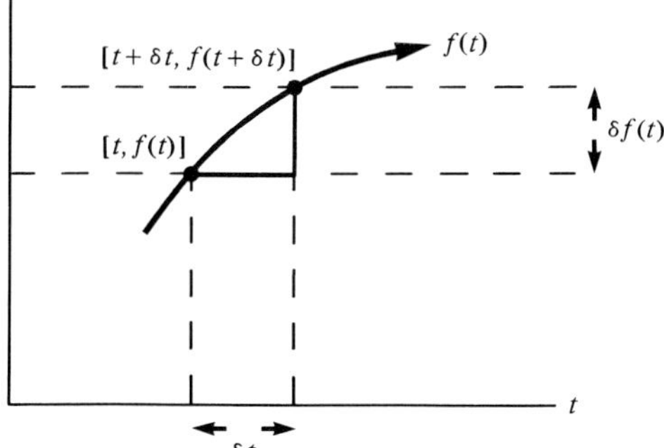

Figure A2.23. The use of differentiation to make a satisfactory approximation to the slope of a curve f over the range δt.

means that complicated expressions can often be more easily differentiated by separating summed terms and differentiating them individually. The notation is in some ways a clumsy one (its main merit is that it indicates in itself the method by which the differential is obtained) and a more concise and versatile one is to use D to represent the differential operator. Thus we can write:

$$\mathrm{D}(kt^2) = 2kt.$$

An extension of this notation is to use $\mathrm{D}^2(f)$ to mean $\mathrm{D}[\mathrm{D}(f)]$, that is, the differential of the differential of f, or its rate of change of slope. Thus since $\mathrm{D}(kt) = k$, $\mathrm{D}^2(kt^2) = 2k$. Comprehensive lists of functions and their differentials (often called derivatives) can be found in many sources (for example Petit Bois, 1961). It is perhaps worthwhile outlining the effects of differentiating the three basic types of function described earlier. Two particular cases of power functions (kt and kt^2) have already been mentioned: the general formula is:

$$\mathrm{D}(kt^n) = nkt^{n-1}.$$

It follows from this that the differential of an odd function will always be even, and vice versa. This formula also enables one to calculate the differentials of functions whose power series expansions are known. Thus:

$$\mathrm{D}\exp t = \mathrm{D}\left(1+x+\frac{x^2}{2!}+\frac{x^3}{3!}+\ldots\right)$$

$$= \quad 1+x+\frac{x^2}{2!}+\ldots = \exp t.$$

In other words, the function $\exp t$ has the remarkable property that it is equal to its own slope at every point. In the same way, one can show that $\mathrm{D}\exp(kt) = k\exp(kt)$, so that—as expected of a growth function

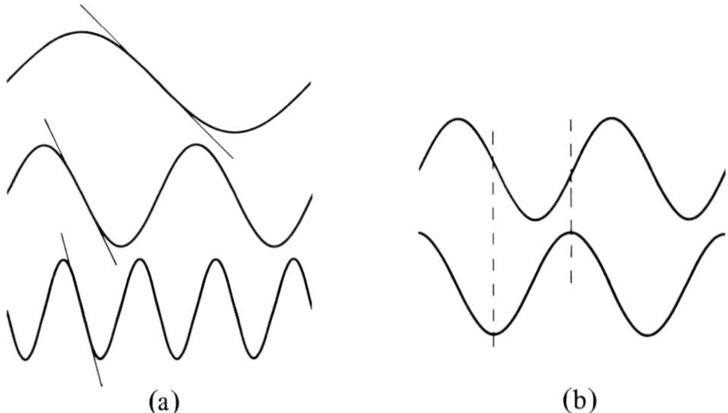

Figure A2.24. Effect of differentiation on sine waves: (a) increasing the frequency of a wave increases its maximum slope, even though the amplitude remains constant; (b) since the maximum slope of a sine wave occurs one quarter cycle before the peak itself, the differential of a sine wave is advanced in phase by 90°.

—its rate of increase is proportional to its instantaneous value. If we express a sine wave in its complex form as $A \exp(\mathrm{i}\omega t)$, we can now immediately obtain its differential as $\mathrm{i}\omega A \exp(\mathrm{i}\omega t)$, so that differentiating a sine wave is identical to multiplying it by $\mathrm{i}\omega$. As we have seen, the i implies a rotation through 90°—that is, a phase advance of $\frac{1}{2}\pi$—whereas the ω term implies that the higher the frequency of the wave, the greater will be the amplitude of the output. This is only to be expected, since the maximum slope of a sine wave must increase as the period decreases (figure A2.24), and occurs one quarter of a cycle ahead of the maximum of the original wave.

Integration

Although integration is normally first encountered as a method of finding the area under functions, from the point of view of the systems analyst it is more convenient to think of it simply as the inverse operation to differentiation. Just as the inverse of a function is what you have to do to arrive back at the original input, so the inverse of an operator is one that restores the original input function. As with inverse functions, there is no guarantee that such an inverse necessarily exists, because the original operator may have thrown away some of the information contained in its input. In the case of differentiation and integration, and also of the linear systems that depend on them, this is true of the original DC level from which the input signal starts, knowledge of which is lost after differentiation. But the point is somewhat academic, since in practice one is always considering spans of time that are short in comparison with the age of the system itself. By a logical extension of the D notation, one can express a single integration as D^{-1}, two successive integrations as D^{-2}, and so on. Integration is generally more awkward to perform from first principles than differentiation, and lists of standard results must often be consulted (for example Petit Bois, 1961). Even so, many extremely important functions [$\exp(-t^2)$ is a good example] have integrals that cannot be expressed analytically, in terms of other known functions, and recourse must be had to tabulated values, or reiterative computation. Fortunately this is not true of the three classes of function that we are mostly concerned with, whose integrals can be deduced immediately by consideration of their differentials. Thus

$$\mathrm{D}^{-1}(kt^n) = \frac{k}{n+1}\, t^{n+1}$$

(except when $n = -1$), and

$$\mathrm{D}^{-1}[A \exp(kt)] = \frac{A}{k} \exp(kt).$$

For sine waves,

$$\mathrm{D}^{-1}[A \exp(\mathrm{i}\omega t)] = \frac{A}{\mathrm{i}\omega} \exp(\mathrm{i}\omega t), \quad \text{or} \quad \frac{-\mathrm{i}}{\omega} A \exp(\mathrm{i}\omega t).$$

In other words, integration introduces a 90° phase *lag*, and the amplitude is *reduced* in proportion to the frequency.

Transfer functions

If a system is known to be linear, so that multiplying the input by a fixed factor will multiply the output by the same factor, then the ratio of the output to the input will be constant whatever the size of the input, and will therefore provide an economical description of the operation it performs. For example, if we apply a sine wave $A \exp(\mathrm{i}\omega t)$ to the input of a differentiator D, we know that the output will be given by $\mathrm{i}\omega A \exp(\mathrm{i}\omega t)$. Thus the ratio of the output to the input is simply $\mathrm{i}\omega$, which is independent of the amplitude of the original wave (but not its frequency). If the input is sinusoidal, this ratio as a function of frequency is called the *frequency transfer function*, and is characteristic of the filter concerned. There are two ways in which a frequency transfer function can be plotted. The first is called the *Bode plot* and consists of a pair of graphs, one being of the ratio of the amplitudes of the output and input waves (disregarding phase), and the other a graph of phase alone, both plotted as a function of frequency. For a reason that will be explained in a moment, it is normal to use logarithmic axes for frequency and for amplitude ratio, but linear axes for phase; amplitude ratio is more commonly called *gain*, although this word is sometimes also used to denote the complex ratio of output to input that also includes a phase component. Figure A2.25 shows the Bode plot of the operator D: it can be seen that the phase is constant and equal to $+\frac{1}{2}\pi$ throughout, whereas the gain increases with frequency on a straight line with slope $+1$. Figure A2.26 shows a similar plot for the operator D^{-1}: here the phase is everywhere $-\frac{1}{2}\pi$, and the gain plot has a slope of -1.

Bode plots are extremely useful in deriving the overall frequency response of a system consisting of a number of filters in series. Suppose we have two such filters, of gains G_1 and G_2 (figure A2.27). Then the output of the first in response to a sine wave of amplitude A will be another wave of amplitude $\mathrm{G}_1 A$; the output of the second will then be of amplitude

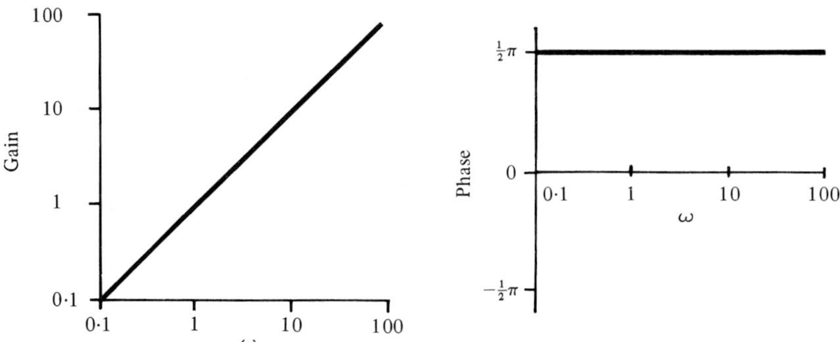

Figure A2.25. Bode plot of the operator D.

G_2G_1A, so that the gain of the whole (G) is simply the product of the two individual gains (G_1G_2). The advantage of using logarithmic gain plots can now be seen, since $\lg G = \lg G_1 + \lg G_2$, so that the Bode gain plot for the two series can be simply obtained by adding their separate responses. On the other hand, any phase change produced by the first filter will be *added* (not multiplied) to any produced by the second, and so phase is plotted with linear rather than logarithmic axes.

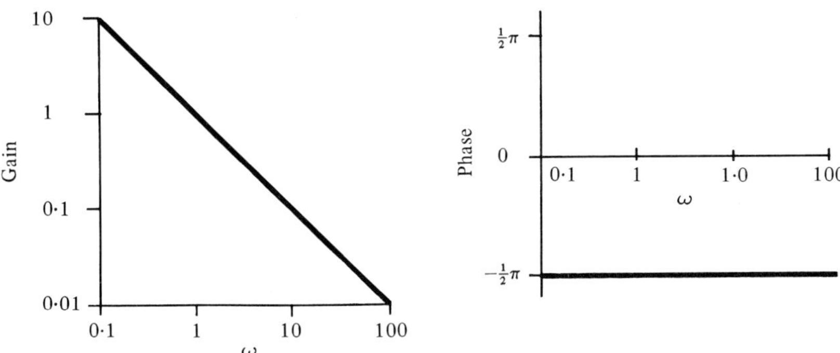

Figure A2.26. Bode plots of the operator D^{-1}.

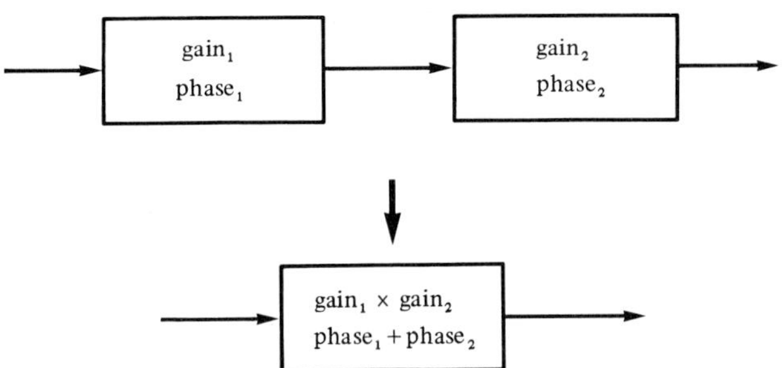

Figure A2.27. Reduction of two filters in series to a single equivalent filter. The overall gain is the *product* of the individual gains: the total phase is the *sum* of that produced by each filter.

The second method of plotting frequency-response functions, the *Nyquist plot*, enables one to show gain and phase in the same diagram. Here the gain is plotted on the complex plane, so that at a particular frequency the amplitude ratio is shown by the distance of the point from the origin, and the phase by its angle to the x axis (figure A2.28). Thus a particular filter will trace out its own characteristic locus as the frequency is varied from $\omega = 0$ to infinity. The Nyquist plots for D and D^{-1} are not particularly interesting (figure A2.29), and this method really comes into its own for very much more complex systems and particularly for the evaluation of feedback devices; this application is described later.

It is common practice—though one that is deprecated by mathematical purists—to use the term 'transfer function' for the expression that represents the ratio of output to input, without specifying the kind of input to be applied. Thus, instead of saying "the output in response to an input $f(t)$ is given by $D[f(t)]$", we can say simply that the transfer function *is* D. The justification for this is, as we shall see, that in such expressions D can be treated exactly as one treats algebraic constants [so that we can write $(D+k)f$ for $D(f)+kf$, and so that D^{-1} can be treated as if it meant $1/D$] and that this leads both to economy in describing and solving complex systems, and also to a better comprehension of their operation: for these reasons the student would be well advised to take the plunge in adopting such procedures despite the purists. [Proofs that D does indeed obey the ordinary laws of algebraic manipulation may be found in Brown (1965)]. Nevertheless, many authors are hesitant about using D in this apparently reckless way and prefer to convert it into an s or a p first—they are effectively equivalent—to save appearances.

Of course, if it is known that the input is only of sinusoidal waves, one need have no hesitation at all since we have already seen that under these circumstances D is simply equivalent to multiplication by $i\omega$.

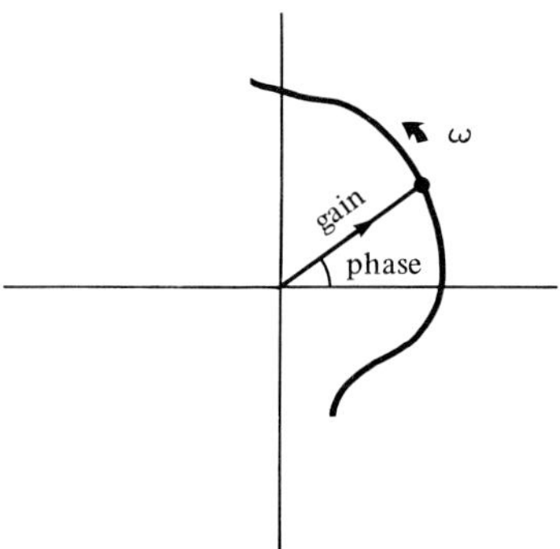

Figure A2.28. The Nyquist plot enables one to show gain and phase in the same diagram.

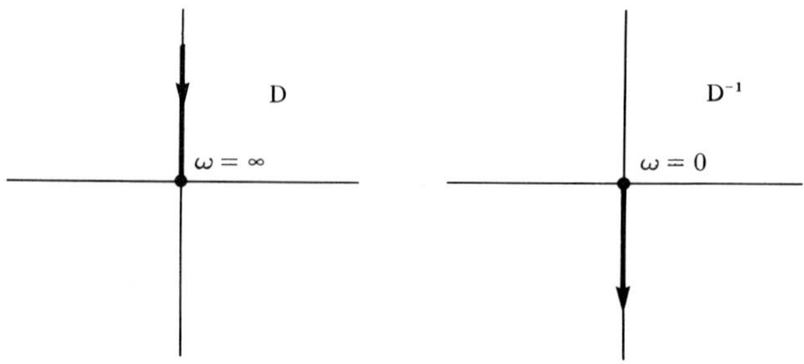

Figure A2.29. Nyquist plots for D and D^{-1}.

It turns out, in fact, that *all* physically realisable signals can be expressed as the sum of a number of sine waves of different frequencies [by a process of *Fourier synthesis*: see for example Bracewell (1965)] in a manner reminiscent of approximation by power series, and so it follows that the operator D can be treated as if it were an algebraic quantity *whatever* the shape out the input signal.

The existence of Fourier synthesis also provides a further justifaction for the measurement of frequency transfer functions as a useful experimental procedure. It is easy to see why the frequency transfer function provides a *complete* description of a linear system, in the sense that it can enable the experimenter to predict the output that will result from any conceivable pattern of input: all we have to do is to analyse the given input signal into its constituent sine waves, calculate from our transfer function how each wave will be treated by the system, and then add the resultant waves together to synthesise the consequent output (figure A2.30). In other words, once we know how a system responds to sine waves, we know at once how it will respond to any other input than can be imagined, within the limits of linearity.

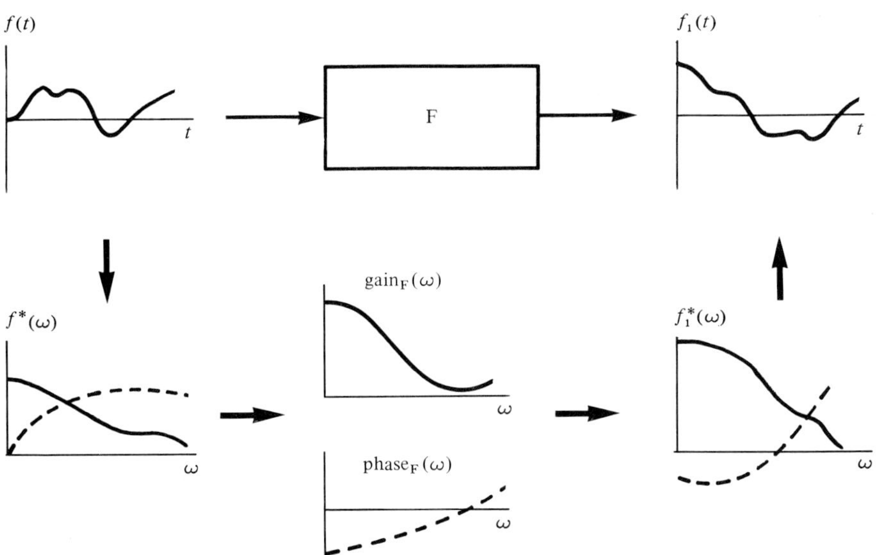

Figure A2.30. Knowledge of the frequency response of a system (F) enables one to predict the output resulting from any conceivable input $f(t)$. The amplitude and phase components of f are first found (f^*) by Fourier analysis: these are then combined, in the usual way, with the gain and phase components G and ϕ of the frequency response of the system, to yield the amplitude and phase components of the output (f_1^*). The output itself can then be found by Fourier synthesis of these frequency components (f_1). Solid lines represent amplitude or gain plots in logarithmic form; broken lines show phase.

Transients

In addition to the three standard types of function whose differentials and integrals have just been considered, one more class must be added that is of particular importance in systems analysis: the class of *transients*. These are functions—typically of time—that show a single discontinuity of some sort at one value of the input variable. The fundamental transient function is the *step* (figure A2.31), which has the value zero for times less than $t = 0$ (an arbitrary origin at the point of discontinuity) and unit value elsewhere. The integral of the step is the *ramp*, which is zero at times less than zero, but thereafter increases linearly with a slope of one. The differential of the step is the *impulse* (delta function), which is vanishingly narrow and infinitely high, yet contrives to have unit area. These three functions (impulse, step, and ramp) form a family related to each other by the operator D; the family can be indefinitely extended in the same way at each end, but, in practice, only the integral of the ramp (the parabolic ramp) and the differential of the impulse (the double impulse) are encountered at all frequently.

In real life, because of the smoothing effects of noise that were mentioned earlier, none of these functions is ever found in its pure form. Real steps are always rounded, real impulses have finite width and height, and the ramp takes a finite time to get going. Nevertheless, the response of a system to one or other of these transient inputs often affords a simple and economical way of assigning it to one of the standard classes of linear filter, as we shall see in the next section. For more complex systems, analysis of

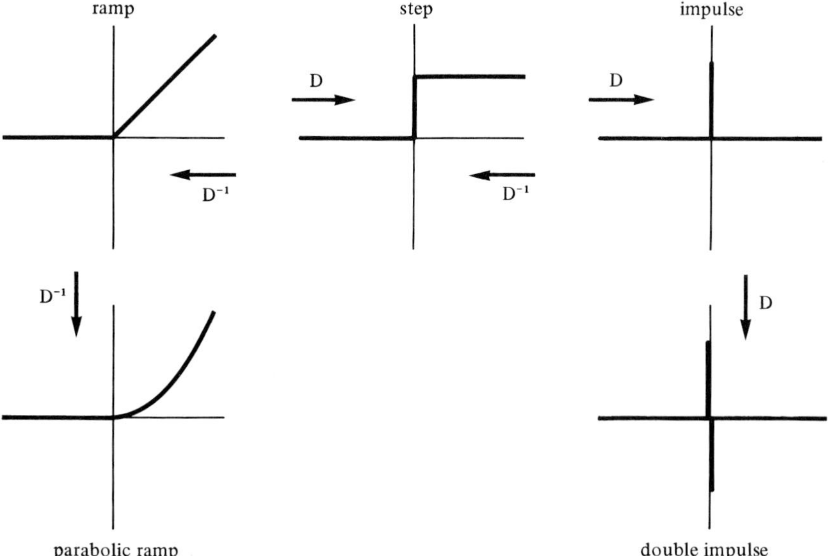

Figure A2.31. Five elementary transient functions, and their interrelationships via the operator D.

transient responses generally proves more difficult than that of frequency transfer functions. A further difficulty is that, since the transient functions have very large higher differentials, they are likely to reveal nonlinearities in in the system, if it contains elements that are sensitive to rate of change.

A2.5 Linear first order building blocks

Consider the transfer function of the system shown in figure A2.32. An input signal $x(t)$ is passed through two filters in parallel: the first is a differentiator, so its output is $\mathrm{D}[x(t)]$; the other is a device having a fixed gain k and so its output is simply $kx(t)$. The two signals are added together (a circle with a Σ sign is commonly used in diagrams to represent a summation point) and so the output of the whole network is given by $y(t) = k[x(t)] + \mathrm{D}[x(t)]$. We can write this as $(k+\mathrm{D})x(t)$, so the transfer function is given by the ratio of the output to the input, which is simply $(k+\mathrm{D})$. If we want to know how this sytem will respond to sinusoidal inputs, we need only substitute $\mathrm{i}\omega$ for D, giving a frequency transfer function of $(k+\mathrm{i}\omega)$. Bode plots of this function are shown in figure A2.33. One can quite often get a rough idea of the form of a frequency response simply by inspection of the expression for the frequency transfer function. What is needed is to ask first what will happen when the frequency is very low, and then what will happen if it is very high.

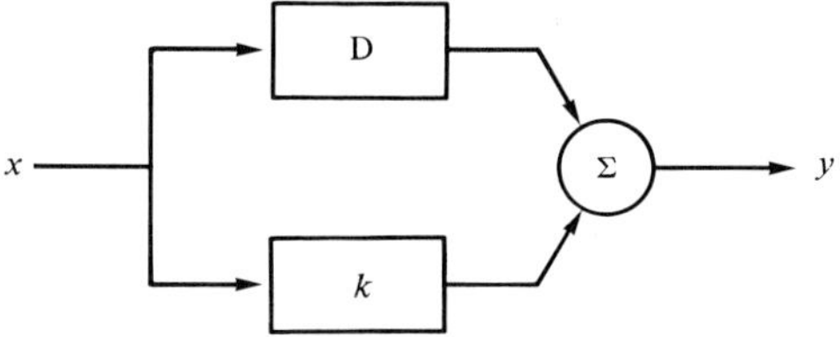

Figure A2.32. A system consisting of a differentiator D in parallel with a filter of constant gain k.

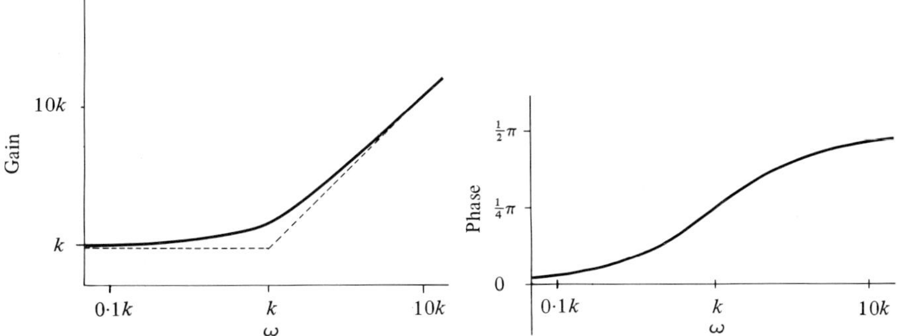

Figure A2.33. Bode plots (gain and phase as a function of ω) of the system $(\mathrm{D}+k)$. The broken lines show asymptotes, meeting at the characteristic frequency k: the right-hand one has unit slope.

In the first case, as ω tends to zero, the contribution of the iω term in the expression will clearly become negligibly small: so that at frequencies much lower than $\omega = k$ the system will behave as if it had a constant gain of k and no phase shift. If ω is much larger than k, the iω term will dominate, and the whole system will behave like a differentiator, with gain proportional to ω, and a $\frac{1}{2}\pi$ phase advance. At intermediate frequencies the gain and phase change smoothly from one condition to the other. In particular, at $\omega = k$, the gain is exactly $\frac{1}{2}$ and the phase lead is equal to $\frac{1}{4}\pi$ (or 45°): this is called the *characteristic frequency* of the filter. These features can be verified in the Bode plots of figure A2.33.

A more commonly occurring linear filter is actually the inverse of the one we have just considered, namely $(k+\mathrm{D})^{-1}$. By exactly similar procedures it is easy to verify that at low frequencies this device has a gain of $1/k$ and no phase lag, while at high frequencies it behaves like an integrator, with a gain that falls off linearly with ω, and a phase lag that ultimately reaches $\frac{1}{2}\pi$ (figure A2.34). This is known as a *first-order low-pass filter*, since it allows low frequencies through intact while attenuating high frequencies, and is probably the commonest of all the first-order filters, as a component of sluggish systems with friction, resistance, or damping: discussion of how these responses arise in practice is reserved for a later section. 'First-order' here simply means that the transfer function contains only terms in D, and not D^2, D^3, etc.

Systems that behave as if they consisted of a first-order low-pass filter and a differentiator in series are common enough to be considered a standard form in their own right, although they could of course be decomposed into their two constituent parts. The transfer function is given by $\mathrm{D}/(k+\mathrm{D})$, and so the frequency response is $\mathrm{i}\omega/(k+\mathrm{i}\omega)$. At high frequencies, the gain approaches unity and the phase tends to zero (the two iω terms cancel out), whereas at low frequencies the gain is proportional to ω, with a phase advance of $\frac{1}{2}\pi$ (figure A2.35). This filter

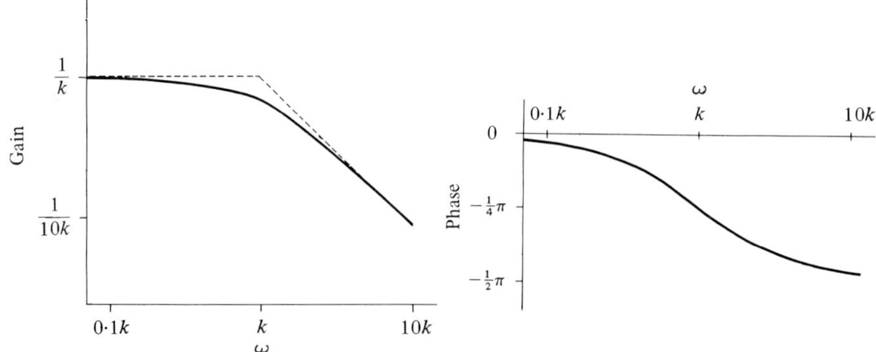

Figure A2.34. Bode plots, as in figure A2.33, of the first-order low-pass system $(\mathrm{D}+k)^{-1}$.

thus tends to suppress low frequencies while passing high frequencies, and is called a *first-order high-pass filter.* It is characteristic of many systems showing adaptation.

These three filters behave in characteristic ways in response to transient inputs such as steps. As might be anticipated, $(k + \mathrm{D})$ shows a step response that is simply the sum of a step of height k and the differential of a step—that is, an impulse (figure A2.36). Its inverse, $(k + \mathrm{D})^{-1}$, responds with what is sometimes called an exponential step: it is a function that rises exponentially from zero to its final value of $1/k$ (figure A2.36). The time constant of the exponential rise is given by $\tau = 1/k$. The high-pass filter $\mathrm{D}/(k + \mathrm{D})$ responds to a step with what can be called an exponential pulse: this function starts with a sudden jump to a value of unity, and then decays exponentially to zero, again with a time constant of $1/k$.

There is often a general relationship for any linear system between its step response and its frequency response. Very low frequencies correspond to the behaviour of the system at times long after the step has occurred: thus if the low-frequency gain of the system is zero, one can be sure that the step response will also eventually decline to zero (as in the case of the high-pass filter). Similarly, the behaviour immediately after the step is closely related to the high-frequency response: thus if the high-frequency response is like that of an integrator (as in the case of the low-pass filter) the step response will start with a ramp; whereas, if the high frequencies are unattenuated, the initial response will be step-like. Finally, bumps on

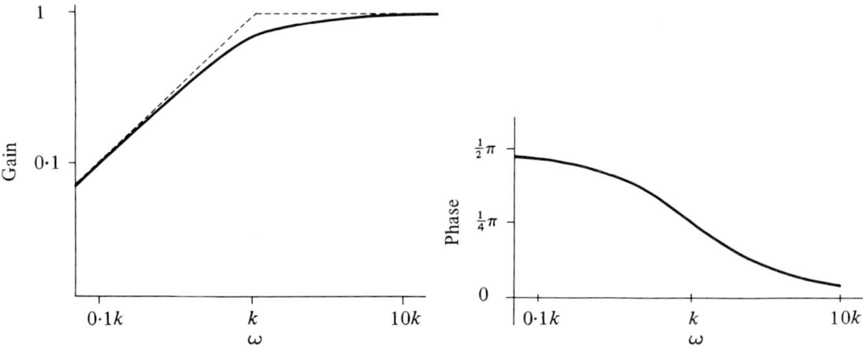

Figure A2.35. Bode plots, as in figure A2.33, of the first-order high-pass system $\mathrm{D}/(k + \mathrm{D})$.

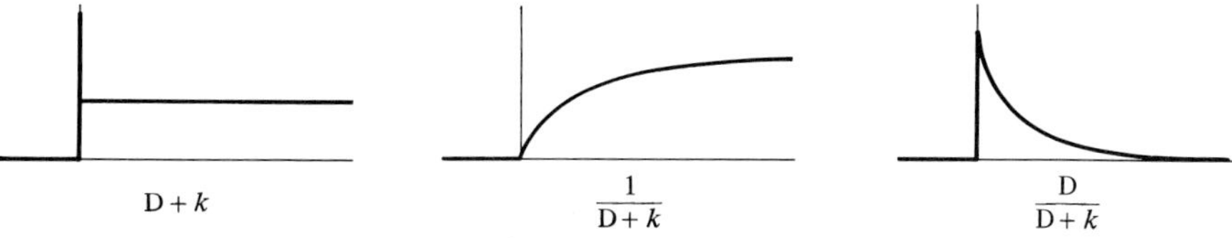

Figure A2.36. Step responses of the three first-order systems.

the frequency transfer function will correspond with transient oscillations in the step response, as we shall see in the next section when we consider second-order systems.

A2.6 Linear second-order systems

Second-order systems are those that contain terms like D^2, as well, possibly, as terms in D and constants. A trivial way in which this can arise is if we have two first-order systems in series (figure A2.37). Here the transfer function is given by $[(k_1+D)(k_2+D)]^{-1}$, and its Bode plots can easily be sketched by summing the frequency responses of its two components, as can be seen in the figure. At low frequencies the gain is $(k_1k_2)^{-1}$ and the phase gradually edges its way down to a final lag, at high frequencies, of 180°. As would be expected, the step response starts as a parabolic ramp, and eventually reaches a height of $(k_1k_2)^{-1}$. Such a system does not show any radically new properties.

The general form for the basic second-order operator is given by $(D^2+2\lambda D+\mu^2)^{-1}$: by choosing the values of the parameters λ and μ appropriately, some novel behaviour becomes apparent. We can try to factorise the expression as $(D+a)^{-1}(D+b)^{-1}$, where $a = \lambda+s$ and $b = \lambda-s$; ($s^2 = \lambda^2-\mu^2$). If $\lambda > \mu$, s is real and the system behaves like the two first-order systems in series that we have just considered. If λ is

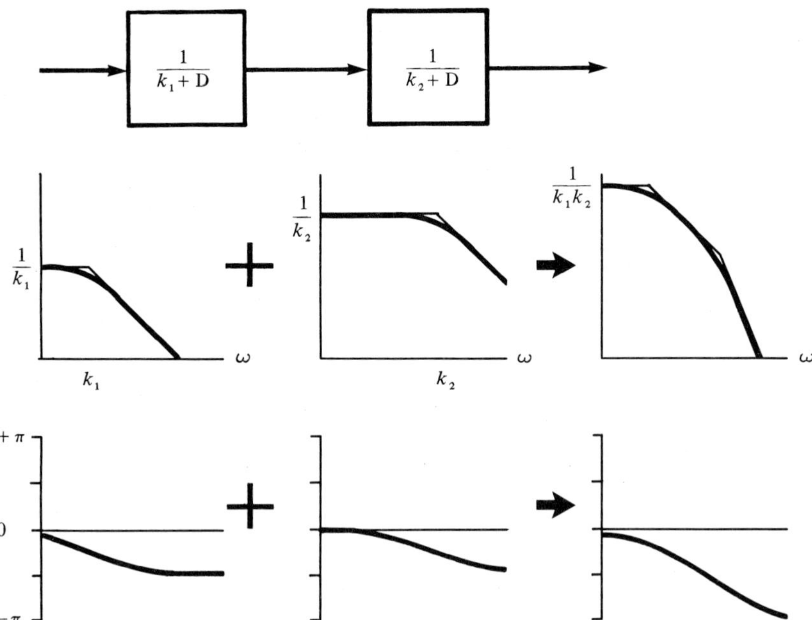

Figure A2.37. Frequency response of a series arrangement of two first-order low-pass systems: at high frequencies the Bode plot of the gain has a slope of −2, and the phase lag approaches $-\pi$.

much greater than μ, so that a and b are widely separated, the frequency response shows three distinct regions: a flat region at low frequencies, a slope of -1 at intermediate frequencies, and a final slope of -2: The step response is then rather sluggish (a, figure A2.38). As λ and μ are made more nearly equal, the frequency response tends to turn over more sharply from the flat region into the final descent, and the step response speeds up, until $\lambda = \mu$, when the system behaves like two identical first-orders in series. But if $\lambda < \mu$, it begins to behave rather differently. s is then imaginary, and may be written as $\mathrm{i}\sigma$, where $\sigma^2 = \mu^2 - \lambda^2$. Thus the frequency response becomes

$$\frac{1}{[\lambda+\mathrm{i}(\omega+\sigma)][\lambda+\mathrm{i}(\omega-\sigma)]},$$

from which it is clear that it will go through a maximum near $\omega = \sigma$, and in fact a plot of the gain shows that it does indeed rise to a peak before the final descent (c, figure A2.38). The step response shows a corresponding transient oscillation of the same frequency, dying away with time constant $1/\lambda$. If λ is made smaller and smaller, the contribution of the $\mathrm{i}(\omega-\sigma)$ term becomes relatively more and more important, and the peak becomes more and more prominent. At the same time, the transient oscillations in the step response take longer and longer to die away. Finally, if λ becomes vanishingly small, so that the frequency response is simply given by $(\mu^2 - \omega^2)^{-1}$, the peak becomes infinitely high and the oscillations in the transient response do not die out at all: the filter has turned into an oscillator of frequency $\omega = \mu$.

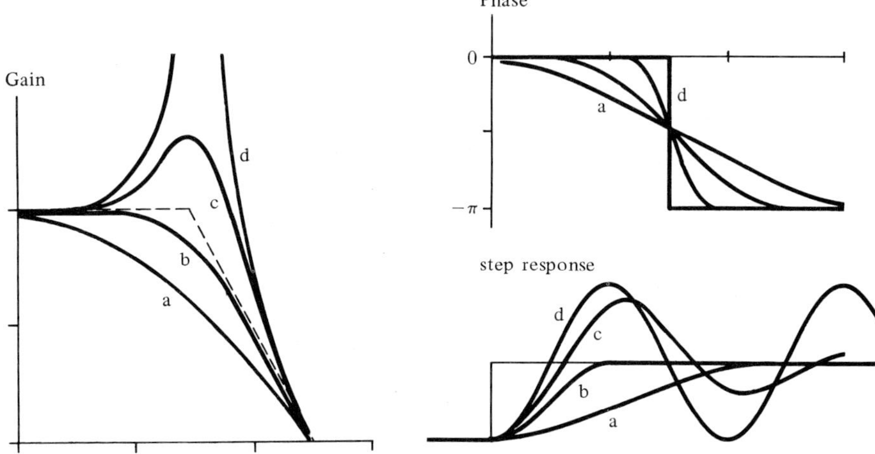

Figure A2.38. Responses of the general second-order system for different relations between λ and μ: Bode plots of gain and phase; step response. The four conditions shown are: a, $\lambda > \mu$ (overdamped); b, $\lambda = \mu$ (critically damped); c, $\lambda < \mu$ (underdamped); d, $\lambda = 0$ (undamped).

Thus, unlike the first-order filters, the behaviour of the basic second-order system depends very critically on the values of its parameters, which have a *qualitative* effect on how it responds.

A2.7 Transfer functions of actual systems

Many kinds of physical systems can be described elegantly and economically by using transfer functions. In this section the transfer functions of the three main types of passive electrical and mechanical components are set out, with methods of analysis for systems in which these components are joined in a network.

Electrical components and systems

There are exactly three linear passive electrical components: the resistor, the capacitor, and the inductor. It is convenient to think of them as devices with an input consisting of the current I that flows through them, and an output voltage U that is developed across them as a consequence. Then the transfer function for the device is given as usual by the ratio of the output to the input, that is by U/I: this transfer function is called the *impedance* of the device, and is often assigned the symbol Z. Each of the three types of device has a characteristic transfer function that can easily be obtained from its known physical properties. Thus the behaviour of a resistor of R ohms is governed by Ohm's law, so that

$$U = IR, \qquad \text{or} \qquad Z = U/I = R.$$

Thus the transfer function or impedance of a resistor is given by its resistance, and is a constant. For a capacitor, we have that the charge it carries is equal to the product of its capacitance C and the voltage across it. The charge is equal to the integral of the current that it has received, and so we can write:

$$CU = \mathrm{D}^{-1}I, \quad \text{or} \quad Z = U/I = (C\mathrm{D})^{-1}.$$

The capacitor thus effectively acts as an integrator. In the case of the inductor, the voltage across it is the product of its inductance L and the rate of change of current. Thus

$$U = L\mathrm{D}I, \qquad \text{or} \quad Z = L\mathrm{D}.$$

The inductor therefore behaves as a differentiator (figure A2.39).

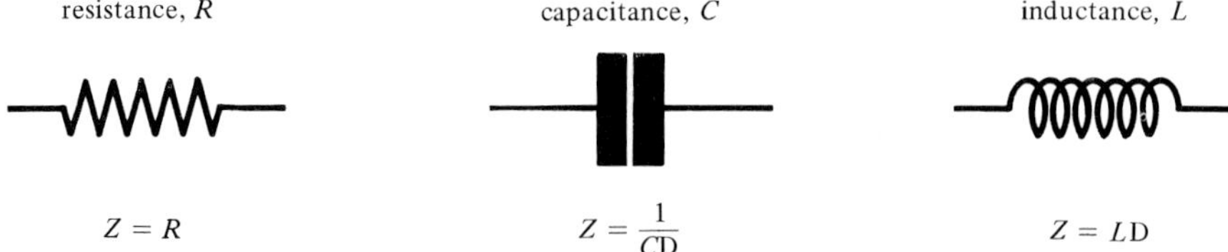

Figure A2.39. The transfer function (impedance, Z) of each of the three linear passive electrical components.

To examine the properties of networks composed of these three components, we need to have rules for combining the impedances of devices that are coupled together. Two rules are sufficient for practically all cases: the *series* rule states that the impedance of two components in series is the sum of their individual impedances, while the *parallel* rule states that the reciprocal of the impedance of two devices in parallel is the sum of the reciprocals of the impedances of the individual components (figure A2.40). Thus a capacitor of capacitance C in series with a resistor of resistance R will have a joint impedance of $R+(1/C\mathrm{D})$, whereas if connected in parallel their impedance will be $1/[(1/R)+C\mathrm{D}]$, or $(1/C)[(1/RC)+\mathrm{D}]^{-1}$, that is of the low-pass form $(k+\mathrm{D})^{-1}$.

Actual electrical filters generally accept a voltage as input, and produce another voltage as output. Such a circuit very often consists of a *voltage divider* (figure A2.41) in which the ratio of output to input is given by

$$\frac{Z_1}{Z_1+Z_2}\,.$$

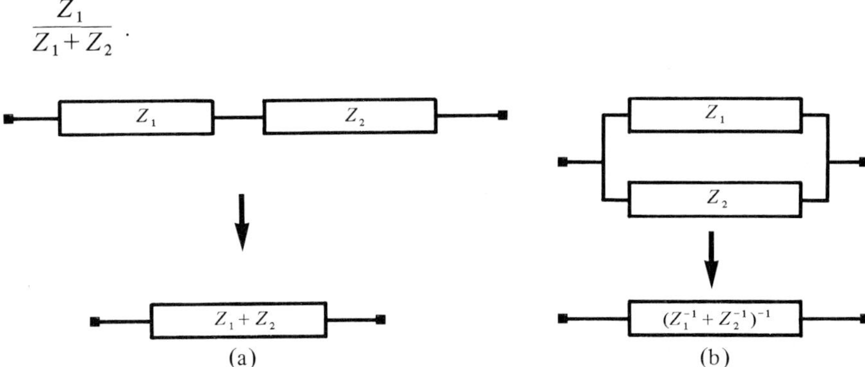

Figure A2.40. (a) The *series* rule and, (b) the *parallel* rule for combining impedances (Z).

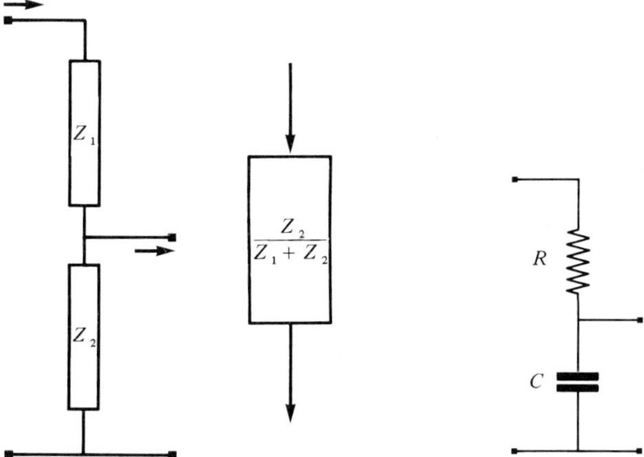

Figure A2.41. The voltage divider and its transfer function.

Figure A2.42. Electrical low-pass filter.

Thus, for the circuit in figure A2.42, the transfer function is given by

$$\frac{(CD)^{-1}}{R+(CD)^{-1}}, \qquad \text{or} \qquad \frac{1}{(RC)[(RC)^{-1}+D]},$$

which is a simple low-pass filter of characteristic frequency $(RC)^{-1}$, and hence of time constant RC. In more complicated cases it is best first to reduce systematically any series or parallel combinations to single impedances and then to evaluate the potential divider: an example is shown in figure A2.43.

$$\text{Transfer function} = \frac{R}{R+(1/R+CD)^{-1}} = \frac{1+RCD}{2+RCD}$$

$$= \frac{1}{RC}\left\{\frac{1}{2/RC+D}+\frac{D}{2/RC+D}\right\}.$$

The transfer function of this system is thus the sum of a low-pass and a high-pass filter. Bode plots and a step response are shown in figure A2.44.

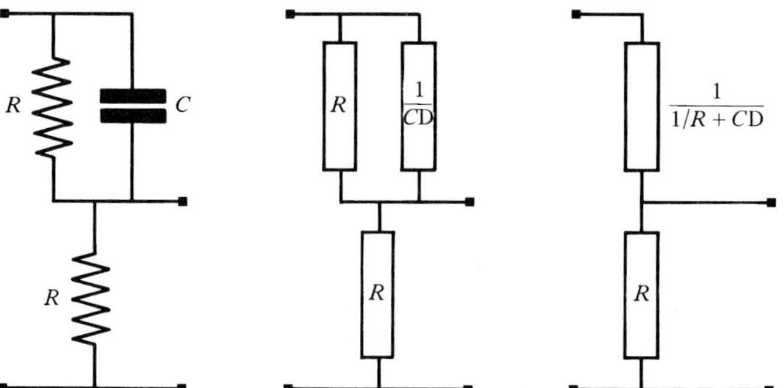

Figure A2.43. The systematic reduction of a circuit to single impedances.

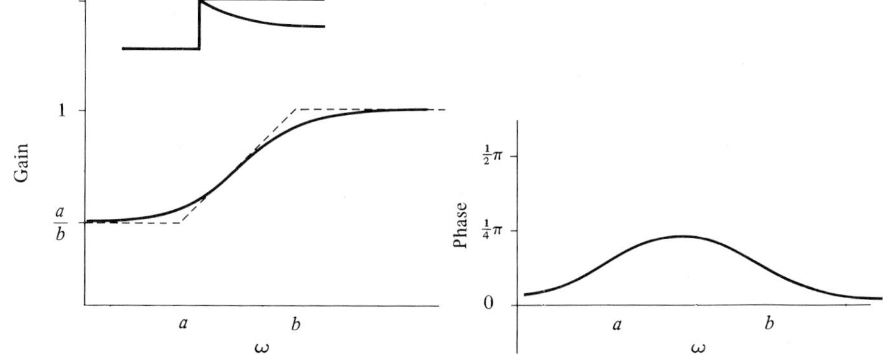

Figure A2.44. Bode plots of the system $(D+a)/(D+b)$, with a step response shown in the inset.

The system can be seen to behave in a way reminiscent of a partially adapting sensory organ like a stretch receptor.

Finally, if a circuit contains all three types of component it will normally give a second-order response (figure A2.45).

$$\text{Transfer function} = \frac{(C\mathrm{D})^{-1}}{[L\mathrm{D} + 2R + (C\mathrm{D})^{-1}]} = \frac{1}{LC\mathrm{D}^2 + 2RC\mathrm{D} + 1}$$

$$= \frac{1}{LC}\left[\frac{1}{\mathrm{D}^2 + 2(R/L)\mathrm{D} + 1/LC}\right].$$

This is the transfer function that was discussed in the previous section, with $\lambda = R/L$ and $\mu^2 = 1/LC$.

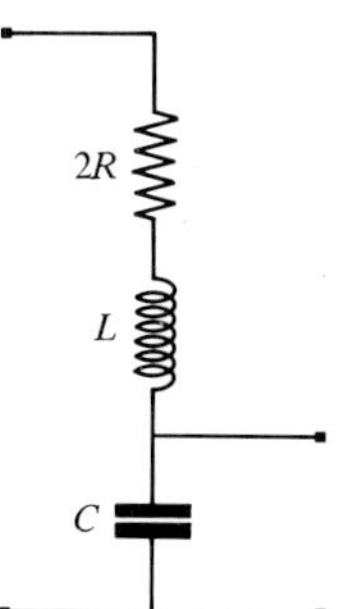

Figure A2.45. A circuit containing all three types of component, resulting in a second-order response.

Mechanical components and systems

It happens that there are also exactly three passive linear mechanical elements: they are the *elastic* element (spring), the *inertial* element (mass), and the dissipative *damping* element (friction or viscosity). For convenience, we shall deal here only with motion along a straight line, although precisely analogous results can be obtained for torsional systems by appropriate changes of unit. It is convenient to treat mechanical components as having a force input F and responding with an output of displacement x. The transfer function describing the component is then given by x/F, and this is often called mechanical *compliance*. It may seem paradoxical that mechanical compliance should thus be equivalent to electrical impedance: but of course a highly compliant spring impedes the transmission of *force* in exactly the same way as a resistor impedes *current*. It may also be objected that from the physical point of view there are certain similarities between voltage and force, and current and velocity: but for the purpose of practical solutions the present formulation is very much more convenient because mechanical networks can, as we shall see, be analysed in this way with exactly the same series and parallel rules as electrical ones: this is not the case if force is taken to be equivalent to voltage. The reason for this is that, if we have two mechanical elements joined in series, the total displacement across them is the sum of their individual displacements, while the force transmitted is equal in both. In the same way, two series electrical components share the same current, but the voltage across the two is the sum of the voltages across each. This functional similarity between voltage and displacement and current and force makes for such increased ease of application that it is undoubtedly preferable to the 'purer' alternative.

A linear elastic element obeying Hooke's law embodies the relation $F = Ex$, where E is the *stiffness*: thus the transfer function is given by $1/E$. With ideal friction or viscosity r the force developed is proportional to the velocity, or rate of change of displacement, so we have:

$$F = r\mathrm{D}x, \qquad \text{or} \quad Z = \frac{x}{F} = \frac{1}{r\mathrm{D}} .$$

Such a device therefore acts as an integrator. Inertia produces forces that are proportional to the acceleration, so that

$$F = M\mathrm{D}^2x, \qquad \text{or} \quad Z = \frac{1}{M\mathrm{D}^2},$$

where M is the inertia of the element.

These results are tabulated in figure A2.46, together with the symbols commonly used to represent them in diagrams. It is important to note that one 'end' of an inertial element is always—quite literally—'earthed', because the forces generated by such an element are normally the result of accelerations relative to the earth's inertial frame of reference.

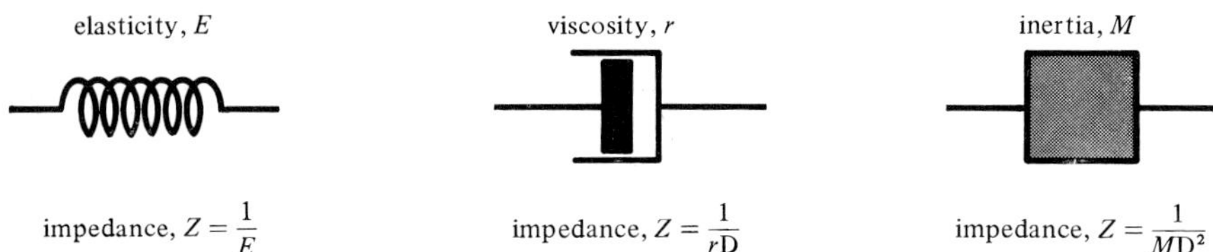

Figure A2.46. Characteristics of the three passive linear mechanical elements.

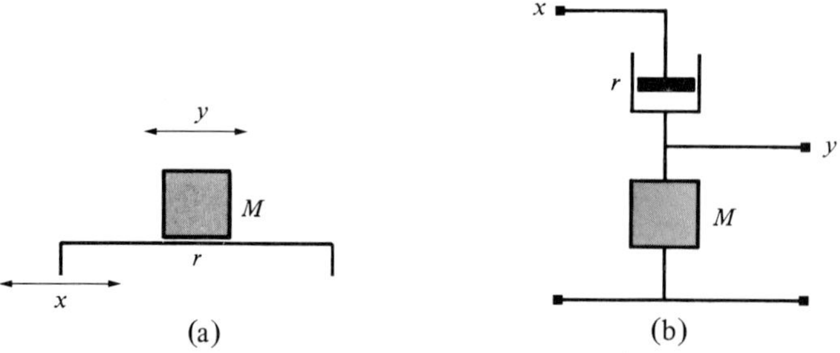

Figure A2.47. (a) A mass M resting frictionally (r) on a movable table. The relationship between the movement of the table (x), and the resultant movement of the mass (y) can be represented by the equivalent mechanical circuit shown in (b).

As mentioned above, the same rules for simplifying and analysing mechanical circuits exist as in the case of electrical ones. As an example, consider the behaviour of a mass M resting frictionally (r) on a movable horizontal surface (figure A2.47). Horizontal movements of the surface—the input—will cause movements of the mass—the output— and the whole arrangement forms a 'potential divider' (strictly, displacement divider) of the form shown in the figure. The transfer function can thus be calculated as:

$$\frac{1/M\mathrm{D}^2}{1/r\mathrm{D}+1/M\mathrm{D}^2}=\frac{r}{M\mathrm{D}+r}=\frac{r}{M}\left(\frac{1}{\mathrm{D}+r/M}\right),$$

and so the whole thing acts as a first-order low-pass filter. Circuits having all three types of mechanical element will be of second order at least: an example is shown in figure A2.48.

$$\text{Transfer function}=\frac{(M\mathrm{D}^2+2r\mathrm{D})^{-1}}{1/E+(M\mathrm{D}^2+2r\mathrm{D})^{-1}}=\frac{E}{M\mathrm{D}^2+2r\mathrm{D}+E}$$

$$=\frac{E}{M}\left[\frac{1}{\mathrm{D}^2+2(r/M)\mathrm{D}+E/M}\right].$$

The exact behaviour of this system will depend on the relationship between r/M and $(E/M)^{1/2}$. If the damping is sufficiently small, so that $(r/M)<(E/M)^{1/2}$, it will tend to show transient oscillations: the 'critical' value of the damping (that is, when transient oscillations just disappear) is when $r^2=EM$. If the damping is further increased, the step response will be slowed and lengthened. In real mechanical problems of this type—the design of motorcar suspensions is a good example—it is often considered desirable to adjust the value of the damping coefficient until the system is critically damped: this affords a compromise between a system that takes a long time to settle because of its sluggishness, and one that takes a long time because it shows transient oscillations (figure A2.38).

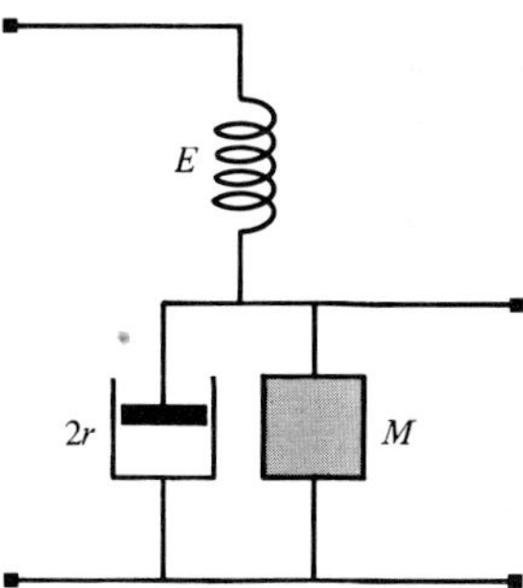

Figure A2.48. An example of a circuit containing all three types of mechanical element, and thus of second order.

A2.8 Feedback systems

Physiologists are of course well aware that feedback of the output of the signal so that it forms part of its own input is a common feature of natural control systems. The benefit of this kind of arrangement is that the desired relationship between the input and output of the system is less easily upset than it would otherwise be by noise and other disturbances that may be added to the output. The behaviour of systems that incorporate this feature can easily be analysed with the techniques already presented: the study of feedback systems is a very important one in its own right, with a huge literature and countless numbers of practical applications: no more than the barest outline can be presented here, and the interested reader could go on to read MacMillan (1955), de Barr (1962), Brown (1965), or Riggs (1970), amongst a host of other useful accounts.

Figure A2.49 shows the essential configuration of a system having a feedback loop: this is a *negative* feedback system, because the output y is subtracted from the input x. So we have: $y = \mathrm{B}(x+y)$, or that the transfer function y/x of the whole system is given by $\mathrm{B}/(\mathrm{B}+1)$. Thus, if for example the element B was actually a differentiator, the transfer function of the system would be given by $\mathrm{D}/(1+\mathrm{D})$: in other words, a first-order high-pass filter with a characteristic frequency of unity. Thus the addition of feedback can make the behaviour of the complete system differ quite markedly from that of the forward pathway—in this case the operator B—usually, as in this case, by limiting the overall gain.

Under some circumstances, however, it may have quite the opposite effect. Consider first what would happen if in figure A2.48 we *added* the output to the input instead of subtracting it, thus making a *positive* feedback system. Let us suppose for the moment that B is simply a device of constant gain k, introducing no phase changes. If a step input were applied, the instantaneous output would be a step of amplitude k; going round the loop, this would be added to the input and multiplied again by k to give a subsequent output $k(1+k)$; and this output would in turn be added to the input, etc, etc. Thus the final output, when everything had reached a steady state, would be given by the extended product

$$k\{1+k[1+k(1+\ldots)]\}\,.$$

If k is greater than unity, the value of this product will be infinite, so that even the smallest input will give an output that grows explosively to an

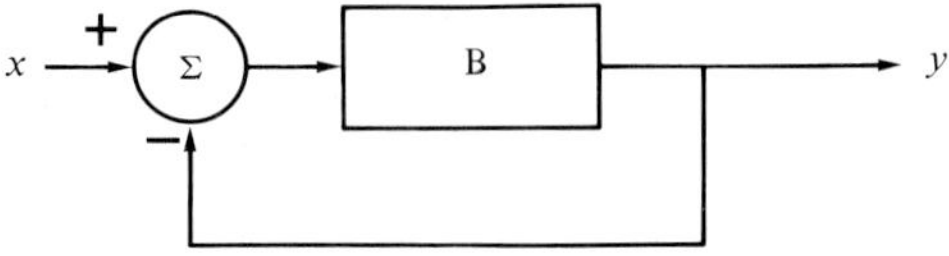

Figure A2.49. A system with a negative feedback loop.

arbitrarily large value—limited in practice by the ever-present saturation of real devices. Positive feedback systems are thus liable, if the forward gain is too large, to produce violent *instability*. This is not a useful process in homeostasis, but can be put to use where it is specifically required that a small input should be able to trigger off a very large output. Thus in the nerve axon a small depolarisation can cause an increased sodium permeability, which causes a further depolarisation, and hence a further increase in permeability, and so on: the net result is an amplification of the original potential change and an explosive propagation of the action potential.

However, in certain circumstances even a negative feedback system can show the same kind of behaviour. Suppose for example that B in figure A2.49 consisted of three low-pass filters in series, as in figure A2.50. Their transfer function would then show a total high-frequency phase lag of $3 \times 90°$, or 270°, so clearly at some intermediate frequency the phase lag must pass through a value of exactly 180°. Now a phase shift of 180° is of course exactly the same thing as an inversion of the original wave, so that at this critical frequency (ω_c) the effect will be essentially to *reverse*, as well as to attenuate, the feedback signal. But, if this inverted sine wave is subtracted from the input, the actual effect will be of addition, since $-(-B) = +B$. Thus, despite the apparent negative sign of the feedback, at ω_c the feedback will in effect be positive, and instability is likely to occur. Whether or not instability does actually occur will depend on the gain of B. If this is less than unity at ω_c, the system will not show an explosive response (although it may well show transient oscillations at around ω_c in frequency), whereas, if the gain of B is greater than unity at this frequency, these oscillations will steadily build up in size to an amplitude that is determined only by the saturation of the components of the system. Such an oscillation is called a *limit cycle*, and is typical of the response of a feedback system with a high gain and large phase lags. A good example is a central-heating system controlled by a simple thermostat, where the on/off nature of the thermostat produces in effect a very high gain around the desired temperature, while the thermal capacity and insulating properties of the ambient air together produce very large phase lags.

There is a simple test that can be applied to a feedback system to see if it is liable to go into unstable oscillation, called the Nyquist criterion.

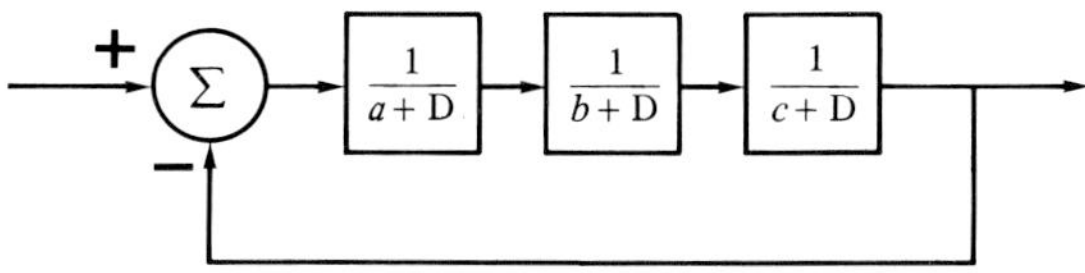

Figure A2.50. Three low-pass filters in series.

If the open-loop response (that is, what the transfer function would be if the feedback were removed: in this case B) is plotted on a Nyquist diagram, one can look to see whether the locus ever crosses the 180° axis (figure A2.51). If it does not, then inversion of the signal round the loop can never occur and the system is said to be unconditionally stable. If it does cross the 180° axis, then one must look to see whether it passes to the right or the left of the point on this axis at unit distance from the origin, facing in the direction of increasing ω. If to the right, then the gain at ω_c is too small to produce more than transient oscillations, and the system is said to be *conditionally stable* (conditional, that is, on the gain remaining sufficiently small). If the locus passes to the left of the point, the system is unstable and will oscillate at a frequency close to ω_c. (The rule requires modification for some complex kinds of feedback systems.)

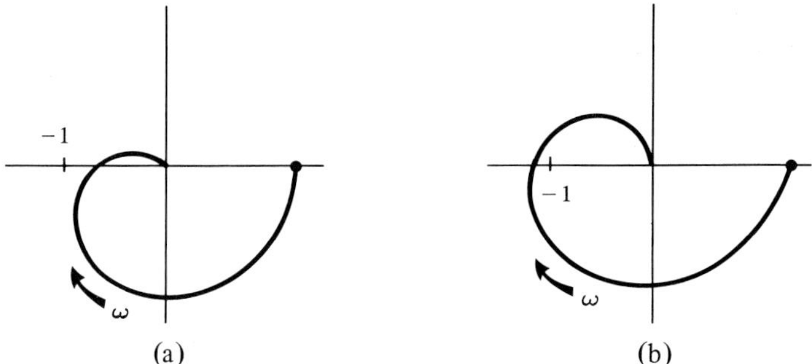

Figure A2.51. Stability of a negative-feedback system from the Nyquist diagram: (a) a conditionally stable system in which the locus passes to the right of the point (−1, 0) as ω increases, (b) an unstable system.

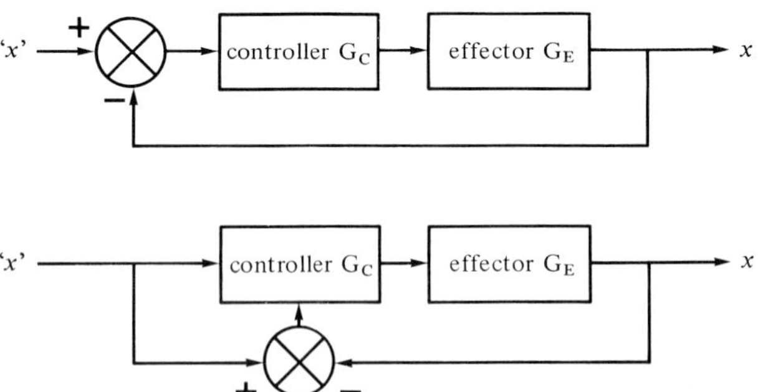

Figure A2.52. Control systems embodying feedback of the output. Above, conventional negative feedback in which the output x is subtracted from the desired input 'x' to provide an error signal that is the input to the controller. Below, parametric feedback, in which the error signal is averaged over a period of time and used to optimise the parameters describing the controller, in such a way that the long-term error is reduced.

Most processes requiring control do in practice contain many phase lags, and efficient controllers are normally designed with a large gain to increase sensitivity. If one thinks of the forward pathway of such a control system as consisting of the controller (whose gain is G_C) and the effector itself (G_E) in series, then the forward gain is given by $G = G_E G_C$ (figure A2.52). The combination of the effector's phase lag and the controller's high gain is thus likely to make the whole arrangement unconditionally unstable, and for this reason a well-designed system will arrange for G_C to introduce phase advance by means of components that perform differentiation, in an effort to cancel the phase lags of the effector and make the system unconditionally stable. Thus an efficient thermostat will take into account the rate of change of temperature as well as the temperature itself in deciding whether or not to turn on the boiler. In the same way, it seems probable that one of the functions of the phase advance that we have seen to be associated with adapting stretch receptors may be to compensate for the delays and phase lags involved in initiating muscular movement.

By a careful design of G_C in relation to the properties of the effector, G_E, in this kind of way, it is possible to make systems that will respond to any required degree of accuracy despite the existence of unwanted noise added to the output: but there is a second source of disturbance that cannot be dealt with like this. If the properties of the effector G_E are themselves subject to random perturbations—if for example the quality of the fuel supplied to our central heating boiler fluctuates unpredictably—it is clear from what has just been said that to maintain optimum performance we must make corresponding alterations in the parameters determining the behaviour of the controller, G_C, so that the two remain correctly matched to one another. One way of doing this is use the average of the error signal—the difference between the desired output and the actual output—over a relatively long period of time to cause slow modifications of G_C such as to maintain performance (figure A2.52). This process is called *parametric feedback*: it is perhaps more usefully discussed in connection with actual examples in the oculomotor system (sections 10.3.3, 11.3.1). A good account of this kind of optimisation is that of Elgerd (1967); a brief but intelligent discussion of its possible contribution to some kinds of human control systems may be found in Craik (1947).

References

Abrahams V C, Richmond F, Rose P K, 1975 "Basic physiology of the head-eye movement system" in *Basic Mechanisms of Ocular Motility* Eds G Lennerstrand, P Bach-y-Rita (Pergamon Press, Oxford) pp 473-476

Adamück E, 1870 "Über die Innervation der Augenbewegungen" *Zentralbl. Med. Wiss.* 8 65-67

Ades H W, Engström H, 1965 "Form and innervation of the vestibular epithelia" in *The Role of the Vestibular Organs in the Exploration of Space* NASA SP-77, National Aeronautic and Space Administration, Washington, DC, pp 23-41

Adler F H, Fliegelman M, 1934 "Influence of fixation on the visual acuity" *Arch. Ophthalmol.* **12** 475-483

Adrian E D, 1943 "Discharges from vestibular receptors in the cat" *J. Physiol (London)* **101** 389-407

Allen R J, 1954 "The dependence of cyclophoria on convergence, elevation, and the system of axes" *Am. J. Optom.* **31** 297-307

Alpern M, 1957 "The position of the eyes during prism vergence" *Am. J. Ophthalmol.* **57** 345-353

Alpern M, 1958 "Vergence and accommodation: I. Can change in size induce vergence movements?" *Arch. Ophthalmol.* **60** 355-357

Alpern M, 1969a "Kinematics of the eye" in *The Eye* (2nd edition) volume III, Ed. H Davson (Academic Press, New York), chapter 3, part I

Alpern M, 1969b "Neurology of movements of the eyes" in *The Eye* (2nd edition) volume III, Ed. H Davson (Academic Press, New York) chapter 4, section V

Alpern M, 1969c "Vergence movements" in *The Eye* (2nd edition) volume III, Ed. H Davson (Academic Press, New York) chapter 5, section VI

Alpern M, Ellen P, 1956 "A quantitative analysis of the horizontal movements of the eyes in the experiment of Johannes Müller" *Am. J. Ophthalmol.* **42** 289-296, 296-303

Alpern M, Wolter J R, 1956 "The relation of horizontal saccadic and vergence movements" *Arch. Ophthalmol.* **56** 685-690

Altman J, Carpenter M B, 1961 "Fibre projection of the superior colliculus in the cat" *J. Comp. Neurol.* **116** 157-178

Alvarado J A, Horn C van, 1975 "Muscle cell types of the cat inferior oblique" in *Basic Mechanisms of Ocular Motility* Eds G Lennerstrand, P Bach-y-Rita (Pergamon Press, Oxford) pp 15-45

Angaut P, Brodal A, 1967 "The projection of the 'vestibulocerebellum' onto the vestibular nuclei in the cat" *Arch. Ital. Biol.* **105** 441-479

Apter J T, 1946 "Eye movements following strychninization of the superior colliculus of cats" *J.Neurophysiol.* **9** 73-86

Arden G B, Kelsey J H, 1962 "Changes produced by light in the standing potential of the human eye" *J.Physiol. (London)* **161** 189-204

Armaly M F, 1959 "Studies on intraocular effects of the orbital parasympathetic pathway" *Arch. Ophthalmol.* **61** 14-29

Aschoff J C, 1968 "Veränderungen rascher Blickbewegungen (Saccaden) beim Menschen unter Diazepam (Valium)" *Arch. Psychiatr. Nervenkr.* **211** 325-332

Aschoff J C, Cohen B, 1971 "Changes in saccadic eye movements produced by cerebellar cortical lesions" *Exp. Neurol.* **32** 123-133

Aschoff J C, Cohen B, 1972 "Cerebellar ablations and spontaneous eye movements in monkeys" in *Cerebral Control of Eye Movements and Motion Perception* Eds J Dichgans, E Bizzi (Karger, Basel), pp 169-177

Aschcroft D W, Hallpike C S, 1934 "On the function of the saccule" *J. Laryngol. Otol.* **49** 450-460

Astruc J, 1971 "Corticofugal projection of area 8 (frontal eye field) in *Malaca Mulatta*" *Brain Res.* **33** 241-256

Atkin A, 1964 "Effect of head movement on gaze velocity" *Physiologist* **7** 82
Atkin A, 1969 "Shifting fixation to another pursuit target: selective and anticipatory control of ocular pursuit initiation" *Exp. Neurol.* **23** 157-173
Atkinson J, 1950 *Telephony* volume II (Pitman, London)
Attneave F, 1954 "Informational aspects of visual perception" *Psychol. Rev.* **61** 183-193
Azzena G D, Desole C, Palmieri G, 1970 "Cerebellar projections of the masticatory and extraocular muscle proprioception" *Expt. Neurol.* **27** 151-161
Baarsma E A, Collewijn H, 1974 "Vestibulo-ocular and optokinetic reactions to rotation and their interaction in the rabbit" *J. Physiol. (London)* **238** 603-625
Baarsma E A, Collewijn H, 1975 "Eye movements due to linear accelerations in the rabbit" *J. Physiol. (London)* **245** 227-247
Bach-y-Rita P, 1971 "Neurophysiology of eye movements" in *The Control of Eye Movements* Eds P Bach-y-Rita, C C Collins, J E Hyde (Academic Press, New York) pp 7-45
Bach-y-Rita P, 1972 "Extraocular muscle inhibitory stretch reflex during active contraction" *Arch. Ital. Biol.* **110** 1-15
Bach-y-Rita P, Ito F, 1966a "In vivo studies on fast and slow muscle fibres in cat extraocular muscles" *J. Gen. Physiol.* **49** 1177-1198
Bach-y-Rita P, Ito F, 1966b "Properties of stretch receptors in cat extraocular muscles" *J. Physiol. (London)* **186** 663-688
Bach-y-Rita P, Lennerstrand G, 1974 "Spindle responses in pig eye muscles" *Acta Physiol. Scand.* **90** 795-797
Bach-y-Rita P, Lennerstrand G, 1975 "Absence of polyneuronal innervation in cat extraocular muscles" *J. Physiol. (London)* **244** 613-624
Bahill A T, Adler D, Stark L, 1975a "Most naturally occurring saccades have magnitudes of 15 degrees or less" *Invest. Ophthalmol.* **14** 468-469
Bahill A T, Clark M R, Stark L, 1975b "Glissades—eye movements generated by mismatched components of the saccadic motoneuronal control signal" *Math. Biosci.* **26** 303-318
Bahill A T, Stark L, 1975 "Overlapping saccades and glissades are produced by fatigue in the saccadic eye movement system" *Exp. Neurol.* **48** 95-106
Baichenko P I, Matyushkin D P, Suvorov V V, 1968 "Participation of fast and tonic oculomotor systems in stretch reflexes and labyrinthine reflexes of extraocular muscles" *Neurosci. Transl.* **3** 350-358
Baizer J S, Glickstein M, 1974 "Role of cerebellum in prism adaptation" *J. Physiol. (London)* **236** 34P-35P
Baker J, Gibson A, Glickstein M, Stein J, 1976 "Visual cells in the pontine nuclei of the cat" *J. Physiol. (London)* **255** 415-433
Baker R, Berthoz A, 1974 "Organization of vestibular nystagmus in oblique oculomotor system" *J. Neurophysiol.* **37** 195-217
Baker R G, Mano N, Shimazu H, 1969 "Postsynaptic potentials in abducens motoneurones induced by vestibular stimulation" *Brain Res.* **15** 577-580
Baker R G, Precht W, Berthoz A, 1973 "Synaptic connections to trochlear motoneurones determined by individual nerve branch stimulation in the cat" *Brain Res.* **64** 402-406
Baker R G, Precht W, Llinas R, 1972 "Cerebellar modulatory action on the vestibulo-trochlear pathway in the cat" *Exp. Brain Res.* **15** 364-385
Barany R, 1906a "Untersuchungen über den vom Vestibularapparat des Ohres reflektorisch ausgelösten rythmischen Nystagmus und seine Begleiterscheinungen" *Monatsschr. für Ohrenheilkd.* **43** 191
Barany R, 1906b "Augenbewegungen, durch Thoraxbewegungen ausgelöst" *Zentralbl. Physiol.* **20** 298-302

Barker D, 1948 "The innervation of the muscle spindle" *Q. J. Microsc. Sci.* **89** 143-186
Barlow H B, 1952 "Eye movements during fixation" *J. Physiol. (London)* **116** 290-306
Barlow H B, 1959 "Possible principles underlying the transformations of sensory messages" in *Sensory Communication* Ed. W A Rosenblith (MIT Press, Cambridge, Mass)
Barlow H B, 1963 "Slippage of contact lenses and other artefacts in relation to fading and regeneration of supposedly stable retinal images" *Q. J. Exp. Psychol.* **15** 36-51
Barlow H B, Blakemore C B, Pettigrew J D, 1967 "The neural mechanism of binocular depth discrimination" *J. Physiol. (London)* **193** 327-342
Barlow H B, Hill R M, 1963 "Evidence for a physiological explanation of the waterfall phenomenon and figural aftereffects" *Nature (London)* **200** 1345-1347
Barmack N H, 1970a "Dynamic visual acuity as an index of eye movement control" *Vision Res.* **10** 1377-1391
Barmack N H, 1970b "Modification of eye movements by instantaneous changes in the velocity of visual targets" *Vision Res.* **10** 1431-1441
Barmack N H, 1974 "Saccadic discharges evoked by intracellular stimulation of extraocular motoneurons" *J. Neurophysiol.* **37** 395-412
Barmack N H, Bell C C, Rence B G, 1971 "Tension and rate of tension development during isometric responses of extra-ocular muscle" *J. Neurophysiol.* **34** 1072-1079
Barnes G R, 1974 "The role of the vestibular system in head-eye coordination" *J. Physiol. (London)* **246** 99P-100P
Barnes G R, Gresty M A, 1973 "Characteristics of eye movements to targets of short duration" *Aerosp. Med.* **44** 1236-1240
Barr A E de, 1962 *Automatic Control* (Chapman and Hall, London)
Barrett Sir James, 1921 "A case of voluntary control of the fusion faculty" *Med. J. Aust.* 12 February, 131
Barry W, Melvill Jones G, 1965 "Influence of eyelid movement upon electro-oculographic recordings of vertical eye movements" *Aerosp. Med.* **36** 855-858
Bartels M, 1911 "Über Regulierung der Augenstellung durch den Ohrapparat. Mitteilung III" *Albrecht von Graefes Arch. Opthalmol.* **78** 129-182
Bartz A, 1962 "Eye movement latency, duration and response time as a function of angular displacement" *J. Exp. Psychol.* **64** 318-324
Basler A, 1906 "Über das Sehen von Bewegungen. I. Die Wahrnehmung kleinster Bewegungen" *Pflügers Arch. Gesamte Physiol. Menschen Tiere* **115** 582-601
Batini C, Buisseret P, 1974 "Sensory peripheral pathway from extrinsic eye muscles" *Arch. Ital. Biol.* **112** 18-32
Batini C, Buisseret P, Buisseret-Delmas C, 1975 "Trigeminal pathway of the extrinsic eye muscle afferents in cat" *Brain Res.* **85** 74-78
Batini C, Buisseret P, Kado R T, 1974 "Extraocular proprioceptive and trigeminal projections to the Purkinje cells of the cerebellar cortex" *Arch. Ital. Biol.* **112** 1-17
Bauer J, Leidler R, 1911 "Über den Einfluss der Ausschaltung verschiedener Hirnabschnitte auf die Vestibulären Augenreflexe" *Arb. Neurol. Inst. Univ. Wien* **29** 155-225
Becker W, 1972 "The control of eye movements in the saccadic system" in *Cerebral Control of Eye Movements and Motion Perception* Eds. J Dichgans, E Bizzi (Karger, Basel) pp 233-243
Becker W, Fuchs A F, 1969 "Further properties of the human saccadic system: eye movements and correction saccades with and without visual fixation points" *Vision Res.* **9** 1247-1258
Becker W, Jürgens R, 1975 "Saccadic reactions to double-step stimuli: Evidence for model feedback and continuous information uptake" in *Basic Mechanisms of Ocular Motility* Eds. G Lennerstrand, P Bach-y-Rita (Pergamon Press, Oxford) pp 519-524

Becker W, Klein H-M, 1973 "Accuracy of saccadic eye movements and maintenance of excentric eye positions in the dark" *Vision Res.* **13** 1021–1034
Beeler G W, 1967 "Visual threshold changes resulting from spontaneous saccadic eye movements" *Vision Res.* **7** 769–775
Belcher S J, 1964 "Ocular torsion" *Br. J. Physiol. Opt.* **21** 1–20
Bell, Sir Charles, 1823 "On the motions of the eye, in the illustration of the uses of the muscles and nerves of the orbit" *Phil. Trans. R. Soc. London Part I* 166–186
Bender M B, 1955 "The eye-centring system" *Arch. Neurol. Psychiatry* **73** 685–699
Bender M B, Shanzer S, 1964 "Oculomotor pathways defined by electrical stimulation and lesions in the brainstem of monkey" in *The Oculomotor System* Ed. M B Bender (Harper and Row, New York) pp 81–140
Bender M B, Weinstein E A, 1943 "Functional representation in the oculomotor and trochlear nuclei" *Arch. Neurol. Psychiatry* **49** 98–106
Bengi H, Thomas J G, 1968a "Three electronic methods for recording ocular tremor" *Med. Biol. Eng.* **6** 171–178
Bengi H, Thomas J G, 1968b "Fixation tremor in relation to eyeball muscle mechanics" *Nature (London)* **217** 773–774
Bennet A G, Francis J L, 1969 "Visual optics" in *The Eye* (2nd edition) volume 4, part I, Ed. H Davson (Academic Press, New York) pp 101–131
Bennet-Clark H C, 1964 "The oculomotor response to small target replacements" *Opt. Acta* **11** 301–314
Benson A J, 1970 "Interactions between semicircular canals and gravireceptors" in *Recent Advances in Aerospace Medicine* Ed. D E Busby (Reidel, Dordrecht) pp 249–261
Benson A J, Bodin M A, 1966a "Interaction of linear and angular accelerations on vestibular receptors in man" *Aerosp. Med.* **37** 144–154
Benson A J, Bodin M A, 1966b "Comparison of the effect of the direction of the gravitational acceleration on post-rotational responses in yaw, pitch and roll" *Aerosp. Med.* **37** 889–897
Benson A J, Guedry F E, Melvill Jones G, 1970 "Response of semi-circular canal dependent units in vestibular nuclei to rotation of a linear acceleration vector without angular acceleration" *J. Physiol. (London)* **210** 475–494
Bergmann P S, Nathanson M, Bender M B, 1952 "Electrical recording of normal and abnormal eye movements modified by drugs" *Arch. Neurol. Psychiatry* **67** 357–374
Berlin E, 1871 "Beitrag zur Mechanik der Augenbewegungen" *Albrecht von Graefes Arch. Ophthalmol.* **17** (Abteilung 2) 154–203
Berthoz A, Baker R, Precht W, 1973 "Labyrinthine control of inferior oblique motoneurones" *Exp. Brain Res.* **18** 225–241
Berthoz A, Llinas R, 1974 "Afferent neck projection to the cat cerebellar cortex" *Exp. Brain Res.* **20** 385–401
Biemond A, de Jong J M B V, 1961 "On cervical nystagmus and related disorders" *Brain* **92** 437–458
Biervliet J van, 1899 "Noyau d'origine du nerf oculo-moteur commun du lapin" *La Cellule* **16** 1–33
Bischof N, Kramer E, 1960 "Investigations and considerations of directional perception during voluntary saccadic eye movements" *Psychol. Forsch.* **32** 185–218
Bisti S, Maffei L, Piccolino M, 1974 "Visuovestibular interactions in the cat superior colliculus" *J. Neurophysiol.* **37** 146–155
Bizzi E, 1966 "Changes in the orthodromic and antidromic response of optic tract during the eye movements of sleep" *J. Neurophysiol.* **29** 861–870
Bizzi E, 1968 "Discharge of frontal eye field neurons during saccadic and following movements in unanaesthetised monkey" *Exp. Brain Res.* **6** 69–80

Bizzi E, Kalil, R E, Morasso P, Tagliasco V, 1972 "Central programming and peripheral feedback during eye-head coordination in monkeys" in *Cerebral Control of Eye Movements and Motion Perception* Eds J Dichgans, E Bizzi (Karger, Basel) pp 220-232

Bizzi E, Schiller P H, 1970 "Single unit activity in the frontal eye fields of unanaesthetized monkeys during head and eye movements" *Exp. Brain Res.* **10** 151-158

Björk A, Kugelberg E, 1953 "Motor unit activity in the human extraocular muscles" *Electroencephalogr. Clin. Neurophysiol.* **5** 271-278

Blakemore C, 1970 "The representation of three-dimensional visual space in the cat's striate cortex" *J. Physiol. (London)* **209** 155-178

Blakemore C B, Carpenter R H S, 1970 "A very simple device to measure human eye movements" *J. Physiol. (London)* **210** 75P-77P

Bles W, Kapteyn T S, 1973 "Separate recording of the movements of human eyes during parallel swing tests" *Acta Oto-Laryngol.* **75** 6-9

Boeder P, 1961 "The co-operation of extraocular muscles" *Am. J.Ophthalmol.* **51** 469-481

Boeder P, 1962 "Co-operative action of extraocular muscles" *Br. J. Ophthalmol.* **46** 397-403

Boeke J, 1926 "Die Beziehungen der Nervenfasern zu den Bindegewebselementen und Tastzellen" *Z. Mikrosk.-Anat. Forsch.* **4** 448-509

Boghen D, Troost B T, Daroff R B, Dellosso L F, Birkett J E, 1974 "Velocity characteristics of normal human saccades" *Invest. Ophthalmol.* **13** 619-622

Borries G V T, 1926 *Fixation and Nystagmus* (Linds, Copenhagen)

Borschke A, Hescheles L, 1902 "Über Bewegungsnachbilder" *Z. Psychol. Physiol. Sinnesorgane* **27** 387-398

Bouma H, Voogd A H de, 1974 "On the control of eye saccades in reading" *Vision Res.* **14** 273-284

Bourdon B, 1902 *La Perception Visuelle de l'Éspace* (Bibliothèque de Pédagogie et de Psychologie, Schleicher, Paris)

Boyce P R, 1965 "The visual perception of movement in the absence of an external frame of reference" *Opt. Acta* **12** 47-54

Boyce P R, 1967 "Monocular fixation in human eye movement" *Proc. R. Soc. London B* **167** 293-315

Boyce P R, West D C, 1968 "The frequency response of contact lens stalk assemblies" *Vision Res.* **8** 475-480

Braak J W G ter, 1936 "Untersuchungen über optokinetischen Nystagmus" *Arch. Néerl. Physiol.* **21** 309-376

Braak J W G ter, 1972 "Ambivalent optokinetic stimulation and motion detection" in *Cerebral Control of Eye Movements and Motion Perception* Eds J Dichgans, E Bizzi (Karger, Basel) pp 308-316

Bracewell R, 1965 *The Fourier Transform and its Applications* (McGraw Hill, New York)

Braitenberg, V, 1961 "Functional interpretation of cerebellar histology" *Nature (London)* **190** 539-540

Braitenberg V, 1967 "Is the cerebellar cortex a biological clock in the millisecond range?" in *The Cerebellum, Prog. Brain Res.* **25** Eds C A Fox, R S Snider (Elsevier, Amsterdam) pp 334-346

Brandt T, Dichgans J, Koenig E, 1973 "Differential effects of central versus peripheral vision on egocentric and exocentric motion perception" *Exp. Brain Res.* **16** 476-491

Brandt T, Wist E, Dichgans J, 1971 "Optisch induzierte Pseudocoriolis-Effekte und Circularvektion" *Arch. Psychiatr. Nervenkr.* **214** 365-389

Brecher G A, Mitchell W G, 1957 "Studies in the role of sympathetic nervous stimulation in extraocular muscle movements" *Am. J. Ophthalmol.* **41** 144-150
Breinin G M, 1957 "Electromyographic evidence for ocular muscle proprioception in man" *Arch. Ophthalmol.* **57** 176-180
Brindley G S, 1962 "Beats produced by simultaneous stimulation of the human eye with intermittent light and intermittent or alternating electric current" *J. Physiol. (London)* **164** 157-167
Brindley G S, 1970 *Physiology of the Retina and Visual Pathway* (2nd edition) (Edward Arnold, London)
Brindley G S, Goodwin G M, Kulikowski J J, Leighton D, 1976 "Stability of vision with a paralysed eye" *J. Physiol. (London)* **258** 65P-66P
Brindley G S, Lewin W D, 1968 "The sensations produced by electrical stimulation of the visual cortex" *J. Physiol. (London)* **196** 479-493
Brindley G S, Merton P A, 1960 "The absence of position sense in the human eye" *J. Physiol. (London)* **153** 127-130
Brodal A, 1967 "Anatomical studies of cerebellar fibre connections with special reference to problems of functional localisation" in *The Cerebellum, Progr. Brain Res.* **25** Eds C A Fox, R S Snider (Elsevier, Amsterdam) pp 135-173
Brodal A, 1969 *Neurological Anatomy in Relation to Clinical Medicine* (Oxford University Press, London)
Brodal A, 1972a "Some features in the anatomical organisation of the vestibular nuclear complex in the cat" in *Basic Aspects of Central Vestibular Mechanisms* Eds A Brodal, O Pompeiano (Elsevier, Amsterdam) pp 31-53
Brodal A, 1972b "Vestibulo-cerebellar input in cat: anatomy" in *Basic Aspects of Central Vestibular Mechanisms* Eds A Brodal, O Pompeiano (Elsevier, Amsterdam) pp 315-327
Brodal A, Høivik B, 1964 "Site and mode of termination of primary vestibulo-cerebellar fibres in the cat" *Arch. Ital. Biol.* **102** 1-21
Brodal A, Pompeiano O, 1957 "The vestibular nuclei in the cat" *J. Anat.* **91** 438-454
Brodal A, Pompeiano O, Walberg F, 1962 *The Vestibular Nuclei and their Connections, Anatomy and Functional Correlations* W R Henderson Trust Lectures (Oliver and Boyd, Edinburgh)
Brodal A, Torvik A, 1957 "Über den Ursprung der sekundären Vestibulocerebellaren Fasern bei der Katze. Eine experimentell-anatomische Studie" *Arch. Psychiatr. Nervenkr.* **195** 550-567
Brodal P, 1972a "The corticopontine projection from the visual cortex of the cat: I. The total projection and the projection from area 17" *Brain Res.* **39** 297-317
Brodal P, 1972b "The corticopontine projection from the visual cortex of the cat: II. The projection from areas 18 and 19" *Brain Res.* **39** 319-335
Brooks V B, 1974 "Some examples of programmed limb movements" *Brain Res.* **71** 299-308
Brooks V B, Cooke J D, Thomas J S, 1974 "The continuity of movements" in *Control of Posture and Locomotion* Eds R B Stein, K B Pearson, R S Smith, J B Redford (Plenum Press, New York)
Brooks V B, Holden A L, 1973 "Suppression of visual signals by rapid image displacement in the pigeon retina: a possible mechanism for 'saccadic' suppression" *Vision Res.* **13** 1387-1390
Brooks V B, Stoney S D, 1971 "Motor mechanisms: the role of the pyramidal system in motor control" *Ann. Rev. Psychol.* **33** 337-392
Brouwer B, 1918 "Klinisch-anatomische Untersuchung über den Oculomotoriuskern" *Z. Gesamte Neurol. Psychiatr.* **40** 152-193
Brown B M, 1965 *The Mathematical Theory of Linear Systems* (Chapman and Hall, London)

Brown J H, Crampton G H, 1966 "Concomitant visual stimulation does not alter habituation of nystagmic, oculogyral or psychophysical responses to angular acceleration" *Acta Oto-Laryngol.* **61** 80-91

Browne J S, 1975 "The responses of muscle spindles in sheep extraocular muscles" *J. Physiol. (London)* **251** 483-496

Browne J S, 1976 "The contractile properties of slow muscle fibres in sheep extraocular muscle" *J. Physiol. (London)* **254** 535-550

Bryngdahl O, 1961 "Effect of retinal image motion on visual acuity" *Opt. Acta* **8** 1-16

Buchtel H A, Iosif G, Marchesi G F, Provini L, Strata P, 1972 "Analysis of the activity evoked in the cerebellar cortex by stimulation of the visual pathways" *Exp. Brain Res.* **15** 278-288

Buchthal F, Kaiser E, 1951 "The rheology of the cross striated muscle fibre" *Biol. Medd. K. Dan. Vidensk. Selske* **21** (7) 1-318

Bülbring E, 1955 "Correlation between membrane potential, spike discharge and tension in smooth muscle" *J. Physiol. (London)* **128** 200-221

Burian H M, Noorden G K van, 1974 *Binocular Vision and Ocular Motility* (Mosby, St Louis, Mo.)

Burnham C A, 1968 "Decrement of the Müller-Lyer illusion with saccadic and tracking eye movements" *Percept. Psychophys.* **3** 424-426

Butler T W, King-Smith P E, Moore R K, Riggs L A, 1976 "Visual sensitivity to retinal image movement" *J. Physiol. (London)* **263** 170P-172P

Büttner U, Fuchs A F, 1973 "Influence of saccadic eye movements on unit activity in simian lateral geniculate and pregeniculate nuclei" *J. Neurophysiol.* **36** 127-141

Buys E, Coppez H, 1909 "Graphic records of nystagmus" *Ophthalmoscope* **7** 808-812

Buzzard F, 1908 "A note on the occurrence of muscle-spindles in ocular muscles" *Proc. R. Soc. Med.* **1** (June) 83-88

Byford G H, 1962 "The fidelity of contact lens eye movement recording" *Opt. Acta* **9** 223-236

Byford G H, 1963 "Non-linear relations between the corneo-retinal potential and horizontal eye movements" *J. Physiol. (London)* **168** 14P-15P

Cajal S, Ramon y, 1908 "El ganglio intersticial del fasciculo longitudinal posterior en el hombre y diversos vertebrados" *Trav. Lab. Rech. Biol. Univ. Madrid* **6** 145-160

Cajal S, Ramon y, 1911 *Histologie du Système Nerveux de l'Homme et des Vertébrés* (Maloine, Paris)

Camarda R, Grupp L A, Pisa M, Rizzolatti G, 1974 "Interaction of visual stimuli in cat superior colliculus: spatial and temporal factors" *Brain Res.* **66** 358-359

Campbell F W, Robson J G, 1961 "A fresh approach to stabilized retinal images" *J. Physiol. (London)* **158** 11P-12P

Carmichael E A, Dix M R, Hallpike C S, 1954 "Lesions of the cerebral hemispheres and their effect upon optokinetic and caloric nystagmus" *Brain* **77** 345-372

Carpenter M B, 1971 "Central oculomotor pathways" in *The Control of Eye Movements* Eds P Bach-y-Rita, C C Collins, J E Hyde (Academic Press, New York) pp 67-103

Carpenter M B, Bard D S, Alling F A, 1959 "Anatomical connections between the fastigial nuclei, the labyrinth and the vestibular nuclei in the cat" *J. Comp. Neurol.* **111** 1-26

Carpenter M B, Hanna G R, 1962 "Lesions of the medial longitudinal fasciculus in the cat" *Am. J. Anat.* **110** 307-332

Carpenter M B, McMasters R E, 1963 "Disturbances of conjugate horizontal eye movements in the monkey. II. Physiological effects and anatomical degeneration resulting from lesions in the medial longitudinal fasciculus" *Arch. Neurol.* **8** 347-368

Carpenter M B, McMasters R, Hanna G, 1963 "Disturbances of conjugate horizontal eye movements in the monkey" *Arch. Neurol.* 8 231-247

Carpenter M B, Nova H R, 1960 "Descending division of the brachium conjunctivum in the cat: A cerebello-reticular system" *J. Comp. Neurol.* **114** 295-305

Carpenter M B, Strominger N L, 1964 "Cerebello-oculomotor fibres in the rhesus monkey" *J. Comp. Neurol.* **123** 211-230

Carpenter M B, Strominger N L, 1965 "The medial longitudinal fasciculus and disturbances of conjugate horizontal eye movements in the monkey" *J. Comp. Neurol.* **125** 41-66

Carpenter R H S, 1972a "Cerebellectomy and the transfer-function of the vestibulo-ocular reflex in the decerebrate cat" *Proc. R. Soc. London B* **181** 353-374

Carpenter R H S 1972b "After-images on backgrounds of different luminance" *J. Physiol. (London)* **226** 713-724

Carr H A, 1910 "The autokinetic sensation" *Psychol. Rev.* **17** 42-75

Chaco J, 1971 "Impairment of function of the extraocular muscles in Parkinson's disease" *Ophthalmologica* **162** 343-347

Chase R, Kalil R E, 1972 "Suppression of visual evoked responses to flashes and pattern shifts during voluntary saccades" *Vision Res.* **12** 215-220

Cheng K, Breinin G M, 1966 "A comparison of the fine structure of extraocular and interosseus muscles in the monkey" *Invest. Ophthalmol.* **5** 535-549

Cheng M, Outerbridge J S, 1974a "Inter-saccadic interval analysis of optokinetic nystagmus" *Vision Res.* **14** 1053-1058

Cheng M, Outerbridge J S, 1974b "Inter-saccadic interval analysis of vestibular nystagmus" *Acta Oto-Laryngol.* **77** 348-353

Childress D S, Jones R W, 1967 "Mechanics of the horizontal movement of the human eye" *J. Physiol. (London)* **188** 273-284

Cilimbaris P A, 1910 "Histologische Untersuchungen über die Muskelspindeln der Augenmuskeln" *Arch. Mikrosk. Anat.* **75** 692-747

Clark B, 1936 "The effect of interfixation distance on binocular fixation movements" *J. Exp. Psychol.* **19** 505-512

Clark G, Lashley K S, 1947 "Visual disturbances following frontal ablations in the monkey" *Anat. Rec.* **97** 326

Clarke F J J, 1957 "Rapid light adaptation of localised areas of the extra-foveal retina" *Opt. Acta* **4** 69-77

Clarke P G H, 1974 "The organisation of visual processing in the pigeon cerebellum" *J. Physiol. (London)* **243** 267-285

Close R I, Luff A R, 1974 "Dynamic properties of inferior rectus muscle of the rat" *J. Physiol. (London)* **236** 259-270

Clowes M B, 1961 "Some factors in brightness discrimination with constraint of retinal image movement" *Opt. Acta* **8** 81-91

Clynes M, 1969 "Rein control, or unidirectional rate sensitivity, a fundamental dynamic and organising function in biology" *Ann. N.Y. Acad. Sci.* **156** (article 2) 627-968

Cogan D C, 1956 *Neurology of the Ocular Muscles* (Charles C Thomas, Springfield, Ill.)

Cogan D C, 1964 "Brain lesions and eye movements in man" in *The Oculomotor System* Ed. M B Bender (Harper and Row, New York) chapter 18, pp 417-423

Cogan D C, 1974 "Paralysis of down-gaze" *Arch. Ophthalmol.* **91** 192-199

Cohen B, 1966 "Functional aspects of lateral geniculate body responses to rapid eye movements" *Fed. Proc. Fed. Am. Soc. Exp. Biol.* **25** 573

Cohen B, 1971 "Vestibulo-ocular relations" in *The Control of Eye Movements* Eds P Bach-y-Rita, C C Collins, J E Hyde (Academic Press, New York) pp 105-148

Cohen B, Feldman M, 1968 "Relationship of electrical activity in pontine reticular formation and lateral geniculate body to rapid eye movements" *J. Neurophysiol.* **31** 806-817

Cohen B, Feldman M, Diamond S P, 1969 "Effects of eye movement, brain-stem stimulation and alertness on transmission through lateral geniculate body of monkey" *J. Neurophysiol.* **32** 583-594

Cohen B, Goto K, Shanzer S, Weis A H, 1965 "Eye movements induced by electrical stimulation of the cerebellum in the alert cat" *Exp. Neurol.* **13** 145-162

Cohen B, Goto K, Tokomasu K, 1967 "Return eye movements; an ocular compensatory reflex in the alert cat and monkey" *Exp. Neurol.* **17** 172-185

Cohen B, Henn V, 1972 "Unit activity in the pontine reticular formation associated with eye movements" *Brain Res.* **46** 403-410

Cohen B, Komatsuzaki A, 1972 "Eye movements induced by stimulation of the pontine reticular formation: evidence for integration in oculomotor pathways" *Exp. Neurol.* **36** 101-117

Cohen B, Komatsuzaki A, Harris H E, 1967 "Characteristics of pontine pathways for conjugate gaze" *Trans. Am. Neurol. Assoc.* **92** 219-220

Cohen B, Suzuki J, Shanzer S, Bender M B, 1964 "Semicircular canal control of eye movements" in *The Oculomotor System* Ed. M B Bender (Harper and Row, New York) chapter 6

Collewijn H, 1969 "Optokinetic eye movements in the rabbit: input-output relations" *Vision Res.* **9** 117-132

Collewijn H, 1970a "Dysmetria of fast phase of optokinetic nystagmus in cerebellectomized rabbits" *Exp. Neurol.* **28** 144-154

Collewijn H, 1970b "The normal range of horizontal eye movements in the rabbit" *Exp. Neurol.* **28** 132-143

Collewijn H, 1972 "An analog model of the rabbit's optokinetic system" *Brain Res.* **36** 71-88

Collewijn H, Kleinschmidt H J, 1975 "Vestibulo-ocular and optokinetic reactions in the rabbit: changes during 24 hours of normal and abnormal interaction" in *Basic Mechanisms of Ocular Motility* Eds G Lennerstrand, P Bach-y-Rita (Pergamon Press, Oxford) pp 477-483

Collewijn H, Mark F van der, 1972 "Ocular stability in variable visual feedback conditions in the rabbit" *Brain Res.* **36** 47-57

Collewijn H, Mark F van der, Jansen T C, 1975 "Precise recording of human eye movements" *Vision Res.* **15** 447-450

Collins C C, 1971 "Orbital mechanics" in *The Control of Eye Movements* Eds P Bach-y-Rita, C C Collins, J E Hyde (Academic Press, New York) pp 283-325

Collins C C, 1975 "The human oculomotor control system" in *Basic Mechanisms of Ocular Motility* Eds G Lennerstrand, P Bach-y-Rita (Pergamon Press, Oxford) pp 145-180

Collins C C, O'Meara D, Scott A B, 1975 "Muscle tension during unrestrained human eye movements" *J. Physiol. (London)* **245** 351-369

Collins C C, Scott A B, 1973 *The Eye Movement Control Signal. Proc. 2nd Bioeng. Conf. Ophthal. Sec., Milan*

Collins C C, Scott A B, O'Meara D, 1969 "Elements of the peripheral oculomotor apparatus" *Am. J. Optom.* **46** 510-515

Collins W E, Updegraff B P, 1966 "A comparison of nystagmus habituation in the cat and the dog" *Acta Oto-Laryngol.* **62** 19-26

Conrad B, Brooks V B, 1974 "Effects of dentate cooling on rapid alternating arm movements" *J. Neurophysiol.* **37** 792-804

Cooper S, Daniel P M, 1949 "Muscle spindles in human extrinsic eye muscles" *Brain* **72** 1-24

Cooper S, Daniel P M, 1957 "Responses from the stretch receptors of the goat's extrinsic eye muscles with an intact motor innervation" *Q. J. Exp. Physiol.* **42** 222-231

Cooper S, Daniel P M, Whitteridge D, 1951 "Afferent impulses in the oculomotor nuclei from the extrinsic eye muscles" *J. Physiol. (London)* **113** 463-474

Cooper S, Daniel P M, Whitteridge D, 1953a "Nerve impulses in the brainstem of the goat: short latency responses obtained by stretching the extrinsic eye muscles and the jaw muscles" *J. Physiol. (London)* **120** 471-490

Cooper S, Daniel P M, Whitteridge D, 1953b "Nerve impulses in the brainstem of the goat: responses with long latencies obtained by stretching the extrinsic eye muscles" *J. Physiol. (London)* **120** 491-513

Cooper S, Daniel P M, Whitteridge D, 1955 "Muscle spindles and other sensory endings in the extrinsic eye muscles; the physiology and anatomy of the receptors and of their connections with the brainstem" *Brain* **78** 564-583

Cooper S, Eccles J C, 1930 "The isometric response of mammalian muscles" *J. Physiol. (London)* **69** 377-385

Cooper S, Fillenz M, 1955 "Afferent discharges in response to stretch from the extraocular muscles of the cat and monkey and the innervation of these muscles" *J. Physiol. (London)* **127** 400-413

Corazza R, Lombroso C T, 1971 "The neuronal dark discharge in awake 'encéphale isolé' cats" *Brain Res.* **34** 345-359

Coren S, Porac C, 1974 "The fading of stabilized images: eye movements and information processing" *Percept. Psychophys.* **16** 529-534

Cornsweet T N, 1956 "Determination of the stimuli for involuntary drifts and saccadic eye movements" *J. Opt. Soc. Am.* **46** 987-993

Cornsweet T N, 1958 "A new technique for the measurement of small eye movements" *J. Opt. Soc. Am.* **48** 808-811

Cornsweet T N, 1962 "A stabilized image requiring no attachments to the eye" *Am. J. Psychol.* **75** 653-656

Cornsweet T N, Crane H D, 1973 "Accurate two-dimensional eye tracker using first and fourth Purkinje images" *J. Opt. Soc. Am.* **63** 921-928

Correia M J, Money K E, 1970 "The effect of blockage of all six semicircular canal ducts on nystagmus produced by dynamic linear acceleration in the cat" *Acta Oto-Laryngol.* **69** 7-16

Craik K J W, 1947 "Theory of the human operator in control systems. 1. The operator as an engineering system" *Br. J. Psychol.* **38** 56-61

Crampton G H, 1964 "Habituation of ocular nystagmus of vestibular origin" in *The Oculomotor System* Ed. M B Bender (Harper and Row, New York) pp 332-346

Crampton G H, Schwann W J, 1961 "Effects of arousal on nystagmus habituation in the cat" *Am. J. Physiol.* **200** 29-33

Crickmar S D, 1969 "Techniques for the measurement of eye movements: a review" report 483, RAF Institute of Aviation Medicine, Farnborough, Hants

Cronly-Dillon J R, 1964 "Units sensitive to direction of movement in goldfish optic tectum" *Nature (London)* **203** 214-215

Crookes T G, 1957 "Television images" *Nature (London)* **179** 1024-1025

Crosby E C, Henderson J W, 1948 "The mammalian midbrain and isthmus regions. II. Fiber connections of the superior colliculus. B. Pathways concerned in automatic eye movements" *J. Comp. Neurol.* **88** 53-91

Crosby E C, Humphrey T, Lauer E, 1962 *Correlative Anatomy of the Nervous System* (MacMillan, London)

Crosby E C, Woodburne R T, 1943 "The nuclear pattern of the non-tectal portions of the midbrain and isthmus in primates" *J. Comp. Neurol.* **78** 441-482

Crosby E C, Yoss R E, Henderson J W, 1952 "The mammalian midbrain and isthmus regions. II. The fiber connections. D. The pattern for eye movements on the frontal eye field and the discharge of specific portions of the field to and through midbrain levels" *J. Comp. Neurol.* **97** 357-383

Cunitz R J, Steinman R M, 1969 "Comparison of saccadic eye movements during fixation and reading" *Vision Res.* **9** 683-693

Cynader M, Berman N, 1972 "Receptive-field organisation of monkey superior colliculus" *J. Neurophysiol.* **35** 187-201

Daley M L, Barmack N H, 1974 "The current-to-frequency conversion of extraocular motoneurones" *Kybernetik* **15** 39-45

Dallos P J, Jones R W, 1963 "Learning behaviour of the eye fixation control system" *IEEE Trans. Autom. Control* **AC-8** 218-227

Daniel P M, 1946 "Spiral nerve endings in the extrinsic eye muscles of man" *J. Anat.* **80** 189-193

Danis P C, 1948 "The functional organisation of the third-nerve nucleus in the cat" *Am. J. Ophthalmol.* **31** 1122-1131

Darkschewitsch L, 1889 "Über den Oberenkern des N. Oculomotrius" *Arch. Anat. Entwicklungsges. Anat. Abt.* 107-116

Darwin E, 1794 *Zoonomia* (2nd edition) (London)

Davies T, Merton P A, 1958 "Recording compensatory rolling of the eyes" *J. Physiol. (London)* **140** 27P-28P

Davis J K, Fernald H G, 1963 "Instruments and methods for locating the sighting-centre of the eye" *Am. J. Optom.* **40** 676-683

De La Barre E B, 1898 "A method of recording eye-movements" *Am. J. Psychol.* **9** 572-574

Dewar J, 1877 "The physiological action of light" *Nature (London)* **15** 433-435

Dichgans J, 1975 "Spinal afferences to the oculomotor system: physiological and clinical aspects" in *Basic Mechanisms of Ocular Motility* Eds G Lennerstrand, P Bach-y-Rita (Pergamon Press, Oxford) pp 299-302

Dichgans J, Bizzi E, Morasso P, Tagliasco V, 1973 "Mechanisms underlying recovery of eye-head coordination following bilateral labyrinthectomy in monkeys" *Exp. Brain Res.* **18** 548-562

Dichgans J, Bizzi E, Morasso P, Tagliasco V, 1974 "The role of vestibular and neck afferents during eye-head co-ordination in the monkey" *Brain Res.* **71** 225-232

Dichgans J, Brandt T, 1972 "Visual-vestibular interaction and motion perception" in *Cerebral Control of Eye Movements and Motion Perception* Eds J Dichgans, E Bizzi (Karger, Basel) pp 327-338

Dichgans J, Jung R, 1975 "Oculomotor abnormalities due to cerebellar lesions" in *Basic Mechanisms of Ocular Motility* Eds G Lennerstrand, P Bach-y-Rita (Pergamon Press, Oxford) pp 281-302

Dichgans J, Körner F, Voigt K, 1969 "Vergleichende Skalierung des afferenten und efferenten Bewegungssehens beim Menschen" *Psychol. Forsch.* **32** 277-295

Dichgans J, Nauck B, Brooks B, 1969 "Blickbewegungen mit sichtbarem Fixationsziel, intendierte Blickbewegungen im Dunkeln und nach Lidschluss. Beziehungen zu den raschen Phasen des optokinetischen und vestibulären Nystagmus" *Pflügers Arch. Gesamte Physiol. Menschen Tiere* **312** R143-R144

Dichgans J, Wist E R, Schmidt C L, 1970 "Modulation neuronaler Spontanaktivität im N. Vestibularis durch optomotorische Impulse beim Kaninchen" *Pflügers Arch. Gesamte Physiol. Menschen Tiere* **319** R154-R155

Dietert S E, 1965 "The demonstration of different types of muscle fibres in human extraocular muscles by electron microscopy and cholinesterase staining" *Invest. Ophthalmol.* **4** 51-63

Ditchburn R W, 1955 "Eye movements in relation to retinal action" *Opt. Acta* **1** 171-176

Ditchburn R W, 1963 "A new apparatus for producing a stabilized retinal image" *Opt. Acta* **10** 325-331

Ditchburn R W, 1973 *Eye-movements and Visual Perception* (Clarendon Press,Oxford)

Ditchburn R W, Fender D H, 1955 "The stabilised retinal image" *Opt. Acta* **2** 128–133
Ditchburn R W, Fender D H, Mayne S M 1959 "Vision with controlled movements of the retinal image" *J. Physiol (London)* **145** 98–107
Ditchburn R W, Ginsborg B L, 1952 "Vision with a stabilised retinal image" *Nature (London)* **170** 36–37
Ditchburn R W, Ginsborg B L, 1953 "Involuntary eye movements during fixation" *J. Physiol. (London)* **119** 1–17
Ditchburn R W, Pritchard R M, 1956 "Stabilised interference fringes on the retina" *Nature (London)* **177** 434
Dix M R, Hallpike C S, 1966 "Observations on the clinical features and neurological mechanism of spontaneous nystagmus resulting from unilateral acoustic neurofibromata" *Acta. Oto-Laryngol.* **61** 1–22
Dix M R, Hood J D, 1969 "Observations upon the nervous mechanisms of vestibular habituation" *Acta Oto-Laryngol.* **67** 310–318
Dobelle W H, Mladejovsky M G, 1974 "Phosphenes produced by electrical stimulation of human occipital cortex, and their application to the development of a prosthesis for the blind" *J. Physiol. (London)* **243** 553–577
Dodge R, 1900 "Visual perception during eye movement" *Psychol. Rev.* **7** 454–465
Dodge R, 1905 "The illusion of clear vision during eye movement" *Psychol. Bull.* **2** 193–199
Dodge R, Cline T S, 1901 "The angle velocity of eye movements" *Psychol. Rev.* **8** 145–157
Dodge R, Travis R C, Fox J C, 1930 "Optic nystagmus. III. Characteristics of the slow phase" *Arch. Neurol. Psychiatry* **24** 21–34
Dohlman G F, Kuehn L A, 1973 "The role of the perilymph in semicircular canal stimulation" *Acta Oto-Laryngol.* **75** 396–404
Donaldson G W K, 1960 "The diameter of the nerve fibres to the extrinsic eye muscles of the goat" *Q. J. Exp. Physiol.* **45** 25–34
Donaldson P E K, 1964 "Error decorrelation. Studies on a human operator performing a balancing task" *Med. Electron. Biol. Eng.* **2** 393–410
Donders F C (Ed.), 1847 *Holländische Beiträge zu den anatomischen und physiologischen Wissenschaften* volume 1 pp 105, 135, 384
Dow R S, 1935 "The relation of the paraflocculus to the movements of the eyes" *Am. J. Physiol.* **133** 296–298
Dow R S, Manni E, 1964 "The relationship of the cerebellum to extraocular movements" in *The Oculomotor System* Ed. M B Bender, (Harper and Row, New York) chapter 11, pp 280–302
Duensing F, Schaefer K P, 1957a "Die Neuronenaktivität in der Formatio Reticularis des Rhombencephalons beim vestibulären Nystagmus" *Arch. Psychiatr. Nervenkr.* **196** 265–290
Duensing F, Schaefer K P, 1957b "Die 'Locker gekoppelten' Neurone der Formatio Reticularis des Rhombencephalons beim vestibulären Nystagmus" *Arch. Psychiatr. Nervenkr.* **196** 402–420
Duensing F, Schaefer K P, 1959 "Über die Konvergenz verschiedener labyrinthärer Afferenzen auf einzelne Neurone des Vestibularis Kerngebietes" *Arch. Psychiatr. Nervenkr.* **199** 345–371
Duffy F H, Lombroso C T, 1968 "Electrophysiological evidence for visual suppression prior to the onset of a voluntary saccadic eye movement" *Nature (London)* **218** 1074–1075
Duke-Elder Sir Stewart, Wybar K, 1973 "Ocular motility and strabismus" in *System of Ophthalmology* volume 6 Ed. Sir Stewart Duke-Elder (Kimpton, London)
Duke-Elder W S, Duke-Elder P M, 1931 "Contraction of extrinsic muscles of the eye by choline and nicotine" *Proc. R. Soc. London B.* **107** 332–343

Duncker K, 1938 "Induced motion" in *Source Book of Gestalt Psychology* Ed. W D Ellis (Routledge and Kegan Paul, London) pp 161-172

Dunlap K, Mowrer O H, 1931 "Head movements and eye functions of birds" *J. Comp. Psychol.* **11** 99-112

Durston J H J, 1974 "Histochemistry of primate extraocular muscles and the changes of denervation" *Br. J. Physiol. Opt.* **58** 193-216

Dusser de Barenne J G, Kleijn A de, 1923 "Über vestibuläre Augenreflexe. V. Vestibular-untersuchungen nach Ausschaltung einer Grosshirnhemisphäre beim Kaninchen" Albrecht von Graefes Arch. Opthalmol. **111** 374-392

Eakins K E, Katz R L, 1971 "The pharmacology of extraocular muscle" in *The Control of Eye Movements* Eds P Bach-y-Rita, C C Collins, J E Hyde (Academic Press, New York) pp 237-258

Easter S S, 1971 "Spontaneous eye movements in restrained goldfish" *Vision Res.* **11** 333-342

Easter S S, 1972 "Pursuit eye movements in goldfish (*Carassius auratus*)" *Vision Res.* **12** 673-688

Easter S S, 1973 "A comment on the 'glissade'" *Vision Res.* **13** 881-882

Easter S S, 1975 "The time course of saccadic eye movements in goldfish" *Vision Res.* **15** 405-409

Ebbers R W, 1965 "Investigations of vision during involuntary saccadic eye movements" *J. Opt. Soc. Am.* **55** 1577

Ebbers R W, 1973 quoted in Ditchburn (1973)

Eccles J C, Ito M, Szentágothai J, 1967 *The Cerebellum as a Neuronal Machine* (Springer, New York)

Eckmiller R, 1974 "Hysteresis in static characteristics of eye position coded neurons in the alert monkey" *Pflügers Arch.* **350** 249-258

Eckmiller R, Blair S M, Westheimer G, 1974 "Oculomotor neuronal correlations shown by simultaneous unit recordings in alert monkeys" *Exp. Brain Res.* **21** 241-250

Economo C F von, 1929 *The Cytoarchitectonics of the Human Cerebral Cortex* (Oxford University Press, London)

Edwards E, 1969 *Information Transmission* (Chapman and Hall, London)

Edwards S B, Rosenquist A C, Palmer L A, 1974 "An autoradiographic study of ventral lateral geniculate projections in the cat" *Brain Res.* **72** 282-287

Egmond A A J von, Groen J J, Jonkees L B W, 1949 "The mechanics of the semi-circular canal" *J. Physiol. (London)* **110** 1-17

Elgerd O I, 1967 *Control Systems Theory* (McGraw-Hill-Kogakusha, Tokyo)

Emmes A B, 1949 "A statistical analysis of the accommodative-convergence gradient" *Am. J. Optom.* **26** 474-482

Engström H, 1965 "Elektronoptische Histologie des Innenohres" *Z. Hals- Nasen-Ohrenheilk.* **3** 148

Engström H, Ades H W, Hawkins J E, 1962 "Structure and functions of the sensory hairs of the inner ear" *J. Acoust. Soc. Am.* **34** 1356-1362

Erdmann D, Dodge R, 1898 *Psychologische Untersuchungen über das Lesen auf experimentelle Grundlage* (Max Niemeyer, Halle an der Saale); quoted in Volkmann (1962)

Evans C R, 1965 "Some studies of pattern perception using a stabilized retinal image" *Br. J. Psychol.* **56** 121-133

Exner S, 1875 "Das Sehen von Bewegungen und die Theorie des zusammengesetzten Auges" *Sitzungsberg. Akad. Wiss. Wien Math. Naturwiss. Kl. Abt. 3* 72

Faraday A, 1969 *Factors Affecting the Experimental Recall of Dreams* PhD Thesis, University College London, London England; quoted in Crickmar (1969)

Feinstein R, Williams W J, 1972a "Interactions of the horizontal and vertical human oculomotor systems: the saccadic system" *Vision Res.* **12** 33-44

Feinstein R, Williams W J, 1972b "Interactions of the horizontal and vertical human oculomotor systems: the vertical smooth pursuit and horizontal saccadic systems" *Vision Res.* **12** 45-52

Feldman M, Bender M B, 1966 "Non-visual responses of the lateral geniculate body with eye movements" *Fed. Proc. Fed. Am. Soc. Exp. Biol.* **25** 573

Feldman M, Cohen B, 1968 "Electrical activity in the lateral geniculate body of the alert monkey associated with eye movements" *J. Neurophysiol.* **31** 455-466

Fender D H, 1955 "Torsional movements of the eyeball" *Br. J. Ophthalmol.* **39** 65-72

Fender D H, Julesz B, 1967 "Extension of Panum's fusional area in binocularly stabilized vision" *J. Opt. Soc. Am.* **57** 819-830

Fender D H, Nye P W, 1961 "An investigation of the mechanisms of eye movement control" *Kybernetik* **1** 81-88

Fernand V S V, Young J Z, 1951 "The sizes of nerve fibres of muscle nerves" *Proc. R. Soc. London B.* **139** 38-58

Fernandez C, Frederickson J M, 1963 "Experimental cerebellar lesions and their effect on vestibular function" *Acta Oto-Laryngol. Suppl.* **192** 52-62

Fernandez C, Goldberg J M, 1971 "Physiology of peripheral neurons innervating semicircular canals of the squirrel monkey. II. Response to sinusoidal stimulation and dynamics of peripheral vestibular system" *J. Neurophysiol.* **34** 661-675

Fernandez C, Goldberg J M, Abend W K, 1973 "Response to static tilts of peripheral neurons innervating otolith organs of the squirrel monkey" *J. Neurophysiol.* **35** 978-997

Fernandez C, Valentinuzzi M, 1968 "A study on the biophysical characteristics of the cat labyrinth" *Acta Oto-Laryngol.* **65** 293-310

Ferraro A, Barrera S E, 1938 "Differential features of 'cerebellar' and 'vestibular' phenomena in *Macacus rhesus*: preliminary report based on experiments on 300 monkeys" *Arch. Neurol. Psychiatry* **39** 902-918

Festinger L, 1971 "Eye movements and perception" in *The Control of Eye Movements* Eds P Bach-y-Rita, C C Collins, J E Hyde (Academic Press, New York) pp 259-273

Festinger L, Burnham C A, Ono H, Bamber D, 1967 "Efference and the conscious experience of perception" *J. Exp. Psychol. Monograph Suppl.* **74** (whole number 637)

Festinger L, Canon L. K, 1965 "Information about spatial location based on knowledge about efference" *Psychol. Rev.* **72** 373-384

Fick A, 1854 "Die Bewegungen des menschlichen Augapfels" *Z. Rat. Med. N. F.* **4** 101-128

Filehne W, 1922 "Über die optische Wahrnehmung von Bewegungen" *Z. Sinnesphysiol.* **53** 134-144

Findlay J M, 1971 "Frequency analysis of human involuntary eye movement" *Kybernetik* **8** 207-214

Findlay J M, 1974 "Direction perception and human fixation eye movements" *Vision Res.* **14** 703-711

Fiorentini A, Ercoles A M, 1966 "Involuntary eye movements during attempted monocular fixation" *Atti Fond. Giorgio Ronchi* **21** 199-217

Fiorentini A, Mazzintini L, 1965 "Inhibition of after-images due to voluntary eye movements" *Atti Fond. Giorgio Ronchi* **20** 307-320

Fisch U, 1973 "The vestibular response following unilateral vestibular neurectomy" *Acta Oto-Laryngol.* **76** 229-238

Fleming D G, Vossius W, Bowman G, Johnson E L, 1969 "Adaptive properties of eye tracking system as revealed by moving head and open loop studies" *Ann. N.Y. Acad. Sci.* **156** 825-850

Flieringa H J, Hoeve J van der, 1924 "Arbeiten aus dem Gebiete der Akkommodation" *Albrecht von Graefes Arch. Opthalmol.* **114** 1-46

Flock Ä, 1964 "Structure of the macula utriculi with special reference to directional interplay of sensory receptors as revealed by morphological polarization" *J. Cell Biol.* **22** 413-431

Flom M C, 1960 "On the relationship between accommodation and accommodative convergence" (in three parts) *Am. J. Optom.* **37** 474-482, 517-523, 619-632

Fluur E, Mellström A, 1970 "Saccular stimulation and oculomotor reactions" *Laryngoscope* **80** 1713-1721

Fluur E, Mellström A, 1971 "The otolith organs and their influence on oculomotor movements" *Exp. Neurol.* **30** 139-147

Fluur E, Mendel L, 1973 "Relation between strength of stimulus and nystagmus frequency in patients with Ménières disease" *Acta Oto-Laryngol.* **76** 32-36

Fluur E, Siegborn J, 1973 "Interaction between the utricles and the horizontal semicircular canals" *Acta Oto-Laryngol.* **75** 17-20, 393-395, 485-488

Fox J C, Couch F H, Dodge R, 1931 "Optic nystagmus. IV. Psychological conditions" *Arch. Neurol. Psychiatry* **26** 23-35

Franck M C, Kuhlo W, 1970 "Die Wirkung des Alkohols auf die raschen Blickziel-bewegungen beim Menschen" *Arch. Psychiatr. Nervenkr.* **213** 238-245

Freeman J A, Nicholson C N, 1970 "Space-time transformation in the frog cerebellum through an intrinsic tapped delay line" *Nature (London)* **226** 640-642

Fritsch G, Hitzig E, 1870 "Über die elektrische Erregbarkeit des Grosshirsn" *Arch. Anat. Physiol. Wiss. Med.* 300-332

Fry G A, 1937 "An experimental analysis of the accommodation-convergence relationship" *Am. J. Optom.* **14** 402-414

Fry G A, 1939 "Further experiments on the accommodation-convergence relationship" *Am. J. Optom.* **16** 325-336

Fry G A, Hill W W, 1962 "The center of rotation of the eye *Am. J. Optom.* **39** 581-595

Fry G A, Hill W W, 1963 "The mechanics of elevating the eye" *Am. J. Optom.* **40** 707-716

Fuchs A F, 1967a "Saccadic and smooth pursuit eye movements in the monkey" *J. Physiol. (London)* **191** 609-631

Fuchs A F, 1967b "Periodic eye tracking in the monkey" *J. Physiol. (London)* **193** 161-171

Fuchs A F, 1971 "The saccadic system" in *The Control of Eye Movements* Eds P Bach-y-Rita, C C Collins, J E Hyde (Academic Press, New York) pp 343-362

Fuchs A F, Kornhuber H H, 1969 "Extraocular muscle afferents to the cerebellum of the cat" *J. Physiol. (London)* **200** 713-722

Fuchs A F, Luschei E S, 1970 "Firing patterns of abducens neurons of alert monkeys in relationship to horizontal eye movements" *J. Neurophysiol.* **33** 382-392

Fuchs A F, Luschei E S, 1971 "The activity of single trochlear nerve fibres during eye movements in the alert monkey" *Exp. Brain Res.* **13** 78-89

Fuchs A F, Luschei E S, 1972 "Unit activity in the brainstem related to eye movement" in *Cerebral Control of Eye Movements and Motion Perception* Eds J Dichgans, E Bizzi (Karger, Basel) pp 17-27

Fuchs A F, Robinson D A, 1966 "A method for measuring horizontal and vertical eye movements chronically in the monkey" *J. Appl. Physiol.* **21** 1068-1070

Fujita Y, Rosenberg J, Segundo J P, 1968 "Activity of cells in the lateral vestibular nucleus as a function of head position" *J. Physiol. (London)* **196** 1-18

Fukuda J, Highstein S M, Ito M, 1972 "Cerebellar inhibitory control of the vestibulo-ocular reflex investigated in rabbit IIIrd nucleus" *Exp. Brain Res.* **14** 511-526

Gaarder K, 1967 "Mechanisms in fixation saccadic eye movements" *Br. J. Physiol. Opt.* **24** 28-44

Gaarder K R, 1970 "Eye movements and perception" in *Early Experience and Visual Information Processing in Perceptual and Reading Disorders* Eds. F A Young, D B Lindsley (National Academy of Sciences, Washington, DC) pp 79-94

Gacek R R, 1961 "Efferent components of the vestibular nerve" in *Neural Mechanisms of the Auditory and Vestibular Systems* Eds G L Rasmussen, W F Windle (Charles C Thomas, Springfield, Ill.)

Gacek R R, 1969 "The course and central termination of first order neurons supplying vestibular endorgans in the cat" *Acta Oto-Laryngol. Suppl.* **254** 1-66

Gentles W, Llewellyn Thomas E, 1971 "Effect of benzodiazepines upon saccadic eye movements in man" *Clin. Pharmacol. Ther.* **12** 563-574

Gernandt B E, 1968 "Interactions between extraocular myotatic and ascending vestibular activities" *Exp. Neurol.* **20** 120-134

Gerrits A J M, Hann B de, Vendrick A J H, 1966 "Experiments with retinal stabilised images: relations between the observations and neural data" *Vision Res.* **6** 427-440

Gilson R D, Stockwell C W, Guedry F E, 1973 "Nystagmus responses during triangular waveforms of angular velocity about the *Y*- and *Z*-axes" *Acta Oto-Laryngol.* **75** 21-26

Ginsborg B L, 1953 "Small voluntary movements of the eye" *Br. J. Ophthalmol.* **37** 746-754

di Giorgio A, 1935 "Comportamento di alcune reazioni labirintiche durante il sonno fisologico (ricerche nei bambini)" *Boll. Soc. Ital. Biol. Sper.* **10** 951-953

Glickstein M, Stein J, King R A, 1972 "Visual input to the pontine nuclei" *Science* **178** 1110-1111

Gogan P, Gueritaud J P, Horcholle-Bossavit G, Tyc-Dumont S, 1973 "Inhibitory nystagmic interneurones: physiological and anatomical identification within the abducens nucleus" *Brain Res.* **59** 410-416

Gogel W C, 1962 "The effect of convergence on perceived size and distance" *J. Psychol.* **53** 475-489

Goldberg J M, Fernandez C, 1971 "Physiology of peripheral neurons innervating semicircular canals of the squirrel monkey. I. Resting discharge and response to constant angular accelerations" *J. Neurophysiol.* **34** 635-660

Goldberg S J, Hull C D, Buchwald N A, 1972 "Intracellular responses of two populations of neurons in cat abducens nucleus" *Anat. Rec.* **172** 316-317

Gonshor A, Melvill Jones G, 1969 "Investigation of habituation to rotational stimulation within the range of natural movement" *Proc. Ann. Sci. Meeting Aerosp. Med. Ass.*, San Francisco, Calif., 94-95

Gonshor A, Melvill Jones G, 1971 "Vestibular habituation induced by mirror vision: an optimising process?" *Proc. Ann. Sci. Meeting Aerosp. Med. Ass.*, Houston, Tex., 253-254

Gonshor A, Melvill Jones G, 1973 "Changes of human vestibulo-ocular response induced by vision-reversal during head rotation" *J. Physiol. (London)* **234** 102P-103P

Gonshor A, Melvill Jones G, 1976a "Short-term adaptive changes in the human vestibulo-ocular reflex arc" *J. Physiol. (London)* **256** 361-379

Gonshor A, Melvill Jones G, 1976b "Extreme vestibulo-ocular adaptation induced by prolonged optical reversal of vision" *J. Physiol. (London)* **256** 381-414

Goodwin A W, Fender D H, 1973a "The interaction between horizontal and vertical eye-rotations in tracking tasks" *Vision Res.* **13** 1701-1712

Goodwin A W, Fender D H, 1973b "Recognition of component differences in two-dimensional oculomotor tracking tasks" *Vision Res.* **13** 1905-1913

Gordon B, 1973 "Receptive fields in deep layers of cat superior colliculus" *J.Neurophysiol.* **36** 157-178

Goto K, Tokumasu K, Cohen B, 1968 "Return eye movements, saccadic movements, and the quick phase of nystagmus" *Acta Oto-Laryngol.* **65** 426-440

Gould J D, Peeples D R, 1970 "Eye movements during visual search and discrimination of meaningless, symbol, and object patterns" *J. Exp. Psychol.* **85** 51-55
Granit R, 1971 "The probable role of muscle spindles and tendon organs in eye movement control" in *The Control of Eye Movements* Eds P Bach-y-Rita, C C Collins, J E Hyde (Academic Press, New York), pp 3-5
Graybiel A M, 1974 "Visuo-cerebellar and cerebello-visual connections involving the ventral lateral geniculate nucleus" *Exp. Brain Res.* **20** 303-306
Graybiel A M, Hartweig E A, 1974 "Some afferent connections of the oculomotor complex in the cat: an experimental study with tracer techniques" *Brain Res.* **81** 543-551
Green D G, 1970 "Regional variations in the visual acuity for interference fringes on the retina" *J. Physiol. (London)* **207** 351-356
Green D G, Campbell F W, 1965 "Effect of focus on the visual response to a sinusoidally modulated spatial stimulus" *J. Opt. Soc. Am.* **55** 1154-1157
Greene T, Jampel R S, 1966 "Muscle spindles in the extraocular muscles of the macaque" *J. Comp. Neurol.* **126** 547-550
Gregory R L, 1959 "A blue filter technique for detecting eye movements during the autokinetic effect" *Q. J. Exp. Psychol.* **11** 113-114
Gregory R L, Ross H E, Moray N, 1964 "The curious eye of *Copilia*" *Nature (London)* **201** 1166-1168
Gregory R L, Zangwill O L, 1963 "The origin of the autokinetic effect" *Q. J. Exp. Psychol.* **15** 252-261
Grey E J, Barnes C D, 1973 "Some observations on the pathway of the vestibular rapid transmission system" *Brain Res.* **57** 213-217
Groen J J, Lowenstein O, Vendrick A J H, 1952 "The mechanical analysis of the responses from the end-organs of the horizontal semicircular canal in the isolated elasmobranch labyrinth" *J. Physiol. (London)* **117** 329-346
Grolman B, 1963 "The sighting centre" *Am. J. Optom.* **40** 666-675
Gross E G, Vaughan H G, Valenstein E, 1967 "Inhibition of visual evoked responses to patterned stimuli during voluntary eye movements" *Electroencephalogr. Clin. Neurophysiol.* **22** 204-209
Gruber E, 1962 "Reading ability, binocular coordination and the ophthalmograph" *Arch. Ophthalmol.* **67** 280-288
Grüsser-Cornehls U, Grüsser O-J, Bullock T H, 1963 "Unit responses in the frog's tectum to moving and non-moving visual stimuli" *Science* **141** 820-822
Guedry F E, 1965 "Orientation of the rotation-axis relative to gravity: its influence on nystagmus and the sensation of rotation" *Acta Oto-Laryngol.* **60** 30-49
Guilford J P, Dallenbach K M, 1928 "A study of the autokinetic sensation" *Am. J. Psychol.* **40** 83-91
Guitton D, Mandl G, 1973 "The effect of frontal eye field stimulation on unit responses in the superior colliculus of the cat" *Brain Res.* **68** 330-334
Gurevich B Kh, 1961 "Universal characteristics of fixation eye jerks: change of fixation as a cybernetic model of directed behaviour" *Biofizika* **6** 377-384
Haddad G M, Steinman R M, 1973 "The smallest voluntary saccade: implications for fixation" *Vision Res.* **13** 1075-1086
Haliska D T, 1973 "The influence of drugs on caloric-induced nystagmus" *Acta Oto-Laryngol.* **75** 477-484
Hallett P E, Lightstone A D, 1973 "Corrective saccades and visual inflow during the prior saccade" *J. Opt. Soc. Am.* **63** 1311
Hallett P E, Lightstone A D, 1976a "Saccadic eye movements towards stimuli triggered by prior saccades" *Vision Res.* **16** 99-106
Hallett P E, Lightstone A D, 1976b "Saccadic eye movements to flashed targets" *Vision Res.* **16** 107-114

Hammond P H, Merton P A, Sutton G G, 1956 "Nervous gradation of muscular contraction" *Br. Med. Bull.* **12** 214-218

Hardy M, 1934 "Observations on the innervation of the macula sacculi in man" *Anat. Rec.* **59** 403-418

Harker D W, 1972 "The structure and innervation of sheep superior rectus and levator palpebrae muscles. I. Extrafusal muscle fibres" *Invest. Ophthalmol.* **11** 956-969

Harris C S, 1963 "Adaptation to displaced vision: visual, motor or proprioceptive change" *Science* **140** 812-813

Harris H E, Komatsuzaki A, Cohen B, 1967 "Oculomotor defects after lesions of the mesencephalic reticular formation in monkeys" *Physiologist* **10** 195

Hartridge H, 1922 "Visual acuity and the resolving power of the eye" *J. Physiol. (London)* **57** 52-67

Hassler R, 1972 "Supranuclear structures regulating binocular eye and head movements" in *Cerebral Control of Eye Movements and Motion Perception* Eds. J Dichgans, E Bizzi (Karger, Basel) pp 207-219

Hay J C, 1968 "Visual adaptation to an altered correlation between eye movement and head movement" *Science* **160** 429-430

Hayashi Y, Nagata T, Iwama K, 1974 "Modulation of synaptic transmission in cat's superior colliculus by saccadic eye movements" *Brain Res.* **72** 162-167

Hebbard F W, Marg E, 1960 "Physiological nystagmus in the cat" *J. Opt. Soc. Am.* **50** 151-155

Held R, 1961 "Exposure-history as a factor in maintaining stability of perception and co-ordination" *J. Nerv. Ment. Dis.* **132** 26-32

Held R, Bossom J, 1961 "Neonatal deprivation and adult rearrangement: complementary techniques for analyzing plastic sensory-motor co-ordinations" *J. Comp. Physiol. Psychol.* **54** 33-37

Held R, Freedman S J, 1963 "Plasticity in human sensorimotor control" *Science* **142** 455-462

Helmholtz H von, 1909 *Handbuch der Physiologischen Optik* (3rd edition) (Voss, Hamburg) English translation by J P C Southall (1924) for the Optical Society of America

Henderson J W, Crosby E C, 1952 "An experimental study of optokinetic responses" *Arch. Ophthalmol.* **47** 43-54

Henn V, Cohen B, 1973 "Quantitative analysis of activity in eye muscle motoneurones during saccadic eye movements and positions of fixation" *J. Neurophysiol.* **36** 115-126

Henn V, Young L R, Finley C, 1974 "Vestibular nucleus units in alert monkeys are also influenced by moving visual fields" *Brain Res.* **71** 144-149

Henriksson N G, 1955 "The correlation between the speed of the eye in the slow phase of nystagmus and vestibular stimulus" *Acta Oto-Laryngol.* **45** 120-135

Henriksson N G, Novotny M, Tjernström Ö, 1974 "Eye movements as a function of active head turnings" *Acta Oto-Laryngol.* **77** 86-91

Hering E, 1868 *Die Lehre vom binocularen Sehen* (Engelmann, Leipzig)

Hering E, 1879a in *Handbuch der Physiologie* Ed. L Hermann, Volum III, Teil 1 (Vogel, Leipzig) pp 343-601

Hering E, 1879b "Über Muskelgeräusche des Auges" *Sitzungsber. Akad. Wiss. Wien Math. Naturwiss. Kl. Abt. 3* **79** 137-154

Hermann H T, 1971 "Saccade correlated potentials in optic tectum and cerebellum of *Carassius auratus*" *Brain Res.* **26** 293-304

Hermann H T, Constantine M M, 1971 "Eye movements in the goldfish" *Vision Res.* **11** 313-331

Hess A, 1961 "The structure of slow and fast extrafusal muscle fibres in the extraocular muscles and their nerve endings in guinea pigs" *J. Cell. Comp. Physiol.* **58** 63-79

Hess A, Pilar G, 1963 "Slow muscle fibres in the extraocular muscles of the cat" *J. Physiol. (London)* **169** 780-798

Heywood S, 1973 "Asymmetries related to cerebral dominance in returning the eyes to specified target positions in the dark" *Vision Res.* **13** 81-94

Heywood S, Ratcliff G, 1975 "Long-term oculomotor consequences of unilateral colliculectomy in man" in *Basic Mechanisms of Ocular Motility* Eds G Lennerstrand, P Bach-y-Rita (Pergamon Press, Oxford) pp 561-564

Highstein S M, 1971 "Organisation of the inhibitory and excitatory vestibulo-ocular reflex pathways to the third and fourth nuclei in rabbits" *Brain Res.* **32** 218-224

Highstein S M, 1972 "Electrophysiological investigation of the organization of the vestibulo-ocular pathways in the rabbit" in *Cerebral Control of Eye Movements and Motion Perception* Eds J Dichgans, E Bizzi (Karger, Basel) pp 89-98

Highstein S M, Cohen B, Matsunami K, 1974 "Monosynaptic projections from the pontine reticular formation to the IIIrd nucleus in the rat" *Brain Res.* **75** 340-344

Hikosaka P, Maeda M, 1973 "Cervical effects on abducens motoneurones and their interaction with vestibulo-ocular reflex" *Exp. Brain Res.* **18** 512-530

Hilding A C, 1954 "Normal vitreous, its attachments and dynamics during ocular movement" *Arch. Ophthalmol.* **52** 497-514

Hill A V, 1970 *First and Last Experiments in Muscle Mechanics* (Cambridge University Press, London)

Hillebrand F, 1893 "Die Stabilität der Raumwerte auf der Netzhaut" *Z. Psychol. Physiol. Sinnesorg.* **5** 1-60

Hines M, 1931 "Studies in the innervation of skeletal muscle III. Innervation of the extrinsic eye muscles of the rabbit" *Am. J. Anat.* **47** 1-53

Hinoki M, Terayama K, 1966a "Studies on optic head nystagmus from the standpoint of body equilibrium" *Acta Oto-Laryngol.* **62** 8-18

Hinoki M, Terayama K, 1966b "Physiological role of neck muscles in the occurrence of optic eye nystagmus" *Acta Oto-Laryngol.* **62** 157-170

Hitzig E, 1874 *Untersuchungen über das Gehirn* (Hirschwald, Berlin)

Hixson W C, Niven J I, Correia M J, 1966 *Kinematics Nomenclature for Physiological Accelerations* monograph 14, Naval Aerospace Medical Institute, Pensacola, Fla

Hofmann F B, 1925 "Die Lehre vom Raumsinn" in *Graefe und Saemischs Handbuch der Gesamten Augenheilkunde* 2nd edition, volume 3, Eds T Axenfeld, A Elsching (Springer, Berlin)

Hofstetter H W, 1942 "The proximal factor in accommodation and convergence" *Am. J. Optom.* **19** 67-76

Hofstetter H W, 1972 "Interpupillary distances in adult populations" *J. Am. Opt. Ass.* **43** 1151-1155

Holmes G, 1917 "The symptoms of acute cerebellar injuries due to gunshot injuries" *Brain* **40** 461-535

Holmes G, 1938 "The cerebral integration of the ocular movements" *Br. Med. J.*, 16 July, 107-112

Holst E von, 1954 "Relations between the central nervous system and peripheral organs" *Br. J. Anim. Behav.* **2** 89-94

Holst E von, 1957 "Aktive Leistungen der menschlichen Gesichtswahrnehmung" *Stud. Gen.* **10** 231-243

Holt E B, 1903, "Eye-movement and central anaesthesia. I. The problem of anaesthesia during eye-movement" *Psychol. Mon.* **4** (17) 3-46

Honrubia V, Downey W L, Mitchell D P, Ward P H, 1968 "Experimental studies on optokinetic nystagmus. II. Normal humans" *Acta Oto-Laryngol.* **65** 441-448

Honrubia V, Scott B J, Ward P H, 1967 "Experimental studies on optokinetic nystagmus. I. Normal cats" *Acta Oto-Laryngol.* **64** 388-402
Hood J D, 1967a "Observations upon the neurological mechanism of optokinetic nystagmus with especial reference to the contribution of peripheral vision" *Acta Oto-Laryngol.* **63** 208-215
Hood J D, 1967b "Recent advances in the electronystagmographic investigation of vestibular and other disorders of ocular movement" in *Ciba Symp., Myotatic, Kinesthetic and Vestibular Mechanisms* Eds A V S de Reuk, J Knight (Churchill, London) pp 252-269
Hood J D, 1975 "Observations upon the role of the peripheral retina in the execution of eye movements" *Oto-Rhino-Laryngol.* **37** 65-73
Hood J D, Kayan A, Leech J, 1973 "Rebound nystagmus" *Brain* **96** 507-526
Hood J D, Leech J, 1974 "The significance of peripheral vision in the perception of movement" *Acta Oto-Laryngol.* **77** 72-79
Hood J D, Pfaltz C R, 1954 "Observations upon the effects of repeated stimulation upon rotational and caloric nystagmus" *J. Physiol. (London)* **124** 130-144
Horcholle-Bossavit G, Tyc-Dumont S, 1971 "Evidence for a rapid transmission system in the cat vestibulo-ocular pathway" *Exp. Brain Res.* **13** 327-338
Horridge G A, 1966 "Study of a system, as illustrated by the optokinetic response" *Symp. Soc. Exp. Biol.* **20** 179-198
Houk J, Henneman E, 1967 "Responses of Golgi tendon organs to active contractions of the soleus muscle of the cat" *J. Neurophysiol.* **30** 466-481
Howe L, 1907 *The Muscles of the Eye* volume 1 (Putnam, New York)
Hoyt W F, Daroff R B, 1971 "Supranuclear disorders of ocular control in man" in *The Control of Eye Movements* Eds P Bach-y-Rita, C C Collins, J E Hyde (Academic Press, New York) pp 175-235
Hubel D H, Wiesel T N, 1962 "Receptive fields, binocular organisation and functional architecture in the cat's visual cortex" *J. Physiol. (London)* **160** 559-568
Hubel D H, Wiesel T N, 1968 "Receptive fields and functional architecture of monkey striate cortex" *J. Physiol. (London)* **195** 215-243
Huber G C, 1900 "Sensory nerve terminations in the tendons of the extrinsic eye-muscles of the cat" *J. Comp. Neurol.* **10** 152-158
Hughes A, 1972 "Vergence in the cat" *Vision Res.* **12** 1961-1994
Hughlings Jackson J, 1932 *Selected Writings* volume 2 (Hodder and Stoughton, London) p 470
Hughlings Jackson J, Paton L, 1909 "On some abnormalities of ocular movements" *Lancet* **176** 900-905
Hunt C C, Kuffler S W, 1951 "Further study of efferent small-nerve fibres to mammalian muscle spindles: muscle spindle innervation and activity during contraction" *J. Physiol. (London)* **113** 283-297
Hyde J E, 1959 "Some characteristics of voluntary human ocular movements in the horizontal plane" *Am. J. Ophthalmol.* **48** 85-94
Hyde J E, Eason R G, 1959 "Characteristics of ocular movements evoked by stimulation of brainstem of cat" *J. Neurophysiol.* **22** 666-678
Hyde J E, Toczek S, 1962 "Functional relation of interstitial nucleus to rotatory movements evoked from zona incerta stimulation" *J. Neurophysiol.* **25** 455-466
Ikeda H, Wright M J, 1972 "The outer disinhibitory surround of the retinal ganglion cell receptive field" *J. Physiol. (London)* **226** 511-544
Irvine S R, Ludvigh E J, 1936 "Is ocular proprioceptive sense concerned in vision?" *Arch. Ophthalmol.* **15** 1037-1049
Ito F, Bach-y-Rita P, 1969 "Afferent discharges from extraocular muscle in the squirrel monkey" *Am. J. Physiol.* **217** 332-335
Ito M, 1972 "Neural design of the cerebellar motor system" *Brain Res.* **40** 81-84

Ito M, Nisimaru N, Yamamoto M, 1973a "The neural pathways mediating reflex contractions of extraocular muscles during semicircular canal stimulation in rabbits" *Brain Res.* **55** 183-188

Ito M, Nisimaru N, Yamamoto M, 1973b "The neural pathways relaying reflex inhibition from semicircular canals to extraocular muscles of rabbits" *Brain Res.* **55** 189-193

Ito M, Nisimaru N, Yamamoto M, 1973c "Specific neural connections for the cerebellar control of vestibulo-ocular reflexes" *Brain Res.* **60** 238-243

Ito M, Shiida T, Yagi N, Yamamoto M, 1974 "Visual influence on rabbit horizontal vestibulo-ocular reflex presumably effected via the cerebellar flocculus" *Brain Res.* **65** 170-174

Ito M, Yoshida M, Obata K, 1964 "Monosynaptic inhibition of the intracerebellar nuclei induced from the cerebellar cortex" *Experientia* **20** 575-576

Ittelson W H, Ames A Jr, 1950 "Accommodation, convergence, and their relation to apparent distance" *J. Psychol.* **30** 43-62

James W, 1950 *Principles of Psychology* volume 2 (Dover, New York)

Jampel R S, 1960 "Convergence, divergence, pupillary reactions and accommodation of the eyes from faradic stimulation of the macaque brain" *J. Comp. Neurol.* **115** 371-400

Jampel R S, 1966 "The action of the superior oblique muscle" *Arch. Opthalmol.* **75** 535-544

Jampolsky A, 1970 "Ocular divergence mechanisms" *Trans. Am. Opthalmol. Soc.* **68** 730-822

Janeke J B, Jonkees C B W, Oosterveld W J, 1969 "Selective suppression of the fast phase of labyrinthine nystagmus by phentanyl (fentanyl)" *Acta Oto-Laryngol.* **68** 468-473

Jeannerod M, 1972 "Saccade correlated events in the lateral geniculate body" in *Cerebral Control of Eye Movements and Motion Perception* Eds J Dichgans, E Bizzi (Karger, Basel) pp 189-198

Jeannerod M, Kiyono S, Mouret J, 1968 "Effets des lesions frontales bilaterales sur le comportement oculo-moteur chez le chat" *Vision Res.* 8 575-583

Jeannerod M, Putkonen P T S, 1971 "Lateral geniculate unit activity and eye movements: saccade-locked changes in dark and in light" *Exp. Brain Res.* **13** 533-546

Johnson W H, Winter N R, 1958 "Eye movement detection" *IRE Canadian Convention Record* 194

Johnstone J R, Mark R F, 1969 "Evidence for efference copy for eye movements in fish" *Comp. Biochem. Physiol.* **30** 931-939

Jones L A, Higgins G C, 1947 "Photographic granularity and graininess. III. Some characteristics of the visual system of importance in the evaluation of graininess and granularity" *J. Opt. Soc. Am.* **37** 217-263

Jones R, 1973 "Two dimensional eye movement recording using a photo-electric matrix method" *Vision Res.* **13** 425-431

de Jong J D, Melvill Jones G, 1971 "Akinesia, hypokinesia and bradykinesia in the oculomotor system of patients with Parkinson's disease" *Exp. Neurol.* **32** 58-68

Jordan S, 1970 "Ocular pursuit movement as a function of visual and proprioceptive stimulation" *Vision Res.* **10** 775-780

Judd C H, 1905 " The Müller-Lyer illusion" *Psychol. Rev.* 7 *Monogr. Suppl.* **29** 55-58

Judge S J, 1973 "Temporal interaction between human voluntary saccades and rapid phases of optokinetic nystagmus" *Exp. Brain Res.* **18** 114-118

Jung R, Kornhuber H H, 1964 "Results of electronystagmography in man: the value of optokinetic, vestibular and spontaneous nystagmus for neurological diagnosis and research" in *The Oculomotor System* Ed. M B Bender (Harper and Row, New York) pp 428-482

Jürgens R, Becker W, 1975 "Is there a linear addition of saccades and pursuit movements?" in *Basic Mechanisms of Ocular Motility* Eds G Lennerstrand, P Bach-y-Rita (Pergamon Press, Oxford) pp 525-529

Karrer E, Stevens H C, 1930 "The response of negative after-images to passive motion of the eyeball and the bearing of these observations on the visual perception of motion" *Am. J. Physiol.* **94** 611-614

Kasahara M, Uchino Y, 1974 "Bilateral semicircular canal inputs to neurons in cat vestibular nuclei" *Exp. Brain Res.* **20** 285-296

Kato T, 1938 "Über histologische Untersuchungen der Augenmuskeln von Menschen und Säugetieren" *Okajimas Folia Anat. Jpn.* **16** 131-145

Katz R L, Eakins K E, 1966a "A comparison of the effects of neuromuscular blocking agents and cholinesterase inhibitors on the tibialis anterior and superior rectus muscles of the cat" *J. Pharmacol. Exp. Ther.* **152** 304-312

Katz R L, Eakins K E, 1966b "The effects of succinylcholine, decamethonium, hexacarbacholine, gallamine and dimethyl tubocurarine on the twitch and tonic neuromuscular systems of the cat" *J. Pharmacol. Exp. Ther.* **154** 303-309

Kaufman L, Richards W, 1969 "Spontaneous fixation tendencies for visual forms" *Percept. Psychophys.* **5** 85-88

Kawamura H, Marchiafava P L, 1968 "Excitability changes along visual pathways during eye tracking movements" *Arch. Ital. Biol.* **106** 141-156

Kawamura H, Brodal A, 1973 "The tectopontine projection in the cat: an experimental anatomical study with comments on pathways for teleceptive impulses to the cerebellum" *J. Comp. Neurol.* **149** 371-390

Kawamura H, Brodal A, Hoddevik G, 1974 "The projection of the superior colliculus onto the reticular formation of the brain stem: an experimental study in the cat" *Exp. Brain Res.* **19** 1-19

Keesey U T, 1960 "Effects of involuntary eye movement on visual acuity" *J. Opt. Soc. Am.* **50** 769-774

Keller E L, 1973 "Accommodative vergence in the alert monkey: motor unit analysis" *Vision Res.* **13** 1565-1575

Keller E L, 1974 "Participation of medial pontine reticular formation in eye movement generation in monkey" *J. Neurophysiol.* **37** 316-332

Keller E L, Robinson D A, 1971 "Absence of a stretch reflex in extraocular muscle of the monkey" *J. Neurophysiol.* **34** 908-919

Keller E L, Robinson D A, 1972 "Abducens unit behaviour in the monkey during vergence movements" *Vision Res.* **12** 369-382

Kelly D H, Crane H D, Hill J W, Cornsweet T N, 1969 "Non-contact method of measuring small eye movements and stabilising the retinal image" *J. Opt. Soc. Am.* **59** 508

Kennard D W, Hartmann R W, Kraft D P, Boshes B, 1970 "Perceptual suppression of after-images" *Vision Res.* **10** 575-585

Kern R, 1965 "A comparative phamacologic-histologic study of slow and twitch fibres in the superior rectus of the rabbit" *Invest. Ophthalmol.* **4** 901-910

Kertesz A E, Jones R W, 1969 "The effect of angular velocity of stimulus on human torsional eye movements" *Vision Res.* **9** 995-998

Kertesz A E, Jones R W, 1970 "Human cyclofusional response" *Vision Res.* **10** 891-896

Kleijn A de, 1921a "Experiments on the quick component phase of vestibular nystagmus in the rabbit" *K. Ned. Akad. Wet. Ges. Physiol. Amst.* **23** 1357-1364

Kleijn A de, 1921 b "Tonische Labyrinth- und Halsreflexe auf die Augen" *Pflügers Archiv. Gesamte Physiol. Menschen Tiere* **186** 82-97

Klinke R, 1970 "Efferent influence on the vestibular organ during active movements of the body" *Pflügers Arch. Gesamte Physiol. Menschen Tiere* **318** 325-332

Klinke R, Schmidt C L, 1968 "Efferente Impulse in Nervus Vestibularis bei Reizung des kontraleteralen Otolithenorgans" *Pflügers Arch. Gesamte Physiol. Menschen Tiere* **304** 183-188

Knoll H A, 1949 "Pupillary changes associated with accommodation and convergence" *Am. J. Optom.* **26** 346-357

Koerner F, Schiller P H, 1972 "The optokinetic response under open and closed loop conditions in the monkey" *Exp. Brain Res.* **14** 318-330

Kommerell G, 1975 "Clinical clues for the organisation of horizontal quick eye movements and subsequent periods of fixation" in *Basic Mechanisms of Ocular Motility* Eds G Lennerstrand, P Bach-y-Rita (Pergamon Press, Oxford) pp 325-335

Kommerell G, Täumer R, 1972 "Investigations of the eye tracking system through stabilised retinal images" in *Cerebral Control of Eye Movements and Motion Perception* Eds J Dichgans, E Bizzi (Karger, Basel) pp 288-297

Komoda M K, Festinger L, Phillips L J, Duckman R H, Young R A, 1973 "Some observations concerning saccadic eye movements" *Vision Res.* **13** 1009-1020

Korn H, Sotelo C, Crepel F, 1973 "Electrotonic coupling between neurons in the rat lateral vestibular nucleus" *Exp. Brain Res.* **16** 255-275

Körner F H, 1975 "Non-visual control of human saccadic eye movements" in *Basic Mechanisms of Ocular Motility* Eds G Lennerstrand, P Bach-y-Rita (Pergamon Press, Oxford) pp 565-569

Kornhuber H H, 1971 "Motor functions of the cerebellum and basal ganglia: the cerebellocortical saccadic (ballistic) clock, the cerebellonuclear hold regulator, and the basal ganglia ramp (voluntary speed smooth movement) generator" *Kybernetik* 8 157-162

Kornmüller A E, 1931 "Eine experimentelle Anästhesie der äusseren Augenmuskeln von Menschen und ihre Auswirkungen" *J. Psychol. Neurol.* **41** 354-366

Krauskopf J, 1957 "Effect of retinal image motion on contrast thresholds for maintained vision" *J. Opt. Soc. Am.* **47** 740-744

Krauskopf J, Cornsweet T N, Riggs L A, 1960 "Analysis of eye movements during monocular and binocular fixation" *J. Opt. Soc. Am.* **50** 572-578

Krauskopf J, Graf V, Gaarder K, 1966 "Lack of inhibition during involuntary saccades" *Am. J. Psychol.* **79** 73-81

Krejcova H, Cohen B, Highstein S, 1973 "Compensatory ocular counter-rolling in the monkey" in *The Oculomotor System and Brain Function* Ed. V Zikmund (Butterworth, London) pp 491-503

Krejcova H, Highstein S, Cohen B, 1971 "Labyrinthine and extralabyrinthine effects on ocular counter-rolling" *Acta Oto-Laryngol.* 72 165-171

Krewson W E, 1950 "The action of the extraocular muscles" *Trans. Am. Ophthalmol. Soc.* **48** 443-486

Krieger H P, Bender M B, 1956 "Optokinetic afternystagmus in the monkey" *Electroencephalogr. Clin. Neurophysiol.* 8 97-106

Kris C, 1958 "Corneo-fundal potential variations during light and dark adaptation" *Nature (London)* **182** 1027-1028

Krishnan V V, Phillips S, Stark L, 1973 "Frequency analysis of accommodation, accommodative vergence and disparity vergence" *Vision Res.* **13** 1545-1554

Krüger P, 1929 "Über einen möglichen Zusammenhang zwischen Struktur, Funktion und chemischer Beschaffenheit der Muskeln" *Biol. Zentralbl.* **49** 616-622

Kuffler S W, Vaughan Williams E M, 1953a "Small-nerve junctional potentials: the distribution of small motor nerves to frog skeletal muscle, and membrane characteristics of the fibres they innervate" *J. Physiol. (London)* **121** 289-317

Kuffler S W, Vaughan Williams E M, 1953b "Properties of the 'slow' skeletal muscle fibres of the frog" *J. Physiol. (London)* **121** 318-340

Kuré K, Sunaga Y, Hatano S, Imagawa T, 1927 "Experimentelle und pathologische Studien über die progressive Muskelatrophie: V. Über die tropische Innervation der äusseren Augenmuskeln" *Z. Gesamte Exp. Med.* **54** 366-381

Kuypers H G J M, 1958 "Corticobulbar connections to the pons and lower brainstem in man: an anatomical study" *Brain* **81** 364-388

Kuypers H G J M, Lawrence D G, 1967 "Cortical projections to the red nucleus and the brain stem in the rhesus monkey" *Brain Res.* **4** 151-188

Ladpli R, Brodal A, 1968 "Experimental studies of commissural and reticular formation projections from the vestibular nuclei in the cat" *Brain Res.* **8** 65-96

Lamansky S, 1869 "Bestimmung der Winkelgeschwindigkeit der Blickbewegung, respective Augenbewegung" *Pflügers Arch. Gesamte Physiol. Menschen Tiere* **2** 418-422

Lamb H, 1919 "The kinematics of the eye" *Phil. Mag.* series 6 **38** 685-695

Lancaster W B, 1943 "Terminology in ocular motility and allied subjects" *Am. J. Ophthalmol.* **26** 122-132

Land M F, 1969 "Movements of the retinae of jumping spiders (*Salticidae dendryphantinae*) in response to visual stimuli" *J. Exp. Biol.* **51** 471-493

Land M F, 1973 "Head movement of flies during visually guided flight" *Nature (London)* **243** 299-300

Landers P H, Taylor A, 1975 "Transfer function analysis of the vestibulo-ocular reflex in the conscious cat" in *Basic Mechanisms of Ocular Motility* Ed. G Lennerstrand, P Bach-y-Rita (Pergamon Press, Oxford) pp 505-508

Landolt E, 1886 "The refraction and accommodation of the eye" translated by C M Culver (Pentland, Edinburgh)

Landolt E, 1891 "Nouvelles récherches sur la physiologie des mouvements des yeux" *Arch. Ophtalmol. Paris* **11** 385-395

Lane R H, Allman J M, Kaas J H, Miezin F M, 1973 "The visuotopic organisation of the superior colliculus of the owl monkey (*Aotus trivirgatus*) and the bush baby (*Galago senegalensis*) *Brain Res.* **60** 335-349

Larmande A, 1973 "The oculomotor role of the occipito-frontal connections" *Arch. Ophtalmol.* **33** 735-738

Latour P L, 1962 "Visual thresholds during eye movements" *Vision Res.* **2** 261-262

Latto R, Cowey A, 1971a "Visual field defects after frontal eye-field lesions in monkeys" *Brain Res.* **30** 1-24

Latto R, Cowey A, 1971b "Fixation changes after frontal eye-field lesions in monkeys" *Brain Res.* **30** 25-36

Laurentius, Andreas (André du Laurens), 1599 *A Discourse of the Preservation of the Sight: of Melancholike Diseases; of Rheumes, and of Old Age* translated by R Surphlet (Ralph Jacson, London) facsimile edition published by the Shakespeare Association, 1938 (Oxford University Press, London)

Le Conte J, 1881 *Sight; an Exposition of the Principles of Monocular and Binocular Vision* (Appleton, New York)

Lederberg V, 1970 "Color recognition during voluntary saccades" *J. Opt. Soc. Am.* **60** 835-842

Le Gros Clark W E, 1926 "The mammalian oculomotor nucleus" *J. Anat.* **60** 426-448

Leibovic K N, Balslev E, Mathieson T A, 1971 "Binocular vision and pattern recognition" *Kybernetik* **8** 14-23

Leinfelder P J, Black N M, 1941 "Experimental transposition of the extraocular muscles in monkeys" *Am. J. Ophthalmol.* **24** 1115-1120
Lemmen L J, Davis J S, Radnor L L, 1959 "Observations on stimulation of the human frontal eye field" *J. Comp. Neurol.* **112** 163-168
Lennerstrand G, 1974 "Mechanical studies on the retractor bulbi muscle and its motor units in the cat" *J. Physiol. (London)* **236** 43-55
Levy J, 1972 "Autokinetic illusion: a systematic review of theories, measures and independent variables" *Psychol. Bull.* **78** 457-474
Lévy-Schoen A, 1973 "Position of stimuli in the visual field and within a pattern, as determinants of the fixation response" in *The Oculomotor System and Brain Function* Ed. V Zikmund (Butterworth, London) pp 243-255
Lippold O C J, Shaw J C, 1971 "Alpha rhythm in the blind" *Nature (London)* **232** 134
Lisberger S G, Fuchs A F, 1974 "Response of flocculus Purkinje cells to adequate vestibular stimulation in the alert monkey: fixation vs. compensatory eye movements" *Brain Res.* **69** 347-353
Listing J B, 1855 The first reference to Listing's Law appears to be in Ruete's *Lehrbuch der Ophthalmologie* 2nd edition, volume 1, p 37
Llinas R, 1974 "Motor aspects of cerebellar control" *Physiologist* **17** 19-46
Llinas R, Precht W, Clarke M, 1971 "Cerebellar Purkinje cell responses to physiological stimulation of the vestibular system" *Exp. Brain Res.* **13** 408-431
Lloyd D P C, 1941 "The spinal mechanisms of the pyramidal system in cats" *J. Neurophysiol.* **4** 525-546
Lockhart R D, Brandt W, 1938 "Length of striated muscle fibres" *J. Anat.* **72** 470
Loe P R, Tomko D L, Werner G, 1973 "The neural signal of angular head position in primary vestibular nerve axons" *J. Physiol. (London)* **230** 29-50
Lord M P, Wright W D, 1948 "Eye movements during monocular fixation" *Nature (London)* **162** 25-26
Lorente de No R, 1933 "Vestibulo-ocular reflex arc" *Arch. Neurol. Psychiat.* **30** 245-291
Lorente de No R, 1949 "The structure of the cerebral cortex" in *Physiology of the Nervous System* Ed. J F Fulton (Oxford University Press, London)
Löwenstein O, 1937 "The tonic function of the horizontal canals in fishes" *J. Exp. Biol.* **14** 473-482
Löwenstein O, Roberts T D M, 1949 "The equilibrium function of the otolith organs of the thornback ray *(Raja clavata)*" *J. Physiol. (London)* **110** 392-415
Löwenstein O, Sand A, 1940 "The mechanism of the semicircular canal: a study of the responses of single-fibre preparations to angular accelerations and to rotation at constant speed" *Proc. R. Soc. London B.* **129** 256-275
Ludvigh E, 1952a "Possible role of proprioception in the extraocular muscles" *Arch. Ophthalmol.* **48** 436-441
Ludvigh E, 1952b "Control of ocular movements and visual interpretation of environment" *Arch. Ophthalmol.* **48** 442-448
Ludvigh E, McKinnon P, 1966 "Relative effectivity of foveal and parafoveal stimuli in eliciting fusion movements of small amplitude" *Arch. Ophthalmol.* **76** 443-449
Ludvigh E, McKinnon P, 1968 "Dependence of the amplitude of fusional convergence movements on the velocity of the eliciting stimulus" *Invest. Ophthalmol.* **7** 347-352
Ludvigh E, McKinnon P, Zaitzeff L, 1965 "Relative effectivity of foveal and parafoveal stimuli in eliciting fusional movements" *Arch. Ophthalmol.* **73** 115-121
Luneburg R K, 1948 *Mathematical Analysis of Binocular Vision* (Princeton University Press, Princeton, NJ)

Luneburg R K, 1950 "The metric of binocular visual space" *J. Opt. Soc. Am.* **40** 627-642

Luschei E S, Fuchs A F, 1972 "Activity of brain stem neurones during eye movements of alert monkeys" *J. Neurophysiol.* **35** 445-461

McCabe B F, 1965 "The quick component of nystagmus" *Laryngoscope* **75** 1619-1646

McCabe B F, Ryu J H, 1973 "Does perilymph modify cupular deflection?" *Acta Oto-Laryngol.* **75** 405-407

McCouch G P, Adler F H, 1932 "Extraocular reflexes" *Am. J. Physiol.* **100** 78-88

McCouch G P, Deering I D, Ling T M, 1951 "Location of receptors for tonic neck reflexes" *J. Neurophysiol.* **14** 191-195

McIlwain J T, 1973 "Retinotopic fidelity of striate cortex-superior colliculus interactions in the cat" *J. Neurophysiol.* **36** 702-710

McIlwain J T, Fields H L, 1971 "Interactions of cortical and retinal projections on single neurones of the cat's superior colliculus" *J. Neurophysiol.* **34** 763-772

McIntyre A K, 1939 "The quick component of nystagmus" *J. Physiol.* **97** 8-16

MacKay D M, 1970a "Elevation of visual threshold by displacement of retinal image" *Nature (London)* **225** 90-92

MacKay D M, 1970b "Mislocation of test flashes during saccadic image dispiacement" *Nature (London)* **227** 731-733

MacKay D M, 1973 "Visual stability and voluntary eye movements" in *Handbook of Sensory Physiology* volume VII/3A, Ed. R Jung (Springer, Berlin)

McLaughlin S C, Kelly M J Jr, 1968 "Parametric feedback in pursuit movements of the eyes" *J. Opt. Soc. Am.* **58** 728

McLaughlin S C, Sisto M J de, Breslow M, 1968 "Directional and nondirectional auditory feedback in control of eye position" *J. Opt. Soc. Am.* **58** 1559

McMasters R E, Weiss A H, Carpenter M B, 1966 "Vestibular projections to the nuclei of the extraocular muscles" *Am. J. Anat.* **118** 163-194

MacMillan R H, 1955 *An Introduction to the Theory of Control in Mechanical Engineering* (Cambridge University Press, London)

Mach E, 1875 *Grundlinien der Lehre von den Bewegungsempfindungen* (Engelmann, Leipzig)

Mach E, 1886 *Beiträge zur Analyse der Empfindungen* (Fischer, Jena) English translation, 1959: *The Analysis of Sensations* (Dover, New York)

Mack A, Bachant J, 1969 "Perceived movement of the afterimage during eye movements" *Percept. Psychophys.* **6** 379-384

Mackensen G, Schumacher J, 1960 "Die Geschwindigkeit der raschen Phase des optokinetischen Nystagmus" *Albrecht von Graefes Arch. Ophthalmol.* **162** 400-415

Mackensen G, Wiegmann O, 1959 "Untersuchungen zur Physiologie des optokinetischen Nachnystagmus. I Mitteilung. Die Abhängigkeit des optokinetischen Nachnystagmus von der Drehrichtung und der Winkelgeschwindigkeit des Reizmusters" *Albrecht von Graefes Arch. Ophthalmol.* **160** 497-509

Mackworth J F, Mackworth N H, 1958 "Eye fixations recorded on changing visual scenes by the television eye-marker" *J. Opt. Soc. Am.* **48** 439-445

Mackworth N H, Thomas E L, 1962 "Head-mounted eye-movement camera" *J. Opt. Soc. Am.* **52** 713-716

Maddox E E, 1907 *The Clinical Use of Prisms; and the Decentring of Lenses* 5th edition (John Wright, Bristol)

Maeda M, Shimazu H, Shinoda Y, 1971 "Rythmic activities of secondary vestibular efferent fibres recorded within the abducens nucleus during vestibular nystagmus" *Brain Res.* **34** 361-365

Maeda M, Shimazu H, Shinoda Y, 1972 "Nature of synaptic events in cat abducens motoneurones at slow and quick phase of vestibular nystagmus" *J. Neurophysiol.* **35** 279-296

Maekawa K, Simpson J I, 1971 "Climbing fibre responses evoked in the flocculus by visual pathway stimulation in the rabbit" *Proc. XXV Int. Congr. Physiol. Sci., Munich* **IX** abstract 1060, p 358

Maekawa K, Simpson J I, 1973 "Climbing fibre responses evoked in vestibulo-cerebellum of rabbit from visual system" *J. Neurophysiol.* **36** 649-666

Magnin M, Jeannerod M, Putkonen P T S, 1974 "Vestibular and saccadic influences on dorsal and ventral nuclei of the lateral geniculate body" *Exp. Brain Res.* **21** 1-18

Magoun H W, Hare W K, Ranson S W, 1937 "Electrical stimulation of the interior of the cerebellum in the monkey" *Am. J. Physiol.* **112** 329-339

Maier A, Eldred E, Edgerton V R, 1972 "Types of muscle fibers in the extraocular muscles of birds" *Exp. Eye Res.* **13** 255-265

Maier A, Santis M de, Eldred E, 1971 "Absence of muscle spindles in avian extraocular muscles" *Exp. Eye Res.* **12** 251-253

Malcolm R, Melvill Jones G, 1970 "A quantitative study of vestibular adaptation in humans" *Acta Oto-Laryngol.* **70** 126-135

Manni E, Bortolami R, Desole C, 1968 "Peripheral pathway of eye muscle proprioception" *Exp. Neurol.* **22** 1-12

Marchiafava P L, Pepeu G C, 1966 "Electrophysiological study of tectal responses to optic nerve volley" *Arch. Ital. Biol.* **104** 406-420

Marg E, 1951 "Development of electro-oculography" *Arch. Ophthalmol.* **45** 169-185

Marg E, Morgan M W Jr, 1949 "The pupillary near reflex: the relation of pupillary diameter to accommodation and the various components of convergence" *Am. J. Optom.* **26** 183-198

Marg E, Morgan M W Jr, 1950 "Further investigation of the pupillary near reflex; the effect of accommodation, fusional convergence and the proximity factor on pupillary diameter" *Am. J. Optom.* **27** 217-225

Marina A, 1915 "Die Relationen des Palaeencephalons (Edinger) sind nicht fix" *Neurol. Zentralbl.* **34** 338-345

Markham C H, 1968 "Midbrain and contralateral labyrinth influences on brain stem vestibular neurons in the cat" *Brain Res.* **9** 312-333

Markham C H, 1972 "Descending control of the vestibular nuclei: physiology" in *Basic Aspects of Central Vestibular Mechanisms* Eds A Brodal, O Pompeiano *Prog. Brain Res.* **37** 589-600

Markham C H, Curthoys I S, 1972 "Labyrinthine convergence on vestibular nuclear neurones using natural and electrical stimulation" in *Basic Aspects of Central Vestibular Mechanims* Eds A Brodal, O Pompeiano *Prog. Brain Res.* **37** 121-137

Markham C H, Precht W, Shimazu H, 1966 "Effect of stimulation of interstitial nucleus of Cajal on vestibular unit activity in the cat" *J. Neurophysiol.* **29** 493-507

Marquez M, 1949 "Supposed torsion of the eye around the visual axis in oblique directions of gaze" *Arch. Ophthalmol.* **41** 704-717

Marr D, 1969 "A theory of cerebellar cortex" *J. Physiol. (London)* **202** 437-470

Martin J P, 1967 *The Basal Ganglia and Posture* (Pitman, London)

Maruo T, 1964 "Electromyographical studies on stretch reflex in human extraocular muscle" *Jpn. J. Ophthalmol.* **8** 96-111

Masland R H, Chow K L, Stewart D L, 1971 "Receptive-field characteristics of superior colliculus neurones in the rabbit" *J. Neurophysiol.* **34** 148-156

Mathog R H, 1972 "Testing of the vestibular system by sinusoidal angular acceleration" *Acta Oto-Laryngol.* **74** 96-103

Matin E, 1974 "Saccadic suppression: a review and an analysis" *Psychol. Bull.* **81** 899-917

Matin L, MacKinnon G E, 1964 "Autokinetic movement: selective manipulation of directional components by image stabilization" *Science* **143** 147-148

Matin L, Matin E, Pearce D G, 1969 "Visual perception of direction when voluntary saccades occur. 1. Relation of visual direction of fixation target extinguished before a saccade to a flash presented during the saccade" *Percept. Psychophys.* **5** 65-80

Matin L, Matin E, Pearce D G, 1970 "Eye movements in the dark during the attempt to maintain a prior fixation position" *Vision Res.* **10** 837-857

Matin L, Pearce D G, 1965 "Visual perception of direction for stimuli flashed during voluntary eye movements" *Science* **148** 1485-1487

Matin L, Pearce D G, Kibler G, 1964 "Roles of local sign and ocular proprioception in the determination of visual direction during eye movements" *J. Opt. Soc. Am.* **54** 1398

Matin L, Pearce D G, Matin E, Kibler G, 1966 "Visual perception of direction in the dark: roles of local sign, eye movements and ocular proprioception" *Vision Res.* **6** 453-469

Matsunami K, 1972 "Saccadic eye movement and neurons in the central gray areas in awake monkeys" *Brain Res.* **38** 217-221

Matthews P B C, 1972 *Mammalian Muscle Receptors and their Central Actions* (Edward Arnold, London)

Matyushkin D P, 1961 "Phasic and tonic neuromotor units in the oculomotor apparatus of the rabbit" *Sechenov Physiol. J.USSR* **47** 65-69

Mayr R, 1971 "Structure and distribution of fibre types in external eye muscles of rat" *Tissue Cell* **3** 433-462

Melvill Jones G, 1960 "Comparison of nystagmoid responses to rotational stimuli about vertical and rolling axes" *J. Physiol. (London)* **154** 32P-33P

Melvill Jones G, 1963 "Ocular nystagmus recorded simultaneously in three orthoganal planes" *Acta Oto-Laryngol.* **56** 619-631

Melvill Jones G, 1964 "Predominance of anti-compensatory oculomotor response during rapid head rotation" *Aerosp. Med.* **35** 965

Melvill Jones G, 1965 "The vestibular contribution to stabilization of the retinal image" in *The Role of the Vestibular Organs in the Exploration of Space* NASA SP-77, National Aeronautics and Space Administration, Washington, DC, pp 163-174

Melvill Jones G, 1970 "Origin, significance and amelioration of Coriolis illusions from the semicircular canals: a non-mathematical appraisal" *Aerosp. Med.* **41** 483-490

Melvill Jones G, Barry W, Kowalsky N, 1964 "Dynamics of the semicircular canals compared in yaw, pitch and roll" *Aerosp. Med.* **35** 984-989

Melvill Jones G, de Jong J D, 1971 "Dynamic characteristics of saccadic eye movements in Parkinson's disease" *Exp. Neurol.* **31** 17-31

Melvill Jones G, Milsum J H, 1970 "Characteristics of neural transmission from the semicircular canal to the vestibular nuclei of cats" *J. Physiol. (London)* **209** 295-316

Melvill Jones G, Milsum J H, 1971 "Frequency-response analysis of central vestibular unit activity resulting from rotational stimulation of the semicircular canals" *J. Physiol. (London)* **219** 191-215

Melvill Jones G, Spells K E, 1963 "A theoretical and comparative study of the functional dependence of the semicircular canal upon its physical dimensions" *Proc. R. Soc. London B.* **157** 403-419

Melvill Jones G, Sugie N, 1965 "Patterns of neuronal response in the region of the VIth nerve nucleus during controlled rotational stimulation of the semicircular canals" *Proc. Can. Fed. Biol. Soc.* **8** 14

Melvill Jones G, Sugie N, 1972 "Vestibulo-ocular responses in man during sleep" *Electroencephalogr. Clin. Neurophysiol.* **32** 43-53

Merrillees N C R, Sutherland S, Hayhow W, 1950 "Neuromuscular spindles in the extraocular muscles in man" *Anat. Rec.* **108** 23-30

Merton P A, 1951 "The silent period in a muscle of the human hand" *J. Physiol. (London)* **114** 183-198

Merton P A, 1956 "Compensatory rolling movements of the eye" *J. Physiol. (London)* **132** 25P–27P
Merton P A, 1959 discussion in *Proc. R. Soc. Med.* **52** 183–184
Merton P A, 1961 "The accuracy of directing the eyes and the hand in the dark" *J. Physiol. (London)* **156** 555–577
Merton P A, 1964 "Human position sense and sense of effort" *Symp. Soc. Exp. Biol.* **18** 387–400
Mettler F A, 1964 "Supratentorial mechanisms influencing the oculomotor apparatus" in *The Oculomotor System* Ed. M B Bender (Harper and Row, New York) pp 1–17
Meyers I L, 1929 "Electronystagmography" *Arch. Neurol. Psychiatry (Chicago)* **21** 901–918
Michael C R, 1970 "Integration of retinal and cortical information in the superior colliculus of the ground squirrel" *Brain Behav. Evol.* **3** 205–209
Michael J A, Melvill Jones G, 1966 "Dependence of visual tracking capability upon stimulus predictability" *Vision Res.* **6** 707–716
Miles F A, 1974 "Single unit firing patterns in the vestibular nuclei related to voluntary eye movements and passive body rotation in conscious monkeys" *Brain Res.* **71** 215–224
Miles F A, Fuller J H, 1974 "Adaptive plasticity in the vestibulo-ocular responses of the rhesus monkey" *Brain Res.* **80** 512–516
Miles W R, 1931 "Elevation of the eye-balls on winking" *J. Exp. Psychol.* **14** 311–332
Miller E F, 1962 "Counter-rolling of the human eyes produced by head tilt with respect to gravity" *Acta Oto-Laryngol.* **54** 479–501
Miller E F, Graybiel A, 1962 "A comparison of ocular counter-rolling movements between normal persons and deaf subjects with bilateral labyrinthine defects" report 68, project MR005-13-6001, US Naval School of Aviation Medicine, Pensacola, Fla
Miller J E, 1958 "Electromyographic pattern of saccadic eye movements" *Am. J. Ophthalmol.* **46** 183–186
Miller J E, 1959 "The electromyography of vergence movement" *Arch. Ophthalmol.* **62** 790–794
Miller J E, 1967 "Cellular organisation of rhesus extraocular muscle" *Invest. Ophthalmol.* **6** 18–39
Millodot M, 1972 "Variation of visual acuity in the central region of the retina" *Br. J. Physiol. Opt.* **27** 24–28
Milsum J H, 1965 *Biological Control Systems Analysis* (McGraw-Hill, New York)
Milsum J H, Melvill Jones G, 1969 "Dynamic asymmetry in neural components of the vestibular system" *Ann. N. Y. Ac. Sci.* **156** 851–871
Mishkin S, Melvill Jones G, 1966 "Predominant direction of gaze during slow head rotation" *Aerosp. Med.* **37** 897–900
Mitrani L, Mateef S, Yakimoff N, 1970 "Smearing of the retinal image during voluntary saccadic eye movements" *Vision Res.* **10** 405–409
Mitrani L, Mateeff S, Yakimoff N, 1971 "Is saccadic suppression really saccadic?" *Vision Res.* **11** 1157–1161
Mitrani L, Yakimoff N, Mateeff S, 1970 "Dependence of visual suppression on the angular size of voluntary saccadic eye movements" *Vision Res.* **10** 411–415
Mittelstaedt H, 1964 "Basic control patterns of orientational homeostasis" *Symp. Soc. Exp. Biol.* **18** 365–385
Miyoshi T, Ohta F, Nakano K, Hashiguchi T, 1970 "Analysis of optokinetic nystagmus using electronic computer" *Pract. Otol. Kyoto* **63** 89–101
Miyoshi T, Pfaltz C R, Piffko P, 1973 "Effect of repetitive optokinetic stimulation upon optokinetic and vestibular responses" *Acta Oto-Laryngol.* **75** 259–265

Mohler C W, Goldberg M E, Wurtz R H, 1973 "Visual receptive fields of frontal eye field neurons" *Brain Res.* **61** 385-389

Money K E, Miles W S, 1974 "Heavy water nystagmus and effects of alcohol" *Nature (London)* **247** 404-405

Morasso P, Bizzi E, Dichgans J, 1973 "Adjustment of saccade characteristics during head movements" *Exp. Brain Res.* **16** 492-500

Morgan M W Jr, 1944 "Accommodation and its relation to convergence" *Am. J. Optom.* **21** 183-195

Morgan M W Jr, 1954 "The ciliary body in accommodation and accommodative convergence" *Am. J. Optom.* **31** 219-229

Morgan M W Jr, Peters H B, 1951 "Accommodative-convergence in presbyopia" *Am. J. Optom.* **28** 3-10

Moses R A, 1950 "Torsion of the eye on oblique gaze" *Arch. Ophthalmol.* **44** 136-139

Moses R A, 1970 *Adler's Physiology of the Eye* 5th edition (Mosby, St Louis, Mo.)

Mountcastle V B, 1957 "Modality and topographic properties of single neurones of cat's somatic sensory cortex" *J. Neurophysiol.* **20** 408-434

Mowrer O M, 1934 "The influence of excitement on the duration of post-rotational nystagmus" *Arch. Oto-Laryngol.* **19** 46-54

Müller J, 1826 *Zur vergleichenden Physiologie der Gesichtssinnes* (Leipzig) p 207

Murphy B J, Haddad G M, Steinman R M, 1974 "Simple forms and fluctuations of the line of sight: implications for motor theories of form processing" *Percept. Psychophys.* **16** 557-563

Nachmias J, 1959 "Two dimensional motion of the retinal image during monocular fixation" *J. Opt. Soc. Am.* **49** 901-908

Nachmias J, 1961 "Determiners of the drift of the eye during monocular fixation" *J. Opt. Soc. Am.* **51** 761-766

Nakayama K, 1974 "Photographic determination of the rotational state of the eye using matrices" *Am. J. Optom. Physiol. Opt.* **51** 736-742

Nakayama K, 1975 "Coordination of extraocular muscles" in *Basic Mechanisms of Ocular Motility* Eds G Lennerstrand, P Bach-y-Rita (Pergamon Press, Oxford) pp 193-207

Namba T, Nakamura T, Takahashi A, Grob D, 1968 "Motor nerve endings in extraocular muscles" *J. Comp. Neurol.* **134** 385-396

Nashold B, Slaughter G, Gills J, 1969 "Ocular reactions in man from deep cerebellar stimulation and lesions" *Arch. Ophthalmol.* **81** 538-543

Nathanson M, Bergmann P, 1958 "Newer methods of evaluation of patients with altered states of consciousness" *Med. Clin. North Am.* **42** 701-710

Nauta W J H, Kuypers H G J M, 1958 "Some ascending pathways in the brain stem reticular formation" in *Reticular Formation of the Brain, Henry Ford Hospital Symposium* Ed. H H Jasper et al (Churchill, London) pp 3-30

Niven J I, Hixson W C, 1961 "Frequency response of the human semicircular canals. I. Steady state ocular nystagmus response to high-level sinusoidal angular rotations" report 58, project MR005-13-6001, US Naval School of Aviation Medicine, Pensacola, Fla

Niven J I, Hixson W C, Correia M J, 1966 "Elicitation of horizontal nystagmus by periodic linear acceleration" *Acta Oto-Laryngol.* **62** 429-441

Noda H, 1975a "Depression in the excitability of relay cells of lateral geniculate nucleus following saccadic eye movements in the cat" *J. Physiol. (London)* **249** 87-102

Noda H, 1975b "Discharges of relay cells in lateral geniculate nucleus of the cat during spontaneous eye movements in light and darkness" *J. Physiol. (London)* **250** 579-595

Noda H, Ross Adey W, 1974 "Retinal ganglion cells of the cat transfer information on saccadic eye movement and quick target motion" *Brain Res.* **70** 340-345

Nowgrodska-Zagórska M, 1974 "The organisation of extraocular muscles in *Anura*" *Acta Anat.* **87** 22-44

Nye P W, 1969 "The monocular eye movements of the pigeon" *Vision Res.* **9** 133-144

Nykiel F, Torok N, 1963 "A simplified nystagmograph" *Ann. Otol. Rhinol. Laryngol.* **72** 647-654

Ogle K N, 1962 "The optical space sense" in *The Eye* 2nd edition, volume 4, part II, Ed. H Davson (Academic Press, New York)

Ogle K N, Ellerbrock V J, 1946 "Cyclofusional movements" *Arch. Ophthalmol.* **30** 700-735

Ogle K N, Martens T G, 1957 "On the accommodative convergence and the proximal convergence" *Arch. Ophthalmol.* **57** 702-715

Ohm J, 1922 "Die klinische Bedeutung des optischen Drehnystagmus" *Klin. Monatsbl. Augenheilk.* **68** 323-355

Ohm J, 1926 "Ist der optische Drehnystagmus von einem unbeweglichen Auge auslösbar?" *Klin. Monatsbl. Augenheilk.* **21** 330-336

Ohm J, 1928 "Die Hebelnystagmographie" *Albrecht von Graefes Arch. Ophthalmol.* **120** 235-252

Ohm J, 1936 "Über Interferenz mehrerer Arten von Nystagmus" *Proc. Acad. Sci. Amst.* **39** 549-558

Olmstead J, Margutti M, Yanagisawa K, 1936 "Adaptation to transposition of eye muscles" *Am. J. Physiol.* **116** 245-251

Oosterveld W H, 1973 "On the origin of positional alcohol nystagmus" *Acta Oto-Laryngol.* **75** 252-258

Oppel O, 1959 "Untersuchungen über den Einfluss der Myo-Sensorik der Augenmuskeln auf die egozentrische Lokalisation beidäugiger optischer Nachbilder" *Albrecht von Graefes Arch. Ophthalmol.* **160** 462-470

Orban G, Duysens J, Callens M, 1973 "Movement perception during voluntary saccadic eye movements" *Vision Res.* **13** 1343-1353

Orem J, Schlag J, 1971 "Direct projections from cat frontal eye field to internal medullary lamina of the thalamus" *Exp. Neurol.* **33** 509-517

Oscarsson O, 1969 "The sagittal organisation of the cerebellar anterior lobe as revealed by the projection patterns of the climbing fibre system" in *Neurobiology of Cerebellar Evolution and Development* Ed. R Llinas (American Medical Association, Chicago, Ill.) pp 525-537

Orschansky J, 1898 "Eine Methode die Augenbewegungen direkt zu untersuchen (Ophthalmographie)" *Zentralbl. Physiol.* **12** 785-790

Outerbridge J S, Melvill Jones G, 1971 "Reflex vestibular control of head movements in man" *Aerosp. Med.* **42** 935-940

Oyster C W, 1968 "The analysis of image motion by the rabbit retina" *J. Physiol.* **199** 613-635

Ozawa T, 1964 "Some electrophysiological properties of rabbit extraocular muscle recorded in vivo with intracellular electrode" *Jpn. J. Ophthalmol.* **8** 47-52

Palmer L A, Rosenquist A C, 1974 "Visual receptive fields of single striate cortical units projecting to the superior colliculus in the cat" *Brain Res.* **67** 27-42

Palmieri G, Oliva G A, Scotto M, 1971 "C.R.T. spot-follower device for eye-movement measurements" *Kybernetik* **8** 23-30

Papaioannou J N, 1973 "Effects of caloric labyrinthine stimulation on the spontaneous activity of lateral geniculate nucleus neurones in the cat" *Exp. Brain Res.* **17** 1-9

Park G E, Park R S, 1940 "Further evidence of change of position of the eyeball during fixation" *Arch. Ophthalmol.* **23** 1216-1230

Park R S, Park G E, 1933 "The center of ocular rotation in the horizontal plane" *Am. J. Physiol.* **104** 545-552

Partridge L D, Kim J H, 1969 "Dynamic characteristics of a vestibulomotor reflex" *J. Neurophysiol.* **32** 485-495

Pasik P, Pasik T, 1964 "Oculomotor functions in monkeys with lesions of the cerebrum and the superior colliculi" in *The Oculomotor System* Ed. M B Bender (Hoeber, New York)

Pasik P, Pasik T, Krieger H P, 1959 "Effects of cerebral lesions upon optokinetic nystagmus in monkeys" *J. Neurophysiol.* **22** 297-304

Pasik T, Pasik P, Bender M B, 1969a "The pretectal syndrome in monkeys. I. Disturbances of gaze and body posture" *Brain* **92** 521-534

Pasik P, Pasik T, Bender M B, 1969b "The pretectal syndrome in monkeys. II. Spontaneous and induced nystagmus, and 'lightning' eye movements" *Brain* **92** 871-884

Peachey L D, 1971 "The structure of the extraocular muscle fibres of mammals" in *The Control of Eye Movements* Eds P Bach-y-Rita, C C Collins, J E Hyde (Academic Press, New York) pp 47-66

Peachey L D, Huxley A F, 1962 "Structural identification of twitch and slow striated muscle fibres of the frog" *J. Biophys. Biochem. Cytol.* **13** 177-180

Pearson A A, 1949a "The development and connections of the mesencephalic root of the trigeminal nerve in man" *J. Comp. Neurol.* **90** 1-46

Pearson A A, 1949b "Further observations on the mesencephalic root of the trigeminal nerve" *J. Comp. Neurol.* **91** 147-194

Peckham R H, 1934 "Foveal projection during duction" *Arch. Ophthalmol.* **12** 562-566

Pernier J, Jeannerod M, Gerin P, 1969 "Elaboration et decision des saccades: adaptation à la trace du stimulus" *Vision Res.* **9** 1149-1165

Perryman J H, Breinin G M, 1971 "Coordination of the extraocular recti muscles in the cat" *Invest. Ophthalmol.* **10** 78-86

Peterson B W, 1970 "Distribution of neural responses to tilting within vestibular nuclei of the cat" *J. Neurophysiol.* **33** 750-767

Peterson B W, 1972 "Responses of vestibular nuclear neurones to macular input" in *Basic Aspects of Central Vestibular Mechanisms* Eds A Brodal, O Pompeiano *Prog. Brain Res.* **37** 109-120

Petit Bois G, 1961 *Tables of Indefinite Integrals* (Dover, New York)

Petrov A P, Zenkin G M, 1973 "Torsional eye movements and constancy of the visual field" *Vision Res.* **13** 2465-2477

Philipszoon A J, 1962 "Compensatory eye movements and nystagmus provoked by stimulation of the vestibular organ and the cervical nerve roots" *Pract. Oto-Rhino-Laryngol.* **24** 193-202

Pickwell L D, 1972 "Hering's law of equal innervation and the position of the binoculus" *Vision Res.* **12** 1499-1507

Pilar G, 1967 "Further study of the electrical and mechanical responses of slow fibres in cat extraocular muscles" *J. Gen. Physiol.* **50** 2289-2300

Pompeiano O, 1972 "Reticular control of the vestibular nuclei: physiology and pharmacology" in *Basic aspects of central vestibular mechanisms* Eds A Brodal, O Pompeiano *Prog. Brain Res.* **37** 601-618

Pompeiano O, Walberg F, 1957 "Descending connections to the vestibular nuclei: an experimental study in the cat" *J. Comp. Neurol.* **108** 465-502

Porterfield W, 1759 *A Treatise on the Eye* volume 1 (Edinburgh) p 416

Precht W, 1972 "Vestibular and cerebellar control of oculomotor functions" in *Cerebral Control of Eye Movements and Motion Perception* Eds J Dichgans, E Bizzi (Karger, Basel) pp 71-88

Precht W, 1974 "Physiological aspects of the efferent vestibular system" in *Handbook of Sensory Physiology, Volume VI/1: Vestibular System Part I: Basic Mechanisms* Ed. H H Kornhuber (Springer, Berlin) pp 221-236

Precht W, 1975 "Cerebellar influences on eye movements" in *Basic Mechanisms of Ocular Motility* Eds G Lennerstrand, P Bach-y-Rita (Pergamon Press, Oxford) pp 261-280

Precht W, Llinas R, 1969 "Functional organization of the vestibular afferents to the cerebellar cortex of frog and cat" *Exp. Brain Res.* **9** 30-52

Precht W, Richter A, Grippo J, 1969 "Responses of neurones in cat's abducens nuclei to horizontal angular acceleration" *Pflügers Arch. Gesamte Physiol. Menschen Tiere* **309** 285-309

Precht W, Shimazu H, 1965 "Functional connections of tonic and kinetic vestibular neurons with primary vestibular afferents" *J. Neurophysiol.* **28** 1014-1028

Precht W, Shimazu H, Markham C H, 1966 "A mechanism of central compensation of vestibular function following hemi-labyrinthectomy" *J. Neurophysiol.* **29** 996-1010

Pringle J W S, 1960 "Models of muscle" *Symp. Soc. Exp. Biol.* **14** 41-68

Pritchard R M, 1958 "Visual illusions viewed as stabilised retinal images" *Q. J. Exp. Psychol.* **10** 77-81

Pritchard R M, 1964 "Physiological nystagmus and vision" in *The Oculomotor System* Ed. M B Bender (Harper and Row, New York) pp 321-331

Pritchard R M, Heron W, 1960 "Small eye movements of the cat" *Can. J. Psychol.* **14** 131-137

Pucket J de W, Steinman R M, 1969 "Tracking eye movements with and without saccadic corrections" *Vision Res.* **9** 695-703

Purkinje J E, 1820 "Beiträge zur näheren Kenntnis des Schwindels aus heautogonostischen Daten" *Med. Jb. (Österreich)* **6** 79-125

Purkinje J E, 1825 *Beobachtungen und Versuche zur Physiologie der Sinne* volume 2 (Prague) p 53

Putkonen P T S, Magnin M, Jeannerod M, 1973 "Directional responses to head rotation in neurones from the ventral nucleus of the lateral geniculate body" *Brain Res.* **61** 407-411

Putnam O A, Quereau J van D, 1951 "The tropophorometer" *Arch. Ophthalmol.* **45** 186-193

Quereau J van D, 1954 "Some aspects of torsion" *Arch. Ophthalmol.* **51** 783-788

Quereau J van D, 1955 "Rolling of the eye around its visual axis during normal movements" *Arch. Ophthalmol.* **53** 807-810

Rademaker G G J, Braak J W G ter, 1948 "On the central mechanisms of some optic reactions" *Brain* **71** 48-76

Raehlmann E, 1878 "Über den Nystagmus und seine Ätiologie" *Arch. für Ophthalmol. Abt. III* **24** 237-317

Rahn A C, Zuber B L, 1971 "Cerebellar evoked potentials resulting from extraocular stretch: evidence against cerebellar origin" *Exp. Neurol.* **31** 230-238

Rashbass C, 1959 "Barbiturate nystagmus and the mechanics of visual fixation" *Nature (London)* **183** 897-898

Rashbass C, 1960 "New method for recording eye movements" *J. Opt. Soc. Am.* **50** 642-644

Rashbass C, 1961 "The relationship between saccadic and smooth tracking eye movements" *J. Physiol. (London)* **159** 326-338

Rashbass C, 1971 "Second thoughts on smooth pursuit" in *The Control of Eye Movements* Eds P Bach-y-Rita, C C Collins, J E Hyde (Academic Press, New York) pp 445-446

Rashbass C, Russell G F M, 1961 "Action of a barbiturate drug (amylobarbitone sodium) on the vestibulo-ocular reflex" *Brain* **84** 329-335

Rashbass C, Westheimer G, 1960 "Recording rotational eye movements independently of lateral displacements" *J. Opt. Soc. Am.* **50** 512
Rashbass C, Westheimer G, 1961a "Disjunctive eye movements" *J. Physiol. (London)* **159** 339–360
Rashbass C, Westheimer G, 1961b "Independence of conjunctive and disjunctive eye movements" *J. Physiol. (London)* **159** 361–364
Ratliff F, 1952 "The role of physiological nystagmus in monocular acuity" *J. Exp. Psychol.* **43** 163–172
Ratliff F, Riggs L A, 1950 "Involuntary motions of the eye during monocular fixation" *J. Exp. Psychol.* **40** 687–701
Reid G, 1949 "The rate of discharge of the extraocular motoneurones" *J. Physiol. (London)* **110** 217–225
Reinecke R D, 1961 "Review of optokinetic nystagmus from 1954–1960" *Arch. Ophthalmol.* **65** 609–615
Reinecke R D, Simons K, 1975 "Phoria and EOM afference: preliminary support for a new theory" in *Basic Mechanisms of Ocular Motility* Eds G Lennerstrand, P Bach-y-Rita (Pergamon Press, Oxford) pp 113–117
Reinhart R J, Zuber B L, 1970 "Horizontal eye movements from abducens nerve stimulation in the cat" *IEEE Trans. Biomed. Eng.* **BME-17** 11–14
Rémond A, Gabersek V, Lesèvre N, 1958 "L'enrégistrement des déplacements du regard: détermination des axes de référence horizontaux et verticaux" *Rev. Neurol.* **99** 186–189
Richard D, Thiery J C, Buser P, 1973 "Cortical control of the superior colliculus in awake non-paralyzed cats" *Brain Res.* **58** 524–528
Richards W A, 1968a "Visual suppression during passive eye movements" *J. Opt. Soc. Am.* **58** 1159–1160
Richards W A, 1968b "Enhanced sensitivity associated with saccades" *J. Opt. Soc. Am.* **58** 1559
Richards W A, 1969 "Saccadic suppression" *J. Opt. Soc. Am.* **59** 617–623
Richards W A, 1972 "Response functions for sine- and square-wave modulations of disparity" *J. Opt. Soc. Am.* **62** 907–911
Richards W, Kaufman L, 1969 "'Center-of-gravity' tendencies for fixations and flow patterns" *Percept. Psychophys.* **5** 81–84
Richards W, Miller J F Jr, 1969 "Convergence as a cue to depth" *Percept. Psychophys.* **5** 317–320
Richter H R, 1956 "Principes de la photo-electro nystagmographie" *Rev. Neurol.* **94** 422–424
Richter H R, Pfaltz C R, 1956 "A propos de l'ectro-oculographie (rapport préliminaire sur une nouvelle méthode)" *Confin. Neurol.* **16** 279–289
Riggs D S, 1970 *Control Theory and Physiological Feedback* (Williams and Wilkins, Baltimore)
Riggs L A, Armington J C, Ratliff F, 1954 "Motions of the retinal image during fixation" *J. Opt. Soc. Am.* **44** 315–321
Riggs L A, Merton P A, Morton H B, 1974 "Suppression of visual phosphenes during saccadic eye movements" *Vision Res.* **14** 997–1011
Riggs L A, Niehl E W, 1960 "Eye movements recorded during convergence and divergence" *J. Opt. Soc. Am.* **50** 913–920
Riggs L A, Ratliff F, 1951 "Visual acuity and the normal tremor of the eyes" *Science* **114** 17–18
Riggs L A, Ratliff F, 1952 "The effects of counteracting the normal movements of the eye" *J. Opt. Soc. Am.* **42** 872–873
Riggs L A, Ratliff F, Cornsweet J C, Cornsweet T N, 1953 "The disappearance of visual test objects" *J. Opt. Soc. Am.* **43** 495–501

Riggs L A, Schick A M L, 1968 "Accuracy of retinal image stabilization achieved with a plane mirror on a tightly fitting contact lens" *Vision Res.* **8** 159-169

Riggs L A, Tulunay S Ü, 1959 "Visual effects of varying the extent of compensation for eye movements" *J. Opt. Soc. Am.* **49** 741-745

Rizzolatti G, Camarda R, Grupp L A, Pisa M, 1973 "Inhibition of visual responses of single units in the cat superior colliculus by the introduction of a second visual stimulus" *Brain Res.* **61** 390-394

Roberts T D M, 1967 *The Neurophysiology of Postural Mechanisms* (Butterworths, London)

Robinson D A, 1963 "A method of measuring eye movements using a search coil in a magnetic field" *IEEE Trans. Bio- Med. Electron* **10** 137-145

Robinson D A, 1964 "The mechanics of human saccadic eye movements" *J. Physiol. (London)* **174** 245-264

Robinson D A, 1965 "The mechanics of human smooth pursuit eye movements" *J. Physiol. (London)* **180** 569-591

Robinson D A, 1966 "The mechanics of human vergence eye movement" *J. Pediatr. Ophthalmol.* **3** 31-37

Robinson D A, 1968a "A note on the oculomotor pathway" *Exp. Neurol.* **22** 130-132

Robinson D A, 1968b "The oculomotor control system: a review" *Proc. IEEE* **56** 1032-1049

Robinson D A, 1970 "Oculomotor unit behaviour in the monkey" *J. Neurophysiol.* **33** 393-404

Robinson D A, 1972 "Eye movements evoked by collicular stimulation in the alert monkey" *Vision Res.* **12** 1795-1808

Robinson D A, 1973 "Models of the saccadic eye movement control system" *Kybernetik* **14** 71-83

Robinson D A, 1974 "The effect of cerebellectomy on the cat's vestibulo-ocular integrator" *Brain Res.* **71** 195-207

Robinson D A, 1975a "A quantitative analysis of extraocular muscle cooperation and squint" *Invest. Ophthalmol.* **14** 801-825

Robinson D A, 1975b "Oculomotor control signals" in *Basic Mechanisms of Ocular Motility* Eds G Lennerstrand, P Bach-y-Rita (Pergamon Press, Oxford) pp 337-378

Robinson D A, Fuchs A F, 1969 "Eye movements evoked by stimulation of frontal eye fields" *J. Neurophysiol.* **32** 637-648

Robinson D A, Keller E L, 1972 "The behaviour of eye movement motoneurones in the alert monkey" in *Cerebral Control of Eye Movements and Motion Perception* Eds J Dichgans, E Bizzi (Karger, Basel) pp 7-16

Robinson D A, O'Meara D M, Scott A B, Collins C C, 1969 "The mechanical components of human eye movements" *J. Appl. Physiol.* **26** 548-553

Robinson D L, Jarvis C D, 1974 "Superior colliculus neurons studied during head and eye movements of the behaving monkey" *J. Neurophysiol.* **37** 533-540

Robson J G, 1966 "Spatial and temporal contrast-sensitivity functions of the visual system" *J. Opt. Soc. Am.* **56** 1141-1142

Rochon-Duvigneaud A, 1943 *Les Yeux et la Vision des Vertébrés* (Masson, Paris)

Ron S, Robinson D A, 1973 "Eye movements evoked by cerebellar stimulation in the alert monkey" *J. Neurophysiol.* **36** 1004-1022

Ron S, Robinson D A, Skavenski A A, 1972 "Saccades and the quick phase of nystagmus" *Vision Res.* **12** 2015-2022

Rosen M J, 1972 "A theoretical neural integrator" *IEEE Trans. Biomed. Eng.* **19** 362-367

Ross Adey W, Noda H, 1973 "Influence of eye movements on geniculo-striate excitability in the cat" *J. Physiol. (London)* **235** 805-821

Rossi G, Cortesini G, 1965 "The 'efferent cochlear and vestibular system' in *Lepus Cuniculus*" *Acta Anat.* **60** 362-381
Ryu J H, McCabe B F, 1973 "Types of neuronal activity in the inferior vestibular nucleus" *Acta Oto-Laryngol.* **76** 11-16
Sansbury R V, Skavenski A A, Haddad G M, Steinman R M, 1973 "Normal fixation of eccentric targets" *J. Opt. Soc. Am.* **63** 612-614
Sas J, Appeltauer C, 1963 "Atypical muscle spindles in the extrinsic eye muscles of man" *Acta Anat.* **55** 311-322
Saslow M G, 1967a "Effects of components of displacement-step stimuli upon latency for saccadic eye movements" *J. Opt. Soc. Am.* **57** 1024-1029
Saslow M G, 1967b "Latency for saccadic eye movement" *J. Opt. Soc. Am.* **57** 1030-1033
Scala N P, Spiegel E A, 1938 "The mechanism of optokinetic nystagmus" *Trans. Am. Acad. Ophthalmol.* **43** 277-299
Schäfer E A, 1888 "Experiments on the electrical excitation of the visual area of the cerebral cortex in the monkey" *Brain* **11** 1-6
Schaefer K-P, 1965 "Die Erregungsmuster einzelner Neurone des Abducens-Kernes beim Kaninchen" *Pflügers Arch. Gesamte Physiol.* **284** 31-52
Schaefer K-P, 1972 "Neuronal elements of the orienting response" in *Cerebral Control of Eye Movements and Motion Perception* Eds J Dichgans, E Bizzi (Karger, Basel) pp 139-148
Schaefer K-P, Meyer D L, Schott D, 1971 "Optic and vestibular influences on ear movements" *Brain Behav. Evol.* **4** 323-333
Scheibel M E, Scheibel A B, 1958 "Structural substrates for integrative patterns in the brain stem reticular core" in *Reticular Formation of the Brain, Henry Ford Hospital Symposium* Ed. H H Jasper (Churchill, London)
Schiller P H, 1970 "The discharge characteristics of single units in the oculomotor and abducens nuclei of the unanaesthetized monkey" *Exp. Brain Res.* **10** 347-362
Schiller P H, 1972 "Some functional characteristics of the superior colliculus of the rhesus monkey" in *Cerebral Control of Eye Movements and Motion Perception* Eds J Dichgans, E Bizzi (Karger, Basel) pp 122-129
Schiller P H, Koerner F, 1971 "Discharge characteristics of single units in the superior colliculus of the alert rhesus monkey" *J. Neurophysiol.* **34** 920-936
Schiller P H, Stryker M, 1972 "Single-unit recording and stimulation in superior colliculus of the alert rhesus monkey" *J. Neurophysiol.* **35** 915-924
Schlag J, Schlag-Rey M, 1971 "Induction of oculomotor responses from thalamic internal medullary lamina in the cat" *Exp. Neurol.* **33** 498-508
Schlag J, Lehtinen I, Schlag-Rey M, 1974 "Neuronal activity before and during eye movements in thalamic internal medullary lamina of cat" *J. Neurophysiol.* **37** 982-995
Schmidt C L, Wist E R, Dichgans J, 1972 "Efferent frequency modulation in the vestibular nerve of goldfish correlated with saccadic eye movements" *Exp. Brain Res.* **15** 1-14
Schöne H, 1954 "Statocystenfunktion und statische Lageorientierung bei decapoden Krebsen" *Z. Vergl. Physiol.* **36** 241-260
Schor R H, 1974 "Responses of cat vestibular neurons to sinusoidal roll tilt" *Exp. Brain Res.* **20** 347-362
Schott E, 1922 "Über die Registrierung des Nystagmus und anderer Augenbewegungen vermittels des Saitengalvanometers" *Dtsch. Arch. Klin. Med.* **140** 79-90
Schwindt P C, Precht W, Richter A, 1974 "Monosynaptic excitatory and inhibitory pathways from medial midbrain nuclei to trochlear motoneurons" *Expt. Brain Res.* **20** 223-238

Schwindt P C, Richter A, Precht W, 1973 "Short latency utricular and canal input to ipsilateral abducens motoneurones" *Brain Res.* **60** 259-292

Sears M L, Teasdall R D, Stone H H, 1959 "Stretch effects in human extraocular muscle" *Bull. Johns Hopkins Hosp.* **104** 174-178

Sekuler R W, Ganz L, 1963 "After-effect of seen motion with a stabilized retinal image" *Science* **139** 419-420

Shackel B, 1959 "Skin-drilling: a method of diminishing galvanic skin potentials" *Am. J. Psychol.* **72** 114-121

Shackel B, 1960a "A pilot study in EOG" *Br. J. Ophthalmol.* **44** 89-113

Shackel B, 1960b "Note on mobile eye viewpoint recording" *J. Opt. Soc. Am.* **50** 763-768

Shackel B, 1967 "Eye movement recording by electro-oculography" in *Manual of Psychophysiological Methods* Eds P H Venables, I Martin (North-Holland, Amsterdam) pp 229-334

Sharpe C R, 1972 "The visibility and fading of thin lines visualized by their controlled movement across the retina" *J. Physiol.* **222** 113-134

Sherrington C S, 1893 "Further experimental note on the correlation of action of antagonistic muscles" *Proc. R. Soc. London B* **53** 407-420

Sherrington C S, 1894 "Experimental note on two movements of the eye" *J. Physiol. (London)* **17** 27-29

Sherrington C S, 1900 "The muscular sense" in *Textbook of Physiology* Ed. E A Schäfer (Pentland, Edinburgh) p 1004

Sherrington C S, 1918 "Observations on the sensual role of the proprioceptive nerve supply of the extrinsic ocular muscles" *Brain* **41** 332-343

Shimazu H, Precht W, 1965 "Tonic and kinetic responses of cat's vestibular neurons to horizontal angular acceleration" *J. Neurophysiol.* **28** 991-1013

Shimazu H, Precht W, 1966 "Inhibition of central vestibular neurones from the contralateral labyrinth and its mediating pathway" *J. Neurophysiol.* **29** 467-492

Shimazu H, Smith C M, 1971 "Cerebellar and labyrinthine influences on single vestibular neurones identified by natural stimuli" *J. Neurophysiol.* **34** 493-508

Shimo-oku M, 1970 "Cerebellar influence on the evoked potential of the oculomotor nucleus induced by stimulation of the oculomotor nerve branches in the cat" *Invest. Ophthalmol.* **9** 236-244

Shinoda Y, Yoshida K, 1974 "Dynamic characteristics of responses to horizontal head angular acceleration in vestibulo-ocular pathway in the cat" *J. Neurophysiol.* **37** 653-673

Shipley T, Rawlings S C, 1970a "The Nonius horopter. I. History and theory" *Vision Res.* **10** 1225-1262

Shipley T, Rawlings S C, 1970b "The Nonius horopter. II. An experimental report" *Vision Res.* **10** 1263-1299

Shortess G K, Krauskopf J, 1961 "Rôle of involuntary eye movements in stereoscopic acuity" *J. Opt. Soc. Am.* **51** 555-559

Siebeck R, 1954 "Wahrnehmungsstörung und Störungswahrnehmung bei Augenmuskellähmungen" *Albrecht von Graefes Arch. Ophthalmol.* **155** 26-34

Silberpfennig J, 1941 "Contributions to the problem of eye movements. III. Disturbances of ocular movements with pseudo-hemianopsia in frontal lobe tumours" *Confin. Neurol.* **42** 1-13

Singer W, Bedworth N, 1974 "Correlation between the effects of brainstem stimulation and saccadic eye movements on transmission in the cat lateral geniculate nucleus" *Brain Res.* **72** 185-202

Singh B M, Ivamoto H, Strobos R J, 1973 "Slow eye movements in spinocerebellar degeneration" *Am. J. Ophthalmol.* **76** 237-240

Skavenski A A, 1971 "Extraretinal correction and memory for target position" *Vision Res.* **11** 743-746

Skavenski A A, 1972 "Inflow as a source of extraretinal eye position information" *Vision Res.* **12** 221-229

Skavenski A A, Robinson D A, 1973 "Role of abducens nucleus in vestibulo-ocular reflex" *J. Neurophysiol.* **36** 724-738

Skavenski A A, Steinman R M, 1970 "Control of eye position in the dark" *Vision Res.* **10** 193-203

Slatt B, Loeffler J D, Hoyt W F, 1966 "Ocular motor disturbances in Parkinson's disease: electromyographic observations" *Can. J. Ophthalmol.* **1** 267-273

Slotnick R S, 1969 "Adaptation to curvature distortion" *J. Exp. Psychol.* **81** 441-448

Smith K V, 1937 "The postoperative effects of removal of the striate cortex upon certain unlearned visually controlled reactions in the cat" *J. Genet. Psychol.* **50** 137-156

Smith W M, Warter P J Jr, 1960 "Eye movement and stimulus movement: new photoelectric electromechanical system for recording and measuring tracking motions of the eye" *J. Opt. Soc. Am.* **50** 245-250

Snider R S, 1950 "Recent contributions to the anatomy and physiology of the cerebellum" *Arch. Neurol. Psychiatry* **64** 196-219

Snider R S, Niemer W T, 1961 *A Stereotaxic Atlas of the Cat Brain* (University of Chicago Press, Chicago, Ill.)

Snider R S, Stowell A, 1944 "Receiving areas of the tactile auditory and visual systems in the cerebellum" *J. Neurophysiol.* **7** 331-357

Sotelo C, Palay S L, 1967 "Synapses avec des contacts étroits (tight junctions) dans le noyau vestibulaire latéral du rat" *J. Microsc. (Paris)* **6** 83a

Sparks D L, Sides J P, 1974 "Brain stem unit activity related to horizontal eye movements occurring during visual tracking" *Brain Res.* **77** 320-325

Sparks D L, Travis R P, 1971 "Firing patterns of reticular formation neurons during horizontal eye movements" *Brain Res.* **33** 477-481

Spekreijse H, Oosting H, 1970 "Linearizing: a method for analyzing and synthesizing nonlinear systems" *Kybernetik* **7** 22-31

Sperling G, Speelman R, 1965 "Visual spatial localisation during object motion, apparent object motion and image motion produced by eye movements" *J. Opt. Soc. Am.* **55** 1576-1577

Sperry R W, 1950 "Neural basis of the spontaneous optokinetic response produced by visual inversion" *J. Comp. Physiol. Psychol.* **43** 482-489

Spiegel E A, 1933 "Role of vestibular nuclei in cortical innervation of the eye muscles" *Arch. Neurol. Psychiatry* **29** 1084-1097

Spiegel E A, Aronson L, 1934 "Interaction of cortical and labyrinthine impulses to ocular muscle movements" *Am. J. Phsyiol.* **109** 693-703

Spiegel E A, Price J B, 1939 "Origin of the quick component of labyrinthine nystagmus" *Arch. Oto-Laryngol.* **30** 576-588

Spoendlin H H, 1965 "Ultrastructural studies of the labyrinth in squirrel monkeys" in *The Role of the Vestibular Organs in the Exploration of Space* NASA SP-77 National Aeronautics and Space Administration, Washington, DC, pp 7-22

Sprague J M, 1963 "Corticofugal projections to the superior colliculus in the cat" *Anat. Rec.* **145** 288

Spyer K M, Ghelarducci B, Pompeiano O, 1974 "Gravity responses of neurons in main reticular formation" *J. Neurophysiol.* **37** 705-721

Stark L, 1968 *Neurological Control Systems* (Plenum Press, New York)

Stark L, 1971 "The control system for versional eye movements" in *The Control of Eye Movements* Eds P Bach-y-Rita, C C Collins, J E Hyde (Academic Press, New York) pp 363-428

Stark L, Sandberg A, 1961 "A simple instrument for measuring eye movements" *Q. Prog. Rep. Res. Lab. Electron. MIT* **62** 268-270 (Massachusetts Institute of Technology, Cambridge, Mass)

Stark L, Vossius G, Young L R, 1962 "Predictive control of eye tracking movements" *IRE Trans. on Hum. Factors Electron.* **HFE-3** 52-57

Starkman S, Kaul S, Fried J, Behrens M, 1972 "Unusual abnormal eye movements in a family with hereditary spinocerebellar degeneration" *Neurology* **22** 402

Starr A, 1967 "A disorder of rapid eye movements in Huntington's chorea *Brain* **90** 545-564

St Cyr G J, 1973 "Signal and noise in the human oculomotor system" *Vision Res.* **13** 1979-1991

St Cyr G J, Fender D H, 1969a "The interplay of drifts and flicks in binocular fixation" *Vision Res.* **9** 245-265

St Cyr G J, Fender D H, 1969b "Nonlinearities of the human oculo-motor system: gain" *Vision Res.* **9** 1235-1246

St Cyr G J, Fender D H, 1969c "Nonlinearities of the human oculo-motor system: time delays" *Vision Res.* **9** 1491-1503

Steers J A, 1953 *An Introduction to the Study of Map Projections* 9th edition (University of London Press, London)

Stein B M, Carpenter M B, 1967 "Central projections of portions of the vestibular ganglia innervating specific parts of the labyrinth in the rhesus monkey" *Am. J. Anat.* **120** 281-318

Steinacker A, Bach-y-Rita P, 1968 "The fibre spectrum of the cat VI nerve to the lateral rectus and retractor bulbi muscles" *Experienta* **24** 1254-1255

Steinbach M J, 1969 "Eye tracking of self-moved targets: the role of efference" *J. Exp. Psychol.* **82** 366-376

Steinbach M J, Angus R G, Money K E, 1974 "Torsional eye movements of the owl" *Vision Res.* **14** 745-746

Steinbach M J, Money K E, 1973 "Eye movements of the owl" *Vision Res.* **13** 889-891

Steinbach M J, Pearce D G, 1972 "Release of pursuit eye movements using after-images" *Vision Res.* **12** 1307-1311

Steinhausen W, 1931 "Über den Nachweis der Bewegung der Cupula in der intakten Bogengangsampulle des Labyrinthes bei der natürlichen rotatorischen und calorischen Reizung" *Pflügers Arch. Gesamte Physiol. Menschen Tiere* **228** 322-328

Steinman R M, 1965 "Effect of target size, luminance and color on monocular fixation" *J. Opt. Soc. Am.* **55** 1158-1165

Steinman R M, Cunitz R J, 1968 "Fixation of targets near the absolute foveal threshold" *Vision Res.* **8** 277-286

Steinman R M, Cunitz R J, Timberlake G T, Herman M, 1967 "Voluntary control of microsaccades during maintained monocular fixation" *Science* **155** 1577-1579

Steinman R M, Haddad G M, Skavenski A A, Wyman D, 1973 "Miniature eye movements" *Science* **181** 810-819

Steinman R M, Skavenski A A, Sansbury R V, 1969 "Effect of lens accommodation on holding the eye in place without saccades" *Vision Res.* **9** 629-631

Stevens J K, Emerson R C, Gerstein R L, Kallos T, Neufeld G R, Nichols C W, Rosenquist A C, 1976 "Paralysis of the awake human: visual perceptions" *Vision Res.* **16** 93-98

Stibbe E P, 1930 "Sensory components of the motor nerves of the eye" *J. Anat.* **64** 112-113

Stockwell C W, Gilson R D, Guedry F E Jr, 1973 "Adaptation of horizontal semicircular canal responses" *Acta Oto-Laryngol.* **75** 471-476

Stone S L, Thomas J G, Zakian V, 1965 "The passive rotatory characteristics of the dog's eye and its attachments" *J. Physiol.* **181** 337-349

Straschill M, Hoffmann K P, 1970 "Activity of movement sensitive neurones of cat's tectum opticum during spontaneous eye movements" *Exp. Brain Res.* **11** 318-326

Straschill M, Rieger P, 1972 "Optomotor integration in the colliculus superior of the cat" in *Cerebral Control of Eye Movements and Motion Perception* Eds J Dichgans, E Bizzi (Karger, Basel) pp 130-138

Straschill M, Rieger P, 1973 "Eye movements evoked by focal stimulation of the cat's superior colliculus" *Brain Res.* **59** 211-227

Straschill M, Schick F, 1974 "Neuronal activity during eye movements in a visual association area of cat cerebral cortex" *Exp. Brain Res.* **19** 467-477

Stryker M, Blakemore C, 1972 "Saccadic and disjunctive eye movements in cats" *Vision Res.* **12** 2005-2013

Sugie N, Melvill Jones G, 1971 "A model of eye movements induced by head rotation" *IEEE Trans. Sys. Man Cybern.* **SMC-1** 251-260

Suzuki J-I, Tokumasu K, Goto K, 1969 "Eye movements from single utricular nerve stimulation in the cat" *Acta Oto-Laryngol.* **68** 350-362

Syka J, Straschill M, Radil-Weiss T, 1973 "On the role of the tectum in eye movements in the cat" in *The Oculomotor System and Brain Function* Ed. V Zikmund (Butterworth, London) pp 33-43

Szentágothai J, 1942 "Die innere Gliederung des Oculomotoriuskernes" *Arch. Neurol. Psychiatry* **115** 127-135

Szentágothai J, 1943 "Die zentrale Innervation der Augenbewegungen" *Arch. Neurol. Psychiatry* **116** 721-760

Szentágothai J, 1950 "The elementary vestibulo-ocular reflex arc" *J. Neurophysiol.* **13** 395-407

Szentágothai J, 1964 "Synaptic articulation in vestibulo-ocular function" in *The Oculomotor System* Ed. M B Bender (Harper and Row, New York)chapter 8

Szentágothai J, Rajkovits K, 1958 "Der Hirnnervenanteil der Pyramidenbahn und der prämotorische Apparat motorischer Hirnnervenkerne" *Arch. Psychiatr. Nervenkr.* **197** 335-354

Szentágothai J, Rajkovits K, 1959 "Über den Ursprung der Kletterfasern des Kleinhirn" *Z. Anat. Entwicklungsgesch.* **121** 130-141

Takemori S, Cohen B, 1974a "Visual suppression of vestibular nystagmus in rhesus monkeys" *Brain Res.* **72** 203-212

Takemori S, Cohen B, 1974b "Loss of visual suppression of vestibular nystagmus after flocculus lesions" *Brain Res.* **72** 213-224

Takemori S, Suzuki J, 1971 "Eye deviations from neck torsion in humans" *Ann. Otol. Rhinol. Laryngol.* **80** 439-444

Tamler E, Jampolsky A, Marg E, 1958 "An electromyographic study of asymmetric convergence" *Am. J. Ophthalmol.* **46** 174-182

Tamler E, Marg E, Jampolsky A, 1959a "An electromyographic study of co-activity of human extraocular muscles in following movements" *Arch. Ophthalmol.* **61** 270-273

Tamler E, Jampolsky A, Marg E, 1959b "Electromyographic study of following movements of the eye between tertiary positions" *Arch. Ophthalmol.* **62** 804-809

Taren J A, 1964 "An anatomic demonstration of afferent fibres in the IV, V and VI cranial nerves of the *Macaca mulatta*" *Am. J. Ophthalmol.* **58** 408-412

Tarkhan A A, 1934 "The innervation of the extrinsic ocular muscle" *J. Anat.* **68** 293-313

Tarlov E, 1972 "Anatomy of two vestibulo-oculomotor projection systems" in *Basic Aspects of Central Vestibular Mechanisms* Eds A Brodal, O Pompeiano *Prog. Brain Res.* **37** 471-491

Tarlov E, Tarlov S R, 1971 "The representation of extraocular muscles in the oculomotor nuclei: experimental studies in the cat" *Brain Res.* **34** 37-52

Täumer R, 1975 "Three reaction mechanisms of the saccadic system in response to a double jump" in *Basic Mechanisms of Ocular Motility* Eds G Lennerstrand, P Bach-y-Rita (Pergamon Press, Oxford) pp 515-518

Taylor A, 1965a "Discharge patterns in the abducens nucleus related to eye movements in the vestibulo-ocular reflex in the cat" *J. Physiol. (London)* **177** 54P

Taylor A, 1965b "The role of sensory feedback in the vestibulo-ocular response in cats" *J. Physiol. (London)* **179** 76P-77P

Teräväinen H, 1968 "Electron microscopic and histochemical observations on different types of nerve endings in the extraocular muscles of the rat" *Z. Zellforsch. Mikrosk. Anat.* **90** 372-388

Theopold H, Kommerell G, 1974 "Phasische und tonische Funktion der Augenmuskeln. Untersuchungen an Patienten mit Oculomotorius- oder Abducens-Paralyse" *Albrecht von Graefes Arch. Ophthalmol.* **192** 247

Thomas J G, 1961 "Subjective analysis of saccadic eye movements *Nature (London)* **189** 842-843

Thomas J G, 1965 "Use of a piezo-accelerometer in studying eye dynamics" *J. Opt. Soc. Am.* **55** 534-537

Thomas J G, 1967 "The torque-angle transfer function of the human eye" *Kybernetik* **3** 254-263

Tibbling L, 1969 "The influence of tobacco smoking, nicotine, CO and CO_2 on vestibular nystagmus" *Acta Oto-Laryngol.* **68** 118-126

Timberlake G T, Wyman D, Skavenski A A, Steinman R M, 1972 "The oculomotor error signal in the fovea" *Vision Res.* **12** 1059-1064

Tokumasu K, Goto K, Cohen B, 1965 "Eye movements produced by the superior oblique muscle" *Arch. Ophthalmol.* **73** 851-862

Torok N, Derbyshire A J, 1968 "Computation of the nystagmogram" *Acta Oto-Laryngol.* **65** 70-78

Tozer F, Sherrington C S, 1910 "Receptors and afferents of the III, IV and VI cranial nerves" *Proc. R. Soc. London B* **82** 450-457

Trimble J L, Zuber B L, Trimble S N, 1974 "Enhancement of single motor unit activity in the human extraocular electromyogram" *Vision Res.* **14** 1327-1332

Troelstra A, 1972 "Intraocular noise: origin and characteristics" *Vision Res.* **12** 1313-1326

Troelstra A, Zuber B L, Simpson J I, Stark L, 1963 "Pupil variation and disjunctive eye position as a result of photic and accommodative stimulation" *Q. Prog. Rep. Res. Lab. Electron. MIT* **69** 250-253 (Massachusetts Institute of Technology, Cambridge, Mass)

Trojanowski J Q, Jacobson S, 1974 "Medial pulvinar afferents to frontal eye fields in rhesus monkey demonstrated by horseradish peroxidase" *Brain Res.* **80** 395-411

Troxler D, 1804 "Über das Verschwinden gegebener Gegenstände innerhalb unseres Gesichtskreises" in *Ophthal. Bibliothek* volume 2 Eds K Himly, J A Schmidt (Jena) pp 51-53

Truex R C, Carpenter M B, 1969 *Human Neuroanatomy* 6th edition (Williams and Wilkins, Baltimore, Md)

Tscherning M H E, 1900 *Physiological Optics* (Keystone Press, Philadelphia, Pa)

Uemara T, Cohen B, 1973 "Effect of vestibular nuclei lesions on vestibulo-ocular reflexes and posture in monkeys" *Acta Oto-Laryngol. Suppl.* **315**

Verheijen F J, 1961 "A simple after image method demonstrating the involuntary multi-directional eye movements during fixation" *Opt. Acta* 8 309-311

Vernon M D, 1931 *The Experimental Study of Reading* (Cambridge University Press, London)
Verveen A A, 1969 "An introduction to the use of time series analysis in physiology" in *Proc. Int. Sch. Phys. "Enrico Fermi"* **43** 291-327 (Academic Press, New York)
Volkmann A W, 1869 "Zur Mechanik der Augenmuskeln" *Ber. Sächs. Gesamte Akad. Wiss.* **21** 28-69
Volkmann F C, 1962 "Vision during voluntary saccadic eye movement" *J. Opt. Soc. Am.* **52** 571-578
Volkmann F C, Schick A M L, Riggs L A, 1969 "Time course of visual inhibition during voluntary saccades" *J. Opt. Soc. Am.* **58** 562-569
Voss H, 1957 "Beiträge zur mikroskopischen Anatomie der Augenmuskeln des Menschen (Faserdicke, Muskelspindeln, Ringbinden)" *Anat. Anz.* **104** 345-355
Wadia N H, Swami R K, 1971 "A new form of heredo-familial spino-cerebellar degeneration with slow eye movements (nine families)" *Brain* **94** 359-374
Wagman I H, Krieger H P, Bender M B, 1958 "Eye movements elicited by surface and depth stimulation of the occipital lobe of *Macaca mulatta*" *J. Comp. Neurol.* **109** 169-193
Wagman I H, Krieger H P, Papatheodorou C A, Bender M B, 1961 "Eye movements elicited by surface and depth stimulation of the frontal lobe of the *Macaca mulatta*" *J. Comp. Neurol.* **117** 179-188
Walberg F, 1956 "Descending connections to the inferior olive: an experimental study in the cat" *J. Comp. Neurol.* **104** 77-173
Walberg F, Bowsher D, Brodal A, 1958 "The termination of primary vestibular fibres in the vestibular nuclei in the cat: an experimental study with silver methods" *J. Comp. Neurol.* **110** 391-419
Walberg F, Pompeiano O, Brodal A, Jansen J, 1962 "The fastigio-vestibular projection in the cat" *J. Comp. Neurol.* **118** 49-76
Walls G L, 1942 "Eye movements and the fovea" in *The Vertebrate Eye* (Cranbrook Institute of Science, Bloomfield Hills, Mich.) chapter 10
Walls G L, 1962 "The evolutionary history of eye movements" *Vision Res.* **2** 69-80
Wang S C, Chinn H I, 1956 "Experimental motion sickness in dogs: importance of labyrinth and vestibular cerebellum" *Am. J. Physiol.* **185** 617-623
Warwick R, 1953 "Representation of the extraocular muscles in the oculomotor nuclei of the monkey" *J. Comp. Neurol.* **98** 449-504
Warwick R, 1955 "The so-called nucleus of convergence" *Brain* **78** 92-114
Warwick R, 1964 "Oculomotor organization" in *The Oculomotor System* Ed. M B Bender (Harper and Row, New York) chapter 7, p 173
Weale R A, 1959 "The problem of false torsion" *Proc. R. Soc. Med.* **52** 183-184
Weber R B, Daroff R B, 1972 "Corrective movements following refixation saccades: type and control system analysis" *Vision Res.* **12** 467-475
Wendt P R, 1952 "Development of an eye camera for use with motion pictures" *Psychol. Monographs* **66** 1-18
Wersäll J, 1956 "Studies on the structure and innervation of the sensory epithelium of the cristae ampullares in the guinea pig" *Acta Oto-Laryngol. Suppl.* **126**
Wertheim T, 1887 "Über die Zahl der Sehnheiten im mittleren Theile der Netzhaut" *Albrecht von Graefes Arch. Ophthalmol.* **33** (2) 137-146
West D C, Boyce P R, 1968 "The effect of flicker on eye movements" *Vision Res.* **8** 171-192
Westheimer G, 1954a "Mechanism of saccadic eye movements" *Arch. Ophthalmol.* **52** 710-724
Westheimer G, 1954b "Eye movement responses to a horizontally moving visual stimulus" *Arch. Ophthalmol.* **52** 932-941
Westheimer G, 1957 "Kinematics of the eye" *J. Opt. Soc. Am.* **47** 967-974

Westheimer G, 1958 "A note on the response characteristics of the extraocular muscle system" *Bull. Math. Biophys.* **20** 149-153

Westheimer G, 1963 "Amphetamine, barbiturates and accommodation convergence" *Arch. Ophthalmol.* **70** 830-836

Westheimer G, 1973 "Saccadic eye movements" in *The Oculomotor System and Brain Function* Ed. V Zikmund (Butterworth, London) pp 59-77

Westheimer G, Blair S M, 1972a "Concerning the supranuclear organization of eye-movements" in *Cerebral Control of Eye Movements and Motion Perception* Eds J Dichgans, E Bizzi (Karger, Basel) pp 28-35

Westheimer G, Blair S M, 1972b "Mapping the visual sensory onto the visual motor system" *Invest. Ophthalmol.* **11** 490-496

Westheimer G, Blair S M, 1973a "Saccadic inhibition induced by brain-stem stimulation in the alert monkey" *Invest. Ophthalmol.* **12** 77-78

Westheimer G, Blair S M, 1973b "Oculomotor defects in cerebellectomised monkeys" *Invest. Ophthalmol.* **12** 618-621

Westheimer G, Blair S M, 1974 "Functional organization of primate oculomotor system, revealed by cerebellectomy" *Exp. Brain Res.* **21** 463-472

Westheimer G, McKee S P, 1973 "Failure of Donders' law during smooth pursuit eye movements" *Vision Res.* **13** 2145-2153

Westheimer G, Mitchell A M, 1956 "Eye movement responses to convergence stimuli" *AMA Arch. Ophthalmol.* **55** 848-856

Westheimer G, Mitchell D E, 1969 "The sensory stimulus for disjunctive eye movements" *Vision Res.* **9** 749-755

Westheimer G, Rashbass C, 1961 "Barbiturates and eye vergence" *Nature (London)* **191** 833-834

Wheeless L L, Boynton R M, Cohen G H, 1966 "Eye-movement responses to step and pulse-step stimuli" *J. Opt. Soc. Am.* **56** 956-960

Wheeless L L, Cohen G H, Boynton R M, 1967 "Luminance as a parameter of the eye-movement control system" *J. Opt. Soc. Am.* **57** 394-400

White C T, Eason R G, Bartlett N R, 1962 "Latency and duration of eye movements in the horizontal plane" *J. Opt. Soc. Am.* **52** 210-213

Whitteridge D, 1955 "A separate afferent nerve supply from the extraocular muscles of goats" *Q. J. Exp. Physiol.* **40** 331-336

Whitteridge D, 1958 "The motor nerve supply to extraocular muscle spindles" *Electroencephalogr. Clin. Neurophysiol.* **10** 353

Whitteridge D, 1959 "The effect of stimulation of intrafusal muscle fibres on sensitivity to stretch of extraocular muscle spindles" *Q.J.Exp. Physiol.* **44** 385-393

Whitteridge D, 1960 "Central control of eye movements" *Handbook of physiology: Neurophysiology* volume II (American Physiological Society, Washington, DC) pp 1089-1109

Wickelgren B G, Sterling P. 1969 "Influence of visual cortex on receptive fields in the superior colliculus of the cat" *J. Neurophysiol.* **32** 16-23

Wiener N, 1961 *Cybernetics, or Control and Communication in the Animal and the Machine* 2nd edition (MIT Press, Cambridge, Mass)

Wilkinson I M S, Kime R, Purnell M, 1974 "Alcohol and human eye movement" *Brain* **97** 785-792

Wilson D, 1973a "A centre for accommodative vergence motor control" *Vision Res.* **13** 2491-2503

Wilson D, 1973b "Noise coupling between accommodation and accommodative vergence" *Vision Res.* **13** 2505-2513

Wilson V J, Felpel L P, 1972 "Specificity of semicircular canal input to neurons in the pigeon vestibular nuclei" *J. Neurophysiol.* **35** 253-264

Wilson V J, Wylie R M, 1970 "A short-latency labyrinthine input to the vestibular nuclei in the pigeon" *Science* **168** 124-127

Winckler G, 1937 "L'innervation sensitive et motrice des muscles extrinsèques de l'oeil chez quelques ongulés" *Arch. Anat. Strasbourg* **23** 217-234

Wohlgemuth A, 1911 "On the after-effect of seen movement" *Br. J. Psychol. Monogr. Suppl.* **1** 1-117

Woinow M, 1870 "Über den Drehpunkt des Auges" *Albrecht von Graefes Arch. Ophthalmol.* **16** 243-250

Wolfe J, 1971 "Relationship of cerebellar potentials to saccadic eye movements" *Brain Res.* **30** 204-207

Wolter J R, 1955 "Morphology of the sensory nerve apparatus in the striated muscles of the human eye" *Arch. Ophthalmol.* **53** 201-217

Wood C C, Spear P D, Braun J J, 1973 "Direction-specific deficits in horizontal optokinetic nystagmus following removal of visual cortex in the cat" *Brain Res.* **60** 231-273

Woodworth R S, 1906 "Vision and localisation during eye movements" *Psychol. Bull.* **3** 68-70

Woolard H H, 1931 "The innervation of the ocular muscles" *J. Anat.* **65** 215-223

Wright J C, Kertesz A E, 1975 "The rôle of positional and orientational disparity cues in human fusional response" *Vision Res.* **15** 427-430

Wundt W, 1862 *Beiträge zur Theorie der Sinneswahrnehmung* (Leipzig)

Wurtz R H, 1969 "Comparison of effects of eye movements and stimulus movements on striate cortex neurons of the monkey" *J. Neurophysiol.* **32** 987-994

Wurtz R H, Goldberg M E, 1972a "The role of the superior colliculus in visually-evoked eye movements" in *Cerebral Control of Eye Movements and Motion Perception* Eds J Dichgans, E Bizzi (Karger, Basel) pp 149-158

Wurtz R H, Goldberg M E, 1972b "Activity of superior colliculus in behaving monkey. III. Cells discharging before eye movements" *J. Neurophysiol.* **35** 575-586

Wurtz R H, Goldberg M E, 1972c "Activity of superior colliculus in behaving monkey. IV. Effects of lesions on eye movements *J. Neurophysiol.* **35** 587-596

Wurtz R H, Mohler C W, 1974 "Selection of visual targets for the initiation of saccadic eye movements" *Brain Res.* **71** 209-214

Wyman D, Steinman R M, 1973a "Small step tracking: implications for the oculomotor 'dead zone' " *Vision Res.* **13** 2165-2172

Wyman D, Steinman R M, 1973b "Latency characteristics of small saccades" *Vision Res.* **13** 2173-2175

Yagi T, 1974 "Spontaneous and evoked behaviour of single units in the oculomotor nucleus of the rabbit" *Jpn. J. Physiol.* **24** 305-316

Yamanaka Y, Bach-y-Rita P, 1968 "Conduction velocity in the abducens nerve correlated with vestibular nystagmus in cats" *Exp. Neurol.* **20** 143-155

Yamazaki A, Ishikawa S, 1972 "The eye movement abnormality in Parkinson's disease" *Jpn. J. Clin. Ophthalmol.* **26** 619-623

Yarbus A L, 1956 "The motion of the eye in the process of changing points of fixation" *Biofizika* **1** 76-78

Yarbus A L, 1957a "Eye movements during changes of the stationary points of fixation" *Biofizika* **2** 698-702

Yarbus A L, 1957b "The perception of an image fixed with respect to the retina" *Biofizika* **2** 703-712

Yarbus A L, 1967 *Eye Movements and Vision* (Plenum Press, New York)

Yoshida T, Watanabe A, 1969 "Analysis of interaction between accommodation and vergence feedback control systems of human eyes" *Bull. NHK Broadcasting Sci. Res. Lab.* **3** 72-80

Young L R, 1963 "Measuring eye movements" *Am. J. Med. Electron.* **2** 300-307

Young L R, Henn V S, 1974 "Selective habituation of vestibular nystagmus by visual stimulation" *Acta Oto-Laryngol.* **77** 159-166

Young L R, Meiry J L, Li T Y, 1966 "Control engineering approaches to human dynamic space orientation" in *The Role of the Vestibular Organs in the Exploration of Space* NASA SP-77 National Aeronautics and Space Administration, Washington, DC, pp 217-227

Young L R, Sheena D, 1975 "Survey of eye movement recording methods" *Behav. Res. Methods Instrum.* **7** 397-429

Young L R, Stark L, 1963 "Variable feedback experiments testing a sampled data model for eye tracking movements" *IEEE Trans. Hum. Factors Electron.* **HFE-4** 38-51

Young T, 1801 "On the mechanism of the eye" *Phil. Trans. R. Soc. London B* 23-88

Zee D S, Friendlich A R, Robinson D A, 1974 "The mechanism of downbeat nystagmus" *Arch. Neurol.* **30** 227-237

Zee D S, Optican L M, Cook J D, Robinson D A, King Engel W, 1976 "Slow saccades in spinocerebellar degeneration" *Arch. Neurol.* **33** 243-251

Zenker W, Anzenbacher H, 1964 "On the different forms of myo-neural junction in two types of muscle fibre from the external ocular muscles of the rhesus monkey" *J. Cell. Comp. Physiol.* **63** 273-285

Zuber B L, 1968a "Eye movement dynamics in the cat: the final motor pathway" *Exp. Neurol.* **20** 255-260

Zuber B L, 1968b "Sinusoidal eye movements from brain stem stimulation in the cat" *Vision Res.* **8** 1073-1079

Zuber B L, Crider A, Stark L, 1964 "Saccadic suppression associated with microsaccades" *MIT Electron. Res. Lab. Q. Prog. Rep.* **74** 244-249

Zuber B L, Horrocks A, Lorber M, Stark L, 1964 "Visual suppression during the fast phase of vestibular nystagmus" *MIT Electron. Res. Lab. Q. Prog. Rep.* **73** 221-223

Zuber B L, Stark L, 1965 "Microsaccades and the velocity-amplitude relationship for saccadic eye movements" *Science* **150** 1459-1460

Zuber B L, Stark L, 1966 "Saccadic suppression: elevation of visual threshold associated with saccadic eye movements" *Exp. Neurol.* **16** 65-79

Zuber B L, Stark L, 1968 "Dynamical characteristics of the fusional vergence eye movement system" *IEEE Trans. Sys. Man Cybern.* **SCC 4** 72-79

Zuber B L, Stark L, Cook G, 1965 "Microsaccades and the velocity-amplitude relationship for saccadic eye movements" *Science* **150** 1459-1460

Zuber B L, Stark L, Lorber M, 1966 "Saccadic suppression of the pupillary light reflex" *Exp. Neurol.* **14** 351-370

Index

A. E. KERTESZ